Applications of Antioxidant Nanoparticles

Applications of Antioxidant Nanoparticles

Guest Editors

Rita Cortesi
Maddalena Sguizzato

MDPI

Basel • Beijing • Wuhan • Barcelona • Belgrade • Novi Sad • Cluj • Manchester

Guest Editors

Rita Cortesi
Department of Chemical, Pharmaceutical and Agricultural Sciences
University of Ferrara
Ferrara
Italy

Maddalena Sguizzato
Department of Chemical, Pharmaceutical and Agricultural Sciences
University of Ferrara
Ferrara
Italy

Editorial Office
MDPI AG
Grosspeteranlage 5
4052 Basel, Switzerland

This is a reprint of the Special Issue, published open access by the journal *Antioxidants* (ISSN 2076-3921), freely accessible at: https://www.mdpi.com/journal/antioxidants/special_issues/antioxidant_nanoparticles.

For citation purposes, cite each article independently as indicated on the article page online and as indicated below:

Lastname, A.A.; Lastname, B.B. Article Title. *Journal Name* **Year**, *Volume Number*, Page Range.

ISBN 978-3-7258-4737-2 (Hbk)
ISBN 978-3-7258-4738-9 (PDF)
https://doi.org/10.3390/books978-3-7258-4738-9

Contents

About the Editors

Rita Cortesi

Rita Cortesi is an Associate Professor at the University of Ferrara, Department of Chemical, Pharmaceutical and Agricultural Sciences. After graduation, she earned a PhD in Pharmaceutical Sciences and attended an HMC post-doc fellowship at Nottingham University (UK), in the Pharmaceutical Sciences Dept. As a Pharmaceutical Technologist, she works on the formulation and development of nanosystems for the controlled release of bioactive molecules, drug delivery systems for gene therapy, and pharmaceutical nanotechnology. Her other interests are in the cosmetic field. She is the author of more than 170 scientific works, including papers in international journals, book chapters, and patents. Her studies are conducted in collaboration with prestigious international research groups throughout the world.

Maddalena Sguizzato

Maddalena Sguizzato is currently a Tenure Track Researcher at the University of Ferrara, in the Department of Chemical, Pharmaceutical and Agricultural Sciences. She earned a PhD in Chemical Sciences, was a Visiting PhD student at NC State University (NC, USA), and a Visiting Researcher at the University of Oslo (Norway) and at the University of Geneva (Switzerland). Her research focuses on the formulation of lipid-based nanosystems for the targeted delivery of poorly soluble molecules, as well as the field of cosmetics. She is a co-author of several publications in the field of drug delivery.

antioxidants

MDPI

Editorial

Applications of Antioxidant Nanoparticles

Rita Cortesi * and Maddalena Sguizzato

Department of Chemical, Pharmaceutical and Agricultural Sciences (DoCPAS), University of Ferrara, 44100 Ferrara, Italy; maddalena.sguizzato@unife.it

* Correspondence: crt@unife.it

The regulation of numerous physiological processes is strictly dependent on the production of reactive oxygen species (ROS). Nonetheless, their overproduction could generate oxidative stress, responsible for the onset of different diseases [1]. Hence, a useful treatment approach for oxidative stress is the delivery of antioxidants. Generally, neutralization of ROS, chelating effect and enzyme inhibition are the three main mechanisms of action exerted by antioxidant molecules to inhibit the effect of ROS and the generation of oxidative stress.

In recent decades, the application of nanoparticles has shown a considerable deal of interest in the fields of pharmaceutics, cosmetics and food [2–4]. For instance, lipid nanoparticles, due to the "green" characteristics related to their biodegradation and non-toxicity, have received significant attention as a carrier for antioxidant molecules [5]. Over the past few decades, considerable achievements have been made in the development of antioxidant nanotherapies, exhibiting multiple advantages.

This Special Issue of *Antioxidants*, entitled "Applications of Antioxidant Nanoparticles", includes thirteen research articles and two reviews, describing recent advances in the design, production, characterization, use, and effect of antioxidant nanoparticles, including polymeric or lipid-based nanoparticles, ROS-scavenging inorganic nanoparticles, organic nanoparticles with intrinsic antioxidant activity and drug-loaded antioxidant nanoparticles. In addition, the use of antioxidant nanoparticles in various fields, such the biomedical, pharmaceutical, cosmetic and food industries, and their administration through different routes have been considered.

Concerning the different routes of administration, the review of Qi and colleagues (contribution 14) focuses on the involvement of different types and delivery of antioxidants in dental procedures. Particularly the study of their mechanisms of action in the treatment of oxidative stress induced by dental restorations is also taken into consideration.

On the other hand, the review of Subroto and colleagues provides information on the current research on solid lipid nanoparticles (SLNs) for the encapsulation and delivery of active and antioxidant compounds. Various synthesis methods and application fields of SLNs were considered. It was underlined that fabrication design, which includes the selection of lipid matrices and surfactants and their preparation methods, determines the characteristics of SLNs. Therefore, an appropriate fabrication design can produce SLNs with stable active compounds and antioxidants that become suitable encapsulation systems for various applications or uses (contribution 15).

With regard to the research papers, they can be divided in some groups on the basis of the type of delivery system proposed, namely nanoparticles (contributions 1, 5, 6, 7, 8, 11 and 12), nanocomposites and nanoclusters (contributions 3 and 10), SEDDS and nanoemulsions (contributions 2, 4 and 9) and vesicles (contribution 13).

Among the nanoparticle group, Bellini et al. demonstrated that poly (lipoic acid)-based nanoparticles stabilized by Pluronic are able to effectively antagonize the formation of radicals and ROS. In addition, these nanoparticles inhibited the overproduction of ROS in tumor cells, human macrophages and rat ventricular myocytes. In addition their capture by macrophages and cardiomyocytes induce a better effect as compared to tumor cells and non-phagocytic leukocytes. Notably, these nanoparticles decreased the mitochondrial ROS generation induced by simulated ischemia/reperfusion injury in isolated cardiomyocytes, hence appearing to be an effective and cardiomyocyte-selective drug to protect against damages induced by post-ischemic reperfusion (contribution 1).

Another study, conducted by the group of Mawed and colleagues, investigated the ultrastructure changes in the ovary in response to exposure to zinc oxide nanoparticles and the effect during egg maturation and ovulation on the fertility of female zebrafish. They found that zinc oxide nanoparticles could induce cytotoxicity in the maturing oocyte by activating autophagy and apoptosis in a caspase-dependent manner and could induce oxidative stress by generating ROS (contribution 5).

The research by Tellechea et al. investigated the characteristics of a recombinant protein from the legume cowpea (*Vigna unguiculata*) immobilized on gold nanoparticles. Notably, the study, conducted as a function of nanoparticle surface chemistry and biofunctionalization methods, evidenced the importance of the interaction between the biomolecule and the gold nanoparticles for the functionality of the hybrid; hence, this strategy can be useful in the development of electrochemical biosensors in biomedical applications (contribution 6).

Otherwise, Kim and colleagues studied the use of α-bisabolol as a natural bioactive compound in bioproducts to minimize oxidative stress. In order to bypass its water-insolubility, α-bisabolol-loaded polyglyceryl-4 caprate nanoparticles were proposed, obtaining an improvement in long-term stability and antioxidant activity, and an outstanding antibacterial effect that could allow for the use of these nanoparticles in treating diseases related to various oxidative stresses as well as in many fields, such as the pharmaceuticals, cosmetics, and food industries (contribution 7).

The research by Ivanova's group focused on the use of an environmentally friendly and cost-effective self-assembly nanoencapsulation technology based on zein to obtain multifunctional essential oil-loaded nanocapsules with antioxidant and bactericidal activity toward *Cutibacterium acnes*. The obtained results demonstrated that once incorporated into creams, the produced nanocapsules led to complete inhibition of *C. acnes* and demonstrated the capacity to scavenge ROS, thus preventing damage to human skin cells (contribution 8).

The study by De Luca and colleagues considered the phytochemical resveratrol loaded onto positive charged polymeric nanoparticles within an in situ gelled matrix to prolong the residence time of the active into the cornea, decrease the administration frequency and enhance the therapeutic effect. The obtained eye drop formulation could be employed to bypass the rapid clearance typical of solutions in the treatment of a number of inflammation- and oxidative stress-related diseases (contribution 11).

The last manuscript belonging to the nanoparticle group is that of Thirupathi and colleagues. The authors evaluated on the palatal wounds of Wistar rats the cytotoxic effect and the activity of gold nanoparticles reduced by the green synthesis method. They found that topical treatment with these nanoparticles potentially remitted the palatal wounds and the mucosal lesions of mouth, preventing inflammation or infections and facilitating the healing process (contribution 12).

The second group of delivery systems including nanocomposites and nanocluster includes the works of Alam et al. (contribution 3) and Ungor and colleagues (contribution 10). The former considers a novel copper–zinc–manganese trimetal oxide nanocomposite synthesized using the co-precipitation method, which was then characterized and tested in vitro, showing potent activity against *Escherichia coli* and a strong antioxidant effect where scavenging activity was observed. In contrast, the latter studied the improvement in antioxidant activity of a simple synthesis method for the preparation of Vitamin B1-stabilized few-atomic gold nanoclusters. The obtained nanostructure carries gold in the zero oxidation state, while Vitamin B1 is able to stabilize the metal core by coordinating pyrimidine-N. In this way the gold nanoclusters is able to enhance its antioxidant property as compared to pure Vitamin B1.

The third group includes SEDDS and nanoemulsions. Notably, self-emulsifying drug delivery systems (SEDDSs) are isotropic mixtures of oils, surfactants, solvents and co-solvents/surfactants, useful for improving the oral absorption of lipophilic drug compounds. Afifi and colleagues loaded β-Sitosterol glucoside on SEDDSs in order to ameliorate insulin resistance, protect against oxidative stress and restore pancreatic β-cell secretory function. The obtained results suggest the possible employment of these systems in diabetes progression (contribution 2).

Concerning nanoemulsions, the study of Das and colleagues investigated a nanosized food-grade quercetin-loaded nanoemulsion for its neuroprotective and cytotoxicity effects against *Caenorhabditis elegans* strains and human cancer cells, respectively. In vivo results showed that the quercetin-nanoemulsion potentially reduced the α-Syn aggregation, increased mitochondrial and fat content, and improved the lifespan in transgenic *C. elegans* strain. Moreover, it significantly down-regulates the ROS levels in wild-type *C. elegans strain*, therefore showing improved solubility, targeting and neuroprotective effects against the parkinsonian-induced model (contribution 4).

The study by Thuy et al. took into consideration the development of a mitochondria-targeting emulsion, using dequalinium and α-tocopherol succinate for cancer treatment. The authors found that this nanoemulsion effectively inhibited spheroid growth in the 3D model, as well as prevented the growth of tumor cells grafted onto zebrafish larvae, and showed promising potential for mitochondria-targeting and cancer treatment (contribution 9).

Lastly, another type of formulation is typified by vesicles, which are described in the study of Sguizzato et al. considering bilosystems to improve the water solubility of budesonide. The obtained systems showed good encapsulation efficiency and dimensional stability. Moreover, immunofluorescence experiments evidenced that bile acid-based vesicles containing the drug effectively decrease the inflammation induced by glucose oxidase stimuli and counteract intestinal cells ox-inflammatory damage (contribution 13).

In summary, with this Special Issue, we have tried to uncover the possible applications of different types of nanoparticles, or more precisely, "nanosystems", in different fields, including the biomedical, pharmaceutical, cosmetic, as well as nutraceutical or food industries. The involvement of oxidative stress in different diseases, ranging from cutaneous damages to systemic pathologies and cancer, clearly suggests that the use of antioxidant nanosystems with targeted and controlled release could enhance the effect of common treatments. Indeed, the results discussed in this Special Issue unveil the multiple modes of action of a potential antioxidant activity performed by some molecules when delivered in different technological systems and support the ongoing research for a better understanding of optimal ways to exploit the activities of antioxidant molecules in everyday life. The correlation between oxidative stress and physiological processes or disease progression is still an appealing topic to be investigated, and the application of antioxidant nanoparticles has proven to be a promising strategy to adopt in particular when endogenous defenses are lacking.

Author Contributions: Conceptualization, writing—original draft, review and editing, R.C. and M.S. All authors have read and agreed to the published version of the manuscript.

Conflicts of Interest: The authors declare no conflicts of interest.

List of Contributions:

1. Bellini, C.; Antonucci, S.; Morillas-Becerril, L.; Scarpa, S.; Tavano, R.; Mancin, F.; Di Lisa, F.; Papini, E. Nanoparticles Based on Cross-Linked Poly(Lipoic Acid) Protect Macrophages and Cardiomyocytes from Oxidative Stress and Ischemia Reperfusion Injury. *Antioxidants* **2022**, *11*, 907. https://doi.org/10.3390/antiox11050907.

2. Afifi, S.M.; Ammar, N.M.; Kamel, R.; Esatbeyoglu, T.; Hassan, H.A. β-Sitosterol Glucoside-Loaded Nanosystem Ameliorates Insulin Resistance and Oxidative Stress in Streptozotocin-Induced Diabetic Rats. *Antioxidants* **2022**, *11*, 1023. https://doi.org/10.3390/antiox11051023.
3. Alam, M.W.; Al Qahtani, H.S.; Souayeh, B.; Ahmed, W.; Albalawi, H.; Farhan, M.; Abuzir, A.; Naeem, S. Novel Copper-Zinc-Manganese Ternary Metal Oxide Nanocomposite as Heterogeneous Catalyst for Glucose Sensor and Antibacterial Activity. *Antioxidants* **2022**, *11*, 1064. https://doi.org/10.3390/antiox11061064.
4. Das, S.S.; Sarkar, A.; Chabattula, S.C.; Verma, P.R.P.; Nazir, A.; Gupta, P.K.; Ruokolainen, J.; Kesari, K.K.; Singh, S.K. Food-Grade Quercetin-Loaded Nanoemulsion Ameliorates Effects Associated with Parkinson's Disease and Cancer: Studies Employing a Transgenic *C. elegans* Model and Human Cancer Cell Lines. *Antioxidants* **2022**, *11*, 1378. https://doi.org/10.3390/antiox11071378.
5. Mawed, S.A.; Marini, C.; Alagawany, M.; Farag, M.R.; Reda, R.M.; El-Saadony, M.T.; Elhady, W.M.; Magi, G.E.; Di Cerbo, A.; El-Nagar, W.G. Zinc Oxide Nanoparticles (ZnO-NPs) Suppress Fertility by Activating Autophagy, Apoptosis, and Oxidative Stress in the Developing Oocytes of Female Zebrafish. *Antioxidants* **2022**, *11*, 1567. https://doi.org/10.3390/antiox11081567.
6. Tellechea, E.; Asensio, A.C.; Ciaurriz, P.; Buezo, J.; López-Gómez, P.; Urra, M.; Moran, J.F. A Study of the Interface of Gold Nanoparticles Conjugated to Cowpea Fe-Superoxide Dismutase. *Antioxidants* **2022**, *11*, 2082. https://doi.org/10.3390/antiox11112082.
7. Kim, S.; Yu, S.; Kim, J.; Khaliq, N.U.; Choi, W.I.; Kim, H.; Sung, D. Facile Fabrication of α-Bisabolol Nanoparticles with Improved Antioxidant and Antibacterial Effects. *Antioxidants* **2023**, *12*, 207. https://doi.org/10.3390/antiox12010207.
8. Ivanova, K.; Ramon, E.; Ivanova, A.; Sanchez-Gomez, S.; Tzanov, T. Bio-Based Nano-Enabled Cosmetic Formulations for the Treatment of *Cutibacterium acnes*-Associated Skin Infections. *Antioxidants* **2023**, *12*, 432. https://doi.org/10.3390/antiox12020432.
9. Thuy, L.T.; Lee, S.; Dongquoc, V.; Choi, J.S. Nanoemulsion Composed of α-Tocopherol Succinate and Dequalinium Shows Mitochondria-Targeting and Anticancer Effects. *Antioxidants* **2023**, *12*, 437. https://doi.org/10.3390/antiox12020437.
10. Ungor, D.; Gombár, G.; Juhász, Á.; Samu, G.F.; Csapó, E. Promising Bioactivity of Vitamin B_1-Au Nanocluster: Structure, Enhanced Antioxidant Behavior, and Serum Protein Interaction. *Antioxidants* **2023**, *12*, 874. https://doi.org/10.3390/antiox12040874.
11. De Luca, I.; Di Cristo, F.; Conte, R.; Peluso, G.; Cerruti, P.; Calarco, A. In-Situ Thermoresponsive Hydrogel Containing Resveratrol-Loaded Nanoparticles as a Localized Drug Delivery Platform for Dry Eye Disease. *Antioxidants* **2023**, *12*, 993. https://doi.org/10.3390/antiox12050993.
12. Thirupathi, A.; Guzzatti, M.F.M.; Corrêa, M.E.A.B.; Venturini, L.M.; Casagrande, L.R.; Lima, I.R.; Da Costa, C.; De Pieri, E.; Tietbohl, L.T.W.; Feuser, P.E.; et al. Green Synthesis of Gold Nanoparticles with Curcumin or Açai in the Tissue Repair of Palatal Wounds. *Antioxidants* **2023**, *12*, 1574. https://doi.org/10.3390/antiox12081574.
13. Sguizzato, M.; Ferrara, F.; Baraldo, N.; Bondi, A.; Guarino, A.; Drechsler, M.; Valacchi, G.; Cortesi, R. Bilosomes and Biloparticles for the Delivery of Lipophilic Drugs: A Preliminary Study. *Antioxidants* **2023**, *12*, 2025. https://doi.org/10.3390/antiox12122025.
14. Qi, F.; Huang, H.; Wang, M.; Rong, W.; Wang, J. Applications of Antioxidants in Dental Procedures. *Antioxidants* **2022**, *11*, 2492. https://doi.org/10.3390/antiox11122492.
15. Subroto, E.; Andoyo, R.; Indiarto, R. Solid Lipid Nanoparticles: Review of the Current Research on Encapsulation and Delivery Systems for Active and Antioxidant Compounds. *Antioxidants* **2023**, *12*, 633. https://doi.org/10.3390/antiox12030633.

References

1. Dizdaroglu, M.; Jaruga, P.; Birincioglu, M.; Rodriguez, H. Free Radical-Induced Damage to DNA: Mechanisms and Measurement. *Free. Radic. Biol. Med.* **2002**, *32*, 1102–1115. [CrossRef] [PubMed]
2. Van Tran, V.; Moon, J.-Y.; Lee, Y.-C. Liposomes for Delivery of Antioxidants in Cosmeceuticals: Challenges and Development Strategies. *J. Control. Release* **2019**, *300*, 114–140. [CrossRef] [PubMed]
3. Da Silva Santos, V.; Badan Ribeiro, A.P.; Andrade Santana, M.H. Solid Lipid Nanoparticles as Carriers for Lipophilic Compounds for Applications in Foods. *Food Res. Int.* **2019**, *122*, 610–626. [CrossRef] [PubMed]

4. Paliwal, R.; Paliwal, S.R.; Kenwat, R.; Kurmi, B.D.; Sahu, M.K. Solid Lipid Nanoparticles: A Review on Recent Perspectives and Patents. *Expert Opin. Ther. Pat.* **2020**, *30*, 179–194. [CrossRef] [PubMed]
5. Borges, A.; de Freitas, V.; Mateus, N.; Fernandes, I.; Oliveira, J. Solid Lipid Nanoparticles as Carriers of Natural Phenolic Compounds. *Antioxidants* **2020**, *9*, 998. [CrossRef] [PubMed]

antioxidants

Article

Bilosomes and Biloparticles for the Delivery of Lipophilic Drugs: A Preliminary Study

Maddalena Sguizzato [1,†], Francesca Ferrara [1,†], Nada Baraldo [1], Agnese Bondi [1], Annunziata Guarino [2], Markus Drechsler [3], Giuseppe Valacchi [4,5,6] and Rita Cortesi [1,7,*]

1 Department of Chemical, Pharmaceutical and Agricultural Sciences (DoCPAS), University of Ferrara, I-44121 Ferrara, Italy; sgzmdl@unife.it (M.S.); frrfnc3@unife.it (F.F.); nada.baraldo@edu.unife.it (N.B.); agnese.bondi@unife.it (A.B.)
2 Department of Neurosciences and Rehabilitation, University of Ferrara, I-44121 Ferrara, Italy; annunziata.guarino@unife.it
3 Bavarian Polymer Institute (BPI), Keylab "Electron and Optical Microscopy", University of Bayreuth, D-95440 Bayreuth, Germany; markus.drechsler@uni-bayreuth.de
4 Department of Environmental Sciences and Prevention, University of Ferrara, I-44121 Ferrara, Italy; giuseppe.valacchi@unife.it or gvalacc@ncsu.edu
5 Animal Science Department NC Research Campus, Plants for Human Health Institute, NC State University, Kannapolis, NC 28081, USA
6 Department of Food and Nutrition, Kyung Hee University, Seoul S02447, Republic of Korea
7 Biotechnology Interuniversity Consortium (C.I.B.), Ferrara Section, University of Ferrara, I-44121 Ferrara, Italy
* Correspondence: crt@unife.it
† These authors contributed equally to this work.

Abstract: In this study, bile acid-based vesicles and nanoparticles (i.e., bilosomes and biloparticles) are studied to improve the water solubility of lipophilic drugs. Ursodeoxycholic acid, sodium cholate, sodium taurocholate and budesonide were used as bile acids and model drugs, respectively. Bilosomes and biloparticles were prepared following standard protocols with minor changes, after a preformulation study. The obtained systems showed good encapsulation efficiency and dimensional stability. Particularly, for biloparticles, the increase in encapsulation efficiency followed the order ursodeoxycholic acid < sodium cholate < sodium taurocholate. The in vitro release of budesonide from both bilosytems was performed by means of dialysis using either a nylon membrane or a portion of Wistar rat small intestine and two receiving solutions (i.e., simulated gastric and intestinal fluids). Both in gastric and intestinal fluid, budesonide was released from bilosystems more slowly than the reference solution, while biloparticles showed a significant improvement in the passage of budesonide into aqueous solution. Immunofluorescence experiments indicated that ursodeoxycholic acid bilosomes containing budesonide are effective in reducing the inflammatory response induced by glucose oxidase stimuli and counteract ox-inflammatory damage within intestinal cells.

Keywords: bile acids; nanovesicles; nanoparticles; SLN; NLC; drug solubility; nanotechnology; poorly water-soluble drugs; immunofluorescence; inflammasome

1. Introduction

In recent years, the number of new molecules for which poor solubility in water represents the main obstacle to absorption has increased [1].

Indeed, the poor water solubility of a drug affects its bioavailability and the route of administration required to produce a therapeutic effect. Particularly, the water solubility of a drug is an important parameter to take into consideration when it comes to oral administration, being the preferred route for administering medicines. Notably, in order to be absorbed after oral administration, an active ingredient must pass into the solution in the aqueous gastrointestinal environment.

In this context, lipids represent a promising solution to this problem. It is known, in fact, that the intake of food rich in fat, together with lipophilic drugs, with poor solubility in water, can facilitate their absorption and therefore improve their bioavailability [1,2], depending on the numerous mechanisms related to the intake of food with a fair amount of lipid, including increased residence time in the intestinal lumen, increased biliary and pancreatic secretions, the stimulation of lymphatic transport, increased permeability of the intestinal wall, the inhibition of metabolic activities and efflux transporters and impaired mesenteric and hepatic blood flow.

With these concepts taken together, lipid-based delivery systems are of great interest to the oral administration of active ingredients, especially for those poorly soluble in aqueous environments. The goal of researchers is to exploit and optimize the ability of lipids to promote the absorption of an active ingredient in the intestine, possibly reducing the dose of drug that must be administered and, at the same time, limiting the dependence between the bioavailability of the drug and food intake [3].

Among the many types of lipid-based formulations that can be advantageously used to transport both hydrophilic and lipophilic drugs, in this preliminary study, lipid-based nanosystems, such as vesicles and nanoparticles containing different bile acids in their composition [4], namely, ursodeoxycholic acid (U), sodium cholate (C) and sodium taurocholate (T), are investigated and compared, with the aim of evaluating technological strategies to promote the bioavailability of poorly water-soluble drugs after oral administration. Indeed, bile salts are physiologically involved in the digestion of lipids; therefore, they can affect the absorption of poorly soluble drugs in different ways, especially if administered orally. Furthermore, many studies have reported that bile salt–phospholipid vesicles are able to transport the drug to the intestinal wall, leading to increased bioavailability [5–8] due to their additional ability to protect drug contents from the harsh environment of the gut [6,9,10].

As a model drug, budesonide was considered [11]. The choice of budesonide was made on the basis that it is considered the anti-inflammatory drug of "first choice" in the treatment of patients with mild to moderate inflammatory bowel disease (IBD) [12–14], but when administered orally, its absorption in the gastrointestinal tract is difficult, resulting in poor bioavailability [15–17], poor release at sites of intestinal inflammation and, therefore, low effectiveness [18]. Furthermore, it is necessary to take into account the high rate of metabolization and hepatic clearance [19]. Therefore, strategies able to improve patient compliance and gastrointestinal efficiency [20,21], such as bilosystems, become interesting in order to expand budesonide's clinical use [21].

The aim of this study is to investigate the ability of formulations to improv the solubility and the intestinal absorption of budesonide, thanks to the presence of bile acids. To address this point, lipids for the production of bilosystems were selected on the basis of the most common components used in the preparation of traditional lipid-based nanosystems such as liposomes, SLN and NLC, as reported in the literature [22–26].

2. Materials and Methods

2.1. Materials

Phosphatidylcholine (Phospholipon 90 G, PC) was purchased from Lipoid GmbH (Ludwigshafen am Rhein, Germany), and cholesterol (CH), tristearin (stearic triglyceride), pluronic F-68, ursodeoxycholic acid (U), sodium cholate hydrate (C), sodium taurocholate (T), porcine lipase and budesonide were purchased from Merck KGaA (Darmstadt, Germany). Caprylic/capric triglycerides (Miglyol 812) were obtained from Sasol Germany GmbH (Witten, Germany). All other materials and solvents of high-performance liquid chromatography (HPLC) grade and of analytical grade were supplied by Carlo Erba (Rodano, Milan, Italy).

2.2. Preparation of Bilosomes

Bilosomes, with 25 mg/mL of final lipid concentration, were prepared via the hot hydration method. This technique involves the formation of a lipid film, consisting of PC,

CH and bile acid (U, T and C) in a ratio of 4:1:1 mol/mol/mol, which was subsequently hydrated with an aqueous phase at 60 °C.

The various organic solutions were placed inside a flask (which was eventually padded with the drug) and subjected to forced evaporation, with the use of a rotary evaporator (70 bar, 200 rpm), until complete elimination of the organic solvent. The obtained thin lipid film was then hydrated with hot water, swirled (VELP scientifica srl, Usmate Velate, Italy) and subjected to 30 min of bath sonication at 40 °C [27,28].

2.3. Preparation of Biloparticles

Biloparticles were produced via hot homogenization followed by a sonication technique [29]. The lipid phase (5% of the total weight of the formulation) consisted of Tristearin, to which Tricaprin was added in the case of NLC. An aqueous solution of Poloxamer 188 (2.5% *w/w*) represented the remaining 95% of the preparation. Bile acids and the drug that would eventually be present were added in the lipid phase. Compositions of the different formulations are summarized in Table S1.

The lipid phase was melted at 80 °C in a water bath. When the fusion was completed, the aqueous phase was rapidly added. Afterwards, the system was subjected to 1 min homogenization at 1500 rpm (IKA T25 digital ultra-turrax, VWR International srl, Milan, Italy). Subsequently the obtained emulsion underwent 15 min of ultrasound treatment (MICROSON Ultrasonic Cell Disruptor-XL MISONIX, VWR International srl, Milan, Italy) and the system was cooled down to room temperature.

2.4. Dimensional Analysis

Dimensional characterization of bilosomes and biloparticles was performed via Photon Correlation Spectroscopy (PCS) using a Zetasizer Nano S90 (Malvern Instr., Malvern, UK) equipped with a 5 Mw He/Ne laser with a wavelength output of λ = 633 nm. Samples were diluted 1:10 (*v/v*) with double distilled water up to 1 mL and poured in polystyrene cuvettes with four transparent faces. The measurements were thrice repeated at 25 °C at a 90° laser angle [30].

At the end of the analysis, a graph of the dimensional distribution of nanoparticles was obtained, giving the Z-Average and PdI. The first parameter represents the mean diameter of the nanoparticle population, while the second is the polydispersity index describing the dimensional homogeneity of the system (with <0.3 being the optimal value for solid nanoparticles) [31].

2.5. Encapsulation Efficiency Evaluation

To evaluate the encapsulation efficiency (EE) of the drug, the bilosystem was subjected to disruption to allow the passage of budesonide into the solution; then, its concentration was measured using a high-performance liquid chromatography (HPLC) system (Agilent Technologies, 1200 Series, Santa Clara, CA, USA) equipped with a UV detector and a 50 µL loop Rheodyne injection valve. The HPLC conditions for analysis are summarized in Table 1.

Table 1. HPLC analysis conditions for samples containing Budesonide.

Column	Mobile Phase	Flow (mL/min)	Wavelength (nm)	Pressure (bar)	Retention Time (min)
Kinetex 5 µm C18 100 Å, RP, 150 × 4.6 mm	Acetonitrile and Phosphate buffer (pH 3.2) 60:40 *v/v*	0.8 (isocratic mode)	245	80	3.4–3.5

Particularly, 100 µL of bilosystem dispersion was mixed with 900 µL of HPLC mobile phase, and the system was kept under magnetic stirring for 3 h in an ice bath; then, the mix was filtered through 0.22 µm pore nylon filters and diluted 1:5 by volume with the mobile phase. Subsequently, each sample was injected twice in the chromatographic HPLC column and the drug concentration was calculated by comparison with a reference standard solution. The EE was calculated using Equation (1):

$$EE = B/TB \times 100 \quad (1)$$

where B is the amount of budesonide determined via HPLC and TB is the total budesonide amount used to prepare the formulation.

2.6. Equilibrium Dialysis Experiments

Budesonide release was evaluated via dialysis using either a nylon membrane (cutoff 10,000–12,000 Da) or a rat small intestine fragment and different receiving phases (i.e., fasted-state simulated gastric fluid, FaSSGF; fasted-state simulated intestinal fluid, FaSSIF; phosphate-buffered saline, PBS), whose composition is reported in Table 2.

Table 2. Composition of receiving phases used in diffusion experiments.

Receiving Phase	Component	Concentration
FaSSGF (pH 1.6)	Sodium cholate Phosphatidylcholine NaCl	80 μM 20 μM 0.32 mM
FaSSIF (pH 6.5)	Sodium taurocholate Phosphatidylcholine porcine lipase	3.0 mM 0.2 mM 100 U/mL
PBS (pH 7.2–7.4)	$NaH_2PO_4 \times H_2O$ $NaHPO_4 \times 2\,H_2O$ NaCl	16.08 mM 80 mM 1.5 M

Wistar rat intestine was used for permeation experiments (OpBA protocol codes CBCC2.50 and 373/2021-PR CBCC2.48). After removal from the animal, the intestine was washed with PBS, cut into 10 cm long fragments, stored at −20 °C until use and submerged in PBS for 12 h before use.

The membrane was filled with 1 mL of formulation, and then, closed at the ends with plastic pincers and submerged in 50 mL of receiving phase inside flasks kept on a tilting agitator (IKA LABORTECHNIK KS250basic). Samples of 500 μL were withdrawn from the receiving phase at predetermined time intervals during the 8 h of the experiment and filtered (nylon filters of 0.22 μm porosity) before HPLC analyses. After each collection, an equal volume of fresh receiving phase was reintegrated into the flask.

2.7. Cell Culture and Treatments

Human colorectal adenocarcinoma CaCo2 cells were cultured in high-glucose Dulbecco's Modified Eagle's Medium (Corning, Corning, NY, USA) supplemented with 10% FBS (Sigma-Aldrich, St. Louis, MO, USA), 100 U/mL penicillin, 100 μg/mL streptomycin (Gibco, Waltham, MA, USA) and 1% non-essential amino acids (Microtech cat. ACL006), as previously described [32]. All cell cultures were performed at 37 °C in 5% CO_2 and 95% air. For the experiment, CaCo2 cells were treated for 24 h with different formulations containing budesonide, such as the ethanol solution (Sol B) and bilosomes (Bilos), at the indicated doses. Before the treatment, all the formulations were subjected to simulated digestion by incubating them for 30 min with FaSSIF. For the glucose oxidase (GO) experiments, cells were exposed to 0.5 U/mL of GO (G2133, Sigma Aldrich, Saint Louis, MO, USA) for 1 h, and then, samples were harvested 0 and 3 h after the end of GO insult for the following immunofluorescence and ELISA analyses.

2.7.1. Cytotoxicity Study (MTT Assay)

To determine the non-toxic treatment dose, an MTT assay was performed on CaCo2 cells as previously described [32]. Briefly, CaCo2 cells were cultured in 96-well plates at a density of 1×10^4 in 200 μL of media and treated for 24 h with the different formulations containing concentrations of budesonide ranging from 1 to 20 μg/mL. Upon removal of treatment, 110 μL of cell medium containing the MTT solution at a concentration of 0.5 mg/mL was added to each well and incubated for 4 h at 37 °C, 5% CO_2. The insoluble purple formazan crystals were then dissolved in 100 μL of DMSO at 37 °C for 15 min and the solution absorbance was measured using a spectrophotometer at 570 nm, using 690 nm as a reference wavelength, and then, converted into percentage of viability.

2.7.2. Immunofluorescence Staining

We seeded 1×10^5 cells/mL of CaCo2 cells in 12-well plates and they were cultured for 24 h. Then, cells were pre-treated with the budesonide formulations (Sol B, Bilos) at a dose of 2.5 μg/mL and the respective unloaded formulations. After 24 h, cells were exposed to 0.5 U/mL of GO for 1 h, and then, collected right after the end of GO exposure (T0) and 3 h later (T3). Cells were washed in PBS, and then, fixed in 4% paraformaldehyde (PFA) in PBS for 10 min at room temperature. Cells were permeabilized with 0.25% Triton X-100 in PBS for 10 min at RT, and then, blocked in PBS-BSA 2% for 45 min at RT. Slides were incubated with primary antibody NLRP3 (NBP2-12446, Novus Biological, Littleton, CO, USA) 1:200 in 0.25% BSA/PBS and ASC (SC-514414, Santa Cruz Biotechnology Inc., Dallas, TX, USA) 1:100 in 0.25% BSA/PBS overnight at 4 °C. The samples were then incubated with fluorochrome-conjugated secondary antibodies (A11004 Alexa Fluor 568, A11008 Alexa Fluor 488) for 1 h at RT, and nuclei were stained with 1 μg/mL of DAPI (Sigma-Aldrich, Merck, Darmstadt, Germany) for 5 min. PermaFluor Aqueous Mounting Medium (TA-006-FM ThermoFisher Scientific, Waltham, MA, USA) was used to mount the coverslips onto glass slides, and the fluorescence signal was examined using a Leica light microscope (Leica, Wetzlar, Germany) equipped with epifluorescence at 40× magnification. Images were quantified using ImageJ software (ImageJ 1.53a, Wayne Rasband National Institute of Health, Bethesda, MD, USA).

2.7.3. IL-1β ELISA Assay

An IL-1β ELISA kit (Cat. DY201-05, Novus Biologicals, Centennial, CO, USA) was employed to measure the levels of IL-1β in media of CaCo2 cells treated with budesonide formulations and collected 3 h post-GO exposure. Absorbance was measured using a spectrophotometer equipped with a filter of 450 nm, using 570 nm as a reference wavelength. IL-1β levels were expressed as pg/mL in culture media according to the manufacturer's instructions.

2.8. Mathematical and Statistical Analysis

Concerning mathematical analysis, a graphical method is used to experimentally obtain the order of release. Indeed, the experimental data were plotted according to the equations of the different orders. Afterwards the coefficient of linear regression was determined and the coefficient of determination (R^2) was then obtained. R^2 values closest to 1 allowed us to obtain the order of reaction. Therefore, the release kinetics were determined via linear regression analysis of the in vitro release curves according to the best mathematical models expressing the kinetic release profile, namely, zero-order (cumulative amount (%) of drug released over time), first order (logarithmic cumulative amount (%) of drug released over time) and second order (Higuchi) (cumulative amount (%) of drug released over the square root of time).

The Shapiro–Wilk test was used to find the normality distribution of data, and statistical analysis was conducted using GraphPad Prism 9 (Version 9.4.1 (458), GraphPad Software Inc., La Jolla, CA, USA). Analysis of variance (1-way or 2-way ANOVA), followed by Tukey's post hoc test, was used for each of the variables tested. Data are expressed as mean ± SD of duplicate determinations obtained in three independent experiments. The probability (p) value was considered non-significant statistically when $p > 0.05$, statistically significant when $p \leq 0.05$ and highly significant when $p \leq 0.01$.

3. Results and Discussion

3.1. Preformulation Studies

3.1.1. Bilosomes

A preformulation study, which aimed to select and to identify the best characteristics of the formulation, in terms of stiffness of the lipid bilayer and its stability, was carried out on bilosomes composed of PC and ursodeoxycholic acid (U) (Bilos_PU) and bilosomes composed of PC, CH and U (Bilos_PCU), as described in Table S2. As expected, Bilos_PCU dispersion was found to be more stable after production; therefore, a technological study was carried out on Bilos_PCU applying the same preparation protocols (i.e., Film hydration, Fh) with a few differences, such as hydration with room temperature solution (FhRT), hydration with room temperature solution followed by sonication (FhRTS), hydration with warm solution (FhW) and hydration with warm solution followed by sonication (FhWS).

The obtained bilosome dispersions were analyzed in terms of size via PCS, considering as dimensional parameters the mean diameter of the vesicles (Z-Average), the polydispersion index (PdI) and the scattering intensity (Intensity). The formulations, periodically analyzed to define their macroscopic and dimensional characteristics, indicated that FhWS is the most effective production process, leading to vesicles becoming stable over time (Figure S1). Indeed, the process carried out using room-temperature hydrating solution led to vesicles increasing in mean diameter and the formation of macroscopically visible aggregates one month after production. On the other hand, hydration conducted with warm solution (60 °C) seemed to favor the formation of stable and well-organized vesicles.

It is well known that the formation of the phospholipid bilayer is not a spontaneous process but requires energy. The phase transition of phospholipids varies according to the type of membrane composition, passing from an ordered "gel" phase to a more fluid and disordered "liquid-crystalline" phase; to reach this phase, characterized by greater molecular freedom of movement, an increase in temperature is needed to form the phospholipid bilayer [33]. Sonication seems to ensure stability over time, avoiding the formation of aggregates. In fact, in FhW preparations, the average diameter increases over time, whereas sonicated preparations show a gradual decrease over time and a gradual decrease in polydispersion to 0.3.

Therefore, the technological preformulation study indicated that warm hydration and subsequent sonication allow the membrane to undergo a thermotropic phase transition, giving greater stability and reducing aggregation phenomena.

The preformulative study was conducted on bilos_PC obtained in the presence of other bile acids, such as T or C. The preformulative study allowed us to identify the most efficient preparation technique and the most stable vesicular composition of the bilosomes. We then proceeded with the preparation of bilosomes containing the active principle budesonide for the following studies.

3.1.2. Biloparticles

In the case of biloparticles, a preformulation study was performed to select the composition of lipid nanoparticles, namely, SLN (BilopS) and NLC (BilopN). Lipid nanoparticles were prepared by adding increasing amounts of bile acids, namely, ursodeoxycholic acid (BilopS_U), sodium cholate (BilopS_C) and sodium taurocholate (BilopS_T), with the aim of finding out the formulation leading to the best dimensional characteristics. Notably, direct proportionality between mean size (Z-Ave) and bile acid content for BilopS_C and BilopS_T was observed, which was not visible for BilopS_U. The type of bile acid induces large variability in terms of the size and polydispersity of nanoparticles at concentrations of 0.2%, 0.4% and 1.2%, while a content 0.8% of bile acid allowed for the maintenance of homogeneity in size and dispersion in all conditions (Figure S2). Therefore, on the basis of the obtained results, a content of 0.8% of bile acid was selected as the quantity to produce biloparticles for this study.

3.2. Production and Characterization of Bilosomes and Biloparticles Containing Budesonide

3.2.1. Bilosomes

Taking into account the results of the preformulation studies, bilosomes were produced in the presence of budesonide, and the vesicles were characterized in terms of morphology, size distribution and encapsulation yield. As an example, in Figure 1 images of empty and budesonide-loaded Bilos_PCU are reported.

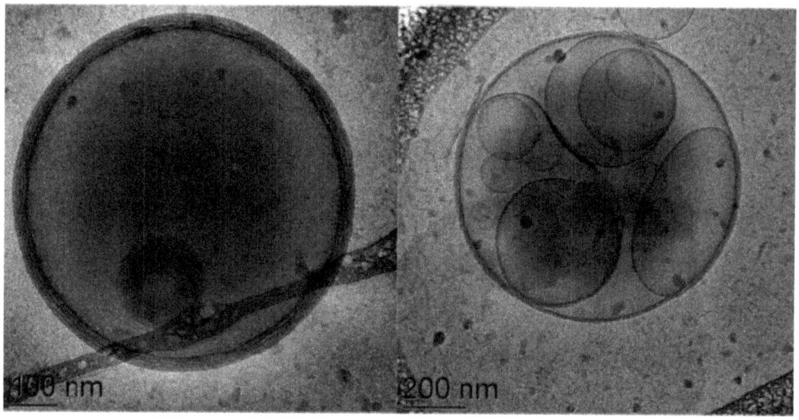

(**a**) (**b**)

Figure 1. Cryo-TEM images of Bilos_PCU without (**a**) and with (**b**) budesonide prepared via a warm film hydration method followed by sonication (FhWS).

The PCS data obtained for the produced bilosomes were compared with those of the corresponding empty preparations. Figure 2 shows the Z-Average and PdI values of the produced bilosomes that were unloaded (Bilos_PCU, Bilos_PCT, Bilos_PCC) and loaded with the drug (Bilos_PCUB, Bilos_PCTB, Bilos_PCCB). In particular, Bilos_PCUB's mean size is 410.8 nm, comparable to that of Bilos_PCU (419.9 nm). Bilos_PCTB (338.4 nm) and Bilos_PCCB (150.4 nm) instead exhibit a much smaller mean diameter than the corresponding empty bilosome dispersions (i.e., Bilos_PCT 458.5 nm and Bilos_PCC 320.82 nm).

Observing the PdI data, it can be seen that budesonide-loaded U bilosomes show slightly different polydispersity values compared to the corresponding unloaded formulation, with 0.31 for Bilos_PCUB and 0.35 for Bilos_PCU. Bilos_PCT (0.48) and Bilos_PCC (0.43) instead present higher PdI values than the corresponding formulations containing budesonide (i.e., Bilos_PCTB 0.35 and Bilos_PCCB 0.32).

From the analysis of the reported results, it emerges that the dimensional variation can be attributed to the presence of the drug. This behavior is more evident for bilos_PCCB as compared to bilos_PCUB or bilos_PCTB. We tentatively hypothesized that the assembling of the drug within the bilayer could be responsible for vesicle size reduction due to the interactions among the lipophilic moieties of phospholipids and bile acids, on the basis of some studies demonstrating that increasing amounts of cholesterol (a steroid molecule similar to budesonide) in the liposome bilayer improves particle uniformity (PDI) [25,34,35], and that a synthetic budesonide derivative assembled into liposomal nanovesicles for oral delivery shows favorable colloidal stability in different media (i.e., PBS, FASSGF, FASSIF) [21].

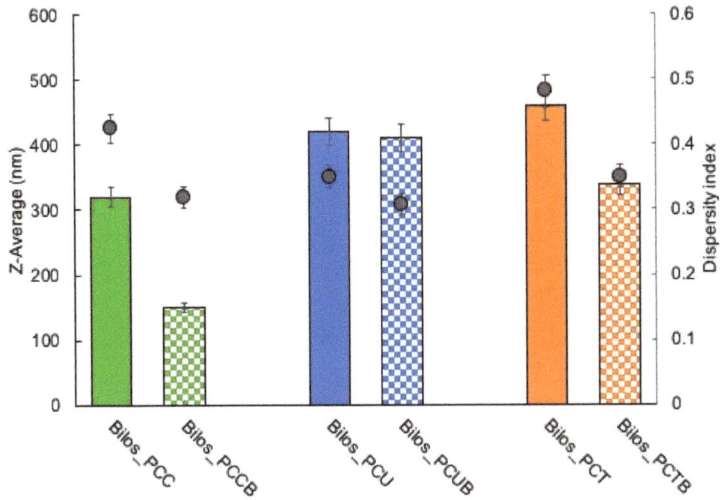

Figure 2. Dimensional parameters of bilosomes with (squares) and without (plain) budesonide, expressed as average diameter (histograms) and dispersity index (circles). Values are the mean of 3 batches ± s.d.

Indeed, the presence of a budesonide steroid nucleus with hydrophilic groups in positions 11β and 17β confers an amphipathic nature to the molecules, allowing the intercalation of the drug within the membrane, possibly improving the characteristics of the bilayer and making the size more homogeneous and monodisperse.

Concerning the efficiency of drug encapsulation (encapsulation efficiency, EE%), an essential parameter to indicate how much drug has actually been encapsulated inside the nanocarrier, it was calculated as the quantity of drug present in the formulation with respect to the drug content weighed for the preparation. The analysis was performed via HPLC the day after production. The percentage yield of the drug was calculated using the mathematical equation described in the Materials and Methods section.

It was found that all the formulations present high encapsulation yields. Notably Bilos_PCUB displays the highest percentage yield (92.76 ± 7.12), while both Bilos_PCTB (88.8 ± 17.9) and Bilos_PCCB (88.7 ± 21.9) display superimposable values. This behavior corroborates studies describing that the film hydration method, leading to multilamellar vesicles, is able to highly incorporate lipophilic drugs due to their intercalation between the alkyl chains of phospholipids [36–39].

3.2.2. Biloparticles

Biloparticles with compositions obtained from the preformulation study were loaded with budesonide, and then, characterized. The biloparticles' morphology was investigated via cryo-TEM, and the exemplificative images of budesonide-loaded BilopS_U and BilopN_U are reported in Figure 3. No differences in terms of morphology are evident in drug-loaded bilopS and bilopN with the presence of different bile acids (i.e., S and T).

In general, the three-dimensional particles are projected in a two-dimensional way. Concerning bilopS, elongated circular platelet-like crystalline particles and electron-dense "needle-like" structures, when viewed edge-on, can be observed due to the tilted position of the particle. On the other hand, bilopN's shape appears roundish, discoid from the top view, or more electron-dense and rod-like from the edge-on view. Some inner ultrastructures are visible, showing several layers [40].

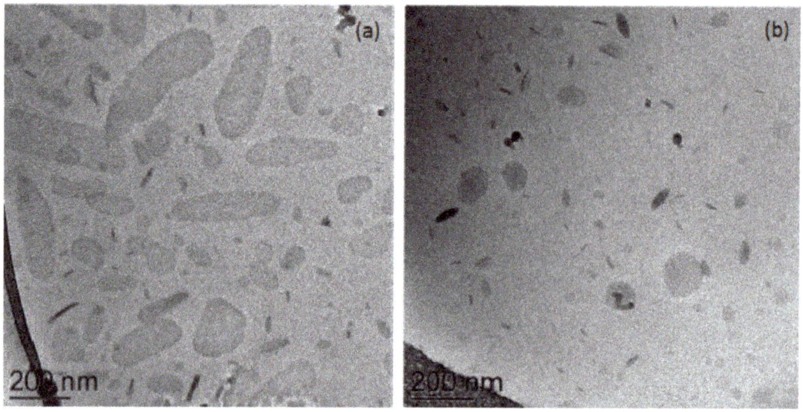

Figure 3. Cryo-TEM images of BilopS_UB (**a**) and BilopN_UB (**b**).

Figure 4 shows the dimensional characteristics of the produced biloparticle dispersions loaded with budesonide. In terms of size, BilopS usually displays a larger mean diameter than BilopN. Additionally, BilopN shows a more homogenous size distribution compared to BilopS; in fact, the difference between the PdI of BilopS and BilopN is very small.

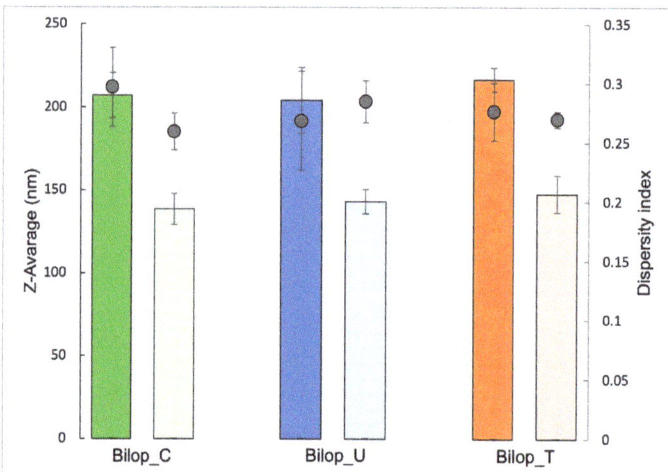

Figure 4. Mean diameter (Z-Average, histograms) and polydispersity (PdI, circles) of BilopS (dark color) and BilopN (light color) containing different bile acids, as determined via PCS. Each value is the average of 5 batches ± s.d.

The encapsulation efficiency of budesonide of both BiolpS and BilopN is summarized in Table 3. In general, BilopS shows higher encapsulation efficiency and lower drug loss in the aggregate compared to BilopN. For both types of biloparticles, the increase in encapsulation efficiency follows the order Bilop_U < Bilop_C < Bilop_T.

Table 3. Encapsulation efficiency of budesonide within the produced biloparticles.

Biloparticles	Encapsulation Efficiency * (%) ± s.d.
BilopS_CB	69.25 ± 6.48
BilopS_UB	59.10 ± 1.96
BilopS_TB	81.96 ± 2.76
BilopN_CB	61.87 ± 9.32
BilopN_UB	57.74 ± 1.66
BilopN_TB	70.20 ± 5.44

* Each value is the average of 5 batches ± standard deviation.

3.3. *In Vitro and Ex Vivo Studies*

The release kinetics of budesonide from bilosomes and biloparticles were studied in vitro via equilibrium dialysis. In particular, two different types of membranes were used, a synthetic one (nylon cutoff 10,000–12,000 Da) and a natural one consisting of a portion of the small intestine of a Wistar rat. Furthermore, two different receiving solutions were considered: FaSSGF, able to simulate gastric fluid, and FaSSIF, able to simulate intestinal fluid (Table 2). The experimental model is described in the Materials and Methods section.

The in vitro study attempts to mimic in vivo oral administration. Once administered, the formulation encounters environments that differ profoundly in terms of pH, the presence of enzymes and electrolytes, fluid viscosity and mucous surface characteristics. All of these factors can affect drug absorption; therefore, through equilibrium dialysis, it is possible to investigate the behavior of the drug by mimicking gastrointestinal transit using artificial gastric and intestinal fluid, with their specific characteristics in terms of pH and composition.

The experiment was conducted for all the bilosystems containing budesonide, namely, Bilos_PCUB, Bilos_PCTB, Bilos_PCCB, BilopS_UB, BilopN_UB, BilopS_CB, BilopN_CB, BilopS_TB and BilopN_TB, which were then compared with a dispersion of the drug in FaSSGF or FaSSIF (Susp B) and with an ethanol solution of the drug (Sol B).

The release kinetics obtained for the different formulations are represented in Figure 5. The left column displays the results of experiments with FaSSGF as the receiving phase, whereas the column on the right reports the release in the FaSSIF receiving phase.

From the obtained results, it is possible to notice that, both in FaSSGF and FaSSIF, budesonide is released from the bilosystems more slowly than from Sol B, which reaches 100% of release after the third hour, with no significant differences between gastric and intestinal environments. On the other hand, the drug released from Susp B (either in FaSSGF or FaSSIF) reaches 4% after 24 h. In the same time interval, most of the bilosystem formulations release a maximum of 20% of the drug. Indeed, comparing the percentage of budesonide released by Bilos_UB in the gastric fluid, it reaches a maximum of 37%, while in the intestinal fluid, the maximum release is 20%. This indicates that in an acidic environment, the presence of U in the bilosome composition causes a greater release than in a basic environment and in the presence of lipase.

The pH-sensitive release may enhance the targeting ability of the drug-loaded bilosomes following the gastrointestinal absorption of intact vesicles. However, this requires further in vivo confirmatory investigations.

Conversely, Bilos_PCTB and Bilos_PCCB in the gastric environment (Figure 5a) show approximately the same trend, with a release of 30% after 8 h and 37% after 24 h. In the intestinal environment (Figure 5b), bilos_PCCB shows a release of 37% after 8 h, which remains constant even at the twenty-fourth hour. In the case of Bilos_PCC, a 25% release and a maximum of 28% after 24 h is evident, lower than Bilos_PCTB.

This experiment indicates that Bilos_PCTB is the formulation able to release higher quantities of budesonide in the intestinal and gastric environments (40% release). Bilos_PCCB, on the other hand, keeps the release superimposable in both receiving phases, increasing by 7% in the gastric fluid after 24 h. In the intestinal environment Bilos_PCUB is lower in terms of percentage release, while in the gastric environment, it surpasses the other preparations up to the eighth hour, and then, remains constant (37%).

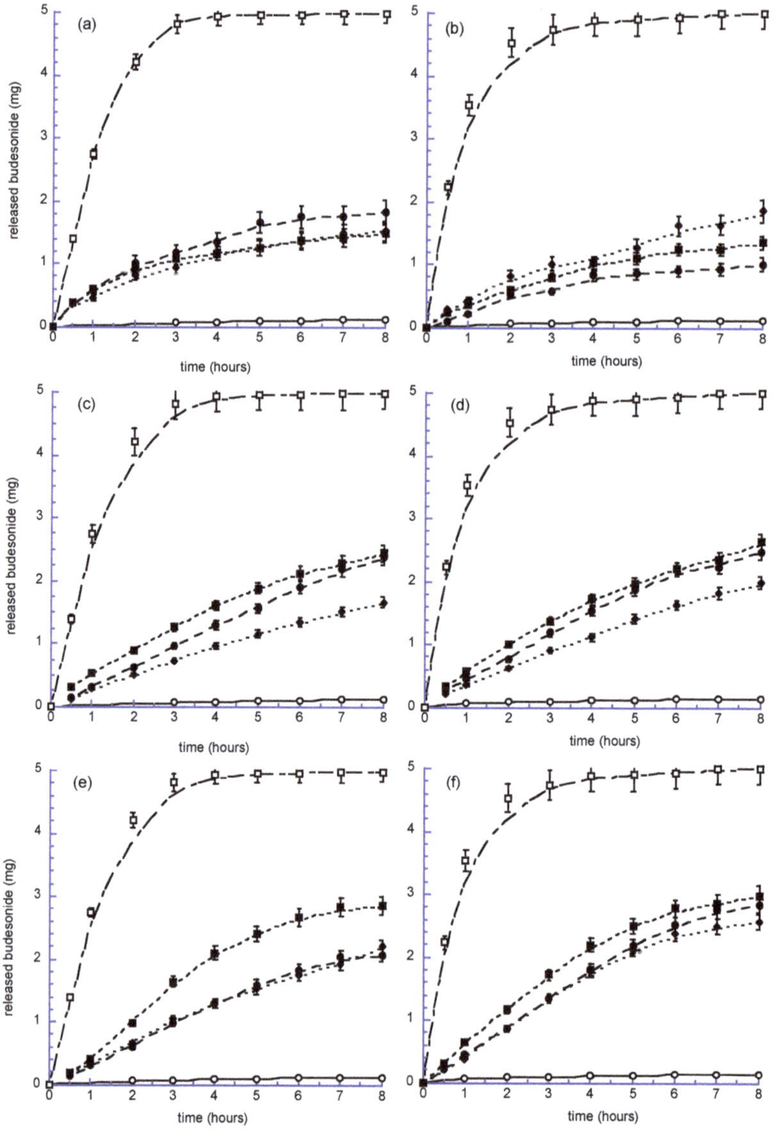

Figure 5. Budesonide release kinetics in FaSSGF (**a**,**c**,**e**) and FaSSIF (**b**,**d**,**f**) from Bilos (**a**,**b**), BilopS (**c**,**d**) and BilopN (**e**,**f**). Bilos_PCUB, BilopS_UB and BilopN_UB: closed circle; Bilos_PCCB, BilopS_CB and BilopN_CB: closed square; Bilos_PCTB, BilopS_TB and BilopN_TB: closed diamond; For comparison, the releases from Susp B in FaSSGF/FaSSIF (open circle) and Sol B (open square) are also reported. Each datum is the average of 2 experiments ± s.d.

The comparison of biloparticle release curves with those of budesonide dispersed in FaSSGF and FaSSIF highlights a significant improvement in budesonide's passage into the aqueous solution when carried by biloparticles. Budesonide is a lipophilic molecule with poor water solubility and cannot solubilize on its own in FaSSIF and FaSSGF, leading to a very low percentage of release even after 24 h (only 3% of the active ingredient released), while its encapsulation in biloparticles increases the release up to 70%.

In addition, it is possible to observe some differences in the release of bilopS and bilopN, depending on the type of bile acid and on the receiving phase. Specifically, for both bilopS and bilopN, greater release percentages were obtained in FaSSIF than in FaSSGF. BilopN_UB, bilopN_CB and bilopN_TB are able to release budesonide faster than the corresponding bilopS in FaSSGF and FaSSIF.

Among bilopN, bilopN_CB shows the highest release kinetics, especially in FaSSGF. In particular, after 24 h, 72% of budesonide was released in FaSSIF and 67% in FaSSGF. Concerning bilopS, BilopS_UB and BilopS_CB show the highest release kinetics both in FaSSGF and FaSSIF, while BilopS_TB has the slowest release; in fact, after 24 h, only 53% of the drug was released in the intestinal environment and 45% in the gastric environment. Percentages greater than 60% were achieved for all other formulations after the same time interval.

Subsequently, in order to have information about how budesonide could cross the intestinal wall, an experiment using an ex vivo model was carried out. The experiment was performed using a rat small intestine fragment as a dialysis tube, and phosphate saline buffer (PBS) as the receiving phase. The bilosomes and biloparticles, namely, Bilos_PCUB, BilopS_UB, BilopN_UB, Bilos_PCCB, BilopS_CB, BilopN_CB, Bilos_PCTB, BilopS_TB and BilopN_TB, diluted 1:1 by volume with FaSSIF, were inserted into the intestinal tube, which was suitably closed at the ends, to mimic the in vivo conditions. As a control, a budesonide suspension in FaSSIF (Susp B) was used.

In general, in agreement with the literature [41], it was found that budesonide loaded into bilosystems reveals remarkable improvement in drug intestinal transport compared to simple budesonide aqueous suspension. Notably, from the analysis of Figure 6a, Bilos_PCUB and Bilos_PCTB display almost the same trend, increasing the release up to 20% at 8 h. The release from Bilos_PCCB is higher than the other Bilos, reaching a release of about 30% of the total drug content.

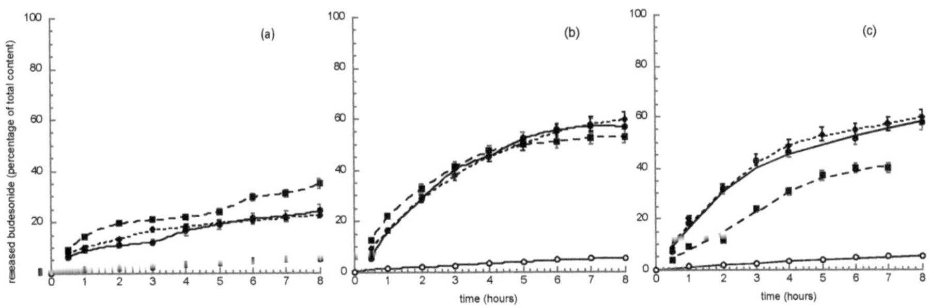

Figure 6. Budesonide releases kinetics through rat small intestine from Bilos (**a**), BilopS (**b**) and BilopN (**c**) suspended in PBS/FaSSIF (50:50 v:v). Bilos_PCUB, BilopS_UB and BilopN_UB: closed circle; Bilos_PCCB, BilopS_CB and BilopN_CB: closed square; Bilos_PCTB, BilopS_TB and BilopN_TB: closed diamond; The release from FaSSIF Susp B (open circle) is also reported for comparison. Each value is the mean of 3 experiments ± s.d.

By comparing bilopS and bilopN (Figure 6b,c), it is evident that both can enhance budesonide intestinal absorption compared to the active ingredient in suspension, which does not exceed 5% of release after 8 h. Notably, for bilopS, after 3 h, at least 40% of budesonide is released from the biloparticles, reaching the 60% after 8 h. Moreover, the presence of different bile acids seems to not affect the release of the drug.

Regarding bilopN (Figure 6c), the expected increase in Budesonide release involves only bilopN_U and bilopN_T.

From the comparison between bilopS and bilopN (Figure 6b,c), the drug release from bilosystems containing U or T displays similar trends, while bilopN_C is characterized by slower release kinetics than the corresponding bilopS_C.

These results indicate that the bilosystem (either bilosome or biloparticle) is able to increase the solubility and to control the release of the incorporated drug. Furthermore, these data revealed the significant dominance of the bilosystem to enhance the intestinal passage of budesonide, possibly due to the ability of these nanocarriers to improve the intestinal permeability of the encapsulated drugs [42–56].

3.3.1. Mathematical Analysis

It is well known that the passage of a molecule from a donor compartment to a recipient increases until it reaches equilibrium, with the transit rate depending on the physico-chemical properties of the drug, the nature of the membrane and the gradient concentration between the two compartments.

On the basis of Fick's laws, it is possible to obtain the release rate of the drug described by kinetic models in which the drug is released as a function of time [57]. Particularly, both the empirical and mechanistic mathematical models based on the Fick's laws are usually employed to describe the drug release from a drug delivery system [58]. The main types of kinetics are the zero-, first- and second-order (or Higuchi).

The zero-order equation (Table 4) describes a release directly proportional to time, such as that from matrices with low solubility and osmotic systems. Notably, the carrier enables the release of the same amount of drug per unit of time, with the release being independent of its concentration in the system. On the other hand, the first-order equation (Table 4) relates to a drug release rate depending on the concentration of the drug remaining within the system, typical, for instance, of the release from a porous matrix.

Table 4. Kinetic parameter R^2 of budesonide released from bilosomes and biloparticles through synthetic and natural membranes.

Formulation	Nylon Membrane			Rat Intestinal Membrane		
	Zero Order $F = K_0\ t$	First Order $\ln(1 - F) = -K_1\ t$	Second Order $F = K_2\ t^{1/2}$	Zero Order $F = K_0\ t$	First Order $\ln(1 - F) = -K_1\ t$	Second Order $F = K_2\ t^{1/2}$
Susp B	0.8753	0.8650	0.9878	0.9703	0.9642	0.9624
Bilos_PCUB	0.9038	0.9160	0.9614	0.9774	0.9584	0.9768
Bilos_PCCB	0.9365	0.9524	0.9850	0.9324	0.9128	0.9256
Bilos_PCTB	0.9634	0.9721	0.9763	0.9815	0.8605	0.9170
BilopS_UB	0.9798	0.9922	0.9601	0.8708	0.9343	0.9577
BilopS_CB	0.9717	0.9940	0.9808	0.8327	0.8776	0.9350
BilopS_TB	0.9922	0.9986	0.9589	0.9289	0.9721	0.9878
BilopN_UB	0.9807	0.9935	0.9531	0.8648	0.9305	0.9524
BilopN_CB	0.9461	0.9793	0.9720	0.9460	0.9643	0.9672
BilopN_TB	0.9632	0.9986	0.9572	0.8682	0.9315	0.9574

Concerning the second-order equation (Higuchi model), being substantially derived from Fick diffusion law [59], a direct relationship between the drug release rate from the matrix and the square root of time is described as typical of a homogeneous non-erodible granular matrix. Particularly, the Higuchi equation (Table 4) [60] refers to systems in which (a) the drug concentration at the beginning is greater than the drug solubility, (b) the matrix is a thin film that is not erodible or degradable, (c) the size of the drug particle is lower than the film thickness and (d) the diffusivity of the drug does not depend on space and time.

As shown in Table 4, the second-order (Higuchi) model expresses the highest value of the R^2 coefficient for all types of bilosome preparations when the synthetic membrane (nylon) is used for the release. On the other hand, the bilosome kinetics obtained from a natural membrane (rat intestine) follow the zero order.

Concerning biloparticles, different behavior was found. Indeed, budesonides' release kinetics followed the first order when a nylon membrane was used for the experiment, whereas in the case of intestinal membrane, a second-order release was detected.

This different behavior between bilosomes and biloparticles is ascribable either to the nature of the nanosystem or to the type of interaction with the membrane.

Indeed, when the vesicular systems are poured into a nylon bag, the bilosomes are stable, acting as a non-degradable system, and the release is independent of space and time. On the other hand, when the vesicles are in contact with the intestinal tube, they interact with the membrane and possibly fuse with it, allowing for a concentration independent of the release by the system.

Regarding biloparticles, the transition from the first to the second order can be due to the solid state of the particles compared to the more fluid vesicles. Notably, when poured in the synthetic membrane, it seems that the drug release from biloparticles mainly depends on the structural conformation of the matrix and the drug concentration loaded within the particles, whereas when the release is carried out within the intestinal membrane, the system becomes more stable and less erodible, possibly due to a firm interaction with the mucous on the tissue surface.

3.3.2. Cell Studies

On the basis of the encapsulation efficiency of the drug (Table 3) and the drug content stability over time, Bilos_PCU and Bilos_PCUB were selected for the experiments on cultured cells.

MTT Assay

To select the non-toxic treatment dose to be used in the experiments, CaCo2 cells were treated for 24 h with formulations containing or not containing budesonide at a concentration ranging from 1 to 20 μg/mL and subjected to an MTT assay. As shown in Figure 7, cells treated with the solution containing budesonide (Sol B) at a dose above 2.5 μg/mL displayed a decrease in viability (less than 80%) compared to untreated controls cells, whereas Bilos_PCUB formulations did not significantly affect cell viability at any selected doses. Considering that the aim of this study was to compare whether Bilos_PCU is a more effective vehicle for budesonide with respect to the solution, we selected 2.5 μg/mL as the safe treatment dose to use in further analysis.

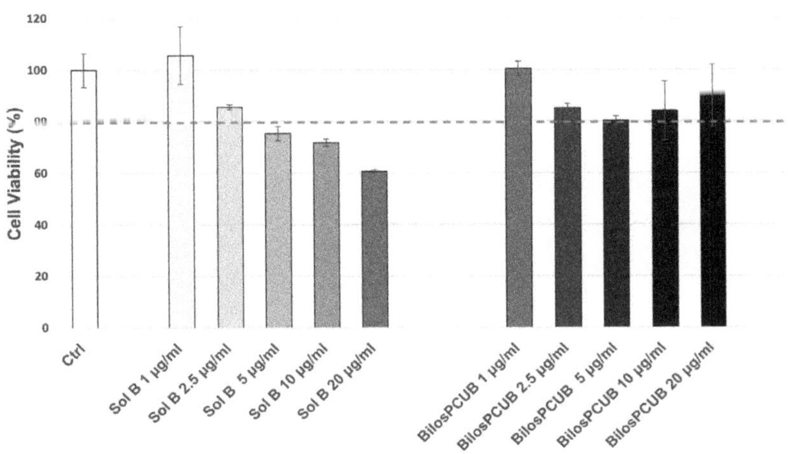

Figure 7. MTT assay on CaCo2 cells treated for 24 h with budesonide formulations (Sol B, Bilos_PCUB) at different doses ranging from 1 to 20 μg/mL. Cell viability is presented as percentage with respect to untreated control cells. Data are given as mean ± SD, representative of three independent experiments with at least three technical replicates each time. A value of 80% (red dotted line) was considered the reference accepted cell viability.

Immunofluorescence NLRP3-ASC and ELISA IL-1β

Budesonide is a corticosteroid used as an anti-inflammatory drug in many gastric and intestinal pathologies [11]. Inflammasomes are multiprotein complexes of the innate immune systems that are currently widely studied due to their role in mediating the inflammatory response in several tissues [61].

These inflammatory pathways can be activated by different stimuli, including pathogens and oxidative stress mediators such as reactive oxygen species (ROS). In particular, stimuli able to induce oxidative stress reactions have been shown to promote the activation of inflammasome pathways, and thus, the inflammatory response [62].

For instance, NLRP3, one of the most well-known inflammasomes, has been shown to mediate the inflammatory response in intestinal disorders via an oxidative stress mechanism [63–65]. Thus, to understand whether the NLRP3 inflammasome could be activated in human intestinal cells in response to an oxidative stimulus, and to evaluate whether formulations containing budesonide could prevent an oxidative stress-related inflammatory response, as already evidenced [66], we triggered CaCo2 cells with the oxidoreductase enzyme glucose oxidase (GO), able to induce the production of hydrogen peroxide (H_2O_2) via glucose oxidation as previously described [67].

Our results show that GO exposure could induce an inflammatory state in CaCo2 cells, represented by increased expression levels of NLRP3 and ASC right after the end of exposure (Figure 8).

Notably, pre-treatment with Bilos_PCUB could significantly prevent the induction of NLRP3 and ASC upon GO insult, whereas Sol B could only partially prevent the damage. Interestingly, CaCo2 cells pretreated with Sol B and not exposed to GO also presented an increase in inflammasome component expression, suggesting that when budesonide is not conveyed/included in a delivery system, it can be irritating for cells.

When activated, the inflammasome pathway results in the production and maturation of inflammatory cytokines such as Interleukin-1β (IL-1β) that can propagate the inflammatory response. Thus, we measured the levels of IL-1β in media of CaCo2 cells exposed to GO and pre-treated with budesonide formulations.

As shown in Figure 9, we found increased levels of IL-1β 3 h after the end of GO exposure. These data confirm the activation of the inflammasome and the establishment of an inflammatory response. When treated with both Sol B and Bilos_PCUB, the levels of IL-1β were completely restored to the basal state. Of note, Bilos_PCUB was even more effective in reducing the inflammatory response induced by GO stimuli compared to Sol B, confirming that this delivery system can serve as a better vehicle for budesonide to counteract ox-inflammatory damage within intestinal cells. As a matter of fact, the interplay between oxidative and inflammatory mediators can promote a phenomenon called ox-inflammation [68], which often occurs in many conditions, including intestinal disorders [69].

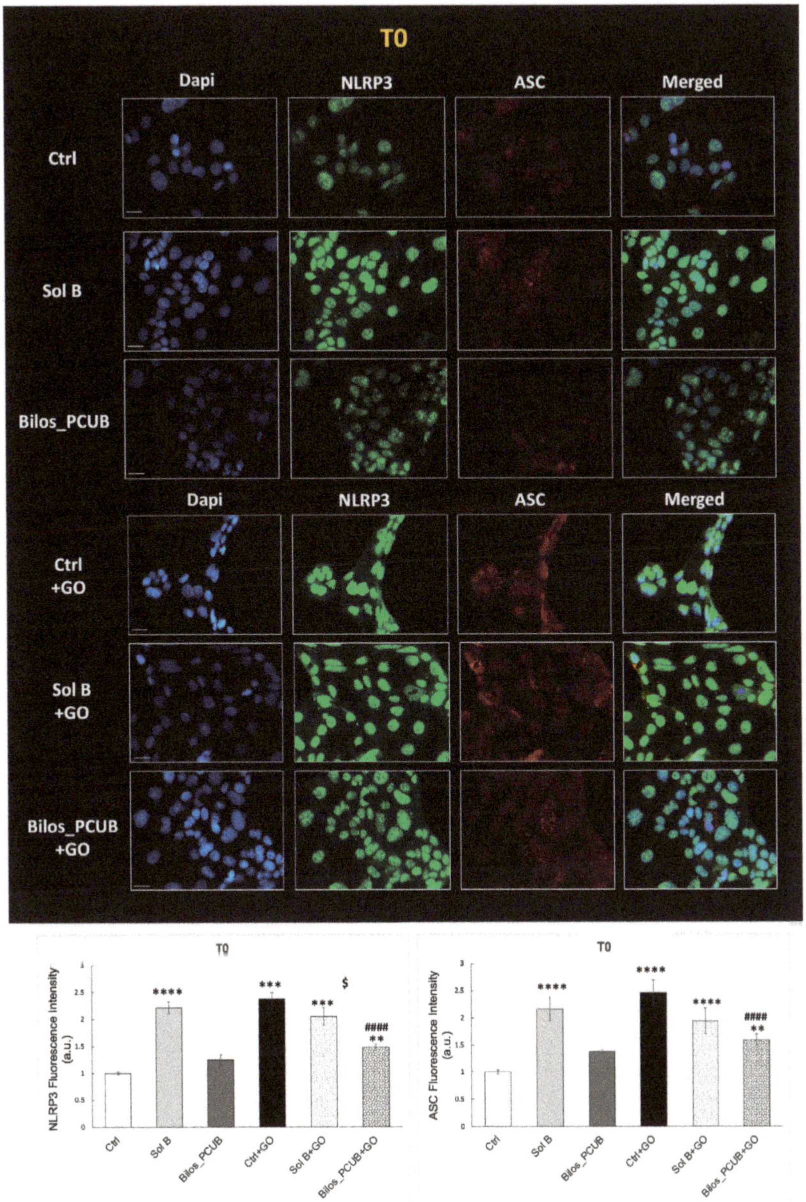

Figure 8. Immunofluorescence staining for NLRP3 (green) and ASC (red) on CaCo2 cells treated with formulations containing budesonide and exposed to 0.5 U/mL of GO for 1 h. Blue staining (DAPI) represents nuclei. Images were taken at 40 × magnification (scale bar = 40 μm), and the fluorescent signal was quantified using ImageJ software. Data are the results of the averages of at least three different experiments, obtained via 2-way ANOVA followed by Tukey's post hoc comparison test. $^{\$}$ $p < 0.05$; ** $p < 0.01$; *** $p < 0.005$; ****,#### $p < 0.0001$ (* with respect to Ctrl and # with respect to Ctrl + GO).

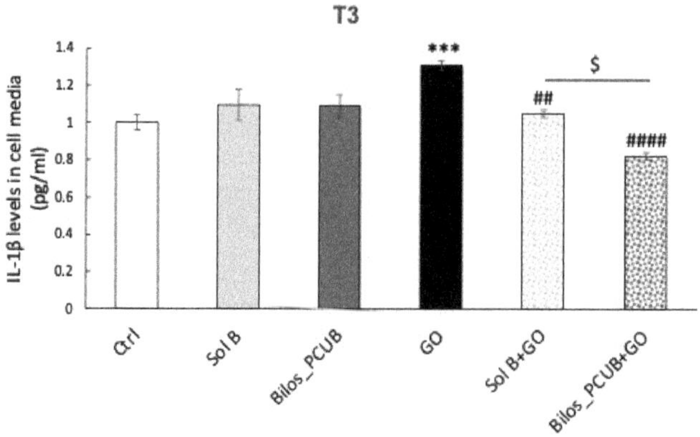

Figure 9. Released levels of IL- 1β in media of CaCo2 cells pre-treated with formulations containing budesonide, exposed to 0.5 U/mL of GO for 1 h and collected after 3 h (T3). Data are the results of the averages of at least three different experiments, obtained via 2-way ANOVA followed by Tukey's post hoc comparison test. $^{\$}$ $p < 0.05$; $^{\#\#}$ $p < 0.01$; *** $p < 0.005$; $^{\#\#\#\#}$ $p < 0.0001$ (* with respect to Ctrl and # with respect to Ctrl + GO).

4. Conclusions

This study proposes and compares different types of bile acid-based nanosystems, namely, bilosomes and biloparticles, as delivery systems to improve the solubility and to preserve the activity of lipophilic drugs. For instance, at present, bilosomes are used to deliver numerous biological macromolecules [45,70–72]. It was found that bilosystems are able to efficiently encapsulate the drug while preserving its properties. However, the influence of different bile acids (i.e., U, C, T) on the performance of the produced bilosystem needs to be studied in depth to try to understand their contribution to specific drug release properties. This study, in fact, being preliminary, focused mainly on macroscopic evidence of the different behaviors of the produced bilosystems. Subsequent studies will be carried out that try to delve deeper into the reasons for the different behaviors expressed by the different bile acids used. In addition, our encouraging results, showing the efficient antioxidant effect of the complete restoration of IL-1β to the basal level after Bilos_PCUB treatment, suggest the possibility of further investigating the use of bilosystems to counteract ox-inflammatory damage within intestinal cells, especially for those intestinal pathologies correlated with the development of an oxidative stress status.

Supplementary Materials: The following supporting information can be downloaded at: https://www.mdpi.com/article/10.3390/antiox12122025/s1, Figure S1. Size after production and after 30 days of storage of Bilos_PCU, obtained following different protocols (FhRT, FhRTS, FhW, FhWS). Size is expressed as average diameter (Z-Average) and dispersity index (PdI). The values are the mean of 3 batches ± s.d. Figure S2. Mean diameter (Z-Average) (a) and polydispersity (PdI) (b) after production of BilopS_C (green), BilopS_U (blue) and Bi-lopS_T (orange) with increasing concentrations of bile acids as determined via PCS. Each value is the average of 2 batches ± s.d. Figure S3. Colocalization expression levels of NLRP3 and ASC (Pearson's correlation coefficient) in CaCo2 cells treated with formulations containing budesonide and exposed to 0.5 U/mL of GO for 1 h. The colocalization expression levels were quantified using ImageJ software. Data are the results of the averages of at least three different experiments, obtained via 2-way ANOVA followed by Tukey's post hoc comparison test. * $p < 0.05$; $^{\#\#}$ $p < 0.01$; (* with respect to Ctrl and # with respect to Ctrl + GO). Table S1. Composition of the produced biloparticles, expressed as percentage of weight. Table S2. Composition of ursodeoxycholic bilosomes used for the preformulation study. Table S3. Composition, in percentage of weight, of biloparticles used in the preformulation study.

Author Contributions: Conceptualization, R.C.; methodology, R.C. and M.S.; investigation, N.B., A.B. and M.D.; data curation R.C., M.S. and F.F.; liposomal analyses, M.S.; in vitro experiments F.F., N.B., A.G., A.B. and M.S.; original draft preparation, R.C. and M.S.; writing and editing, R.C., F.F., M.S. and G.V.; funding acquisition, R.C. All authors have read and agreed to the published version of the manuscript.

Funding: This research was funded by the University of Ferrara (FAR2020 and FAR2021).

Institutional Review Board Statement: The animal study protocol was approved by the Institutional Review Board of Ferrara University (Organismo preposto al Benessere Animale, OpBA, protocol code CBCC2.50 and 373/2021-PR CBCC2.48, 23 January 2023) for studies involving animals.

Informed Consent Statement: Not applicable.

Data Availability Statement: Data are contained within the article and Supplementary Materials.

Acknowledgments: We acknowledge Silvia Zucchini of the Laboratory for Preclinical Research (LARP) of Ferrara University.

Conflicts of Interest: The authors declare no conflict of interest. The funders had no role in the design of the study; in the collection, analyses, or interpretation of the data; in the writing of the manuscript; or in the decision to publish the results.

References

1. Porter, C.J.H.; Pouton, C.W.; Cuine, J.F.; Charman, W.N. Enhancing Intestinal Drug Solubilisation Using Lipid-Based Delivery Systems. *Adv. Drug Deliv. Rev.* **2008**, *60*, 673–691. [CrossRef]
2. Charman, W.N. Lipids, Lipophilic Drugs, and Oral Drug Delivery-Some Emerging Concepts. *J. Pharm. Sci.* **2000**, *89*, 967–978. [CrossRef]
3. Porter, C.J.H.; Trevaskis, N.L.; Charman, W.N. Lipids and Lipid-Based Formulations: Optimizing the Oral Delivery of Lipophilic Drugs. *Nat. Rev. Drug Discov.* **2007**, *6*, 231–248. [CrossRef]
4. Stojančević, M.; Pavlović, N.; Goločorbin-Kon, S.; Mikov, M. Application of Bile Acids in Drug Formulation and Delivery. *Front. Life Sci.* **2013**, *7*, 112–122. [CrossRef]
5. Holm, R.; Müllertz, A.; Mu, H. Bile Salts and Their Importance for Drug Absorption. *Int. J. Pharm.* **2013**, *453*, 44–55. [CrossRef]
6. Zarenezhad, E.; Marzi, M.; Abdulabbas, H.T.; Jasim, S.A.; Kouhpayeh, S.A.; Barbaresi, S.; Ahmadi, S.; Ghasemian, A. Bilosomes as Nanocarriers for the Drug and Vaccine Delivery against Gastrointestinal Infections: Opportunities and Challenges. *J. Funct. Biomater.* **2023**, *14*, 453. [CrossRef]
7. Gupta, D.K.; Ahad, A.; Waheed, A.; Aqil, M.; Al-Jenoobi, F.I.; Al-Mohizea, A.M. Bilosomes: A Novel Platform for Drug Delivery. In *Systems of Nanovesicular Drug Delivery*; Elsevier: Amsterdam, The Netherlands, 2022; pp. 293–309, ISBN 978-0-323-91864-0.
8. Ahmad, J.; Singhal, M.; Amin, S.; Rizwanullah, M.; Akhter, S.; Kamal, M.A.; Haider, N.; Midoux, P.; Pichon, C. Bile Salt Stabilized Vesicles (Bilosomes): A Novel Nano-Pharmaceutical Design for Oral Delivery of Proteins and Peptides. *Curr. Pharm. Des.* **2017**, *23*, 1575–1588. [CrossRef]
9. Shukla, A.; Mishra, V.; Kesharwani, P. Bilosomes in the Context of Oral Immunization: Development, Challenges and Opportunities. *Drug Discov. Today* **2016**, *21*, 888–899. [CrossRef]
10. Mohsen, A.M.; Asfour, M.H.; Salama, A.A.A. Improved Hepatoprotective Activity of Silymarin via Encapsulation in the Novel Vesicular Nanosystem Bilosomes. *Drug Dev. Ind. Pharm.* **2017**, *43*, 2043–2054. [CrossRef]
11. Miehlke, S.; Acosta, M.B.; Bouma, G.; Carpio, D.; Magro, F.; Moreels, T.; Probert, C. Oral Budesonide in Gastrointestinal and Liver Disease: A Practical Guide for the Clinician. *J. Gastroenterol. Hepatol.* **2018**, *33*, 1574–1581. [CrossRef]
12. Kozuch, P.L.; Hanauer, S.B. Treatment of Inflammatory Bowel Disease: A Review of Medical Therapy. *WJG* **2008**, *14*, 354. [CrossRef]
13. Molodecky, N.A.; Soon, I.S.; Rabi, D.M.; Ghali, W.A.; Ferris, M.; Chernoff, G.; Benchimol, E.I.; Panaccione, R.; Ghosh, S.; Barkema, H.W.; et al. Increasing Incidence and Prevalence of the Inflammatory Bowel Diseases With Time, Based on Systematic Review. *Gastroenterology* **2012**, *142*, 46–54.e42. [CrossRef]
14. Hanauer, S.B. New Steroids for IBD: Progress Report. *Gut* **2002**, *51*, 182–183. [CrossRef]
15. Martinez, M.N.; Amidon, G.L. A Mechanistic Approach to Understanding the Factors Affecting Drug Absorption: A Review of Fundamentals. *J. Clin. Pharmacol.* **2002**, *42*, 620–643. [CrossRef]
16. Stegemann, S.; Leveiller, F.; Franchi, D.; De Jong, H.; Lindén, H. When Poor Solubility Becomes an Issue: From Early Stage to Proof of Concept. *Eur. J. Pharm. Sci.* **2007**, *31*, 249–261. [CrossRef]
17. Liu, L.; Yao, W.; Rao, Y.; Lu, X.; Gao, J. pH-Responsive Carriers for Oral Drug Delivery: Challenges and Opportunities of Current Platforms. *Drug Deliv.* **2017**, *24*, 569–581. [CrossRef]

18. Lautenschläger, C.; Schmidt, C.; Fischer, D.; Stallmach, A. Drug Delivery Strategies in the Therapy of Inflammatory Bowel Disease. *Adv. Drug Deliv. Rev.* **2014**, *71*, 58–76. [CrossRef]
19. Derendorf, H.; Meltzer, E.O. Molecular and Clinical Pharmacology of Intranasal Corticosteroids: Clinical and Therapeutic Implications. *Allergy* **2008**, *63*, 1292–1300. [CrossRef]
20. Vrettos, N.-N.; Roberts, C.J.; Zhu, Z. Gastroretentive Technologies in Tandem with Controlled-Release Strategies: A Potent Answer to Oral Drug Bioavailability and Patient Compliance Implications. *Pharmaceutics* **2021**, *13*, 1591. [CrossRef]
21. Xian, S.; Zhu, J.; Wang, Y.; Song, H.; Wang, H. Oral Liposomal Delivery of an Activatable Budesonide Prodrug Reduces Colitis in Experimental Mice. *Drug Deliv.* **2023**, *30*, 2183821. [CrossRef]
22. Muller, R.H.; Shegokar, R.; Keck, C.M. 20 Years of Lipid Nanoparticles (SLN & NLC): Present State of Development & Industrial Applications. *Curr. Drug Discov. Technol.* **2011**, *8*, 207–227. [CrossRef]
23. Mu, H.; Holm, R. Solid Lipid Nanocarriers in Drug Delivery: Characterization and Design. *Expert. Opin. Drug Deliv.* **2018**, *15*, 771–785. [CrossRef]
24. Talegaonkar, S.; Bhattacharyya, A. Potential of Lipid Nanoparticles (SLNs and NLCs) in Enhancing Oral Bioavailability of Drugs with Poor Intestinal Permeability. *AAPS PharmSciTech* **2019**, *20*, 121. [CrossRef]
25. Maritim, S.; Boulas, P.; Lin, Y. Comprehensive Analysis of Liposome Formulation Parameters and Their Influence on Encapsulation, Stability and Drug Release in Glibenclamide Liposomes. *Int. J. Pharm.* **2021**, *592*, 120051. [CrossRef]
26. Da Silva Santos, V.; Badan Ribeiro, A.P.; Andrade Santana, M.H. Solid Lipid Nanoparticles as Carriers for Lipophilic Compounds for Applications in Foods. *Food Res. Int.* **2019**, *122*, 610–626. [CrossRef]
27. Sguizzato, M.; Pepe, A.; Baldisserotto, A.; Barbari, R.; Montesi, L.; Drechsler, M.; Mariani, P.; Cortesi, R. Niosomes for Topical Application of Antioxidant Molecules: Design and In Vitro Behavior. *Gels* **2023**, *9*, 107. [CrossRef]
28. Sguizzato, M.; Ferrara, F.; Drechsler, M.; Baldisserotto, A.; Montesi, L.; Manfredini, S.; Valacchi, G.; Cortesi, R. Lipid-Based Nanosystems for the Topical Application of Ferulic Acid: A Comparative Study. *Pharmaceutics* **2023**, *15*, 1940. [CrossRef]
29. Esposito, E.; Sguizzato, M.; Drechsler, M.; Mariani, P.; Carducci, F.; Nastruzzi, C.; Cortesi, R. Progesterone Lipid Nanoparticles: Scaling up and in Vivo Human Study. *Eur. J. Pharm. Biopharm.* **2017**, *119*, 437–446. [CrossRef]
30. Pecora, R. Dynamic Light Scattering Measurement of Nanometer Particles in Liquids. *J. Nanoparticle Res.* **2000**, *2*, 123–131. [CrossRef]
31. Danaei, M.; Dehghankhold, M.; Ataei, S.; Hasanzadeh Davarani, F.; Javanmard, R.; Dokhani, A.; Khorasani, S.; Mozafari, M. Impact of Particle Size and Polydispersity Index on the Clinical Applications of Lipidic Nanocarrier Systems. *Pharmaceutics* **2018**, *10*, 57. [CrossRef]
32. Pozzetti, L.; Ferrara, F.; Marotta, L.; Gemma, S.; Butini, S.; Benedusi, M.; Fusi, F.; Ahmed, A.; Pomponi, S.; Ferrari, S.; et al. Extra Virgin Olive Oil Extracts of Indigenous Southern Tuscany Cultivar Act as Anti-Inflammatory and Vasorelaxant Nutraceuticals. *Antioxidants* **2022**, *11*, 437. [CrossRef]
33. M'Baye, G.; Mély, Y.; Duportail, G.; Klymchenko, A.S. Liquid Ordered and Gel Phases of Lipid Bilayers: Fluorescent Probes Reveal Close Fluidity but Different Hydration. *Biophys. J.* **2008**, *95*, 1217–1225. [CrossRef]
34. Ali Mohammadi, Z.; Foad Aghamiri, S.; Zarrabi, A.; Reza Talaie, M. Liposomal Doxorubicin Delivery Systems: Effects of Formulation and Processing Parameters on Drug Loading and Release Behavior. *Curr. Drug Deliv.* **2016**, *13*, 1065–1070. [CrossRef]
35. Farzaneh, H.; Ebrahimi Nik, M.; Mashreghi, M.; Saberi, Z.; Jaafari, M.R.; Teymouri, M. A Study on the Role of Cholesterol and Phosphatidylcholine in Various Features of Liposomal Doxorubicin: From Liposomal Preparation to Therapy. *Int. J. Pharm.* **2018**, *551*, 300–308. [CrossRef]
36. Liposome Technology: Interactions of Liposomes with the Biological Milieu. Available online: https://www.routledge.com/Liposome-Technology-Interactions-of-Liposomes-with-the-Biological-Milieu/Gregoriadis/p/book/9780367390389 (accessed on 20 October 2023).
37. Perrie, Y. Gregory Gregoriadis: Introducing Liposomes to Drug Delivery. *J. Drug Target.* **2008**, *16*, 518–519. [CrossRef]
38. Gregoriadis, G. Drug Entrapment in Liposomes. *FEBS Lett.* **1973**, *36*, 292–296. [CrossRef]
39. Gregoriadis, G. Engineering Liposomes for Drug Delivery: Progress and Problems. *Trends Biotechnol.* **1995**, *13*, 527–537. [CrossRef]
40. Cortesi, R.; Esposito, E.; Drechsler, M.; Pavoni, G.; Cacciatore, I.; Sguizzato, M.; Di Stefano, A. L-Dopa Co-Drugs in Nanostructured Lipid Carriers: A Comparative Study. *Mater. Sci. Eng. C* **2017**, *72*, 168–176. [CrossRef]
41. Sultan, A.A.; Saad, G.A.; El Maghraby, G.M. Permeation Enhancers Loaded Bilosomes for Improved Intestinal Absorption and Cytotoxic Activity of Doxorubicin. *Int. J. Pharm.* **2023**, *630*, 122427. [CrossRef]
42. Aditya, N.P.; Espinosa, Y.G.; Norton, I.T. Encapsulation Systems for the Delivery of Hydrophilic Nutraceuticals: Food Application. *Biotechnol. Adv.* **2017**, *35*, 450–457. [CrossRef]
43. Ahmed, S.; Kassem, M.A.; Sayed, S. Bilosomes as Promising Nanovesicular Carriers for Improved Transdermal Delivery: Construction, in Vitro Optimization, Ex Vivo Permeation and in Vivo Evaluation. *Int. J. Nanomed.* **2020**, *15*, 9783–9798. [CrossRef]
44. Binsuwaidan, R.; Sultan, A.A.; Negm, W.A.; Attallah, N.G.M.; Alqahtani, M.J.; Hussein, I.A.; Shaldam, M.A.; El-Sherbeni, S.A.; Elekhnawy, E. Bilosomes as Nanoplatform for Oral Delivery and Modulated In Vivo Antimicrobial Activity of Lycopene. *Pharmaceuticals* **2022**, *15*, 1043. [CrossRef]

45. Saifi, Z.; Rizwanullah, M.; Mir, S.R.; Amin, S. Bilosomes Nanocarriers for Improved Oral Bioavailability of Acyclovir: A Complete Characterization through in Vitro, Ex-Vivo and in Vivo Assessment. *J. Drug Deliv. Sci. Technol.* **2020**, *57*, 101634. [CrossRef]
46. Elnaggar, Y.S.R.; Omran, S.; Hazzah, H.A.; Abdallah, O.Y. Anionic versus Cationic Bilosomes as Oral Nanocarriers for Enhanced Delivery of the Hydrophilic Drug Risedronate. *Int. J. Pharm.* **2019**, *564*, 410–425. [CrossRef]
47. Dadashzadeh, S.; Haeri, A.; Daeihamed, M.; Arzani, G.; Bakhtiari Kaboutaraki, H. Niosomal Carriers Enhance Oral Bioavailability of Carvedilol: Effects of Bile Salt-Enriched Vesicles and Carrier Surface Charge. *Int. J. Nanomed.* **2015**, *10*, 4797. [CrossRef]
48. Islam, N.; Zahoor, A.F.; Syed, H.K.; Iqbal, M.S.; Khan, I.U.; Abbas, G.; Mushtaq, M.; Rehman, M.U.; Rasul, A.; Ikram, M.; et al. Improvement of Solubility and Dissolution of Ebastine by Fabricating Phosphatidylcholine/ Bile Salt Bilosomes. *Pak. J. Pharm. Sci.* **2020**, *33*, 2301–2306.
49. Elkomy, M.H.; Eid, H.M.; Elmowafy, M.; Shalaby, K.; Zafar, A.; Abdelgawad, M.A.; Rateb, M.E.; Ali, M.R.A.; Alsalahat, I.; Abou-Taleb, H.A. Bilosomes as a Promising Nanoplatform for Oral Delivery of an Alkaloid Nutraceutical: Improved Pharmacokinetic Profile and Snowballed Hypoglycemic Effect in Diabetic Rats. *Drug Deliv.* **2022**, *29*, 2694–2704. [CrossRef]
50. Aburahma, M.H. Bile Salts-Containing Vesicles: Promising Pharmaceutical Carriers for Oral Delivery of Poorly Water-Soluble Drugs and Peptide/Protein-Based Therapeutics or Vaccines. *Drug Deliv.* **2016**, *23*, 1847–1867. [CrossRef]
51. Liu, C.; Liu, Y.; Wang, C.; Guo, Y.; Cheng, Y.; Qian, H.; Zhao, Y. Lycopene-Loaded Bilosomes Ameliorate High-Fat Diet-Induced Chronic Nephritis in Mice through the TLR4/MyD88 Inflammatory Pathway. *Foods* **2022**, *11*, 3042. [CrossRef]
52. Wilkhu, J.S.; McNeil, S.E.; Anderson, D.E.; Perrie, Y. Characterization and Optimization of Bilosomes for Oral Vaccine Delivery. *J. Drug Target.* **2013**, *21*, 291–299. [CrossRef]
53. Paes Dutra, J.A.; Gonçalves Carvalho, S.; Soares de Oliveira, A.; Borges Monteiro, J.R.; Rodrigues Pereira de Oliveira Borlot, J.; Tavares Luiz, M.; Bauab, T.M.; Rezende Kitagawa, R.; Chorilli, M. Microparticles and Nanoparticles-Based Approaches to Improve Oral Treatment of Helicobacter Pylori Infection. *Crit. Rev. Microbiol.* **2023**, 1–22. [CrossRef]
54. Faustino, C.; Serafim, C.; Rijo, P.; Reis, C.P. Bile Acids and Bile Acid Derivatives: Use in Drug Delivery Systems and as Therapeutic Agents. *Expert Opin. Drug Deliv.* **2016**, *13*, 1133–1148. [CrossRef]
55. Yao, W.; Xu, Z.; Sun, J.; Luo, J.; Wei, Y.; Zou, J. Deoxycholic Acid-Functionalised Nanoparticles for Oral Delivery of Rhein. *Eur. J. Pharm. Sci.* **2021**, *159*, 105713. [CrossRef]
56. Mooranian, A.; Raj Wagle, S.; Kovacevic, B.; Takechi, R.; Mamo, J.; Lam, V.; Watts, G.F.; Mikov, M.; Golocorbin-Kon, S.; Stojanovic, G.; et al. Bile Acid Bio-Nanoencapsulation Improved Drug Targeted-Delivery and Pharmacological Effects via Cellular Flux: 6-Months Diabetes Preclinical Study. *Sci. Rep.* **2020**, *10*, 106. [CrossRef]
57. Siepmann, J.; Siepmann, F. Mathematical Modeling of Drug Dissolution. *Int. J. Pharm.* **2013**, *453*, 12–24. [CrossRef]
58. Lao, L.L.; Peppas, N.A.; Boey, F.Y.C.; Venkatraman, S.S. Modeling of Drug Release from Bulk-Degrading Polymers. *Int. J. Pharm.* **2011**, *418*, 28–41. [CrossRef]
59. Siepmann, J.; Peppas, N.A. Higuchi Equation: Derivation, Applications, Use and Misuse. *Int. J. Pharm.* **2011**, *418*, 6–12. [CrossRef]
60. Higuchi, T. Rate of Release of Medicaments from Ointment Bases Containing Drugs in Suspension. *J. Pharm. Sci.* **1961**, *50*, 874–875. [CrossRef]
61. Paerewijck, O.; Lamkanfi, M. The Human Inflammasomes. *Mol. Asp. Med.* **2022**, *88*, 101100. [CrossRef]
62. Ferrara, F.; Pecorelli, A.; Valacchi, G. Redox Regulation of Nucleotide-Binding and Oligomerization Domain-Like Receptors Inflammasome. *Antioxid. Redox Signal.* **2023**, *39*, 744–770. [CrossRef]
63. Abbasi-Oshaghi, E.; Mirzaei, F.; Pourjafar, M. NLRP3 Inflammasome, Oxidative Stress, and Apoptosis Induced in the Intestine and Liver of Rats Treated with Titanium Dioxide Nanoparticles: In Vivo and in Vitro Study. *Int. J. Nanomed.* **2019**, *14*, 1919–1936. [CrossRef]
64. Lv, Q.; Xu, D.; Ma, J.; Wang, Y.; Yang, X.; Zhao, P.; Ma, L.; Li, Z.; Yang, W.; Liu, X.; et al. Uric Acid Drives Intestinal Barrier Dysfunction through TSPO-Mediated NLRP3 Inflammasome Activation. *Inflamm. Res.* **2021**, *70*, 127–137. [CrossRef]
65. He, Y.; Li, Z.; Xu, T.; Luo, D.; Chi, Q.; Zhang, Y.; Li, S. Polystyrene Nanoplastics Deteriorate LPS-Modulated Duodenal Permeability and Inflammation in Mice via ROS Drived-NF-κB/NLRP3 Pathway. *Chemosphere* **2022**, *307*, 135662. [CrossRef]
66. Bayiha, J.C.; Evrard, B.; Cataldo, D.; De Tullio, P.; Mingeot-Leclercq, M.-P. The Budesonide-Hydroxypropyl-β-Cyclodextrin Complex Attenuates ROS Generation, IL-8 Release and Cell Death Induced by Oxidant and Inflammatory Stress. Study on A549 and A-THP-1 Cells. *Molecules* **2020**, *25*, 4882. [CrossRef]
67. Valacchi, G.; Sticozzi, C.; Belmonte, G.; Cervellati, F.; Pecorelli, A.; Signorini, C.; Leoncini, S.; Ciccoli, L.; De Felice, C.; Della Ragione, F.; et al. Scavenger Receptor B1 Oxidative Post-Translational Modifications Are Responsible for Its Loss in Rett Syndrome. *Free Radic. Biol. Med.* **2014**, *75*, S10–S11. [CrossRef]
68. Valacchi, G.; Virgili, F.; Cervellati, C.; Pecorelli, A. OxInflammation: From Subclinical Condition to Pathological Biomarker. *Front. Physiol.* **2018**, *9*, 858. [CrossRef]
69. Pérez, S.; Taléns-Visconti, R.; Rius-Pérez, S.; Finamor, I.; Sastre, J. Redox Signaling in the Gastrointestinal Tract. *Free Radic. Biol. Med.* **2017**, *104*, 75–103. [CrossRef]
70. Ahmad, R.; Srivastava, S.; Ghosh, S.; Khare, S.K. Phytochemical Delivery through Nanocarriers: A Review. *Colloids Surf. B Biointerfaces* **2021**, *197*, 111389. [CrossRef]

71. D'Elia, R.V.; Woods, S.; Butcher, W.; McGahon, J.; Khadke, S.; Perrie, Y.; Williamson, E.D.; Roberts, C.W. Exploitation of the Bilosome Platform Technology to Formulate Antibiotics and Enhance Efficacy of Melioidosis Treatments. *J. Control. Release* **2019**, *298*, 202–212. [CrossRef]
72. Mohsen, A.M.; Salama, A.; Kassem, A.A. Development of Acetazolamide Loaded Bilosomes for Improved Ocular Delivery: Preparation, Characterization and in Vivo Evaluation. *J. Drug Deliv. Sci. Technol.* **2020**, *59*, 101910. [CrossRef]

antioxidants

MDPI

Article

Green Synthesis of Gold Nanoparticles with Curcumin or Açai in the Tissue Repair of Palatal Wounds

Anand Thirupathi [1], Morgana Francisco Machado Guzzatti [2], Maria Eduarda Anastácio Borges Corrêa [2], Ligia Milanez Venturini [2], Laura de Roch Casagrande [2], Igor Ramos Lima [2], Camila Da Costa [2], Ellen De Pieri [2], Lariani Tamires Witt Tietbohl [2], Paulo Emilio Feuser [2], Ricardo Andrez Machado-de-Ávila [2], Yaodong Gu [1] and Paulo Cesar Lock Silveira [2,*]

1 Research Academy of Medicine Combining Sports, Ningbo No. 2 Hospital, Ningbo 315099, China; anand@nbu.edu.cn (A.T.); guyaodong@nbu.edu.cn (Y.G.)

2 Laboratory of Experimental Physiopathology, Program of Postgraduate in Science of Health, Universidade do Extremo-Sul Catarinense, Criciúma 88806-000, SC, Brazil; morganamachado@unesc.net (M.F.M.G.); meabcorrea@unesc.net (M.E.A.B.C.); ligia.milanez@posgrad.ufsc.br (L.M.V.); lauracasag@unesc.net (L.d.R.C.); igor.mamp@unesc.net (I.R.L.); camiladacosta49@unesc.net (C.D.C.); ellen.bn@unesc.net (E.D.P.); lariani.tietbohl@unesc.net (L.T.W.T.); paulo.feuser@posgrad.ufsc.br (P.E.F.); r_andrez@unesc.net (R.A.M.-d.-Á.)

* Correspondence: psilveira@unesc.net; Tel.: +55-48-34312773

Abstract: This study aimed to evaluate and compare the effects of treatment with gold nanoparticles (GNPs) reduced with Curcumin (*Curcuma longa* L.) or Açai (*Euterpe oleracea*) to a standard commercial treatment of the pharmacological type (Omcilon®) and an electrophysical agent (photobiomodulation) in the palatal wounds of rats. As for the in vitro assay, a cell viability test was performed to assess the toxicity of the synthesized nanoparticles. In vivo assay: 60 Wistar rats were divided into five groups (n = 12): I. Palatal Wound (PW); II. PW + Photobiomodulation (PBM); III. PW + Omcilon®; IV. PW + GNPs-Cur (0.025 mg/mL); V. PW + GNPs-Açai (0.025 mg/mL). Animals were first anesthetized, and circular lesions in the palatine mucosa were induced using a 4 mm-diameter punch. The first treatment session started 24 h after the injury and occurred daily for 5 days. The animals were euthanized, and the palatal mucosa tissue was removed for histological, biochemical, and molecular analysis. GNPs-Açai were able to significantly reduce pro-inflammatory cytokines and increase anti-inflammatory ones, reduce oxidant markers, and reduce inflammatory infiltrate while increasing the collagen area and contraction rate of the wound, along with an improved visual qualification. The present study demonstrated that the proposed therapies of GNPs synthesized greenly, thus associating their effects with those of plants, favor the tissue repair process in palatal wounds.

Keywords: palatal wounds; inflammation; gold nanoparticles; curcumin; açai; green synthesis

1. Introduction

The integrity of the oral mucosa is important in preventing infections [1]. Oral ulcers are a type of lesion with a high prevalence rate in the oral mucosa. Oral disease hurts the patient's well-being and quality of life [2].

Different treatments have been tested to avoid such complications and minimize the patient's discomfort, but so far without absolute success. Advances in nanodentistry and innovations in oral health-related diagnostics, prevention, and therapeutic methods needed to maintain and achieve perfect oral health have been showcased. Recent advances in nanotechnology may bring about a paradigm shift in dentistry [3].

Among nanomaterials, metallic nanoparticles (NPs) have been considered for clinical application due to their low cost, high surface-to-volume ratio, high stability, and safety. Gold nanoparticles (GNPs) have many applications for therapeutic use in the biological detection of drugs and the delivery of proteins, genes, and drugs. These NPs have distinct properties and are being used in the areas of restorative dentistry, periodontology, dental implants, tissue engineering, and cancer diagnosis [4]. Gold-based nanoparticles exhibit unique electronic and optical properties, biostability, low cytotoxicity, and enhanced drug delivery capabilities, which open the possibility of their use in diverse fields. GNPs can penetrate the stratum corneum, and their drug delivery property makes them ideal as carriers for both large and small biomolecules [5].

The anti-inflammatory effects of GNPs are shown in the inhibition of the formation of pro-inflammatory cytokines in macrophages, a mechanism that is due to their ability to suppress the action of NF-κB in addition to their strong catalytic activity in the process of scavenging free radicals [6]. A recent study has observed that the topical application of GNPs in rats significantly accelerates the healing processes, performing wound closure four times faster, suggesting that gold nanoparticles are also capable of generating an increased proliferation of fibroblasts, which are important in the contraction of wounds [7].

Currently, the synthesis of nanoparticles from plant extracts is receiving increased attention due to its environmentally friendly behavior. The plant extract works as a reducing agent and a covering agent in the synthesis of nanoparticles [8]. Green synthesis, as it is called, is defined as the practice of using biologically friendly elements such as plants, bacteria, and fungi to synthesize nanoparticles. It is environmentally friendly and has no toxicity effects compared to chemical reduction methods. Biomolecules in the plant extract, such as amino acids, vitamins, enzymes, and proteins, work to reduce the concentration of metal ions [9].

Curcumin (*Curcuma longa* L.), a polyphenol extracted from the plant's rhizome, is a pleiotropic molecule that can interact with several molecular targets related to inflammation. This molecule proved to be able to trigger early re-epithelialization, improve neovascularization, and increase the migration of various cells, including dermal myofibroblasts, fibroblasts, and macrophages, to the wound bed [10]. Açai (*Euterpe oleracea*) is a purple tropical fruit with many antioxidant nutrients and excellent anti-inflammatory and healing effects on the skin. Studies have shown that this fruit has effects in reversing mitochondrial dysfunction and anti-aging properties, in addition to also presenting an effect suppressor in the generation of reactive oxygen species and the activation of cyclooxygenase-2 (COX-2) and TNF-α in vitro [11].

Given what was presented above, the objective of this work was to evaluate the cytotoxicity and effects of treatment with gold nanoparticles reduced by the green synthesis method with Curcumin (*Curcuma longa* L.) or Açai (*Euterpe oleracea*) in the palatal wounds of Wistar rats compared to a commercial standard pharmacological treatment (Omcilon®) and an electrophysical agent (photobiomodulation).

2. Methods

All animal experiments were conducted in accordance with the National Institutes of Health's (Bethesda, MD, USA) Guide for the Care and Use of Laboratory Animals and with the Ethics Committee of Universidade do Extremo Sul Catarinense—UNESC under protocol number 81/2022 in October 2021. Every animal experiment complies with the ARRIVE guidelines [12].

2.1. Green Synthesis of Gold Nanoparticles

GNPs were obtained by reducing different extracts. A stock solution of *Curcuma longa* L. (Sigma, São Paulo, Brazil) and/or *Euterpe oleracea* (Zona Cerealista, São Paulo, Brazil) extract was prepared in absolute ethanol. Stock solutions of chloroauric acid (HAuCl4) (4 mM) were prepared in Milli-Q water. Next, a pre-defined extract solution was added to Milli-Q water and kept under stirring and heating until reaching a temperature of 90 °C. Sodium hydroxide (NaOH) (0.1 M) was used to adjust the pH between 10 and 11. Next, a 1 mM solution of HAuCl4 was added dropwise under simultaneous stirring. The reaction was kept under stirring until reaching room temperature and the subsequent formation of GNPs (schematic representation in Supplementary Material).

The GNP solutions were characterized by ultraviolet-visible (UV-Vis) spectroscopy in a SpectraMax Plus model. Nanoparticles were measured in the visible region (390–700 nm). The size and morphology of nanoparticles were determined by transmission electron microscopy (TEM) using a JEM-1011 (100 kV). A drop of the nanoparticle solution was added to a copper grid (300 mesh) covered with a thin layer of carbon. Drying was performed at room temperature (24 h), and later images were obtained. Hydrodynamic size and surface charge at pH 7.4 (25 °C) were investigated by dynamic light scattering (DLS) and zeta potential measurements using a Zetasizer Nano ZS. The nanoparticle solutions were placed in a folded capillary cell. All analyses were performed in triplicate to obtain the mean and standard deviation (SD). The stability of the solutions was evaluated by UV-Vis and Zetasizer spectroscopy.

2.2. *In Vitro Assay*

2.2.1. Cell Viability

For cell culture assays, an immortalized murine fibroblast cell line (NIH3T3) was used (Cell Bank of Rio de Janeiro, RJ, Brazil). Immortalized NIH3T3 cells were cultured in 25 cm^2 plastic bottles with Dulbecco's Modified Eagle (DMEM) medium supplemented with 1% penicillin and streptomycin antibiotics (10 U.L/mL) and 10% inactivated fetal bovine serum (complete DMEM).

For cell growth and adhesion, the cells were kept in a humidified incubator with an atmosphere of 5% CO_2 at 37 °C. Medium changes were performed on alternate days, with the possibility of adaptations, until a sufficient cell confluence was obtained, around 80%, for the development of in vitro experiments. When the necessary confluence was obtained, the cells were trypsinized, the DMEM was removed from the bottle, and 4 mL of trypsin was added for 5 min, or until the cells were in suspension, detaching from the bottom of the bottle. Then, 4 mL of DMEM is added to neutralize the trypsin.

Then, the total number of cells was counted in the Neubauer chamber. After counting, these cells were diluted in a complete DMEM medium at the desired concentration. A total of 500 μL/well was added to a 24-well plate, with a final concentration of 1×10^5 cells/well. Finally, they were incubated for 24 h in a humidified incubator with an atmosphere of 5% CO_2 at 37 °C to ensure the adherence of the cells to the surface of the plate and then perform the cell assays.

After the cell adherence period, the complete DMEM medium was removed from all wells, and the following treatments were added to NIH3T3 cells: GNPs-Cur and GNPs-Açai at concentrations of 5%, 10%, 20%, and 30%. The solutions were diluted in DMEM. After the treatments for each group were added, the plate was incubated for 24 h in a humidified incubator with an atmosphere of 5% CO_2 at 37 °C. The next day, the treatment was withdrawn, and then the reagent (3-(4,5-Dimethylthiazol-2-yl)-2,5-diphenyltetrazolium) (MTT) was added for the cell viability assay.

2.2.2. Cell Viability Test—MTT

This method aims to evaluate cell viability by reducing MTT, which, in its oxidized form, is soluble in water and has a yellow color.

After incubating the cells with the specific treatments for 24 h, a solution of 0.5 mg/mL of MTT diluted in PBS was prepared. The treatments were removed from the wells, and 100 μL/well of the MTT solution was added and incubated for 3 h (5% CO_2 at 37 °C) to allow for the formation of formazan crystals. After the incubation period, the MTT solution was removed from all wells, and 100 μL/well of isopropyl alcohol was added to solubilize the formazan crystals. Finally, the plate was analyzed in a plate reader by absorbance at a wavelength of 570 nm.

Cell viability is determined by comparing the absorbance results of the test groups (GNPs-Cur and GNPs-Açai) with the absorbances of the control group, that is, the group that has only viable cells. Therefore, the results are presented in percentages of cell viability, where the control group mimics 100% of live cells. Given this, calculations were performed to obtain the percentage of viable cells in each group, so that in this way the toxicity of the proposed molecule could be evaluated.

2.3. *In Vivo Assay*

2.3.1. Animals

For this experiment, sixty Wistar rats (200–300 g, age 60 days) were needed. The rats were housed in particular cages with an ambient temperature between 20 and 22 ± /°C, a 12-hour light-dark cycle, a standard rodent diet, and water *ad libitum*.

The animals were randomly divided into the following 5 groups (n = 12):

I. Palatal Wound (PW)—without local or systemic treatment;
II. PW + Photobiomodulation (PBM)—standard treatment with Laser 660 nm 2 J;
III. PW + Omcilon®—standard Omcilon® treatment;
IV. PW + GNPs-Cur—treatment with gold nanoparticles reduced with curcumin (0.025 mg/mL);
V. PW + GNPs-Açai—treatment with gold nanoparticles reduced with açai (0.025 mg/mL).

2.3.2. Palatal Wound Model

The animals were anesthetized and maintained under anesthesia using ketamine 100 mg/kg and xylazine 0.5 mg/kg intraperitoneally. When the effect of the anesthetic was verified, each rat was stabilized, and the mouth was kept open using a retractor. The palatine mucosa close to the molar teeth was removed using a 4 mm-diameter stainless steel dermatological punch. The palatal mucosa involved in the circular incision was completely excised, and the periosteum remained exposed within this diameter. After bleeding control, the excised area was left exposed to simulate second-intention wound healing.

2.3.3. Treatment

Twenty-four hours after injury induction, the animals in groups II, III, IV, and V were sedated with 4% isoflurane by inhalation and received their treatments. Group II underwent the first treatment session of photobiomodulation with an application of LBP AlGaInP with continuous emission (wavelength 660 nm; peak power 30 mW; beam size of 0.10 cm^2, 2 J) from the company Laserpulse-Ibramed (São Paulo, Brazil). Irradiation was performed on the wound (five points around the wound), with the laser pen perpendicular to the palate at a distance of 0.5 cm per point, as described by Mendes et al. [7].

In the animals of group III, topical treatment (50 μL) with Omcilon® was applied with a disposable micro-brush-type microapplicator on the palatal wounds. Groups IV and V received applications of GNPs-Cur or GNPs-Açai (50 μL hydrogel, dose of 0.025 mg/mL, and mean size of 20 nm), also with the disposable microbrush on the wounds. Treatments occurred daily for 5 days.

2.4. *Macroscopic Analysis and Inflammatory Score*

Macroscopic assessment of the wound relied on an overall visual score of the level of inflammation, with a protocol adapted from Marques Neto et al. [13], under blinding procedures by the applicators.

The following parameters were included in the inflammation score:

I. No change
II. Irritation
III. Shallow ulcer (1–2 mm) with clean edges
IV. Shallow ulcer (1–2 mm) with necrotic edges
V. Shallow ulcer (3–4 mm) with clean edges
VI. Shallow ulcer (3–4 mm) with necrotic edges
VII. Deep ulcer (1–2 mm) with clean edges
VIII. Deep ulcer (1–2 mm) with necrotic edges
IX. Deep ulcer (3–4 mm) with clean edges
X. Deep ulcer (3–4 mm) with necrotic edges

XI. Necrotic tissue with increased margins

2.5. Euthanasia

Five days after injury induction and the daily application of treatments, the animals were anesthetized with 4% isoflurane and euthanized by decapitation. Next, the area of the injured palatal mucosa was excised with a remaining margin using a 5 mm-diameter stainless steel dermatological punch. The samples were then stored in individual flasks at 80 °C for further biochemical and histopathological analysis.

2.6. Wound Size Analysis

The photographic method is an accurate alternative to measuring the wound area. Images of the wounds were taken at a resolution of 3264 × 2448 pixels and analyzed using the ImageJ® 1.51 software [14]. Images of the lesions were obtained on days 0 and 6 for visual verification of the evolution of the healing process and measurement of size (area in mm^2) by calculating the variation in wound areas in this period in %. These measurements were made by the same researcher, with 3 measurements being performed for each wound and using the average value.

2.7. Histomorphometry

Tissue samples from the soft palate (n = 5 animals/group) were soaked in a 10% paraformaldehyde (PFA) solution in 0.1 M phosphate buffer (pH 7.4) for 24 h. Subsequently embedded in paraffin after dehydration and bleaching and sectioned into 5 µm thick sections. To evaluate the quantification of the inflammatory infiltrate, hematoxylin and eosin (H&E) staining was used, and to assess and quantify collagenesis, staining with Gomori's trichrome was used. The slides were read under an optical microscope (Eclipse 50i, Nikon, Melville, NY, USA) with a magnification of 600×. Images were recorded using a Nikon camera (Sight DS-5M-L1, Melville, NY, USA) and analyzed using NIH ImageJ 1.36b software (NIH, Bethesda, MD, USA). The count of the inflammatory infiltrate was performed using the Plugin "Cell Counter" of the software, considering the nuclear staining of inflammatory cells. To quantify collagenesis, the Plugin "Colour Deconvolution" of the software was used, which quantifies the percentage of blue color in the total area of the image.

2.8. Determination of Cytokine Content Using ELISA

The enzyme-linked immunoabsorbent assay (Duoset ELISA) capture method (R&D System, Inc., Minneapolis, MN, USA) was used to measure cytokines (TNF-α, IL1-β, IL4, and TGF-β). The samples were processed, and then the plate was sensitized for further incubation (at room temperature) with the antibody.

2.9. Biochemical Analysis

- Intracellular determination of reactive oxygen species (ROS) and nitric oxide: The production of hydroperoxides was determined by the intracellular formation of 2′,7′-dichlorofluorescein (DCF) from the oxidation of 2′,7′-dichlorodihydrofluorescein diacetate (DCFHDA) by ROS according to the method previously described by Dong et al. [15] with some modifications. The production of nitric oxide (NO) was evaluated spectrophotometrically through the stable metabolite nitrite. The nitrite content was calculated based on a standard curve from 0 to 100 nM performed with the metabolite sodium nitrite ($NaNO_2$). The results were calculated in µmol Nitrite/mg protein [16].
- Antioxidant defenses: Glutathione (GSH) levels were determined as described by Hissin and Hilf [17], with some adaptations. GSH was measured in the palatal mucosa homogenate after protein precipitation with 1 mL of 10% trichloroacetic acid. An 800 mM phosphate buffer, pH 7.4, and 500 µm DTNB were added to part of the sample. Absorbance was read at 412 nm after 10 min. A reduced glutathione standard curve was used to calculate the GSH levels in the samples.

- Protein Content: The protein content of the palatal mucosa homogenate was assayed using bovine serum albumin as a standard, according to Lowry et al. [18]. Phosphomolybdic phosphotungstic reagent (Folin phenol) was added to bind to the protein. Absorbance was read at 750 nm.

2.10. Statistical Analysis

The macroscopic data collected were analyzed using the IBM Statistical Package for Social Sciences (SPSS) version 21.0 software (IBM, 2012). Quantitative variables were expressed through mean and standard deviation, as they presented a normal distribution, and minimum and maximum values [19].

Statistical tests were performed with a significance level of $\alpha = 0.05$ and 95% confidence. The distribution of data regarding normality was assessed using the Shapiro-Wilk test [20].

The comparison of the mean of the quantitative variables between the categories of dichotomous qualitative variables was performed using the Mann-Whitney U test, as the variable did not present a normal distribution. In turn, in the comparison of the mean of the quantitative variables between the categories of polyatomic qualitative variables, as they do not present a normal distribution, the Kruskal-Wallis H test was used, followed by the post hoc Dunn test when statistical significance was observed [21]. The investigation of the existence of an association between the qualitative variables was carried out by applying the Likelihood Ratio test, followed by residual analysis when statistical significance was observed [22].

The rest of the biochemical and molecular data were expressed as mean and mean standard error and statistically analyzed by two-way analysis of variance (ANOVA), followed by the post hoc Tukey test. The significance level established for the statistical test is $p < 0.05$. SPSS (Statistical Package for the Social Sciences) version 17.0 was used as a statistical package.

3. Results

3.1. Characterization of GNPs

The morphology and size distribution of the particles were analyzed using TEM, showing a spherical morphology and a size distribution in the range of 10–30 nm. Particle size distribution (PSD) and surface charge were determined by DLS. PSD was similar to the data presented using TEM. The zeta potential of the different nanoparticles was >-25 mV (pH 7), giving good stability to the different nanoparticles. A UV-Vis Spectrophotometer Analysis was performed, confirming the formation of different GNPs with curcumin and açai. Nanoparticles with different extracts do not show a significant difference (ANOVA $p < 0.5$) in the maximum wavelength. The obtained wavelengths confirm the formation of metallic nanoparticles. In addition, the stability of the GNPs was evaluated by UV-Vis for six months. The UV-Vis analyses showed that different GNPs remained stable over the six-month period.

Figure 1A shows the maximum wavelength of both GNPs. Below are images of the nanoparticles obtained by TEM, in which Figure 1B is GNPs-Cur and Figure 1C is GNPs-Açai. Table 1 shows the results of the different nanoparticles' mean size distribution and zeta potential.

Table 1. Average size distribution and zeta potential of different nanoparticles.

Samples	SD (nm)	Zeta Potential (mV)	Maximum Wavelength
GNPs-Cur	39 ± 4	-22 ± 3	524 nm
GNPs-Açai	34 ± 2	-28 ± 3	526 nm

$\pm$ Mean standard deviation of 3 determinations.

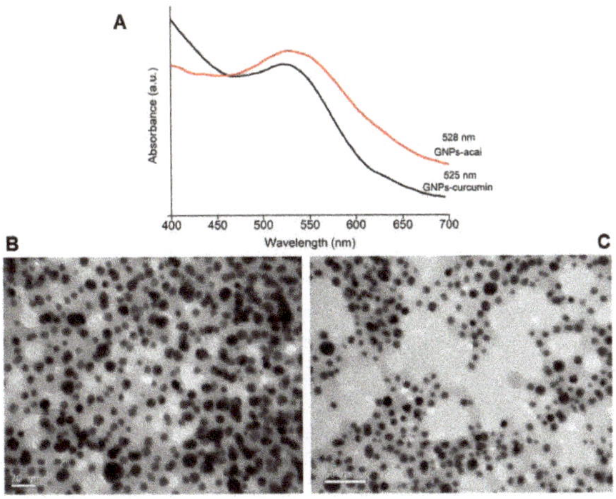

Figure 1. UV-Vis analysis (**A**) and TEM images of GNPs-Cur (**B**) and GNPs-Açai (**C**).

3.2. Cell Viability Test

NIH3T3 fibroblast cells were exposed to four different concentrations of GNPs-Cur and GNPs-Açai. The tested concentrations were 5%, 10%, 20%, and 30%. The treatments occurred for an exposure period of 24 h.

Regarding GNPs-Cur, as can be seen in Figure 2A, at a concentration of 10%, there is a significant reduction when compared to the control; however, the viability is still above 80%. At concentrations of 20% and 30%, the viability is below 80%.

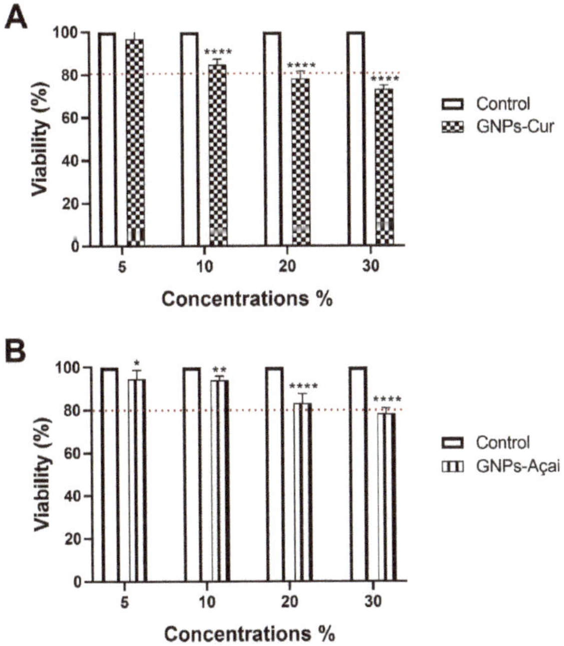

Figure 2. In vitro cytotoxicity of GNPs-Cur (**A**) and GNPs-Açai (**B**) at different concentrations evaluated in NIH3T3 cells within 24 h. Data are presented as mean + SEM, where: * $p < 0.05$ vs. Control; ** $p < 0.01$ vs. Control; **** $p < 0.0001$ vs. Control; (Two-way ANOVA followed by Tukey's post hoc test).

As for GNPs-Açai, in Figure 2B, concentrations of 5, 10, and 20% all presented significant reductions in relation to the control, although only at 30% the viability is below 80%.

It is noteworthy that in both treatments, the concentration of 30% showed the lowest cell viability; that is, it was the most cytotoxic concentration for NIH3T3 cells.

3.3. Macroscopic Analysis and Inflammatory Score

In Table 2, the value of * $p = 0.027$ in the comparison of treatments with GNPs reveals that this event did not occur by chance, indicating that the GNPs-Açai group obtained a better index of visual inflammatory condition than the other treatments.

Table 2. Macroscopic analysis and inflammatory score.

GNPs	n	Mean ±	Minimum	Maximum	*p* Value
PW	9	3.22 ± 1.39	1	6	
PW + PBM	12	4.42 ± 3.11	1	10	
PW + Omcilon®	12	3.67 ± 2.06	2	9	
PW + GNPs-Cur	12	3.33 ± 1.96	1	7	
PW + GNPs-Açai	12	1.92 ± 0.79 *	1	4	0.027

3.4. Wound Contraction

Figure 3 represents the rate of wound contraction in %. There is a significant increase in wound contraction only in the PW + GNPs-Açai ($p < 0.05$) group in relation to the PW group.

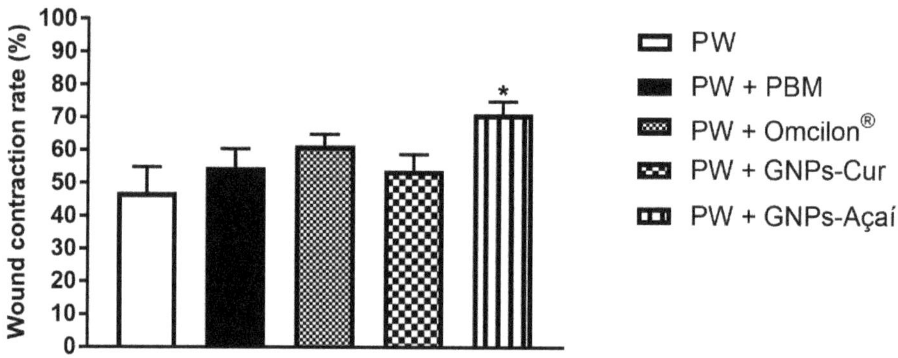

Figure 3. Effects of treatment with PBM, Omcilon®, GNPs-Cur, and GNPs-Açai on the wound contraction rate in %. Data are presented as mean + SEM, where: * $p < 0.05$ vs. Palatal Wound Group (PW); (One-way ANOVA followed by Tukey's post hoc test).

3.5. Histological Analysis

In Figure 4A, representative images of histological sections of the palatine mucosa stained with H&E are observed. In Figure 4B, quantifications of the average number of inflammatory infiltrates were performed, with a significant reduction observed in the PW + GNPs-Cur group in relation to the PW group ($p < 0.05$).

Figure 4C shows representative images of histological sections of the palatine mucosa that were stained with Gomori's trichrome to visualize collagen, and Figure 4D shows a significant increase in the area of collagen in the PW + GNPs-Açai group in relation to the PW group ($p < 0.05$).

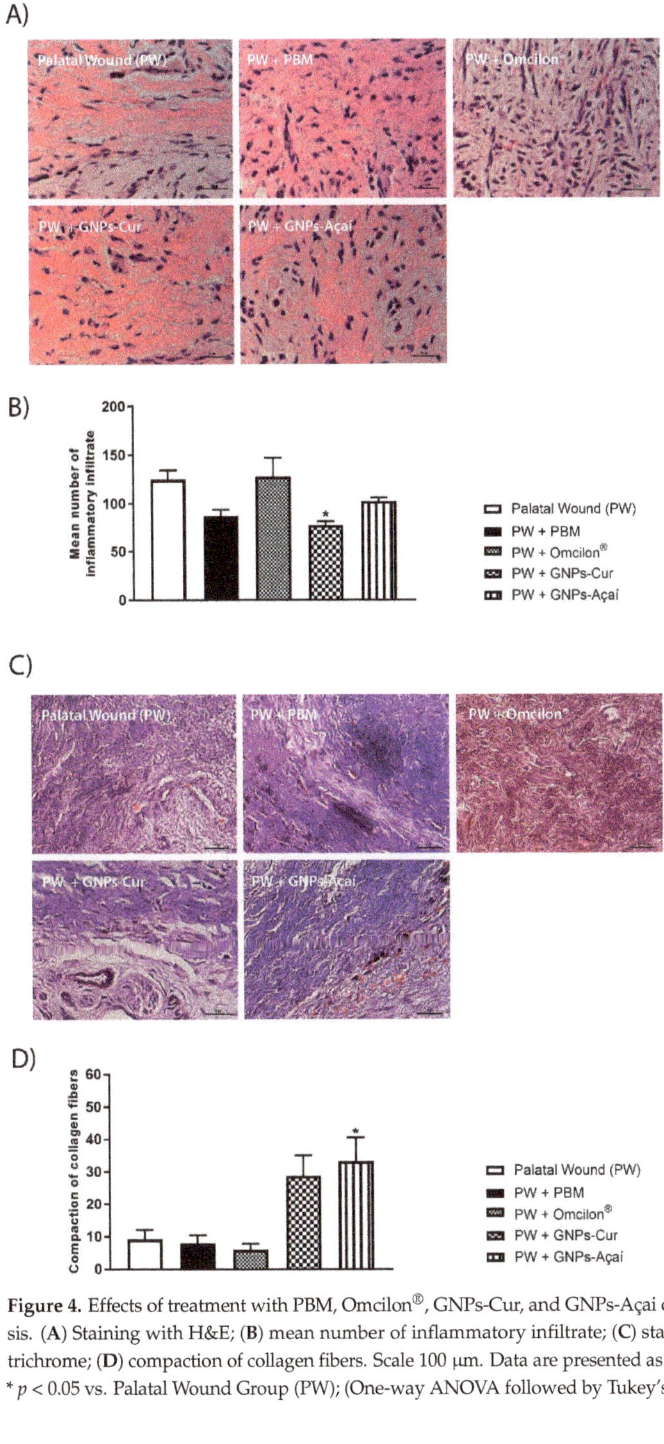

Figure 4. Effects of treatment with PBM, Omcilon®, GNPs-Cur, and GNPs-Açai on histological analysis. (**A**) Staining with H&E; (**B**) mean number of inflammatory infiltrate; (**C**) staining with Gomori's trichrome; (**D**) compaction of collagen fibers. Scale 100 µm. Data are presented as mean + SEM, where: * $p < 0.05$ vs. Palatal Wound Group (PW); (One-way ANOVA followed by Tukey's post hoc test).

3.6. Pro- and Anti-Inflammatory Cytokines

Figure 5 shows the protein levels of the cytokines TNF-α, IL-1β, IL4, and TGF-β. Representing the pro-inflammatory cytokines, when evaluating the levels of TNF-α, the PW + FBM, PW + GNPs-Cur, and PW + GNPs-Açai groups showed a significant decrease in relation to the PW group ($p < 0.05$). In Figure 5B, a significant reduction in IL-1β levels is observed in the PW + GNPs-Açai group when compared to the PW group ($p < 0.05$).

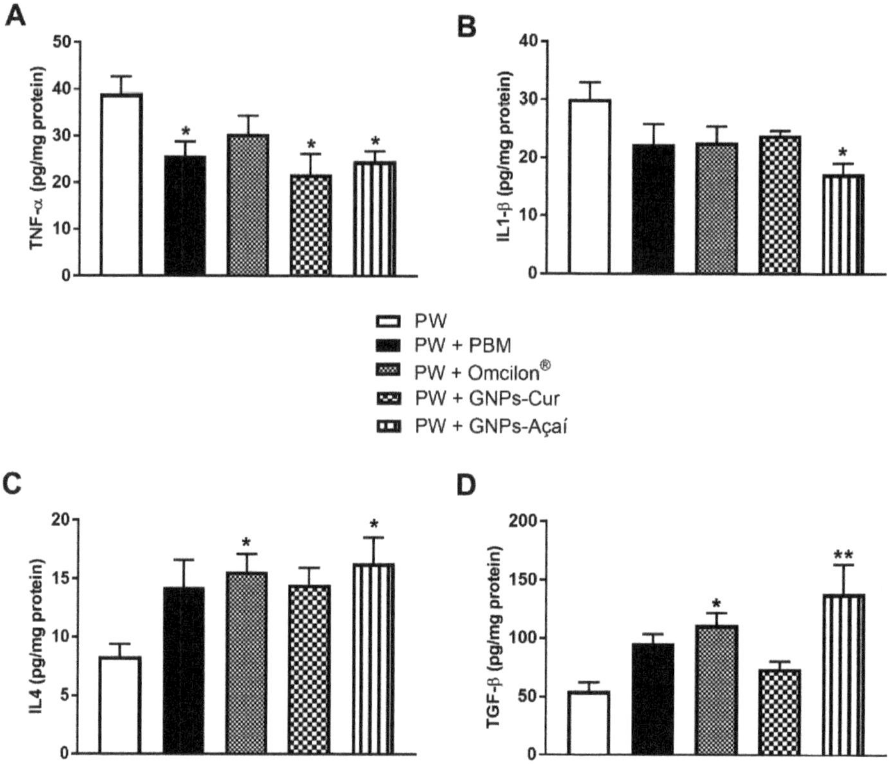

Figure 5. Effects of treatment with PBM, Omcilon®, GNPs-Cur, and GNPs-Açai on the levels of pro- and (TNF-α (**A**) and IL1-β (**B**)) anti-inflammatory cytokines (IL4 (**C**) and TGF-β (**D**)). Data are presented as mean + SEM, where: * $p < 0.05$ vs. Palatal Wound Group (PW); ** $p < 0.01$ vs. Palatal Wound Group (PW); (One-way ANOVA followed by Tukey's post hoc test).

Regarding anti-inflammatory cytokines, Figure 5C shows the results of IL4, which showed a significant increase in the PW + Omcilon® and PW + GNPs-Açai groups in relation to the PW group ($p < 0.05$), as well as what happened with TGF-β levels (Figure 5D), with a difference of $p < 0.01$ in the PW + GNPs-Açai group in relation to the PW group.

3.7. Levels of Oxidants and Antioxidants

For the evaluation of oxidative parameters, the levels of DCF and Nitrite were analyzed, as was GSH as an antioxidant. In Figure 6A, DCF levels were reduced in the PW + GNPs-Açai group when compared to the PW group ($p < 0.05$), as was the case with nitrite levels (Figure 6B). GSH levels, on the other hand, showed no significant difference between groups.

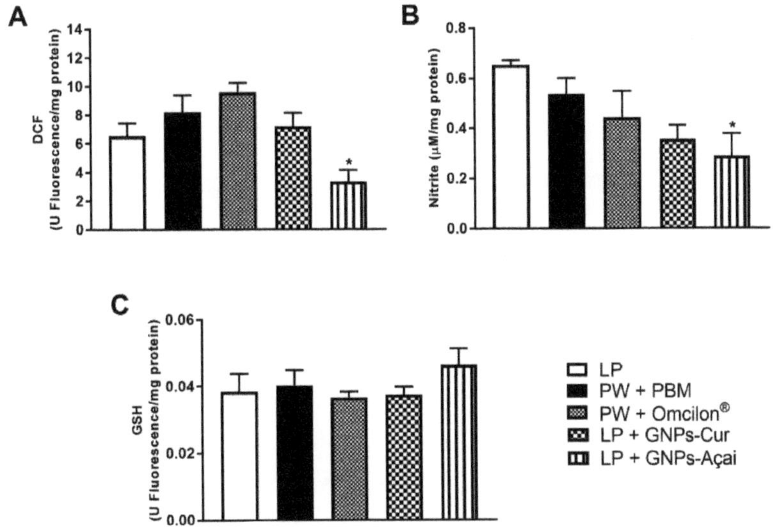

Figure 6. Effects of treatment with PBM, Omcilon®, GNPs-Cur, and GNPs-Açai on levels of oxidants (DCF (**A**) and Nitrite (**B**)) and antioxidants (GSH (**C**)). Data are presented as mean + SEM, where: * $p < 0.05$ vs. Palatal Wound Group (PW); (One-way ANOVA followed by Tukey's post hoc test).

4. Discussion

Due to the particularities and sensitivities that occur in the oral mucosa, causing some possible healing problems in the mouth, the literature is currently gaining attention to the development of biomaterials, such as nanoparticles, which may help trigger faster and more efficient healing. Because they have exceptional properties, a higher surface area/volume ratio, and different formats, NPs find applications in several fields of dentistry due to their mechanical, chemical, and optical properties. Gold is inert in nature, has low toxicity, and has also been used as a medicine. GNPs have many applications for therapeutic use due to their biostability, low cytotoxicity, and improved drug delivery capabilities, which enhance their use in various fields in addition to their potent anti-inflammatory and antioxidant effects [5].

The use of plant-based materials for the green synthesis of metallic nanoparticles has aroused much interest due to their lower toxicity, shorter processing times, and added benefit of being natural coating agents [23]. Curcumin, by limiting inflammation, allows damaged tissue to begin the later stages of healing sooner. The lack of proliferation and migration of fibroblasts will lead to impaired wound healing; curcumin upregulates fibroblast infiltration at wound sites [24]. Açai has antioxidant, anti-inflammatory, and anti-apoptotic effects in addition to promoting fibroblast proliferation; its supplementation can also protect against oxidative damage by reducing the formation of lipid peroxidation products, thus suggesting a potential protective effect promoted by the present antioxidants [25].

Thus, the present study evaluated the effects of treatment with GNPs reduced by the green synthesis method with curcumin and açai on the palatine wounds of Wistar rats. First, the inflammatory process of palatine wounds was evaluated using pro- and anti-inflammatory cytokines. Epithelial cells in inflamed regions express pro-inflammatory cytokines such as IL1-β, IL6, and TNF-α. This release leads to the activation of immune cells that accumulate in the inflamed sites and to the production and release of more cytokines [26]. Pro-inflammatory reactions after tissue injury are mainly triggered by IL1, which is associated with the innate immune system, and TNF-α, which is significantly involved in all inflammatory processes and whose release leads to vasodilation, accompanied by redness, swelling, and increased vascular permeability [27].

Both GNPs synthesized with curcumin and açai were able to significantly reduce the TNF-α marker in relation to the control, while only GNPs-Açai was able to reduce IL1-β. Regarding the anti-inflammatory cytokines, IL4, and the TGF-β growth factor, a significant increase was seen in relation to the control in the GNPs-Açai group, indicating that this therapy modulated and accelerated the inflammatory process, favoring the transition to the proliferative phase.

Controlling the overexpression of cytokines such as TNF-α may be useful in reducing pain and accelerating the healing of oral ulcers in rats, as it reduces acute inflammation [28]. In the case of GNPs, this anti-inflammatory action may be associated with their ability to suppress NF-κB [6], since it is known that inhibition of NF-κB activation leads to downregulation of the expression of COX-2 and inducible nitric oxide synthase (iNOS), suppressing the inflammatory response [29]. Another suggested mechanism is the direct binding of GNPs to IL1-β, inhibiting the binding of this cytokine to its receptor, as stated by Mendes et al. [7], who used gold nanoparticles in wound healing and also obtained a reduction in pro-inflammatory cytokines and an increase in anti-inflammatory cytokines, corroborating the present study.

In addition, in the recent study carried out by Ni et al. [30], it was demonstrated that GNPs can control the inflammatory response through the regulation of macrophage phenotypes (M1 and M2) and therefore generate a microenvironment with reduced levels of pro-inflammatory cytokines and an increased number of anti-inflammatory cytokines.

Wang et al. [31] synthesized curcumin solid lipid nanoparticles (Cur-SLNs) and increased their solubility compared to their native form and significantly reduced pro-inflammatory mediators by obstructing NF-κB activation, demonstrating the anti-inflammatory activity of this molecule. In vitro studies have also shown that Açai (*Euterpe oleracea*) extract downregulates NF-κB and its target genes, such as TNF-α, IL6, IL8, and IL1-β [32–34].

In the repair process, the inflammatory phase is accompanied by extensive phagocytosis, increased oxygen consumption, and mitochondrial dysfunction, which favor the formation of reactive species and enable a state of oxidative stress, which leads to a delay in the repair process. That is why, in this study, parameters of oxidative stress were evaluated. It was observed that GNPs-Açai were able to reduce both oxidant markers, DCF and nitrite, when compared to the control.

A benefit of açai is the ability to reduce the expression of the iNOS, contributing to the attenuation of the inflammatory response, in addition to the scavenging action (neutralizing free radicals) and the increase in the production and activity of antioxidant enzymes, such as superoxide dismutase (SOD), glutathione peroxidase (GPx), and catalase, which work in reducing ROS. Systemically, açai supplementation has been shown to influence the prevention of oxidative damage by a direct mechanism that reduces the formation of lipid peroxidation products, thus suggesting a potential protective effect promoted by the antioxidants present in açai (orientin, homoorientin, vitexin, luteolin, chrysoberyl, and quercetin [32,35].

The effective role of GNPs as antioxidant agents by inhibiting ROS formation, having a scavenger function (neutralizing free radicals), and potentiating the action of antioxidant enzymes has been demonstrated [7]. Li et al. [36] also demonstrated that GNPs increase levels of NRF2, which induces the signaling of antioxidant genes, in a study of endothelial cells. This increase was caused by the action of GNPs affecting the thiol bonds of KEAP1, thus changing its conformation and releasing NRF2 for subsequent transcription of cytoprotective genes, contributing to the antioxidant effect.

After the inflammatory process that takes place until the complete repair of a wound, it is expected that the repaired site will be restored to its normal anatomical condition as well as to its level of functionality. Collagen is the main element of the extracellular matrix and plays an important role in supporting mechanical loads by being a platform for re-epithelialization; therefore, its regeneration after injury is an essential process [37,38]. For this reason, in this study, the structure of the remodeled tissue was evaluated by histological analysis.

As in the studies carried out by BinShabaib et al. [39], Ning et al. [40], and Pona et al. [41], where there was a stimulus to collagen deposition, epithelialization, and wound contraction when evaluating the effects of *Euterpe oleracea* extracts on the healing process, the present study resulted in a significant increase in the area of collagen by GNPs-Açai in relation to the control. Raghuwanshi et al. [42] also demonstrated that GNPs were able to regulate collagen deposition, organize the extracellular matrix, and generate blood vessels, leading to rapid wound healing and closure.

Kang and Kim [11] show that there was a greater production and concentration of collagen in the oral mucosa of the group that received açai application, indicating that this molecule can prevent inflammation of the wound in the oral mucosa and promote re-epithelialization. In addition, it can help with mucosal regeneration and collagen synthesis at the time of remodeling.

As a result, in the results of the macroscopic analysis carried out in the present study to verify and record the visual perception of the inflammatory process, it was verified that the wounds treated with GNPs-Açai obtained an improved visual qualification, with an apparent reduction in the size of the wound and of the degree of inflammation and formation of necrotic tissue, corroborating with Weinberg et al. [43], who macroscopically evaluated the dimensional pattern related to the time taken to close an excisional palatine wound in rats, and obtained a macroscopic decrease in the dimensions of the wound in a temporal manner, which can be explained, as in the present study, by an acceleration of the inflammatory reaction and activity of myofibroblasts.

In this case, wound contraction is essential for reducing wound exposure to constant trauma and bacteria, which are characteristic of the oral environment. This contraction minimizes the open area by pulling neighboring tissue toward the center of the wound. Myofibroblasts, which arise by differentiation from fibroblasts, generate the contractile force by which the wound area contracts during wound healing [44]. However, a balance must be maintained, as although the contraction of the wound is beneficial in leading to its closure, excessive action can result in unwanted scars [45].

In the present study, the GNPs-Açai group was able to satisfactorily increase the wound contraction rate, which can be explained by the concomitant significant increase in the collagen area and the levels of the TGF-β growth factor, representing the potential of this cytokine to lead to re-epithelialization. Van Beurden et al. [46] point out that TGF-β has a biphasic role during the healing of palatal wounds since, at the beginning of healing, it stimulates myofibroblast differentiation and, after re-epithelialization, it stimulates myofibroblast apoptosis. Ratifying such findings, in the study by Kang and Kim [11], the aqueous extract of açai significantly reduced the surgical wound area performed on the backs of animals, showing a significantly potent wound healing effect in vivo based on macroscopic and histological observation.

Correlating the histological, macroscopic, and wound contraction results, it can be seen that only the groups treated with açai obtained satisfactory results in all these parameters. It is thought that this substance may have some mechanism that allows it to present better visual results than at the biochemical level, since in the histological analysis when associated with GNPs, it significantly increased the area of collagen but was not able to significantly reduce the inflammatory infiltrate.

Importantly, the oral microbiota plays a dual role in both wound recovery and oral damage [47]. Lesions on the oral mucosa, despite suffering a relatively brief healing process compared to the skin, can still result in inflammatory responses that hinder the regeneration process. Current treatment models available on the market, such as interventions with "photobiomodulation" and topical use of synthetic corticosteroids, are not completely effective.

Lesions, however small they may be, are painful, making chewing, food intake, and communication very difficult. The present study pointed out that topical treatment with green synthesized nanoparticles is a potential resource for the recovery of palatal wounds and the treatment of oral mucosa lesions (such as ulcers), preventing exacerbated inflammatory responses or infections, and thus facilitating the healing process.

5. Conclusions

We believe that taken together, with the anti-inflammatory, antioxidant, and re-epithelializing effects of GNPs and açai, these associated substances could present statistically more significant results than the other treatments discussed, just as it is possible to state that the proposed treatment has better efficiency when compared to standard treatments used in clinical practice. However, future studies are needed to evaluate other mechanisms involved in palatal tissue repair and the use of these therapies in other experimental models of the oral mucosa.

Supplementary Materials: The following supporting information can be downloaded at: https://www.mdpi.com/article/10.3390/antiox12081574/s1. Green synthesis of gold nanoparticles.

Author Contributions: A.T.: Validation, Investigation, Review and Editing, Funding Acquisition; M.F.M.G.: Conceptualization, Validation, Formal Analysis, Investigation, Data Curation, Writing; M.E.A.B.C.: Validation, Formal Analysis, Investigation, Writing, Review and Editing; L.M.V.: Investigation and Formal Analysis; L.d.R.C.: Investigation, Validation, Formal Analysis; I.R.L.: Investigation and Formal Analysis; C.D.C.: Investigation and Formal Analysis; E.D.P.: Data Curation; L.T.W.T.: Data Curation; P.E.F.: Validation and Resources; R.A.M.-d.-Á.: Validation and Resources; Y.G.: Funding Acquisition and Validation; P.C.L.S.: Supervision, Project Administration, Funding Acquisition. All authors reviewed the manuscript. All authors have read and agreed to the published version of the manuscript.

Funding: This work was supported by grants from the Conselho Nacional de Desenvolvimento Científico e Tecnológico (CNPq), the Fundação de Amparo à Pesquisa e Inovação do Estado de Santa Catarina (FAPESC), Universidade do Extremo Sul Catarinense (UNESC) and Research Academy of Medicine Combining Sports, Ningbo (No. 2023001), the Project of NINGBO Leading Medical & Health Discipline (No. 2022-F15, No. 2022-F22).

Institutional Review Board Statement: Not applicable.

Data Availability Statement: Data available on request from the authors.

Conflicts of Interest: The authors declare no conflict of interest.

References

1. Leoni, G.; Neumann, P.-A.; Sumagin, R.; Denning, T.L.; Nusrat, A. Wound repair: Role of immune–epithelial interactions. *Mucosal Immunol.* **2015**, *8*, 959–968. [CrossRef] [PubMed]
2. Scully, C.; Felix, D.H. Oral medicine—Update for the dental practitioner Aphthous and other common ulcers. *Br. Dent. J.* **2005**, *199*, 259–264. [CrossRef]
3. Abou Neel, E.A.; Bozec, L.; Perez, R.A.; Kim, H.W.; Knowles, J.C. Nanotechnology in dentistry: Prevention, diagnosis, and therapy. *Int. J. Nanomed.* **2015**, *10*, 6371. [CrossRef] [PubMed]
4. Upadhyay, A.; Pillai, S.; Khayambashi, P.; Sabri, H.; Lee, K.T.; Tarar, M.; Zhou, S.; Harb, I.; Tran, S.D. Biomimetic aspects of oral and dentofacial regeneration. *Biomimetics* **2020**, *5*, 51. [CrossRef]
5. Paiva-Santos, A.C.; Herdade, A.M.; Guerra, C.; Peixoto, D.; Pereira-Silva, M.; Zeinali, M.; Mascarenhas-Melo, F.; Paranhos, A.; Veiga, F. Plant-mediated green synthesis of metal-based nanoparticles for dermopharmaceutical and cosmetic applications. *Int. J. Pharm.* **2021**, *597*, 120311. [CrossRef] [PubMed]
6. Wang, X.; Chang, J.; Wu, C. Bioactive inorganic/organic nanocomposites for wound healing. *J. Appl. Mater. Today* **2018**, *11*, 308–319. [CrossRef]
7. Mendes, C.; Dos Santos Haupenthal, D.P.; Zaccaron, R.P.; Silveira, G.D.B.; Corrêa, M.E.A.B.; Casagrande, L.D.R.; Mariano, S.D.S.; Silva, J.I.D.S.; de Andrade, T.A.M.; Feuser, P.E.; et al. Effects of the association between photobiomodulation and hyaluronic acid linked gold nanoparticles in wound healing. *J. ACS Biomater. Sci. Eng.* **2020**, *6*, 5132–5144. [CrossRef]
8. Singh, J.; Dutta, T.; Kim, K.-H.; Rawat, M.; Samddar, P.; Kumar, P. 'Green' synthesis of metals and their oxide nanoparticles: Applications for environmental remediation. *J. Nanobiotechnol.* **2018**, *16*, 84. [CrossRef]
9. Asif, M.; Yasmin, R.; Asif, R.; Ambreen, A.; Mustafa, M.; Umbreen, S. Green Synthesis of Silver Nanoparticles (AgNPs), Structural Characterization, and their Antibacterial Potential. *Dose-Response* **2022**, *20*, 15593258221088709. [CrossRef]
10. Sohn, S.-I.; Priya, A.; Balasubramaniam, B.; Muthuramalingam, P.; Sivasankar, C.; Selvaraj, A.; Valliammai, A.; Jothi, R.; Pandian, S. Biomedical Applications and Bioavailability of Curcumin-An Updated Overview. *Pharmaceutics* **2021**, *13*, 2102. [CrossRef]

11. Kang, M.H.; Kim, B.H. Oral wound healing effects of acai berry water extracts in rat oral mucosa. *Toxicol. Res.* **2018**, *34*, 97–102. [CrossRef] [PubMed]
12. Percie Du Sert, N.; Hurst, V.; Ahluwalia, A.; Alam, S.; Avey, M.T.; Baker, M.; Browne, W.J.; Clark, A.; Cuthill, I.C.; Dirnagl, U.; et al. The ARRIVE guidelines 2.0: Updated guidelines for reporting animal research. *J. Cereb. Blood Flow Metab.* **2020**, *40*, 1769–1777. [CrossRef] [PubMed]
13. Marques Neto, R.; Lima Junior, R.; Vale, M.; Souza, M.; Brito, G. Mucosite Oral: Patogênese e manuseio clínico. *Rev. Bras. Oncol. Clínica* **2008**, *5*, 18–24.
14. Singh, A.V.; Bansod, G.; Mahajan, M.; Dietrich, P.; Singh, S.P.; Rav, K.; Thissen, A.; Bharde, A.M.; Rothenstein, D.; Kulkarni, S.; et al. Digital Transformation in Toxicology: Improving Communication and Efficiency in Risk Assessment. *ACS Omega* **2023**, *8*, 21377–21390. [CrossRef] [PubMed]
15. Dong, J.; Sulik, K.K.; Chen, S.-Y. The role of NOX enzymes in ethanol-induced oxidative stress and apoptosis in mouse embryos. Research Support, N I H, Extramural. *Toxicol. Lett.* **2010**, *193*, 94–100. [CrossRef] [PubMed]
16. Chae, S.Y.; Lee, M.; Kim, S.W.; Bae, Y.H. Protection of insulin secreting cells from nitric oxide induced cellular damage by crosslinked hemoglobin. *Biomaterials* **2004**, *25*, 843–850. [CrossRef]
17. Hissin, P.J.; Hilf, R. A fluorometric method for determination of oxidized and reduced glutathione in tissues. *Anal. Biochem.* **1976**, *74*, 214–226. [CrossRef]
18. Lowry, O.; Rosebrough, N.; Farr, A.L.; Randall, R. Protein measurement with the Folin phenol reagent. *J. Biol. Chem.* **1951**, *193*, 265–275. [CrossRef]
19. Callegari-Jacques, S.M. *Bioestatística: Princípios e Aplicações*; Artmed Editora: Porto Alegre, Brazil, 2009.
20. Field, A. *Discovering Statistics Using SPSS (3. Baskı)*; Sage Publications Ltd.: London, UK, 2009.
21. Vieira, S. *Bioestatística: Tópicos Avançados*, 3rd ed.; RJ; Elsevier: Amsterdam, The Netherlands, 2010.
22. Zar, J. *Biostatistical Analysis*, 5th ed.; Prentice-Hall: Hoboken, NJ, USA, 2010.
23. Peralta-Videa, J.R.; Huang, Y.; Parsons, J.G.; Zhao, L.; Lopez-Moreno, L.; Hernandez-Viezcas, J.A.; Gardea-Torresdey, J.L. Plant-based green synthesis of metallic nanoparticles: Scientific curiosity or a realistic alternative to chemical synthesis? *Nanotechnol. Environ. Eng.* **2016**, *1*, 4. [CrossRef]
24. Chaushu, L.; Rahmanov Gavrielov, M.; Chaushu, G.; Zar, K.; Vered, M. Curcumin Promotes Primary Oral Wound Healing in a Rat Model. *J. Med. Food* **2021**, *24*, 422–430. [CrossRef]
25. Felin, F.D.; Maia-Ribeiro, E.A.; Felin, C.D.; Bonotto, N.A.C.; Turra, B.O.; Roggia, I.; Azzolin, V.F.; Teixeira, C.F.; Mastella, M.H.; de Freitas, C.R.; et al. Amazonian Guarana-and Açai-Conjugated Extracts Improve Scratched Fibroblast Healing and Eisenia fetida Surgical Tail Amputation by Modulating Oxidative Metabolism. *Oxidative Med. Cell. Longev.* **2022**, *2022*, 3094362. [CrossRef] [PubMed]
26. Sugawara, S.; Uehara, A.; Tamai, R.; Takada, H. Innate immune responses in oral mucosa. *J. Endotoxin Res.* **2002**, *8*, 465–468. [CrossRef] [PubMed]
27. Tetyczka, C.; Hartl, S.; Jeitler, R.; Absenger-Novak, M.; Meindl, C.; Fröhlich, E.; Riedl, S.; Zweytick, D.; Roblegg, E. Cytokine-Mediated Inflammation in the Oral Cavity and Its Effect on Lipid Nanocarriers. *Nanomaterials* **2021**, *11*, 1330. [CrossRef]
28. Freitas, M.O.; Fonseca, A.P.R.; de Aguiar, M.T.; Dias, C.C.; Avelar, R.L.; Sousa, F.B.; Alves, A.P.N.N.; Silva, P.G.d.B. Tumor necrosis factor alpha (TNF-α) blockage reduces acute inflammation and delayed wound healing in oral ulcer of rats. *Inflammopharmacology* **2022**, *30*, 1781–1798. [CrossRef] [PubMed]
29. Karthikeyan, A.; Senthil, N.; Min, T. Nanocurcumin: A Promising Candidate for Therapeutic Applications. *Front. Pharmacol.* **2020**, *11*, 487. [CrossRef]
30. Ni, C.; Zhou, J.; Kong, N.; Bian, T.; Zhang, Y.; Huang, X.; Xiao, Y.; Yang, W.; Yan, F. Gold nanoparticles modulate the crosstalk between macrophages and periodontal ligament cells for periodontitis treatment. *Biomaterials* **2019**, *206*, 115–132. [CrossRef]
31. Wang, W.; Chen, T.; Xu, H.; Ren, B.; Cheng, X.; Qi, R.; Liu, H.; Wang, Y.; Yan, L.; Chen, S.; et al. Curcumin-Loaded Solid Lipid Nanoparticles Enhanced Anticancer Efficiency in Breast Cancer. *Molecules* **2018**, *23*, 1578. [CrossRef]
32. Dos Santos, V.R.N.; Frazão, D.R.; Ferreira, R.d.O.; Mendes, P.F.S.; Baia-Da-Silva, D.C.; Souza-Monteiro, D.; Bittencourt, L.O.; de Moura, J.D.M.; Perdigão, J.M.; Teixeira, B.J.B.; et al. Açaí (*Euterpe oleracea* Mart.) Attenuates Oxidative Stress and Alveolar Bone Damage in Experimental Periodontitis in Rats. *Antioxidants* **2022**, *11*, 1902. [CrossRef]
33. de Oliveira, A.C.; Miyagawa, L.M.; Monteiro, K.M.; Dias, A.L.; Longato, G.B.; Spindola, H.; Vendramini-Costa, D.B.; Quetin-Leclercq, J.; Carvalho, J.E.; Rogez, H. Phenolic composition, antiproliferative and antiulcerogenic activities of a polyphenol-rich purified extract from açai (*Euterpe oleracea*) fruits. *Int. J. Food Sci. Technol.* **2021**, *56*, 6626–6634. [CrossRef]
34. Brito, C.; Stavroullakis, A.; Ferreira, A.; Li, K.; Oliveira, T.; Nogueira-Filho, G.; Prakki, A. Extract of acai-berry inhibits osteoclast differentiation and activity. *Arch. Oral Biol.* **2016**, *68*, 29–34. [CrossRef]
35. Barbosa, P.O.; Souza, M.O.; Silva, M.P.; Santos, G.T.; Silva, M.E.; Bermano, G.; Freitas, R.N. Açaí (*Euterpe oleracea* Martius) supplementation improves oxidative stress biomarkers in liver tissue of dams fed a high-fat diet and increases antioxidant enzymes' gene expression in offspring. *Biomed. Pharmacother.* **2021**, *139*, 111627. [CrossRef] [PubMed]
36. Li, X.; Xu, H.; Chen, Z.-S.; Chen, G. Biosynthesis of nanoparticles by microorganisms and their applications. *J. Nanomater.* **2011**, *2011*, 270974. [CrossRef]
37. Kwan, K.H.; Liu, X.; To, M.K.; Yeung, K.W.; Ho, C.-M.; Wong, K.K. Modulation of collagen alignment by silver nanoparticles results in better mechanical properties in wound healing. *Biol. Med.* **2011**, *7*, 497–504. [CrossRef] [PubMed]

38. Fratzl, P.; Misof, K.; Zizak, I.; Rapp, G.; Amenitsch, H.; Bernstorff, S. Fibrillar structure and mechanical properties of collagen. *J. Struct. Biol.* **1998**, *122*, 119–122. [CrossRef]
39. BinShabaib, M.S.; Alharthi, S.S.; Helaby, B.S.; AlHefdhi, M.H.; Mohammed, A.E.; Aabed, K. Comparison of the Anti-bacterial Efficacy of *Saussurea costus* and *Melaleuca alternifolia* against *Porphyromonas gingivalis*, *Streptococcus mutans*, and *Enterococcus faecalis*: An in-vitro Study. *Front. Oral Health* **2022**, *3*, 950840. [CrossRef]
40. Ning, S.; Zang, J.; Zhang, B.; Feng, X.; Qiu, F. Botanical Drugs in Traditional Chinese Medicine With Wound Healing Properties. *Front. Pharmacol.* **2022**, *13*, 885484. [CrossRef]
41. Pona, A.; Cline, A.; Kolli, S.S.; Taylor, S.L.; Feldman, S.R. Review of future insights of Dragon's Blood in dermatology. *Dermatol. Ther.* **2019**, *32*, e12786. [CrossRef]
42. Raghuwanshi, N.; Kumari, P.; Srivastava, A.K.; Vashisth, P.; Yadav, T.C.; Prasad, R.; Pruthi, V. Synergistic effects of Woodfordia fruticosa gold nanoparticles in preventing microbial adhesion and accelerating wound healing in Wistar albino rats in vivo. *Mater. Sci. Eng. C* **2017**, *80*, 252–262. [CrossRef]
43. Weinberg, E.; Vered, M.; Atzil, S.; Chaushu, G.; Chaushu, L. The dynamics of closure following excisional mid-palatal mucoperiosteal wound in a rat model. *Clin. Oral Investig.* **2020**, *24*, 4385–4393. [CrossRef]
44. Feugate, J.E.; Li, Q.J.; Wong, L.; Martins-Green, M. The cxc chemokine cCAF stimulates differentiation of fibroblasts into myofibroblasts and accelerates wound closure. *J. Cell Biol.* **2002**, *156*, 161–172. [CrossRef]
45. Chitturi, R.T.; Murali Balasubramaniam, A.; Arjun Parameswar, R.; Kesavan, G.; Muhamed Haris, K.T.; Mohideen, K. The role of myofibroblasts in wound healing, contraction and its clinical implications in cleft palate repair. *J. Int. Oral Heal.* **2015**, *7*, 75–80.
46. van Beurden, H.; Von den Hoff, J.; Torensma, R.; Maltha, J.; Kuijpers-Jagtman, A. Myofibroblasts in palatal wound healing: Prospects for the reduction of wound contraction after cleft palate repair. *J. Dent. Res.* **2005**, *84*, 871–880. [CrossRef] [PubMed]
47. Vanlancker, E.; Vanhoecke, B.; Sieprath, T.; Bourgeois, J.; Beterams, A.; De Moerloose, B.; De Vos, W.H.; Van de Wiele, T. Oral microbiota reduce wound healing capacity of epithelial monolayers, irrespective of the presence of 5-fluorouracil. *Exp. Biol. Med.* **2018**, *243*, 350–360. [CrossRef] [PubMed]

antioxidants

MDPI

Article

In-Situ Thermoresponsive Hydrogel Containing Resveratrol-Loaded Nanoparticles as a Localized Drug Delivery Platform for Dry Eye Disease

Ilenia De Luca [1,†], Francesca Di Cristo [2,†], Raffaele Conte [2], Gianfranco Peluso [1,3], Pierfrancesco Cerruti [4,*] and Anna Calarco [1,*]

1 Research Institute on Terrestrial Ecosystems (IRET)—CNR, Via Pietro Castellino 111, 80131 Napoli, Italy; ilenia.deluca@iret.cnr.it (I.D.L.)
2 Elleva Pharma s.r.l., Via P. Castellino 111, 80131 Napoli, Italy; francesca.dicristo2@gmail.com (F.D.C.); raffaele.conte86@tiscali.it (R.C.)
3 Faculty of Medicine and Surgery, UniCamillus-Saint Camillus International University of Health Sciences, Via di Sant'Alessandro 8, 00131 Rome, Italy
4 Institute for Polymers, Composites and Biomaterials (IPCB-CNR), Via Campi Flegrei 34, 80078 Pozzuoli, Italy
* Correspondence: cerruti@ipcb.cnr.it (P.C.); anna.calarco@cnr.it (A.C.)
† These authors contributed equally to this work.

Abstract: Dry eye disease (DED) is a dynamic and complex disease that can cause significant damage to the ocular surface and discomfort, compromising the patient's quality of life. Phytochemicals such as resveratrol have received increasing attention due to their ability to interfere with multiple pathways related to these diseases. However, the low bioavailability and the poor therapeutic response of resveratrol hinder its clinical applications. Cationic polymeric nanoparticles, in combination with in situ gelling polymers, could represent a promising strategy to prolong drug corneal residence time reducing the frequency of administration and increasing the therapeutic response. Eyedrop formulations, based on acetylated polyethyleneimine-modified polylactic-co-glicolyc acid- (PLGA-PEI) nanoparticles loaded with resveratrol (RSV-NPs) were dispersed into poloxamer 407 hydrogel and characterized in terms of pH, gelation time, rheological properties, in vitro drugs release, and biocompatibility. Moreover, the antioxidant and anti-inflammatory effects of RSV were assessed in vitro by mimicking a DED condition through the exposition of epithelial corneal cells to a hyperosmotic state. This formulation exhibited sustained release of RSV for up to 3 days, exerting potent antioxidant and anti-inflammatory effects on corneal epithelial cells. In addition, RSV reversed the mitochondrial dysfunction mediated by high osmotic pressure, leading to upregulated sirtuin 1 (SIRT1) expression, an essential regulator of mitochondrial function. These results suggest the potential of eyedrop formulation as a platform to overcome the rapid clearance of current solutions for treating various inflammation- and oxidative stress-related diseases such as DED.

Keywords: eye dry disease; resveratrol; acetylated nanoparticles; hydrogel; epithelial corneal cells; antioxidant; anti-inflammatory

1. Introduction

Eyes are constantly exposed to environmental factors (e.g., air pollutants or adverse indoor and/or outdoor environmental conditions, light exposure, ultraviolet rays, ionizing radiation) that compromise tear film composition and ocular surface components [1]. Prolonged exposure to these insults triggers oxidative damage of the ocular surface through the production of reactive oxygen species (ROS) and activation of pro-inflammatory signaling pathways [2,3]. Overproduction of ROS in tear and ocular surface structures represents one of the main characteristics of Dry Eye Disease (DED) [3], a multifactorial disease quite frequent in the elderly population, and growing rapidly in young people as well [4]. The loss of tear film homeostasis and the damage of the affected eye area up to the cornea causes visual discomfort and disturbance to the patient often compromising daily life [5]. DED symptoms include burning, inflammation, foreign body sensation, blurred vision, heaviness and tear film instability. According to the multifactorial and wide spectrum of DED etiology, the treatment must be tailored specifically to each patient by targeting the specific mechanisms in accordance with disease severity. Mild DED cases are treated with artificial tears to reduce tear evaporation and corneal surface inflammation. More serious cases require treatment with anti-inflammatory agents, such as topical corticosteroids, systemic cholinergic agents, and autologous serum tears [6]. However, long-lasting application of ocular preparations containing preservatives (e.g., benzalkonium chloride (BAK), chlorobutanol, sodium perborate), may cause side effects due to the disruption of the ocular epithelial cell-cell junction and toxic epitheliopathy in the case of preserved products Hence, there is still a demand for novel therapeutic approaches.

Plant polyphenols are vegetable secondary metabolites able to promote beneficial health effects, such as anti-inflammatory, antioxidant and antimicrobial [7]. In particular, their bioactivity is able to influence both the production of ROS, IL (interleukins), ELAM-1 (endothelial leucocyte adhesion molecule-1), the expression of the TNF-α (tumor necrosis factor-α), and VEGF (vascular endothelial growth factor) pathways in ocular tissues. Moreover, some polyphenols could increase antioxidant defense systems and inhibit p53-dependent apoptosis involved in age-related eye disease [8,9]. Moreover, it has been reported that oxidative stress may directly affect ocular surface health, inducing DED. Therefore, topical/systemic use of antioxidants represents a promising approach to the treatment of DED [10].

Recent in vivo and in vitro studies demonstrated that curcumin, epigallocatechin gallate, resveratrol, quercetin, betaine and pterostilbene polyphenols are effective in DED pathology treatment [11]. Among all polyphenols, increasing attention is being paid to Resveratrol (RSV, 3,5,4′-trihydroxy-trans-stilbene) due to its strong antioxidant and anti-inflammatory effects also in ophthalmologic diseases [12,13]. Further, RSV regulates inflammatory responses via various signaling pathways in a dose-dependent manner. Moreover, RSV acts as an antioxidant by controlling antioxidant enzymes and blocking free radical damage to DNA [14].

Even though several studies demonstrated RSV's potential applicability as a treatment for DED, its low water solubility, low stability and poor ocular bioavailability limit clinical efficacy. Recent studies focused on nanotechnology approaches to overcame these limits and produce ophthalmic polyphenols-enriched formulations [15]. Compared to currently available approaches for administering eye drops, nanostructured polymers with bioadhesive properties (e.g., cationic nanoparticles) represent a more efficient approach to delivering the appropriate concentrations of bioactive molecules to the eye. Positively charged nanocarriers could interact with negatively charged cells of the ocular surface prolonging the residence time of the administered eye drops [16]. Hence, the present study aims to design an in situ thermogelling formulation containing RSV-loaded polymeric nanoparticles able to ameliorate the clearance of current eye drop solutions. To this purpose, cationic acetylated lactide/glycolide-polyethyleneimine (PLGA-PEI) nanoparticles (AcPEI-NPs) loaded with RSV were prepared by nanoprecipitation and incorporated in the Poloxamer 407 thermoresponsive hydrogel (RSV@Tgel) to develop novel devices for the treatment of ocular diseases. Poloxamer 407 is a member of the Pluronics® triblock copolymers, made of polyethylene glycol-*b*-polypropylene glycol-*b*-polyethylene glycol, which are non-ionic, water-soluble materials widely used as pharmaceutical excipients [17]. It has been demonstrated that the use of polymers that exhibit thermoresponsive sol-to-gel phase transition in the cul-de-sac could overcome the loss of drug in precorneal tissue caused by eye drainage, thereby extending drug-cornea contact time. Indeed, these ophthalmic formulations, by changing their structure and viscosity upon heating, can be administered as a liquid, and then form a gel in specific environmental circumstances, such as in contact with the eye [18]. The RSV@Tgel formulation was physiochemically characterized, and the release profiles of RSV were evaluated in simulated tear fluid. Moreover, the role of released RSV in preventing oxidative stress and cytokine release was explored in human corneal epithelial cells (HCECs) under hyperosmotic stress, as an in vitro dry eye model. The reported results demonstrated the ability of RSV@Tgel to attenuate hyperosmolar-induced mitochondrial dysfunction in HCECs, restoring mitochondrial function by inducing SIRT1 expression. For these reasons, RSV@Tgel could be an excellent adjuvant in dry eye disease due to its protective effect against inflammation and oxidative stress, as well as the reduced number of eye drop instillations.

2. Materials and Methods

2.1. Materials

D,L-Lactide/glycolide copolymer (PLGA, PURASORB®, inherent viscosity 0.20 dL/g) was a generous gift from PURAC (Gorinchem, The Netherlands). Branched polyethylenimine (PEI, MW: 25 kDa), acetic anhydride, dicyclohexylcarbodiimide (DCC), N-hydroxysuccinimide (NHS), acetone, resveratrol (RSV), polyvinyl alcohol (PVA, average mol wt. 30,000–70,000), Poloxamer 407, phenylmethylsulfonyl fluoride (PMSF), benzamidine, and hydroquinone (HQ) were obtained from Sigma-Aldrich (Milan, Italy). All HPLC analytical grade solvents were purchased from Fisher Scientific (Milan, Italy). Dulbecco's modified Eagle medium (DMEM; Euroclone, Milan, Italy) containing 10% fetal bovine serum (FBS; Euroclone), 100 U/mL penicillin, and 100 µg/mL streptomycin (Euroclone), in 5% CO_2 at 37 °C and 95% humidified room air.

2.2. Physico-Chemical Characterization of RSV-Loaded Nanoparticles (RSV-NPs)

Acetylated nanoparticles (AcPEI-PLGA) were prepared using a two-step procedure as reported by Conte et al. with modifications [19]. Briefly, AcPEI-PLGA copolymer (50 mg) and different quantities of RSV (1–10 mg) were completely dissolved in 10 mL of acetone under ultrasound to form a homogeneous mixed system (Digital Sonifier S-250D, BRANSON, Milan, Italy). The resultant solution was added dropwise into the aqueous phase, containing 100 mL PVA (0.5% *w*/*v*), and stirred overnight on a magnetic stir plate (at 300 rpm) to allow evaporation of the organic solvent. The RSV-NPs were collected by centrifugation for 45 min at 14,810× *g*, 4 °C (5718R, OHAUS, Milan, Italy), washed with ultrapure water (Milli-Q® IQ 7000, Merk Life Science S.r.l., Milan, Italy) and lyophilized. Control nanoparticles (NPs) were prepared following a similar procedure omitting RSV. The hydrodynamic diameter, zeta potential, and polydispersity index (PDI) were measured using Dynamic Light Scattering (DLS, Malvern Zetasizer, Malvern Instruments Ltd., Malvern, UK), and the particle concentration was assessed by Nanoparticles Tracking Analysis (NTA-NanoSight NS300, Malvern Instruments Ltd., Malvern, UK) as reported by Valentino et al. [20]. For both analyses, experiments were performed at 25 °C using a sample volume of 1 mL. The average values were obtained with the data from six separate measurements.

The amount of drug entrapped in NPs was determined indirectly, in triplicate, by analyzing the amount of free RSV in the supernatant (18,620× *g* for 30 min; 5718R, OHAUS, Milan, Italy) as described in Section 2.6. The encapsulation efficiency of RSV-NPs was determined based on the following equation:

$$EE\% = \frac{\text{Total amount of drug} - \text{Amount of drug in supernatant}}{\text{Total amount of drug}} \times 100 \quad (1)$$

2.3. Mucoadhesion of RSV-NPs

The interaction between mucin and RSV-NPs was evaluated by mixing equal volumes of mucin (0.5 mg/mL in PBS) and NPs (2.53×10^9 particles/mL) at 35 °C for 2 h [21]. The suspension was, then, centrifuged at 15,600× *g* (Corning LSE high speed microcentrifuge; Fisher Scientific Italia, Milan, Italy) for 1h at room temperature (25 °C). UV-Visible spectrophotometer (UV-1650 PC, Shimadzu, Milan, Italy) at 255 nm was used to quantify the amount of free mucin. All nanoformulations were analyzed in triplicate ($n = 3$). The mucin-binding efficiency of NPs (%) or mucoadhesive strength of NPs was calculated by using the equation stated as follows:

$$\text{Mucoadhesive efficiency } (\%) = \frac{\text{Total amoun of mucin} - \text{Free amount of mucin}}{\text{Total amount of mucin}} \times 100 \quad (2)$$

2.4. Preparation of RSV-Loaded Hydrogels (RSV@Tgels)

Poloxamer gels were prepared by the cold method as described by Matthew et al. [22] with slight modifications. Briefly, an appropriate amount of polymer was accurately weighed and dispersed in purified distilled water with continuous mild stirring (until polymer dissolution) to prepare solutions at varying polymer concentrations (15–22% w/v). The poloxamer 407 concentration was chosen based on gelation temperature and gelation time. To obtain RSV-NPs dispersion in gel (RSV@Tgel), weighed amounts of lyophilized RSV-NPs (0.1, 0.5, and 1 mg/10 mL solution) were homogeneously mixed with cold poloxamer 407 overnight in an ice bath.

2.5. RSV@Tgels Characterization

2.5.1. Rheological and Mechanical Studies

The sol-gel transition of the RSV@Tgels containing 1 mg/10 mL RSV-NPs was determined by non-isothermal oscillatory rotational rheometry, by means of a Thermo Scientific Mars III device equipped with steel parallel plates (20 mm, plate gap = 1.0 mm). The measurements were carried out at an angular frequency of 10 rad/s and varying deformation from 0.5 to 5%, with a heating rate of 1 °C/min from 20 to 50 °C. Storage (G′) and viscous moduli (G″) were recorded as a function of temperature. The temperature at which G′ attained the plateau value was considered as the gelling temperature, T_{gel}. At least three replicates were performed. Compressive stress–strain tests were performed using the same equipment, with a loading-unloading strain rate of 0.6 mm/min, and a strain level of up to ≈20% of the original plate gap. The compressive moduli were obtained by linear fitting of the stress–strain curves in a strain range of 2–5%. In the cyclic loading–unloading tests, compression and load were recorded for 10 cycles. Each reported value was the mean of at least three measurements.

2.5.2. Gelation Time

The gelation time ($t_{sol\text{-}gel}$) of RSV@Tgels was determined by a modified test tube inversion method using simulated tear fluid (0.67 g NaCl, 0.2 g $NaHCO_3$, and 0.008 $CaCl_2{\cdot}2H_2O$ in 100 g of purified water, STF) as gelation solution [23]. Briefly, a glass vial containing 1.0 mL of sample was kept at the storage temperature of 4 °C for 2 h, then withdrawn and placed in a water bath set at 34 °C. The glass vial was then repeatedly turned upside down to check for gelling of the sample. The gelation time represents the temperature at which the gel did not exhibit gravitational flow during a period of 2 min when the tube was reversed.

2.5.3. Short-Term Stability Studies

The physicochemical stability of RSV@Tgels was monitored over a period of 14 days of storage at different temperatures (4.0 ± 0.5 °C and 25.0 ± 0.5 °C) by visual observation and pH determination. At predetermined times (0 and 14 days), nanoparticles were separated from the hydrogel by centrifugation (12,000× g, 2 h; Corning LSE high speed microcentrifuge; Fisher Scientific Italia, Milan, Italy). The physical stability of the formulation was visually examined for its dispersion parameters such as the presence of aggregates and the occurrence of coalescence phenomena. Further, all samples were analyzed for particle size, PDI, and % drug entrapment efficiency, and the results were compared with the initial values. The RSV stability during storage was confirmed by HPLC analysis as described in Section 2.6.

2.6. *In Vitro RSV Release and Permeation Studies*

The cumulative RSV release was assessed in 5 mL of freshly prepared STF at two different osmolarity values, namely 312 and 500 mOsm/L. During the release test, the temperature was maintained at 34.0 $\pm$ 0.5 °C under continuous magnetic stirring (200 rpm). At given time intervals, 0.5 mL of release media was withdrawn and replenished with fresh media. Samples were centrifuged for 45 min at 21,380$\times$ g (Corning LSE high speed microcentrifuge; Fisher Scientific Italia, Milan, Italy) and the amount of RSV in the samples was determined by liquid chromatography–tandem mass spectrometry (LC-MS/MS), as indicated by Amaghnouje et al. [24].

The permeation studies were performed using vertical Franz diffusion cells with a volume of 12 mL (contact area: 1.77 cm^2, PermeGear Inc., Hellertown, PA, USA) as reported by Bao et al. [25]. Cellulose acetate membranes were placed on top of the receptor chambers of the cells following the addition of freshly prepared STF as release media. During the release test, the temperature was maintained at 34.0 $\pm$ 0.5 °C. To simulate the small amount of tear secreted on the eye surface, 0.25 mL of the release medium was added to the top of the samples loaded into the donor chambers. At specified time intervals, aliquots (0.15 mL) of fresh media were used to replace the same volume withdrawn from the receptor chambers. Then, the supernatants were directly assayed by LC-MS/MS after centrifugation at 21,380$\times$ g (Corning LSE high speed microcentrifuge; Fisher Scientific Italia, Milan, Italy), 4 °C for 45 min.

2.7. *In Vitro Cell Studies*

2.7.1. Cells Culture and In Vitro Dry Eye Model

Human Corneal Epithelial Cells (HCECs) were obtained from the American Type Culture Collection (CRL-11135, ATCC, Milan, Italy) and maintained in DMEM supplemented with 10% FBS, 4.5 mg/mL glucose, 2.0 mM glutamine, 100 U/mL penicillin, 100 μg/mL streptomycin, and 10 ng/mL human epidermal growth factor in a humidified atmosphere of 5% CO_2–95% air and 37 °C. HCECs from the third to tenth passages that exhibited good morphology were used for experiments. The cell viability of HCECs on RSV@Tgel was assessed following the international standard ISO 10993 by cell counting kit (CCK-8) according to the manufacturer's protocol (Sigma-Aldrich, Milan, Italy). Briefly, the gel samples were immersed and incubated in DMEM at 37 °C for 24 h to obtain the "conditioned medium" (CM). Following the adherence of HCECs, the culture medium was removed and replaced with 200 μL CM for 6, 12, and 24 h. Then, 10 μL of CCK-8 solution was added to each well and the absorbance was measured at 450 nm. Cell viability was determined as a percentage compared to the untreated cells.

Cellular death by membrane damage was measured using Lactate Dehydrogenase (LDH) assay (Sigma-Aldrich) as per the manufacturer's instructions. Cells were treated as previously described and LDH released in the culture medium was measured at 490 nm. Triton X-100 solutions (1%) and culture media only were used as positive and negative controls, respectively.

For Dry Eye Cell Model, HCECs were treated with culture medium at different osmolarities ranging from 312 to 500 mOsm/L as reported by Shetty et al. [26]. The protective effects of RSV were studied with the acute toxicity model by pre-treating cells with RSV@Tgel for 24 h. A shorter exposure (4 h) was used to investigate the effects on mRNA expression.

2.7.2. Intracellular Antioxidant Activities

As previously reported [27], the CM-H_2DCFDA assay kit (Sigma-Aldrich) was used to determine intracellular ROS production according to the manufacturer's protocol.

To assess antioxidant enzyme activities, HCECs were treated as reported above and resuspended in 0.5 mL PBS buffer containing 0.5 mM phenylmethylsulfonyl fluoride (PMSF) and 0.2 mM benzamidine. Measurements of Catalase (CAT) and Superoxide dismutases (SODs) activities were carried out on cell lysates after sonication (three intervals of 5 s).

Hydrogen peroxide (H_2O_2) decomposition (at 240 nm) was followed to determine CAT activity (EC 1.11.1.6). Results were normalized to total protein content and expressed as a percentage of control (100% of activity). SOD (EC 1.15.1.1) activity was measured using the standard assay mixture containing an enzymatic sample as per the manufacturer's instructions (Sigma-Aldrich). Samples were exposed for 5 min to intense cool white light. One SOD unit was defined as the amount of enzyme necessary to inhibit 50% of the reaction rate. Samples were measured at 560 nm in a Cytation 3 microplate reader. Results were normalized to total protein content and expressed as a percentage of control. Experiments were performed four times.

2.7.3. Enzyme-Linked Immunosorbent Assay (ELISA)

The levels of human interleukin-6 (IL-6), human interleukin-8 (IL-8), and tumor necrosis factor (TNF-α) were measured in supernatants using an Enzyme-Linked Immunosorbent Assay (ELISA) as reported by Conte et al. [28].

2.7.4. RNA Isolation, Reverse Transcription, and Quantitative Real-Time PCR (qRT-PCR)

Total RNA was extracted from cell cultures using TriFast (EuroClone, Milan, Italy), according to the manufacturer's protocol, and mRNA levels were measured by RT-PCR amplification as reported by De Luca et al. [29]. Specific primers for Human Matrix Metallopeptidase 9 (*MMP-9*), Interleukin-6 (*IL-6*), Interleukin-8 (*IL-8*), tumor necrosis factor (*TNF)-α*, Sirtuin 1 *(Sirt1)* and β-Actin (*ACTB*) were used and listed in Table 1. All reactions were run in triplicate, normalized to the housekeeping gene (*ACTB*), and the results were expressed as mean ± SD. The $2^{-\Delta\Delta Ct}$ method was used to determine the relative quantification.

Table 1. Primers used for qRT-PCR.

Gene	Accession Number	Forward (5′-3′)	Reverse (5′-3′)
IL-6	NM_000600.5	CGCCTTCGGTCCAGTTGCC	GCCAGTGCCTCTTTGCTGCTTT
IL-8	NM_000584.4	CTCTTGGCAGCCTTCCTGATTTC	TTTTCCTTGGGGTCCAGACAGAG
TNF-α	NM_000594.4	AACATCCAACCTTCCCAAACGC	TGGTCTCCAGATTCCAGATGTCAGG
Sirt1	NM_012238.2	GCCTCACATGCAAGCTCTAGTGAC	TTCGAGGATCTGTGCCAATCATAA
ACTB	NM_001101.5	ACTCTTCCAGCCTTCCTTCC	CGTACAGGTCTTTGCGGATG

2.8. Measurement of Cellular Respiration

Analysis of mitochondrial function was performed on live cells using a Seahorse Biosciences XFe24 Flux Analyzer (Seahorse Biosciences, Milan, Italy) according to the manufacturer's protocol. HCECs (2×10^4/well) were seeded in an XF 24-well plate and grown until confluence. Then, cells were treated with a hyperosmotic medium with or without RSV@Tgels CM (100 μL) for 2 h. The cells were washed twice with XF base medium supplemented and incubated in a CO_2-free environment for 60 min at 37 °C and then placed in the XFe24 Flux Analyzer [30]. Oxygen consumption rate (OCR) was measured under basal conditions followed by the sequential addition of 1 μM oligomycin to inhibit adenosine triphosphatase (ATP) synthase activity, 1 μM tri-fluorocarbonylcyanide phenylhydrazone (FCCP) to uncouple mitochondrial oxidative phosphorylation, and 1 μM antimycin A and rotenone to inhibit electron transport in complex I and III, respectively. ATP turnover rate was the difference in OCR between the last measurement before the oligomycin injection and the minimum OCR after the oligomycin injection. Maximal respiration was the difference in OCR between FCCP-induced respiration and OCR after the injection of antimycin A. Spare respiratory capacity was the difference between maximal respiration and basal OCR. OCRs were normalized to total protein content quantified with a BCA protein assay.

2.9. Western Blotting

Total proteins of HCECs were extracted in ice-cold RIPA buffer (1:10 w/v) containing protease inhibitor. Then, Western blot analysis was carried out as described in our previous studies [31,32] using a mouse monoclonal Sirt1 antibody (sc-74465, 1:500, Santa Cruz Biotechnology, Milan, Italy), followed by a secondary antibody conjugated with horseradish peroxidase. The bands were quantified using ImageJ analyzing software. β-actin (ACTB) was used as an internal reference.

2.10. Statistical Analysis

Data were presented in means ± SD of at least three independent experiments. Statistical comparisons between the different experimental groups and their corresponding controls were made with a one-way analysis of variance (ANOVA) followed by Tukey's post hoc test and Student's *t*-test, considering $p < 0.05$ as statistically significant. All the data were analyzed with the GraphPad Prism version 8.01 statistical software package (GraphPad Software, San Diego, CA, USA).

3. Results and Discussion

3.1. Preparation and Characterization of RSV-NPs

Eye-drops and gels represent the most common and convenient topical ophthalmic formulations for ocular delivery, owing to the simple fabrication and the easy/noninvasive administration route. Despite their popularity among patients, drugs delivered through this route are usually poorly absorbed because of the short residence time in the mucosa and corneal permeability [33]. Nanocarrier-based therapeutic delivery systems have been developed to increase the corneal retention of drugs with the final goal of improving the efficacy of treatments for different ocular diseases.

To accomplish prolonged contact time and hence increased residence time in the eye, in this study, PLGA was functionalized with PEI, a biocompatible, biodegradable cationic polymer. Several studies report that positively charged nanoparticles can enhance drug residence time by interacting with anionic tear-film mucins and with the negatively charged surface of cornea and conjunctiva, improving drug bioavailability [16,34,35]. The tertiary amines of PEI were partially acetylated (AcPEI) to improve PEI tolerability while maintaining a positive zeta potential. Indeed, particle size and surface charge are the most important parameters in ophthalmic formulations to warrant low irritation, sufficient bioavailability, and good compatibility with ocular tissues. AcPEI-PLGA nanoparticles loaded with RSV (RSV-NPs) were prepared by a modified nanoprecipitation method, using acetone as a suitable solvent. Nanoprecipitation represents a simple and reproducible technique that possesses a limited number of controllable variables and can be easily scaled up [35]. The prepared NPs were characterized by DLS, zeta potential measurements, and NTA (Figure 1a–c). As reported in Table 2, the lower drug/polymer ratio led to small nanoparticle sizes (89.2 ± 0.9), whereas the higher drug/polymer ratio tended to increase nanoparticle sizes (148.7 ± 2.2) and reduce the EE% (66.4 ± 5.9). This indicated that there was an optimal drug/polymer ratio to reach the maximum EE%, set at 1:10. Moreover, the different drug/polymer ratios have no significant effect on the polydispersity index and zeta potential. Furthermore, the polydispersity of all batches was below 0.3, indicating uniform particle size distribution, while the zeta potential greater than 20 mV suggested a high colloidal stability of RSV-NPs due to the electrostatic repulsion. Indeed, the higher the absolute value of zeta potential, the more stable the system [36].

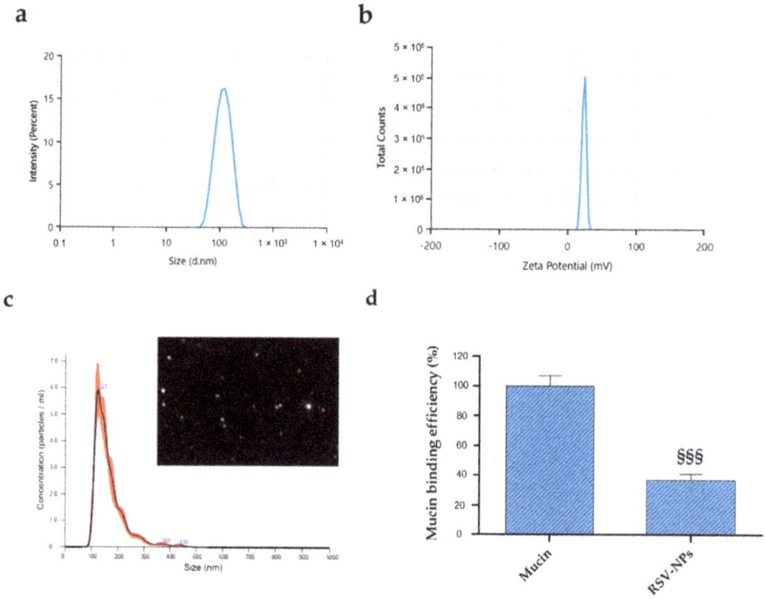

Figure 1. Physico-chemical properties of RSV-NPs. (**a**) Intensity-based size distribution, and (**b**) zeta potential profile of RSV-NPs. (**c**) NTA measurements for RSV-NPs in suspension and screenshot of representative NTA video. Hydrodynamic diameter distribution curves and zeta potential are average of three measurements. (**d**) Mucin binding efficiency (n = 3 ± S.D.—Student's t-test. §§§ $p < 0.001$ shows significant difference with respect to mucin alone.

Table 2. Particle size, zeta potential, polydispersity index, as measured by DLS, and encapsulation efficiency of nanoparticles.

Sample	Polymer (mg)	RSV (mg)	Z-Average (nm)	Zeta Potential (mV)	Polydispersity Index (PDI)	Encapsulation Efficiency (EE %)
NPs	100	0	96.3 ± 0.8	21.9 ± 1.6	0.21 ± 0.6	
RSV_1-NPs	100	5	89.2 ± 0.9	20.7 ± 1.9	0.19 ± 0.9	46.8 ± 2.8
RSV_2-NPs	100	10	125.4 ± 1.3	22.1 ± 1.3	0.16 ± 0.3	78.3 ± 4.9
RSV_3-NPs	100	20	148.7 ± 2.2	21.6 ± 1.8	0.22 ± 1.2	66.4 ± 5.9

Although the size obtained for all formulations agreed with ocular drug release requirements (≤200 nm), RSV_2-NP (coded RSV-NPs), was the formulation selected for further characterization because of the higher EE (Figure 1). The RSV-NPs intensity-based size curve showed a monomodal and narrow distribution (Figure 1a), confirmed by NTA results which also provided the NPs concentration (Figure 1c). In particular, more than 50% of NPs were in a size range between 100 and 150 nm, and the concentration of the NPs with a 100 to 123 nm hydrodynamic diameter was about 2×10^8 particles/mL.

The blink reflex and tear turnover rate are the main contributing factors to a short ocular retention time [37]. The use of cationic nanoparticles represents a possible strategy to extend the residence time and improve the bioavailability of the encapsulated molecule on the ocular surface. Whereas the mucin-aqueous layer of the tear film is commonly reduced in DED patients, leading to inflammation, and patient discomfort [38,39], the cationic nature of RSV-NPs could prolong the residence time in the ocular region and consequently improve RSV bioavailability and therapeutic action. As shown in Figure 1d, cationic RSV-NPs are able to interact with negatively charged sialic acid residues in the mucus with a mucin-binding efficiency of 63% at the ocular pH.

3.2. Rheological and Mechanical Characterization of Hydrogel Formulations (RSV@Tgel)

Liquid formulations based on polymers able to undergo a thermally induced sol-to-gel phase transition can overcome the issue related to removal from the eye through blinking, tear production, and nasolacrimal drainage. In the case of ophthalmic formulation, an optimal gelation temperature should be in the 32–34 °C range. Formation of the hydrogel at temperatures lower than 30 °C limits manufacturing, and handling, and causes difficulty in administration. In contrast, a gelation temperature higher than 36 °C entails that the formulation maintains its liquid state at body temperature, resulting in rapid elimination after administration [40]. Additionally, values of storage modulus G′ above 1000 Pa provide evidence of a pronounced elastic, solid-like character, which is highly sought in formulations employed for ocular administration to avoid washout from the corneal surface [41].

Therefore, the evaluation of the gelling temperature (T_{gel}) is a fundamental prerequisite for the development of an effective ophthalmic formulation. In this respect, several formulations of RSV-NPs in the form of in-situ gelling solutions were prepared by varying the concentration of poloxamer 407 (15–22% w/v) aiming at protracting drug release and increasing ocular bioavailability. The T_{gel} of the prepared formulations was assessed by rotational rheometry. The gelation temperature was evaluated by oscillation measurements performed at a constant frequency value, in a temperature range spanning the physiological temperature. All formulations displayed a stepwise increase in G' and G'', from a liquid ($G' \leq G''$) to a gel state ($G' > G''$), where both moduli reached a plateau (Figure S1). The formulation containing 22% w/v poloxamer 407 displayed a crossover of G' and G'' at 24 °C (Figure S1a). However, the crossover could not be noticed for all samples, as demonstrated in Figure S1b for the formulation containing 17% w/v poloxamer 407. Therefore, the temperature at which the elastic modulus G' attained the plateau value was considered as the T_{gel}. Figure 2a shows the change in elastic modulus (G') with the temperature for all the concentrations tested. The T_{gel} and G' values remarkably depended on the polymer concentration (Figure 2b), ranging from 40 to 26 °C, and 300 to about 10,000 Pa, respectively, thus indicating that the formulation properties could be easily tuned to achieve viscoelastic properties more suitable to facilitate ocular application.

Compressive stress-strain measurements were carried out on the polymer solutions at 37 °C to evaluate the compressive strength and moduli, and the stability of the hydrogel formulations over repeated mechanical solicitations. The stress-strain curves (Figure 2c) showed a region of elastic deformation at low strain, followed by a plastic deformation zone, in which the stress did not change with increasing deformation values. Indeed, deformation caused chains to flow due to the absence of chemical crosslinks between the polymer segments. The compressive properties also depended strongly on the poloxamer 407 concentration, and the maximum stress values recorded varied from 0.5 (15% w/v) to 4 kPa (22% w/v). Similarly, the compressive modulus varied from 4.35 kPa (15% and 17% w/v), up to 23.5 and 52.5 kPa calculated for 19% and 22% w/v, respectively. As a comparison, the compressive modulus of the human cornea is about 1.7 MPa [42]. Cyclic compression tests indicated that the hydrogels had good mechanical stability upon repeated compression, as they maintained over 90% of the initial stress. Interestingly, all formulations showed a reproducible behavior upon unloading, attaining negative stress values, which demonstrate the cohesion of the solution and remarkable adhesive properties.

In the case of ocular administration, a shorter gelling time is preferred for faster onset of drug delivery. The gelling time depicts, in fact, the time required for the formation of the gel after administration, and this is fundamental for preventing its removal from the injection site, and prolonging the retention of the active substance in situ. The gelling time of all prepared batches was determined, by visual observation in simulated tear fluid at 34 °C. Gels with lower polymer concentration (15–17% w/v) had a longer gelation time of about 80 s, while gelation time was considerably shorter for those with higher polymer concentration (19–22% w/v) diminishing to 28.5 s. Figure 2e reports the visual observation of the gelling behavior of the poloxamer 407 at the optimized concentration of 19% w/v.

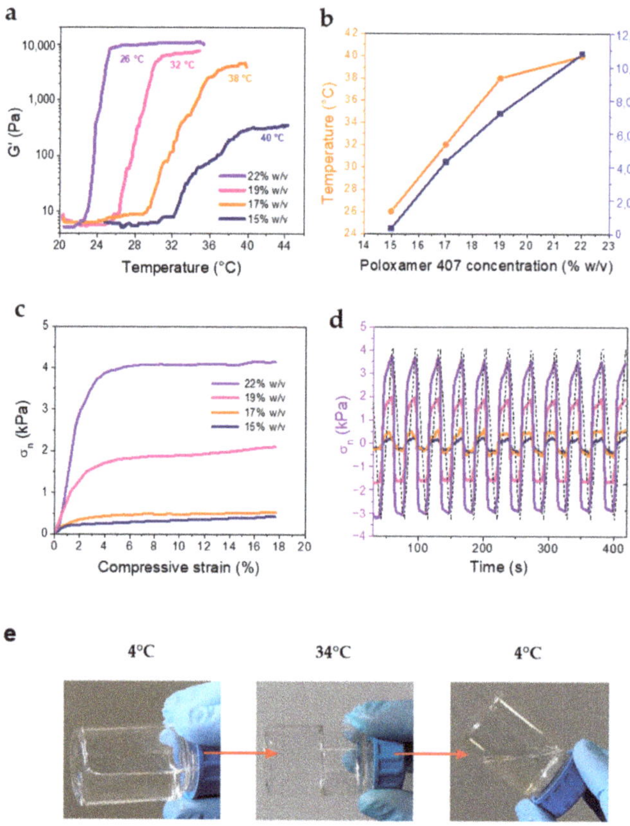

Figure 2. Rheological and mechanical characterization of the RSV@Tgel formulations containing 15, 17, 19, or 22% *w*/*v* poloxamer 407. (**a**) Evolution of the dynamic storage modulus G′ in non-isothermal oscillatory shear experiments. (**b**) T_{gel} and related G′ values as a function of poloxamer 407 concentration. (**c**) Representative compressive stress/strain curves, and (**d**) cyclic loading-unloading curves of the RSV@Tgel formulations. (**e**) Visual observation of the reversible gelling behavior of RSV@Tgel (19%) at 4 and 34 °C.

Based on rheological and gelling data, the RSV@Tgel formulation dispersing 1 mg RSV-NPs in 10 mL of 19% *w*/*v* poloxamer 407 (coded RSV@Tgel from here onward) was considered for further characterization. The physiological pH of the tears is approximately 7.4. Although eyes can tolerate a wide pH range (i.e., 4.5–8.5), the closer the pH of the formulation is to the physiological pH, the better it is tolerated. The pH values of all batches were around 6.8 and storage conditions, conducted at 4 and 25 °C for 14 days, had no significant influence on the corresponding pH of the preparation at different time points (Table 3). Moreover, the stability study of optimized in situ gel (RSV@Tgel) demonstrated that particle size and PDI were not influenced by storage temperature or time and were comparable with the initial values. In addition, the developed formulations remained clear throughout the stability storage period. On the contrary, RSV-NPs stored in free form showed a tendency to aggregate.

Table 3. Stability studies of RSV-NPs and RSV@Tgel before and after 14-day storage.

	RSV-NPs (0 Day)		RSV-NPs (14 Days)		RSV@Tgel (0 Day)		RSV@Tgel (14 Days)	
	4 °C	25 °C	4 °C	25 °C	4 °C	25 °C	4 °C	25 °C
Average particle size (nm ± S.D.)	126.7 ± 9.1	129.6 ± 3.1	169.18 ± 19.2	176.6 ± 11.4	135.4 ± 9.0	138.7 ± 6.4	137.6 ± 5.3	139.1 ± 4.3
PDI	0.15 ± 0.0	0.17 ± 0.0	0.4 ± 0.0	0.5 ± 0.0	0.11 ± 0.0	0.14 ± 0.0	0.13 ± 0.0	0.12 ± 0.0
pH	6.7 ± 0.2	6.6 ± 0.2	6.6 ± 0.1	6.7 ± 0.1	6.8 ± 0.2	6.7 ± 0.3	6.7 ± 0.2	6.7 ± 0.6

Note: Data were expressed as mean ± standard deviation, $n = 3$.

3.3. RSV Release from RSV@Tgel

Tear hyperosmolarity is one of the key pathogenesis mechanisms of DED. Therefore, to mimic in vivo dry eye conditions, the cumulative RSV release profiles were performed at 34 °C in an isosmolar medium (ISO, 312 mOsM) or hyperosmolar medium (HYPER, 400 mOsM). As depicted in Figure 3a, about 15% of the drug was released within 30 min by RSV@Tgel, reaching about 65% after 12 h in ISO condition. Furthermore, the RSV releasing rate from RSV-NPs was two-fold higher, with about 30% of RSV released after the same period, with a cumulative release percent almost achieving 85% at the end of the experiment. The low drug release from RSV@Tgel is probably due to the presence of a gel matrix formed at 35 °C that entraps the nanoparticles, slowing down drug diffusion from PLGA to the gel matrix, and subsequently through the gel into the medium [43]. In the case of nanoparticles alone, the small size led to the burst release of the majority of the encapsulated drugs over the first hours and slow release afterward. Despite the RSV-NPs high initial burst, it may be helpful to counteract inflammation in a short time, the following low RSV release requires repeated and close applications to maintain the therapeutic concentration. On the other hand, the sustained and long-term release phase of RSV@Tgel offers the possibility to steadily provide the bioactive response.

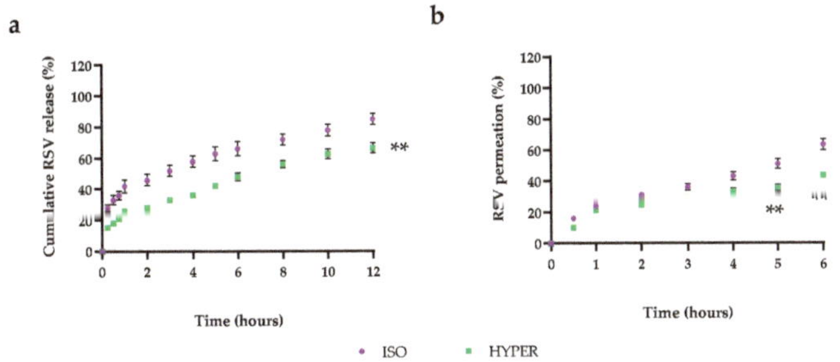

Figure 3. (**a**) Cumulative RSV release profile from RSV@tgel at 34 °C in isosmolar medium (ISO, 312 mOsM) or hyperosmolar medium (HYPER, 400 mOsM); Data were expressed as mean ± SD, $n = 3$. (Student's t-test). ** $p < 0.01$ versus isosmolar medium at each point examined; (**b**) RSV permeation profile obtained from RSV@tgel in the above conditions. Data were expressed as mean ± SD, $n = 3$. (Student's t-test). ** $p < 0.01$ versus isosmolar medium at 5 and 6 h time points.

To obtain information about in vivo epithelium permeation, a Franz diffusion cell study was performed by using cellulose membrane simulating human cornea. The cumulative percentage of RSV in the receptor compartment was about 65% and 48% for RSV-NPs and RSV@Tgel, respectively, after 6 h (Figure 3b). The low corneal permeation of RSV@Tgel could be attributed to the presence of a hydrogel network that slowed down the permeation process. Similar results were obtained by Alruwaili et al. for gentamycin-loaded chitosan nanoparticles embedded into the carbopol hydrogel [44].

3.4. RSV@Tgel Protection of Corneal Cells from Oxidative Damage

The first prerequisite for a new ocular drug vehicle is to be innocuous or show quite low cellular toxicity. In this context, human corneal epithelial cells (HCECs) were incubated in the presence of different concentrations of RSV@Tgel conditioned medium (CM; 1:1, 1:2, and 1:5 v/v) for 24 h. As demonstrated in Figure S2a, the cell viability was around 98% for all tested concentrations. Moreover, less than 10% of lactate dehydrogenase (LDH) was detected in the culture medium (Figure S2b), confirming the negligible toxicity of the ocular gel to the cell membrane. As expected, Triton X-100, which was used as a positive control of membrane damage, dramatically decreased HCECs viability. Taken together, the results suggest an excellent safety profile of RSV@Tgel.

The ROS overproduction is induced on the ocular surface as a consequence of prolonged exposure to atmospheric oxygen and/or environmental factors (e.g., air pollution, wind, low humidity) leading to the loss of physiological balance between the production of free radicals and the ocular defense mechanisms [45–47]. Consequently, ROS accumulation can be responsible for damage to the ocular tissues. Recent studies have confirmed, both in vitro and in vivo, the involvement of oxidative stress in DED reporting the increase in ROS, lipid oxidative stress markers and inflammatory cells [48,49].

To test whether RSV@Tgel was effective in reducing intracellular ROS production, an in vitro hyperosmolarity-induced dry eye model was used [46,50]. The hyperosmolarity of tear film has been recognized as a pro-inflammatory stress factor for the corneal epithelium, leading to cell apoptosis. According to a preliminary assessment, hyperosmolarity of 400 mOsm/L was identified as the correct balance between cell survival and death. The amount of intracellular ROS was defined based on the relative concentration of fluorescent 2′,7′-dichlorodihydrofluorescein (DCF). As shown in Figure 4a, hyperosmolar stress (400 mOsm/L) induces a substantial increase in HCE intracellular oxidants production approximately 2.4 times with respect to untreated cells (control). Pre-incubation with RSV alone (30 μM) induces a slight reduction in the DCF fluorescence intensity (around 20%, $p < 0.05$) with respect to the hyperosmotic group, whereas, in the presence of RSV@Tgel, ROS formation was markedly reduced (about 45%, $p < 0.01$) with a slight increase with respect to the normal isosmotic group.

Under oxidative stress, cellular membrane lipids are the prime targets of ROS attack. Lipid peroxidation leads to the formation of chemically reactive lipid aldehydes, such as MDA, capable of causing severe damage to nucleic acids and proteins, altering their functions and leading to the loss of both structural and metabolic function of cells [51]. As reported in Figure 4b, intracellular lipid peroxidation increased under hyperosmotic conditions by 1.9 times compared with the control. On the contrary, the amount of MDA diminished by 20% in cells treated with RSV alone, while a decrease of about 40% was noted in presence of RSV@Tgel.

Several clinical studies report that patients with ocular diseases have lower levels of SOD, catalase, and glutathione peroxidase (GPx) [52]. Indeed, SOD and CAT constitute, along with glutathione peroxidase, the first antioxidant defense system in cells acting as scavengers for $O_2^{\bullet -}$ and H_2O_2. SOD converts superoxide to oxygen and hydrogen peroxide, and then CAT acts as a catalyst in the reaction of hydrogen peroxide decomposition to water and oxygen [53]. In normal eyes, antioxidant enzymes are highly expressed in the corneal and conjunctival epithelium, while in dry eye syndrome their expression is much less pronounced and is strongly related to the increasing severity of dry eye symptoms [54]. To further validate the role of released RSV in protecting corneal epithelial cells against oxidative damage triggered by hyperosmolarity, the activities of SOD and CAT were evaluated (Figure 4c,d). Hyperosmotic stress caused the reduction of both anti-oxidative enzymes (47% SOD, 52% CAT, respectively) compared to the control cells cultured in an isotonic environment, whereas the changes of activities were partially reversed by the pre-treatment with RSV@Tgel (32% SOD, 39% CAT, respectively) demonstrating a good ability to protect mitochondria from oxidative damage.

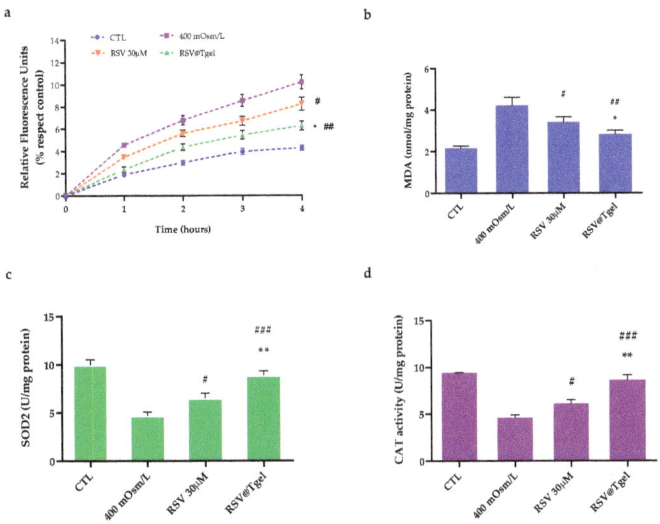

Figure 4. Effect of RSV@Tgel on ROS production. HCECs were cultured under hyperosmotic stress (400 mOsM) in presence of RSV (30 μM) or RSV@Tgel for 24 h. (**a**) Intracellular ROS release determined by oxidized H2DCFDA (DCF). (**b**) Quantification of Malondialdehyde used as a marker of lipid peroxidation. (**c**) Superoxide dismutase (SOD2) and (**d**) Catalase (CAT) activities measured by assay kit. Results are expressed as the means of three independent experiments ± S.D. (n = 3). Statistical analysis was performed by One-way ANOVA, * $p < 0.05$ and ** $p < 0.01$ versus RSV 30 μM; # $p < 0.05$, ## $p < 0.01$, and ### $p < 0.001$ versus 400 mOsM-treated cells.

Pintea et al. have reported on the ability of resveratrol to prevent retinal pigment epithelium cell degeneration induced by oxidative stress [55]. Pretreatment with resveratrol at micromolar concentrations led to a dose-dependent increase in ROS-related enzyme activities (SOD, CAT and GHS), supporting the hypothesis that this polyphenol elicits antioxidant effects by directly scavenging the ROS in retinal pigment epithelium (RPE) cells. In another study, RSV significantly enhanced cell viability and promoted cell growth, by modulating superoxide dismutase (SOD)/malondialdehyde MDA) activity in RPE cells exposed to H_2O_2 [56].

3.5. *Effect of RSV@Tgel on HCEC Mitochondrial Bioenergetics*

Mitochondria are the major site of intracellular ROS production as well as the target of oxidative damage [57]. Since various research accounts report the involvement of mitochondrial dysfunction in DED progression [58], a real-time measurement of HCECs oxygen consumption rate (OCR) was performed using the seahorse XFp analyzer. In particular, key mitochondrial activities were evaluated, including basal respiration (detected as the baseline OCR before the addition of oligomycin), maximal respiration (evaluated as the OCR after the addition of FCCP), spare respiratory capacity (the difference between the maximal and basal respiration), and ATP turnover (the oligomycin-sensitive OCR).

As expected, hyperosmotic conditions induced a reduction of about 50% ($p < 0.01$) in HCE cell mitochondrial bioenergetics with respect to untreated cells (Figure 5a–d). The presence of RSV alone is capable of partially protecting the mitochondrial function of HCE cells under hyperosmotic stress, with a recovery of about 30%. On the other hand, the treatment with RSV@Tgel led to a substantial increase of OCR in the measured respiration functions. In particular, in the case of ATP turnover rate, basal respiration, and maximal respiration, RSV@Tgel treatment restored the OCR at a level similar to that of untreated cells.

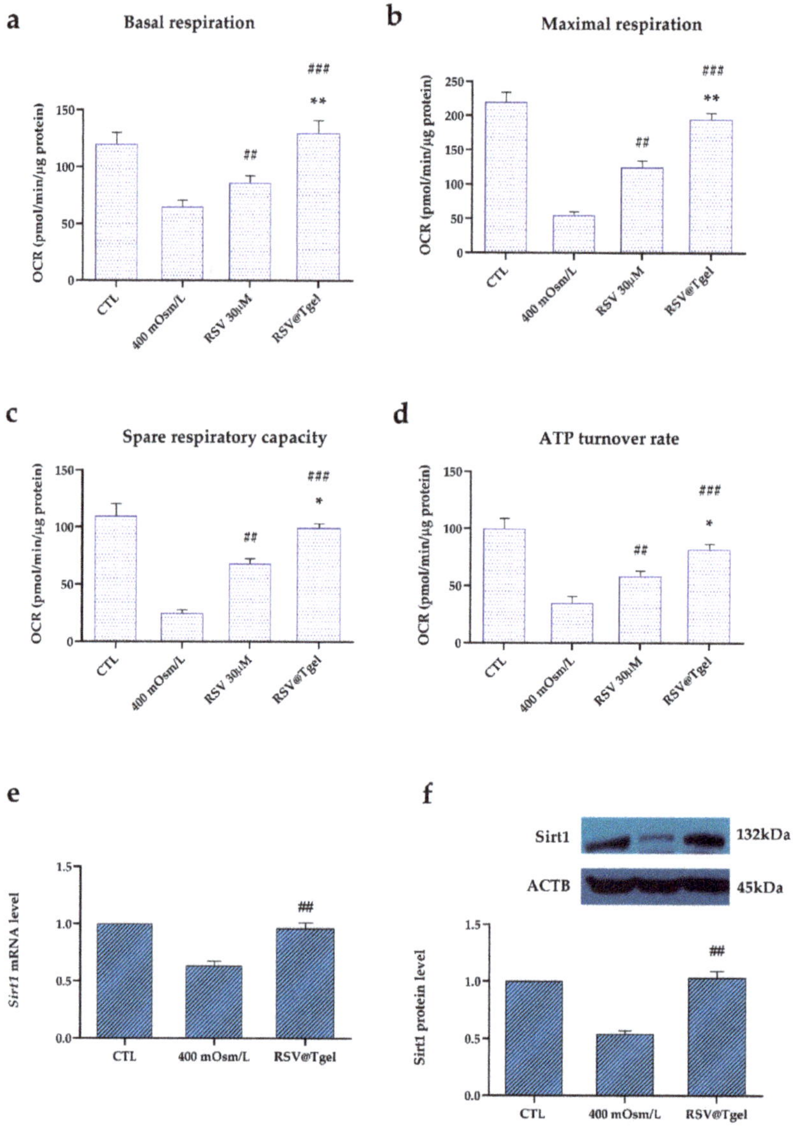

Figure 5. RSV@Tgel improves mitochondrial bioenergetics (**a**–**d**). HCECs were cultured in serum-free DMEM under hyperosmotic stress (400 mOsM) in presence of RSV (30 µM) or RSV@Tgel for 2 h. Measurements of OCR were taken in real-time using an XFe24 Flux Analyzer. OCRs were normalized to total protein content. Data are an average of three separate experiments. Statistical analysis was performed by One-way ANOVA, * $p < 0.05$ and ** $p < 0.01$ versus RSV 30 µM; ## $p < 0.01$, and ### $p < 0.001$ versus 400 mOsM-treated cells. Determination of Sirt1 gene expression (**e**) and protein (**f**) in HCECs under hyperosmotic stress or in presence of RSV@Tgel. Sirt1 mRNA levels were assessed by real-time PCR and calculated after normalization to *ACTB* mRNA levels. The protein levels of Sirt1 were quantified by Western blotting, and β-actin was used as the control protein. The protein levels were quantified using ImageJ. Statistical analysis was performed by the Student *t*-test ## $p < 0.01$ versus 400 mOsM-treated cells.

It has been demonstrated that RSV enhanced mitochondrial function by activating Sirt1, a highly conserved NAD$^+$-dependent histone deacetylase [59] which regulates a wide range of cellular processes, including antioxidation, anti-apoptosis, DNA repair, antiaging, and life-span extension [60]. Recently, it has been found that abnormal Sirt1 expression provokes mitochondrial dysfunction, leading to ocular diseases, including cataracts, age-associated macular degeneration, diabetic retinopathy and glaucoma [61]. Under the hyperosmotic conditions, HCECs revealed a significant downregulation of Sirt1 at both mRNA and protein levels, of about 38% and 49%, respectively, compared to untreated cells (Figure 5e,f). The presence of RSV@Tgel restores the expression of Sirt1 (mRNA and protein) at levels not significantly different from untreated cells. Our results are in line with the literature reporting that RSV promotes mitochondrial protection against oxidation-induced toxicity through the increase in mitochondrial bioenergetics [62,63]. Moreover, Chen et al. demonstrated that high osmotic-induced mitochondrial dysfunction was reduced after treatment with RSV 50 μM by inducing Sirt1 upregulation [64].

3.6. RSV@Tgel Suppression of Inflammatory Response under Hyperosmotic Stress

Recent studies in both animal- and cell-based DED models identify hyperosmotic stress as a principal pathogenic factor responsible for the production of inflammatory signaling molecules, including interleukin, tumor necrosis factor, and matrix metalloproteinases [65,66]. The induced-inflammatory state gives rise to further cell damage, such as apoptosis of conjunctival, corneal, and lacrimal gland epithelial cells, initiating a cycle of events that perpetuate the DED condition. In this context, molecules able to interrupt the vicious circle of DED pathologies, such as polyphenols, and RSV in particular, could be relevant.

As shown in Figure 6a, exposure of HCECs to the hyperosmotic medium resulted in a significant increase in IL-1β, IL-6, and TNF-α production (three-fold, $p < 0.001$). Pre-incubation of cells with 30 μM RSV and RSV@Tgel significantly reduced the amount of released cytokines under hyperosmotic stress by about 30% and 41% for IL-6; about 20% and 50% for IL-8 and TNF-α, respectively. In response to stress stimulation, the mRNA levels of all tested cytokines (relative to the housekeeping gene) were significantly upregulated (two-fold $p < 0.01$) in damage caused by treatment with cells, compared with the control group (Figure 6b). Consistently, the protective effects of RSV result in a reduction in the expression levels of all interleukins tested, by around 30% for RSV alone, which reaches 65% in the presence of RSV@Tgel.

These results suggest that RSV has a suppressive effect on inflammatory biomarkers at both mRNA and protein levels in ocular surface epithelial cells. Our results are in agreement with several studies that demonstrate RSV involvement, both in vitro and in animal experimentation, in reducing pro-inflammatory mediators and cellular pathways involved in inflammation [67,68]. Hsu and colleagues demonstrated the anti-inflammatory effects of RSV on a myopia animal model with a reduction of the expression levels of matrix metalloproteinase 2 (MMP2), transforming growth factor (TGF)-β, and nuclear factor (NF)-κB [69]. Moreover, the treatment with RSV induced the downregulation of inflammatory cytokine production, and the inhibition of AKT, c-Raf, Stat3, and NFκB phosphorylation in ARPE19 cells. Luna et al. investigated the therapeutic effects of RSV administration in chronic oxidative stress-induced trabecular meshwork cells [70]. Their results demonstrated that resveratrol effectively decreased the production of intracellular ROS (iROS) and inflammatory markers such as interleukin-1 alpha (IL-1α), interleukin (IL)-6, and IL-8. Moreover, RSV, via vitamin D receptors, was able to reduce oxidative stress in human corneal epithelial cells under hyperosmolar conditions through the activation of Notch signaling.

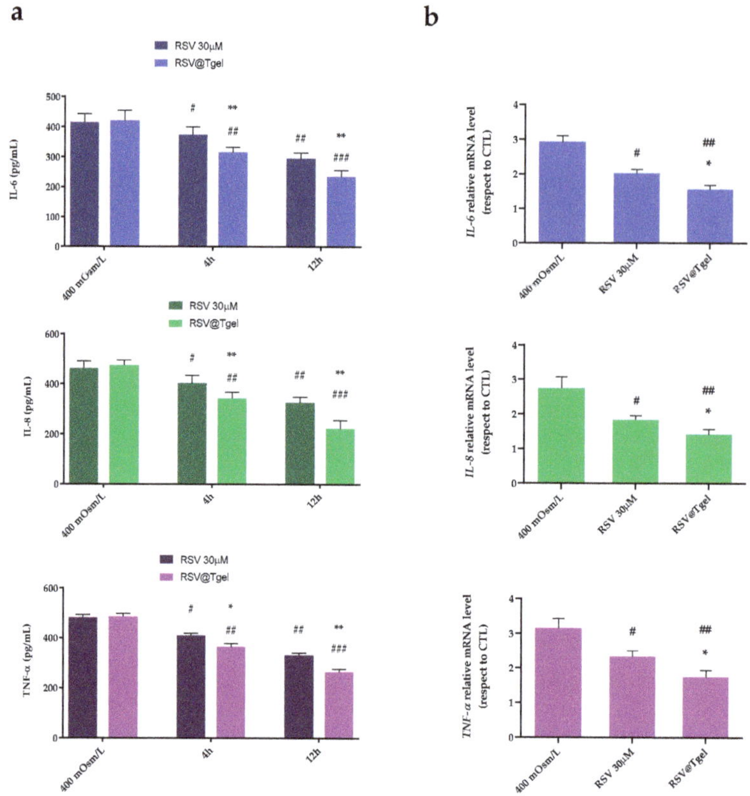

Figure 6. RSV suppressed expression of pro-inflammatory cytokines IL-1 β, IL-6, and TNF-α in HCECs exposed to hyperosmotic medium. HCECs were cultured in isomolar (292 mOsm/L) medium, then switched to hyperosmotic medium (400 mOsm/L) alone or in the presence of RSV and RSV@Tgel for 24 h to measure protein level by ELISA (**a**); or for 4 h to evaluate mRNA level by RT-qPCR (**b**). Data were summarized as mean ± SD from three separate experiments. * $p < 0.05$, ** $p < 0.01$ vs. cells exposed to 400 mOsM/L; # $p < 0.05$, ## $p < 0.01$, and ### $p < 0.001$ vs. RSV@Tgel (Student's *t*-test).

4. Conclusions

DED is a dynamic and complex disease that can cause significant damage to the ocular surface. Several studies demonstrated the potential applicability of RSV as a treatment for DED. However, the low RSV water solubility and stability, and its poor ocular bioavailability limit its clinical application. This study provides new insights into the therapeutic effects of intra-ocular instillation of thermosensitive hydrogels (RSV@Tgel) loaded with acetylated PLGA-PEI nanoparticles able to allow the sustained delivery of resveratrol (RSV-NPs). RSV released from the hydrogel protects HCECs from ROS damage and reverts the activation of inflammatory factors, limiting the damage caused by hyperosmotic conditions. Moreover, RSV@Tgel protects mitochondria from oxidation-induced toxicity through the increase in mitochondrial bioenergetics and Sirt1 upregulation. Overall, the reported results indicate that RSV@Tgel acts as an adjuvant in dry eye disease because of its effect against inflammation and oxidative stress. Furthermore, the thermosensitive formulation extends the residence time in the eye, thus allowing to reduce the number of eye drop instillations, and increasing patient compliance.

Supplementary Materials: The following supporting information can be downloaded at: https://www.mdpi.com/article/10.3390/antiox12050993/s1, Figure S1: Evolution of the dynamic storage and dissipative moduli (G′ and G″) in non-isothermal oscillatory shear experiments of RSV@Tgel formulations containing (a) 22%, and (b) 17% *w*/*v* poloxamer 407. Figure S2: In vitro biocompatibility of RSV@Tgel after 24, 48, and 72 h. Cell viability (a) and Lactate Dehydrogenase (LDH) release (b) were assessed in HCECs incubated with different concentrations of RSV@Tgel conditioned medium (CM; 1:1, 1:2, and 1:5 *v*/*v*). Untreated cells and Triton X-100 treated cells were considered as a negative and positive control, respectively. Results are expressed as the mean of three independent experiments ± S.D. ($n = 3$).

Author Contributions: Conceptualization, P.C., G.P. and A.C.; investigation, I.D.L., F.D.C. and R.C.; writing original draft preparation, I.D.L., F.D.C. and R.C.; writing—review and editing, P.C. and A.C.; supervision, A.C.; funding acquisition, P.C, G.P. and A.C. All authors have read and agreed to the published version of the manuscript.

Funding: This work was financially supported by the PON 03 PE_00110_1/ptd1_000410 Titolo: Sviluppo di nanotecnologie Orientate alla Rigenerazione e Ricostruzione tissutale, Implantologia e Sensoristica in Odontoiatria/oculistica (SORRISO); POR Campania FESR 2014_2020 "Tecnologie abilitanti per la sintesi eco-sostenibile di nuovi materiali per la restaurativa dentale"—ABILTECH; EU funding within the Horizon 2020 Program, under the MSCA-RISE 2016 Project "VAHVISTUS" (Grant 734759).

Institutional Review Board Statement: Not applicable.

Informed Consent Statement: Not applicable.

Data Availability Statement: The data presented in this study are available in the article.

Acknowledgments: The authors gratefully acknowledge Orsolina Petillo for her assistance with cell culture (IRET-CNR).

Conflicts of Interest: The authors declare no conflict of interest.

References

1. Berg, E.J.; Ying, G.S.; Maguire, M.G.; Sheffield, P.E.; Szczotka-Flynn, L.B.; Asbell, P.A.; Shen, J.F.; Group, D.S.R. Climatic and Environmental Correlates of Dry Eye Disease Severity: A Report From the Dry Eye Assessment and Management (DREAM) Study. *Transl. Vis. Sci. Technol.* **2020**, *9*, 25. [CrossRef] [PubMed]
2. Dogru, M.; Kojima, T.; Simsek, C.; Tsubota, K. Potential Role of Oxidative Stress in Ocular Surface Inflammation and Dry Eye Disease. *Investig. Ophthalmol. Vis. Sci.* **2018**, *59*, DES163–DES168. [CrossRef] [PubMed]
3. Yamaguchi, T. Inflammatory Response in Dry Eye. *Investig. Ophthalmol. Vis. Sci.* **2018**, *59*, DES192–DES199. [CrossRef]
4. Shimazaki, J. Definition and Diagnostic Criteria of Dry Eye Disease: Historical Overview and Future Directions. *Investig. Ophthalmol. Vis. Sci.* **2018**, *59*, DES7–DES12. [CrossRef] [PubMed]
5. Gurnani, B.; Kaur, K. Current approach in surgical management of dry eyes—Dry eye review II. *TNOA J. Ophthalmic Sci. Res.* **2021**, *59*, 241–249. [CrossRef]
6. Mohamed, H.B.; Abd El-Hamid, B.N.; Fathalla, D.; Fouad, E.A. Current trends in pharmaceutical treatment of dry eye disease: A review. *Eur. J. Pharm.Sci. Off. J. Eur. Fed. Pharm. Sci.* **2022**, *175*, 106206. [CrossRef]
7. De Luca, I.; Di Cristo, F.; Valentino, A.; Peluso, G.; Di Salle, A.; Calarco, A. Food-Derived Bioactive Molecules from Mediterranean Diet: Nanotechnological Approaches and Waste Valorization as Strategies to Improve Human Wellness. *Polymers* **2022**, *14*, 1726. [CrossRef]
8. Xu, Z.; Sun, T.; Li, W.; Sun, X. Inhibiting effects of dietary polyphenols on chronic eye diseases. *J. Funct. Foods* **2017**, *39*, 186–197. [CrossRef]
9. Bungau, S.; Abdel-Daim, M.M.; Tit, D.M.; Ghanem, E.; Sato, S.; Maruyama-Inoue, M.; Yamane, S.; Kadonosono, K. Health Benefits of Polyphenols and Carotenoids in Age-Related Eye Diseases. *Oxidative Med. Cell. Longev.* **2019**, *2019*, 9783429. [CrossRef]
10. Choi, W.; Lee, J.B.; Cui, L.; Li, Y.; Li, Z.; Choi, J.S.; Lee, H.S.; Yoon, K.C. Therapeutic Efficacy of Topically Applied Antioxidant Medicinal Plant Extracts in a Mouse Model of Experimental Dry Eye. *Oxidative Med. Cell. Longev.* **2016**, *2016*, 4727415. [CrossRef]
11. Favero, G.; Moretti, E.; Krajčíková, K.; Tomečková, V.; Rezzani, R. Evidence of Polyphenols Efficacy against Dry Eye Disease. *Antioxidants* **2021**, *10*, 190. [CrossRef]
12. Abu-Amero, K.K.; Kondkar, A.A.; Chalam, K.V. Resveratrol and Ophthalmic Diseases. *Nutrients* **2016**, *8*, 200. [CrossRef]
13. Bryl, A.; Falkowski, M.; Zorena, K. The Role of Resveratrol in Eye Diseases-A Review of the Literature. *Nutrients* **2022**, *14*, 2974. [CrossRef]
14. Gao, Y.; Fu, R.; Wang, J.; Yang, X.; Wen, L.; Feng, J. Resveratrol mitigates the oxidative stress mediated by hypoxic-ischemic brain injury in neonatal rats via Nrf2/HO-1 pathway. *Pharm. Biol.* **2018**, *56*, 440–449. [CrossRef]

15. Vivero-Lopez, M.; Sparacino, C.; Quelle-Regaldie, A.; Sánchez, L.; Candal, E.; Barreiro-Iglesias, A.; Huete-Toral, F.; Carracedo, G.; Otero, A.; Concheiro, A.; et al. Pluronic®/casein micelles for ophthalmic delivery of resveratrol: In vitro, ex vivo, and in vivo tests. *Int. J. Pharm.* **2022**, *628*, 122281. [CrossRef]
16. Castro, B.F.M.; Fulgêncio, G.D.O.; Domingos, L.C.; Cotta, O.A.L.; Silva-Cunha, A.; Fialho, S.L. Positively charged polymeric nanoparticles improve ocular penetration of tacrolimus after topical administration. *J. Drug Deliv. Sci. Technol.* **2020**, *60*, 101912. [CrossRef]
17. Conte, R.; De Luise, A.; Valentino, A.; Di Cristo, F.; Petillo, O.; Riccitiello, F.; Di Salle, A.; Calarco, A.; Peluso, G. Hydrogel Nanocomposite Systems: Characterization and Application in Drug-Delivery Systems. In *Nanocarriers for Drug Delivery: Nanoscience and Nanotechnology in Drug Delivery*; Elsevier: Amsterdam, The Netherlands, 2018; pp. 319–349.
18. Hamcerencu, M.; Desbrieres, J.; Popa, M.; Riess, G. Thermo-sensitive gellan maleate/N-isopropylacrylamide hydrogels: Initial "in vitro" and "in vivo" evaluation as ocular inserts. *Polym. Bull.* **2020**, *77*, 741–755. [CrossRef]
19. Conte, R.; Finicelli, M.; Borrone, A.; Margarucci, S.; Peluso, G.; Calarco, A.; Bosetti, M. MMP-2 Silencing through siRNA Loaded Positively-Charged Nanoparticles (AcPEI-NPs) Counteracts Chondrocyte De-Differentiation. *Polymers* **2023**, *15*, 1172. [CrossRef]
20. Valentino, A.; Conte, R.; De Luca, I.; Di Cristo, F.; Peluso, G.; Bosetti, M.; Calarco, A. Thermo-Responsive Gel Containing Hydroxytyrosol-Chitosan Nanoparticles (Hyt@tgel) Counteracts the Increase of Osteoarthritis Biomarkers in Human Chondrocytes. *Antioxidants* **2022**, *11*, 1210. [CrossRef]
21. Dyawanapelly, S.; Koli, U.; Dharamdasani, V.; Jain, R.; Dandekar, P. Improved mucoadhesion and cell uptake of chitosan and chitosan oligosaccharide surface-modified polymer nanoparticles for mucosal delivery of proteins. *Drug Deliv. Transl. Res.* **2016**, *6*, 365–379. [CrossRef]
22. Matthew, J.E.; Nazario, Y.L.; Roberts, S.C.; Bhatia, S.R. Effect of mammalian cell culture medium on the gelation properties of Pluronic F127. *Biomaterials* **2002**, *23*, 4615–4619. [CrossRef]
23. Khattab, A.; Marzok, S.; Ibrahim, M. Development of optimized mucoadhesive thermosensitive pluronic based in situ gel for controlled delivery of Latanoprost: Antiglaucoma efficacy and stability approaches. *J. Drug Deliv. Sci. Technol.* **2019**, *53*, 101134. [CrossRef]
24. Amaghnouje, A.; Mechchate, H.; Es-Safi, I.; Boukhira, S.; Aliqahtani, S.A.; MNoman, O.; ANasr, F.; Conte, R.; Calarco, A.; Bousta, D. Subacute Assessment of the Toxicity and Antidepressant-Like Effects of *Origanum majorana* L. Polyphenols in Swiss Albino Mice. *Molecules* **2020**, *25*, 5653. [CrossRef]
25. Bao, Q.; Newman, B.; Wang, Y.; Choi, S.; Burgess, D.J. In vitro and ex vivo correlation of drug release from ophthalmic ointments. *J. Control. Release* **2018**, *276*, 93–101. [CrossRef]
26. Shetty, R.; Subramani, M.; Murugeswari, P.; Anandula, V.R.; Matalia, H.; Jayadev, C.; Ghosh, A.; Das, D. Resveratrol Rescues Human Corneal Epithelial Cells Cultured in Hyperosmolar Conditions: Potential for Dry Eye Disease Treatment. *Cornea* **2020**, *39*, 1520–1532. [CrossRef]
27. Di Cristo, F.; Valentino, A.; De Luca, I.; Peluso, G.; Bonadies, I.; Calarco, A.; Di Salle, A. PLA Nanofibers for Microenvironmental-Responsive Quercetin Release in Local Periodontal Treatment. *Molecules* **2022**, *27*, 2205. [CrossRef]
28. Conte, R.; De Luca, I.; Valentino, A.; Cerruti, P.; Pedram, P.; Cabrera-Barjas, G.; Moeini, A.; Calarco, A. Hyaluronic Acid Hydrogel Containing Resveratrol-Loaded Chitosan Nanoparticles as an Adjuvant in Atopic Dermatitis Treatment. *J. Funct. Biomater.* **2023**, *14*, 82. [CrossRef]
29. De Luca, I.; Di Salle, A.; Alessio, N.; Margarucci, S.; Simeone, M.; Galderisi, U.; Calarco, A.; Peluso, G. Positively charged polymers modulate the fate of human mesenchymal stromal cells via ephrinB2/EphB4 signaling. *Stem Cell Res.* **2016**, *17*, 248–255. [CrossRef]
30. Di Cristo, F.; Calarco, A.; Digilio, F.A.; Sinicropi, M.S.; Rosano, C.; Galderisi, U.; Melone, M.A.B.; Saturnino, C.; Peluso, G. The Discovery of Highly Potent THP Derivatives as OCTN2 Inhibitors: From Structure-Based Virtual Screening to In Vivo Biological Activity. *Int. J. Mol. Sci.* **2020**, *21*, 7431. [CrossRef]
31. Melone, M.A.B.; Calarco, A.; Petillo, O.; Margarucci, S.; Colucci-D'Amato, L.; Galderisi, U.; Koverech, G.; Peluso, G. Mutant huntingtin regulates EGF receptor fate in non-neuronal cells lacking wild-type protein. *Biochim. Biophys. Acta (BBA)—Mol. Basis Dis.* **2013**, *1832*, 105–113. [CrossRef]
32. Di Cristo, F.; Finicelli, M.; Digilio, F.A.; Paladino, S.; Valentino, A.; Scialò, F.; D'Apolito, M.; Saturnino, C.; Galderisi, U. Meldonium improves Huntington's disease mitochondrial dysfunction by restoring peroxisome proliferator-activated receptor γ coactivator 1α expression. *J. Cell. Physiol.* **2019**, *234*, 9233–9246. [CrossRef] [PubMed]
33. Gorantla, S.; Rapalli, V.K.; Waghule, T.; Singh, P.P.; Dubey, S.K.; Saha, R.N.; Singhvi, G. Nanocarriers for ocular drug delivery: Current status and translational opportunity. *RSC Adv.* **2020**, *10*, 27835–27855. [CrossRef] [PubMed]
34. Mohsen, A.M. Cationic Polymeric Nanoparticles for Improved Ocular Delivery and Antimycotic Activity of Terconazole. *J. Pharm. Sci.* **2022**, *111*, 458–468. [CrossRef] [PubMed]
35. Rivas, C.; Tarhini, M.; Badri, W.; Miladi, K.; Greige-Gerges, H.; Nazari, Q.A.; Galindo, S.; Alvarez Roman, R.; Fessi, H.; Elaissari, A. Nanoprecipitation process: From encapsulation to drug delivery. *Int. J. Pharm.* **2017**, *532*, 66–81. [CrossRef]
36. Chen, Z.; Tai, Z.; Gu, F.; Hu, C.; Zhu, Q.; Gao, S. Aptamer-mediated delivery of docetaxel to prostate cancer through polymeric nanoparticles for enhancement of antitumor efficacy. *Eur. J. Pharm. Biopharm.* **2016**, *107*, 130–141. [CrossRef]
37. Chhonker, Y.S.; Prasad, Y.D.; Chandasana, H.; Vishvkarma, A.; Mitra, K.; Shukla, P.K.; Bhatta, R.S. Amphotericin-B entrapped lecithin/chitosan nanoparticles for prolonged ocular application. *Int. J. Biol. Macromol.* **2015**, *72*, 1451–1458. [CrossRef]

38. Georgiev, G.A.; Eftimov, P.; Yokoi, N. Contribution of Mucins towards the Physical Properties of the Tear Film: A Modern Update. *Int. J. Mol. Sci.* **2019**, *20*, 6132. [CrossRef]
39. Holland, E.J.; Darvish, M.; Nichols, K.K.; Jones, L.; Karpecki, P.M. Efficacy of topical ophthalmic drugs in the treatment of dry eye disease: A systematic literature review. *Ocul. Surf.* **2019**, *17*, 412–423. [CrossRef]
40. Pereira, G.G.; Dimer, F.A.; Guterres, S.S.; Kechinski, C.P.; Granada, J.E.; Cardozo, N.S.M. Formulation and characterization of poloxamer 407®: Thermoreversible gel containing polymeric microparticles and hyaluronic acid. *Química Nova* **2013**, *36*, 1121–1125. [CrossRef]
41. Carlfors, J.; Edsman, K.; Petersson, R.; Jörnving, K. Rheological evaluation of Gelrite in situ gels for ophthalmic use. *Eur. J. Pharm. Sci. Off. J. Eur. Fed. Pharm. Sci.* **1998**, *6*, 113–119. [CrossRef]
42. Sharifi, S.; Islam, M.M.; Sharifi, H.; Islam, R.; Koza, D.; Reyes-Ortega, F.; Alba-Molina, D.; Nilsson, P.H.; Dohlman, C.H.; Mollnes, T.E.; et al. Tuning gelatin-based hydrogel towards bioadhesive ocular tissue engineering applications. *Bioact. Mater.* **2021**, *6*, 3947–3961. [CrossRef] [PubMed]
43. Rupenthal, I.D.; Green, C.R.; Alany, R.G. Comparison of ion-activated in situ gelling systems for ocular drug delivery. Part 1: Physicochemical characterisation and in vitro release. *Int. J. Pharm.* **2011**, *411*, 69–77. [CrossRef]
44. Alruwaili, N.K.; Zafar, A.; Imam, S.S. Stimulus Responsive Ocular Gentamycin-Ferrying Chitosan Nanoparticles Hydrogel: Formulation Optimization, Ocular Safety and Antibacterial Assessment. *Int. J. Nanomed.* **2020**, *15*, 4717–4737. [CrossRef]
45. Mandell, J.T.; Idarraga, M.; Kumar, N.; Galor, A. Impact of Air Pollution and Weather on Dry Eye. *J. Clin. Med.* **2020**, *9*, 3740. [CrossRef]
46. Park, B.; Jo, K.; Lee, T.G. Polydatin Inhibits NLRP3 Inflammasome in Dry Eye Disease by Attenuating Oxidative Stress and Inhibiting the NF-κB Pathway. *Nutrients* **2019**, *11*, 2792. [CrossRef] [PubMed]
47. Deng, R.; Hua, X.; Li, J.; Chi, W.; Zhang, Z.; Lu, F.; Zhang, L.; Pflugfelder, S.C.; Li, D.Q. Oxidative stress markers induced by hyperosmolarity in primary human corneal epithelial cells. *PLoS ONE* **2015**, *10*, e0126561. [CrossRef]
48. Wakamatsu, T.H.; Dogru, M.; Ayako, I.; Takano, Y.; Matsumoto, Y.; Ibrahim, O.M.; Okada, N.; Satake, Y.; Fukagawa, K.; Shimazaki, J.; et al. Evaluation of lipid oxidative stress status and inflammation in atopic ocular surface disease. *Mol. Vis.* **2010**, *16*, 2465–2475. [PubMed]
49. Zheng, Q.; Ren, Y.; Reinach, P.S.; She, Y.; Xiao, B.; Hua, S.; Qu, J.; Chen, W. Reactive oxygen species activated NLRP3 inflammasomes prime environment-induced murine dry eye. *Exp. Eye Res.* **2014**, *125*, 1–8. [CrossRef]
50. Wang, H.H.; Chen, W.Y.; Huang, Y.H.; Hsu, S.M.; Tsao, Y.P.; Hsu, Y.H.; Chang, M.S. Interleukin-20 is involved in dry eye disease and is a potential therapeutic target. *J. Biomed. Sci.* **2022**, *29*, 36. [CrossRef] [PubMed]
51. Shi, Q.; Vaillancourt, F.; Côté, V.; Fahmi, H.; Lavigne, P.; Afif, H.; Di Battista, J.A.; Fernandes, J.C.; Benderdour, M. Alterations of metabolic activity in human osteoarthritic osteoblasts by lipid peroxidation end product 4-hydroxynonenal. *Arthritis Res. Ther.* **2006**, *8*, R159. [CrossRef]
52. Cabrera, M.P.; Chihuailaf, R.H. Antioxidants and the integrity of ocular tissues. *Vet. Med. Int.* **2011**, *2011*, 905153. [CrossRef]
53. Bhuyan, K.C.; Bhuyan, D.K. Catalase in Ocular Tissue and Its Intracellular Distribution in Corneal Epithelium. *Am. J. Ophthalmol.* **1970**, *69*, 147–153. [CrossRef] [PubMed]
54. Cejková, J.; Ardan, T.; Simonová, Z.; Cejka, C.; Malec, J.; Dotrelová, D.; Brunová, B. Decreased expression of antioxidant enzymes in the conjunctival epithelium of dry eye (Sjögren's syndrome) and its possible contribution to the development of ocular surface oxidative injuries. *Histol. Histopathol.* **2008**, *23*, 1477–1483. [CrossRef] [PubMed]
55. Pintea, A.; Rugină, D.; Pop, R.; Bunea, A.; Socaciu, C.; Diehl, H.A. Antioxidant effect of trans-resveratrol in cultured human retinal pigment epithelial cells. *J. Ocul. Pharmacol. Ther. Off. J. Assoc. Ocul. Pharmacol. Ther.* **2011**, *27*, 315–321. [CrossRef]
56. Yang, Y.; Wu, Z.Z.; Cheng, Y.L.; Lin, W.; Qu, C. Resveratrol protects against oxidative damage of retinal pigment epithelium cells by modulating SOD/MDA activity and activating Bcl-2 expression. *Eur. Rev. Med. Pharmacol. Sci.* **2019**, *23*, 378–388. [CrossRef]
57. Uchino, Y.; Kawakita, T.; Miyazawa, M.; Ishii, T.; Onouchi, H.; Yasuda, K.; Ogawa, Y.; Shimmura, S.; Ishii, N.; Tsubota, K. Oxidative stress induced inflammation initiates functional decline of tear production. *PLoS ONE* **2012**, *7*, e45805. [CrossRef]
58. Seen, S.; Tong, L. Dry eye disease and oxidative stress. *Acta Ophthalmol.* **2018**, *96*, e412–e420. [CrossRef]
59. Chen, Y.; Zhang, H.; Ji, S.; Jia, P.; Chen, Y.; Li, Y.; Wang, T. Resveratrol and its derivative pterostilbene attenuate oxidative stress-induced intestinal injury by improving mitochondrial redox homeostasis and function via SIRT1 signaling. *Free Radic. Biol. Med.* **2021**, *177*, 1–14. [CrossRef] [PubMed]
60. Mimura, T.; Kaji, Y.; Noma, H.; Funatsu, H.; Okamoto, S. The role of SIRT1 in ocular aging. *Exp. Eye Res.* **2013**, *116*, 17–26. [CrossRef]
61. Zhou, M.; Luo, J.; Zhang, H. Role of Sirtuin 1 in the pathogenesis of ocular disease (Review). *Int. J. Mol. Med.* **2018**, *42*, 13–20. [CrossRef]
62. Sheu, S.J.; Liu, N.C.; Ou, C.C.; Bee, Y.S.; Chen, S.C.; Lin, H.C.; Chan, J.Y. Resveratrol stimulates mitochondrial bioenergetics to protect retinal pigment epithelial cells from oxidative damage. *Investig. Ophthalmol. Vis. Sci.* **2013**, *54*, 6426–6438. [CrossRef] [PubMed]
63. Averilla, J.N.; Oh, J.; Kim, J.-S. Carbon Monoxide Partially Mediates Protective Effect of Resveratrol Against UVB-Induced Oxidative Stress in Human Keratinocytes. *Antioxidants* **2019**, *8*, 432. [CrossRef] [PubMed]
64. Chen, J.; Zhang, W.; Zheng, Y.; Xu, Y. Ameliorative Potential of Resveratrol in Dry Eye Disease by Restoring Mitochondrial Function. *Evid.-Based Complement. Altern. Med.* **2022**, *2022*, 1013444. [CrossRef]

65. Corrales, R.M.; Luo, L.; Chang, E.Y.; Pflugfelder, S.C. Effects of osmoprotectants on hyperosmolar stress in cultured human corneal epithelial cells. *Cornea* **2008**, *27*, 574–579. [CrossRef]
66. Baudouin, C.; Aragona, P.; Messmer, E.M.; Tomlinson, A.; Calonge, M.; Boboridis, K.G.; Akova, Y.A.; Geerling, G.; Labetoulle, M.; Rolando, M. Role of hyperosmolarity in the pathogenesis and management of dry eye disease: Proceedings of the OCEAN group meeting. *Ocul. Surf.* **2013**, *11*, 246–258. [CrossRef]
67. Minagawa, T.; Okui, T.; Takahashi, N.; Nakajima, T.; Tabeta, K.; Murakami, S.; Yamazaki, K. Resveratrol suppresses the inflammatory responses of human gingival epithelial cells in a SIRT1 independent manner. *J. Periodontal Res.* **2015**, *50*, 586–593. [CrossRef]
68. Goutham, G.; Manikandan, R.; Beulaja, M.; Thiagarajan, R.; Arulvasu, C.; Arumugam, M.; Setzer, W.N.; Daglia, M.; Nabavi, S.F.; Nabavi, S.M. A focus on resveratrol and ocular problems, especially cataract: From chemistry to medical uses and clinical relevance. *Biomed. Pharmacother.* **2017**, *86*, 232–241. [CrossRef] [PubMed]
69. Hsu, Y.A.; Chen, C.S.; Wang, Y.C.; Lin, E.S.; Chang, C.Y.; Chen, J.J.; Wu, M.Y.; Lin, H.J.; Wan, L. Anti-Inflammatory Effects of Resveratrol on Human Retinal Pigment Cells and a Myopia Animal Model. *Curr. Issues Mol. Biol.* **2021**, *43*, 716–727. [CrossRef]
70. Luna, C.; Li, G.; Liton, P.B.; Qiu, J.; Epstein, D.L.; Challa, P.; Gonzalez, P. Resveratrol prevents the expression of glaucoma markers induced by chronic oxidative stress in trabecular meshwork cells. *Food Chem. Toxicol.* **2009**, *47*, 198–204. [CrossRef]

antioxidants

MDPI

Article

Promising Bioactivity of Vitamin B_1-Au Nanocluster: Structure, Enhanced Antioxidant Behavior, and Serum Protein Interaction

Ditta Ungor [1,2,*], Gyöngyi Gombár [1], Ádám Juhász [1,2], Gergely F. Samu [2] and Edit Csapó [1,2,*]

1 MTA-SZTE Lendület "Momentum" Noble Metal Nanostructures Research Group, University of Szeged, Rerrich B. sqr. 1, H-6720 Szeged, Hungary

2 Interdisciplinary Excellence Center, Department of Physical Chemistry and Materials Science, University of Szeged, Rerrich B. sqr. 1, H-6720 Szeged, Hungary

* Correspondence: ungord@chem.u-szeged.hu (D.U.); juhaszne@chem.u-szeged.hu (E.C.)

Abstract: In the current work, we first present a simple synthesis method for the preparation of novel Vitamin-B_1-stabilized few-atomic gold nanoclusters with few atomic layers. The formed nanostructure contains ca. eight Au atoms and shows intensive blue emissions at 450 nm. The absolute quantum yield is 3%. The average lifetime is in the nanosecond range and three main components are separated and assigned to the metal–metal and ligand–metal charge transfers. Based on the structural characterization, the formed clusters contain Au in zero oxidation state, and Vitamin B_1 stabilizes the metal cores via the coordination of pyrimidine-N. The antioxidant property of the Au nanoclusters is more prominent than that of the pure Vitamin B_1, which is confirmed by two different colorimetric assays. For the investigation into their potential bioactivity, interactions with bovine serum albumin were carried out and quantified. The determined stoichiometry indicates a self-catalyzed binding, which is almost the same value based on the fluorometric and calorimetric measurements. The calculated thermodynamic parameters verify the spontaneous bond of the clusters along the protein chain by hydrogen bonds and electrostatic interactions.

Keywords: thiamine; gold nanocluster; ORAC; ABTS assay; bovine serum albumin binding

1. Introduction

In recent years, the biomedical applications of noble metal nanostructures, especially gold (Au), silver (Ag), and copper (Cu), have been of interest to researchers. These have several advantages, such as chemical inertness and tunable optical or surface properties. There are many syntheses that can produce particles with different sizes and morphologies, but for most of them, several other components can also be identified in the resulting suspension. Therefore, the purification and additional surface functionalization of the formed nano-objects are necessary to satisfy strict medical requirements. As a result, biocompatible syntheses offer us an outstanding opportunity to simultaneously reduce the metal ions and stabilize/functionalize the formed particles with only one biomolecule (e.g., proteins, nucleotides, amino acids) [1,2]. The character of this molecule, which predominantly contains nitrogen- or sulfur-containing donor groups, has a large effect on the size of the formed particles, therefore also influencing the optical features. In the case of the application of small molar ratios between the ligand and metal ions, the classical plasmonic particle is synthesized [3]. In contrast, noble metal nanoclusters (NCs) with molecular-like optical properties can be prepared when the reducing ligands are present in an excessive amount relative to the metal ions [4].

Due to the biocompatible shell on NCs, several articles can be found related to their potential application in biomedical fields. Thanks to their environment-sensitive luminescence, they are prominent raw materials for biosensors and light emitters [5]. The detection of biologically important molecules (e.g., glutathione [6], dopamine [7], folic acid [8], *L*-kynurenine [9]), pH [10], and intracellular temperature [11] have been previously studied in several articles. Moreover, they have been successfully applied as theragnostic agents. For example, Zheng and co-workers examined the potential application of mercaptobenzoic acid-, cysteine-, and cysteamine-stabilized Au NCs as a potential antimicrobial agent thanks to their more effective production of harmful reactive oxygen species (ROS) [12] in different bacteria. In their article, S. Jindal and P. Gopinath clearly demonstrated the success of an anti-proliferative agent, a chitosan–Ag nanocluster/4-phenylbutyrate hydrogel, as a histone deacetylase inhibitor for breast cancer cells [13]. For the inhibition of neurodegenerative diseases, Li and co-workers have produced several works focused on the potential anti-amyloid usability of noble metal NCs for the treatment of brain-centered hazards [14].

Due to fast and unhealthy daily routines, stress, and chemicals, several types of ROS (peroxynitrite/ONOO•/, nitric oxide/NO•/, peroxyl radical/ROO•/, superoxide radical/$O_2{\bullet}^-$/, etc.) can be formed in living organisms, which can cause dysfunction and damage the tissues by facilitating cell death [15,16]. Apart from the generally used antioxidant lipid-based vesicles [17,18], niosomes [19], gels [20], and composite materials [21], ultra-small NCs are potential devices to prevent these issues because their composition is easily tuned by the selection of the appropriate metal and surface ligand to precisely design smart biomimetic materials [22]. Based on the above-mentioned utilization of few-atomic NCs with few atomic layers, antioxidant and enzyme-like applications should be a priority in future research.

In this present work, a one-pot synthesis of blue-emitting Vitamin B_1-stabilized gold nanoclusters (B_1-Au NCs) is demonstrated for the first time due to the possible antioxidant application of this hybrid nanostructure. Furthermore, the experimental results for the exact optical and structural characterizations of their potential bioactivity are also presented. It is well known that the Vitamin B molecular family shows an intensive inhibition capacity against ROS; therefore, antioxidant behavior was measured by standard 2,2′-azino-bis(3-ethylbenzothiazoline-6-sulfonic acid) (ABTS) and Oxygen Radical Antioxidant Capacity (ORAC) assays, and protein interactions with bovine serum albumin (BSA) were also investigated and interpreted.

2. Materials and Methods

2.1. Chemicals

To synthesize blue-emitting B_1-Au NCs, thiamine hydrochloride (Vitamin B_1; $C_{12}H_{17}ClN_4OS{\cdot}HCl$; ≥99.9%; Sigma, Budapest, Hungary), hydrogen tetrachloroaurate(III) hydrate ($HAuCl_4 \times H_2O$; 99.9% (metal basis); Sigma, Budapest Hungary), and sodium hydroxide (NaOH; 99%; Molar, Budapest, Hungary) were used. During the antioxidant measurements, 2,2′-azino-bis(3-ethylbenzothiazoline-6-sulfonic acid) diammonium salt (ABTS; $C_{18}H_{24}N_6O_6S_4$; ≥98%; Alfa Aesar, Ward Hill, MA, USA), potassium persulfate ($K_2S_2O_8$; 99.99%; Sigma, Budapest, Hungary), 2,2′-azobis(2-methylpropionamidine) dihydrochloride (AAPH; $[=NC(CH_3)_2C(=NH)NH_2]_2 \times 2$ HCl; 97%; Sigma, Budapest, Hungary), 6-Hydroxy-2,5,7,8-tetramethylchromane-2-carboxylic acid (Trolox; $C_{14}H_{18}O_4$; 97%; Sigma, Budapest, Hungary), and fluorescein sodium salt ($C_{20}H_{10}Na_2O_5$; analytical standard; VWR, Debrecen, Hungary) were selected. The buffers and the protein solutions were made by using bovine serum albumin (BSA; lyophilized powder, essentially globulin free; ≥99%; Sigma, Budapest, Hungary), hydrochloric acid (HCl; 37%; Molar, Budapest, Hungary), sodium dihydrogen phosphate 2-hydrate ($NaH_2PO_4 \times 2\ H_2O$; 99%; Molar, Budapest, Hungary), disodium hydrogen phosphate dodecahydrate ($Na_2HPO_4 \times 12\ H_2O$; ≥99.99%; Molar, Budapest, Hungary), and sodium chloride (NaCl; 99.98%; Molar, Budapest, Hungary). The reagents were used without further purification. The fresh stock solutions were prepared with Milli-Q (Merck Millipore, Darmstadt, Germany) ultrapure water (conductivity: 18.2 MΩ·cm). For the purification, a Pur-A-LyzerTM dialysis kit (Sigma, Budapest, Hungary) with a 1 kDa cut-off value was chosen.

2.2. Preparation Protocol of B_1-Au NCs

For the synthesis of blue-emitting NCs, a B_1:$[AuCl_4]^-$/25:1 molar ratio was applied, while the final concentration of the Au in the dispersion was 1.0 mM, and the Vitamin B_1 concentration was 25 mM. In the first step of the synthesis, an adequate amount of the ligand and metal solutions was mixed in ultrapure water. The pH of the reaction mixture was adjusted to pH = 3.5 by using 0.1 M NaOH. After 3 min of stirring, 1 mL of 0.01 M $HAuCl_4$ solution was pipetted into the reaction mixture, and then the solution was incubated at 25.0 ± 0.1 °C. After 24 h, the intensive yellow color of the $[AuCl_4]^-$ ions disappeared, and the solution turned pale brownish. A few larger aggregates were formed at the end of the synthesis, which were removed from the sample by centrifugation at 13,000 rpm for 30 min, and the supernatant was further used. The unnecessary synthesis components and the unreacted salts were removed by dialysis for 1 h in a Pur-A-LyzerTM Mega 1000 dialysis kit (MWCO = 1 kDa, Sigma, Budapest, Hungary).

2.3. Antioxidant Measurements

For the ABTS and ORAC assays, the stock and working solutions were prepared according to Ref. [23]. For ABTS test, the sample solutions were prepared by mixing 200.0 μL ABTS working solution and 10.0 μL sample solution, which contained the Vitamin B_1 or the B_1-Au NCs with a suitable (the same) ligand concentration. The samples were kept in dark for 5 min at 25 °C, then they were diluted to 3 mL and the absorbance of the diluted samples was registered at 734 nm. The inhibition ratio was calculated by the following, Equation (1) [23]:

$$Inhibition\ \% = \left(\frac{A_c - A_s}{A_c}\right) \times 100 \quad (1)$$

where the A_c and A_s are the absorbance at 734 nm of the control and sample after 5 min, respectively. The antioxidant behavior was evaluated by the calculation of IC_{50} value, where the inhibition extent reached 50%. The samples were investigated in the 5–100 μM concentration range.

In the case of the ORAC test, the fluorescence spectra of fluorescein dye were registered between 500 and 650 nm, in which the emission maxima were located at 500 nm, and the excitation wavelength was 485 nm. An adequate volume of antioxidant material and 78 μL of fluorescein solution (c = 1 μM) were pipetted in phosphate-buffered saline (PBS, c_{NaCl} = 0.15 M, pH = 7.4). The incubation took place at 37 °C for 15 min in the dark. After the incubation, 100 μL of 200 mM AAPH solution was also added to start the reaction. Before the measurements, the volume of the samples was completed with a 2 mL buffer to reach the appropriate fluorescence signal. The hydrophilic Vitamin E derivative Trolox molecule served as a reference. To compare and quantify the activity, the ORAC value [24] was determined by the following formula (Equation (2)):

$$ORAC\ value = \frac{c_{Trolox} \times Net_{AUC\ of\ sample} \times k}{Net_{AUC\ of\ Trolox}} \quad (2)$$

where the c_{Trolox} is 50 μM, and the $Net_{AUC\ of\ sample}$ and $Net_{AUC\ of\ Trolox}$ values are the net areas under kinetic curves for the 50 μM B_1 content in the sample and 50 μM in the Trolox solution. Each Net_{AUC} value was calculated after the blank correction by the integration of the time-dependent decay curves. The k is the dilution factor of the sample, which was 4-fold in our case.

2.4. Experimental Conditions for the Investigation of Protein Interaction by Spectrofluorometry and Isotherm Titration Calorimetry

For the optical measurements, the solutions were mixed in PBS buffer. In the case of *L*-tryptophane (*Trp*) quenching, the BSA concentration was fixed at 0.5 mM, while the concentration of the NCs was varied between 0 and 1 mM. The samples were stirred for

2 min at 25 °C. The excitation and emission wavelengths were 280 and 348 nm, respectively. For the calorimetric studies, a room temperature of 25 °C was also selected, and the measurements were carried out with a computer-controlled instrument. The sample cell of the calorimeter with 1.4 mL volume was filled with 0.1 mM concentration of Vitamin B_1 or B_1-Au NCs, while the syringe contained 280 μL BSA solution in 1.5 mM concentration. The titration speed was 8 μL/step/5 min. For the calculation of the thermodynamic parameters, the one- and two-site binding models were selected. The theoretical background of the evaluation can be found in the Supporting Information section.

2.5. Instruments

Fluorescence spectra were registered on the ABL&E JASCO FP-8500 spectrofluorometer in a standard 1 cm quartz cuvette. The measurement was carried out by using 395 nm as excitation wavelength, 2.5–2.5 nm bandwidths, 1 nm resolution, and 200 nm/min scan speed. For the calculation of the absolute internal quantum yield (QY %), the same instrument was used, which was equipped with the ABL&E JASCO ILF-835 integrating sphere. For the calibration, WI light source (ABL&E JASCO ESC-842) was applied; thus, other references were not needed. The evaluation of the spectra was completed in the ABL&E JASCO SpectraManager 2.0 software. The fluorescence lifetime of the NCs was determined by time-correlated single-photon counting (TCSPC) measurements on a Horiba DeltaFlex apparatus using a 1 cm optical length. A DeltaDiode pulsed laser (λ_{laser} = 371 nm) served as an excitation light source. The emitted light was detected at 450 nm with a 6 nm slit. The number of counts on the peak channel was 10,000, and for the instrument response function (IRF), standard LUDOX® SiO_2 colloids (Horiba) were applied. The lifetime components were calculated by exponential fitting with χ^2 goodness values of the registered decay curves in the EZTime program from Horiba. For the determination of the binding energies in the main elements in the B_1-Au NCs, X-ray photoelectron spectra were registered in survey scan (40 eV pass energy) and high-resolution modes (20 eV pass energy). The spectra were collected by a SPECS device equipped with a PHOIBOS 150MCD9 hemispherical analyzer. The sample was deposited on a 0.5 mm thick titanium foil (Sigma) by multistep cyclic freeze-drying. The Al K_α X-ray source was operated at 200 W power and the carbon 1s peak (284.80 eV) was used for charge referencing. Spectra were evaluated by CasaXPS software. To identify the possible coordination between the stabilizing Vitamin B_1 and Au metal cores, Fourier-transformed infrared spectroscopy (FT-IR) was used based on measurement with a JASCO FT/IR-4700 instrument equipped with an ATR PRO ONE single-reflection accessory. The spectra were collected in the range of 500 to 4000 cm^{-1} by 128 interferograms with 1 cm^{-1} resolution on lyophilized powder samples. For the reference thiamine spectra, the powder was prepared at the same concentrations and similar pH to those of the cluster dispersions. The stability of the fluorescent nano-objects was studied on a Malvern Zetasizer NanoZS ZEN 4003 apparatus equipped with a He-Ne laser (λ = 633 nm) at 25 ± 0.1 °C. The ionic strength was regulated by 0.1 M NaCl, and the hydrodynamic diameters (d_H) were calculated by the Smoluchowski model. The secondary structure of the BSA before and after the addition of NCs was investigated by circular dichroism (CD). For this purpose, ABL&E JASCO J-1100 CD spectrometer was applied, equipped a high-energy Xenon lamp (450 W) and a water-cooled ABL&E JASCO PTC-514 Peltier sample holder. The measurements were carried out at 25 °C in a 1 cm quartz cuvette with 200 nm/min scan speed and 1 nm resolution. The spectra were determined by the Secondary Structure Estimation module of the ABL&E JASCO SpectraManager 2.0 software. The thermodynamic characterization of the BSA/NCs complex system's formation was investigated by isotherm titration calorimetry using MicroCal VP-ITC power-compensation microcalorimeter equipped with MicroCal 7.1 Origin®-based software.

3. Results and Discussion

3.1. Structural Characterization of the Fluorescent B_1-Au NCs

The optimization of the synthetic process was carried out to find the ideal parameters for production of nanosized objects with the highest fluorescence intensity. For this purpose, the applied molar ratio between the Vitamin B_1 and $AuCl_4^-$ ions, the pH of the reaction mixture, the concentration of the precursor metal salt, the temperature, and the synthesis time were examined in individual samples. The final parameters were selected based on the highest emission yield of the samples and the measured data are shown in Figure S1. After the optimization process, it was found that the most fluorescent product was prepared by using a B_1:$[AuCl_4]^-$/25:1 molar ratio with a 1.0 mM initial aurate ion concentration (Figure S1a,b). The best fluorescent response (as seen in (Figure S1c)) was achieved by a reaction mixture with an initial pH = 3.5. Under more acidic conditions, the pyrimidine-N1 of the thiamine is still protonated [25], which might facilitate the direct coordination of gold(III) ions to the pyrimidine ring of the Vitamin B_1 molecule via electrostatic interactions. In the case of the deprotonated pseudobase thiamine formed at pH = 4–9, the positive charge is only on the thiazole-N3 nitrogen, which is not able to coordinate to the precursor $[AuCl_4]^-$; thus, this form is not favorable for cluster formation. Under alkaline conditions, the formation of the thiochrome form is the dominant species, which also shows the formation of nanohybrid systems with low fluorescent yields. For the further optimization process, the temperature and the synthesis time were also investigated (Figure S1d,e), in which the samples prepared at 25 °C for 24 h with the previously optimized parameters had superior emissive properties. Before the exact structural characterization, purification via 13,000 rpm centrifugation for 30 min and dialysis were performed to remove the larger aggregates, the unreacted metal salt, and the excess vitamin B_1. After the purification, the final metal concentration was c_{Au} = 0.75 mM, as measured by inductively coupled plasma mass spectrometry (ICP-MS), while the B_1 concentration (c_{B1} = 17 mM) was determined based on spectrophotometric data; the final molar ratio was ca. B_1:Au/22.5:1 in the product, which refers to the total concentrations of the t.

After purification, optical and structural characterizations of the synthesized fluorescent nanomaterial were carried out. As Figure 1a clearly shows, the prepared B_1-stabilized Au nanohybrid system showed intensive blue emissions under a UV lamp. Based on the steady-state spectrofluorometric measurements, the excitation and the emission maxima were found at 395 and 450 nm, respectively. The absolute internal quantum yield was 3.1 ± 0.2%. The determined optical characteristics refer to the formation of few-atomic NCs and ca. eight Au atoms in the primer cores [26,27]. We determined the average lifetime (τ) and the main lifetime components of the prepared system. As can be seen in Figure 1b, the fluorescence lifetime of the Au-containing nano-object is in the nanosecond range, which can indicate the presence of ultra-small metal cores [28]. In the case of the biomolecule-stabilized few-atomic NCs, two to three main τ components can predominantly be separated from the nanosecond-range average lifetime, in which case the shorter components are only metal- or size-dependent, while the longer components show the ligand-dependent charge transfer [29]. By fitting the decay curves, three main lifetime components (τ_1–τ_3) can be identified. The τ_1 is 1.26 ± 0.38 ns (31%), which is in good agreement with the previously published data on the charge transfer to the oxidized form of Vitamin B_1 (thiochrome) [30,31]. This component can form by metal reduction during the synthesis (Scheme S1), and it is presumably on the surface via $\pi \cdots \pi$ stacking to take part in the stabilization of the final metal cores [32]. The τ_2 is 2.46 ± 0.13 ns, which contributes the largest amount (ca. 49%) to the total fluorescence of the sample. Based on the literature data, the τ_2 belongs to the ligand-to-metal charge transfers. In contrast, the shortest component (τ_3 = 0.24 ± 0.01, 20%) can be assigned to the metal–metal transitions in the cluster cores.

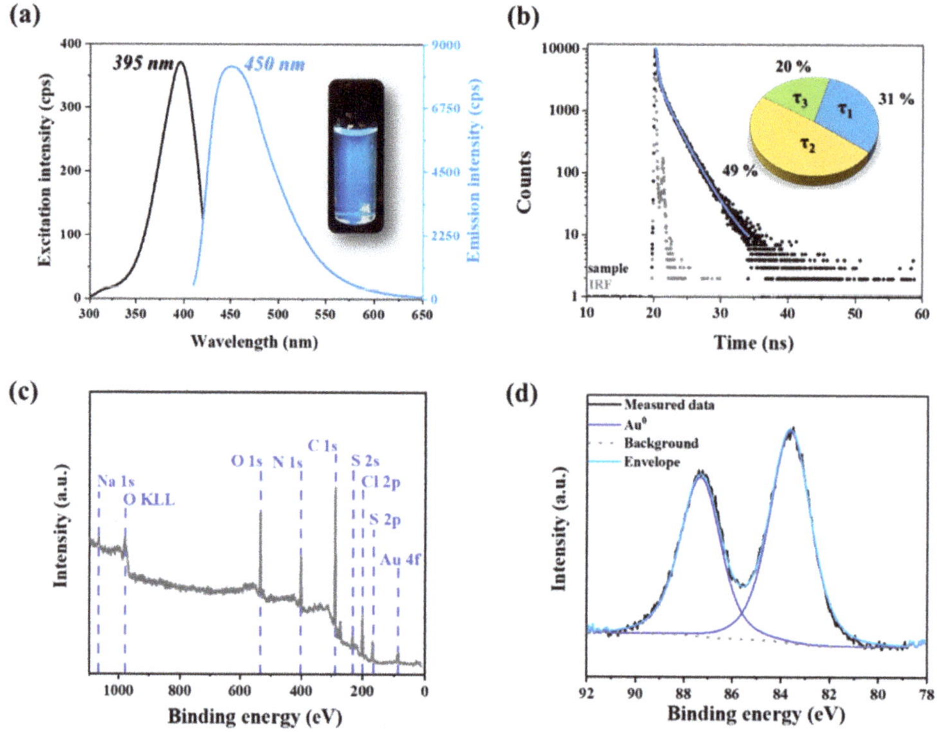

Figure 1. (**a**) The excitation and emission spectra of the B_1-Au NCs with the photo of the sample under UV lamp (λ_{max} = 365 nm). (**b**) The typical fluorescence decay curve of the B_1-Au NCs with the distribution percentage of the main lifetime components (λ_{ex} = 371 nm). (**c**) The survey scan and (**d**) the XPS spectra of the Au content in B_1-Au NCs.

To determine the surface chemical composition, the XPS spectra were recorded in the case of the powder samples. On the survey scan (Figure 1c), the presence of O, N, C, S, and Cl from the stabilizing ligand are observable, together with the presence of Au from the metal cores. The Au 4f region can be fitted with an asymmetric line shape that is characteristic of metals (Figure 1d). The determined binding energies of the $4f_{5/2}$ and $4f_{7/2}$ core-level transitions are located at 87.3 and 83.6 eV, respectively, which shows the presence of metallic Au. The slight negative shift to the $4f_{7/2}$ of the bulk Au (84.0 eV) might be the result of the ultra-small size of the metal cores with strong ligand–metal electron-donating interactions [33], which was also previously shown in the results of the fluorescence lifetime measurements. The other regions on the XP spectra (Figure S2) indicate the presence of the thiamine molecule on the surface of the Au metal cores. In the case of the C 1s region, the following three main binding energy components were identified: C-C and C-H bindings at 284.8 eV; C-OH and C-N bindings at 286.3 eV; and C=O and C=N bindings at 287.8 eV [34], which clearly refer to the presence of the thiamine molecule on the NCs' surface. For the S 2p region, the $2p_{3/2}$ transition at 164.6 eV might be assigned to the sulfur atoms in the thiazole aromatic ring of Vitamin B_1. In the case of the N 1s region, four different types of nitrogen were detected: pyrimidine N at 398.7 eV, the amino group at 400.0 eV, the larger amount of thiazone-N at 401.0 eV, and some oxidized nitrogen at the 406.2 eV peak position [35]. While the stabilizing ligand was applied in the form of hydrochloride, some chloride contaminations were also discovered. Finally, the signal from the oxygen content originated mainly from the -OH form (531.7 eV) and a small amount of adsorbed H_2O (533.4 eV).

To support the coordination of N-donor(s) to the metal cores, the IR spectra of the purified NCs in powder form were registered. Based on the registered FT-IR spectra (Figure S3), it can be concluded that the vibration of the primer -NH_2 stretching at 3426 cm^{-1}, the aromatic C=N in the pyrimidine ring at 1658 cm^{-1} and 1600 cm^{-1}, and the characteristic vibrations of the thiazole rings in the far-middle IR region between 1000–500 cm^{-1} have shifted [36,37]. It should be noted that due to the gold reduction, some oxidized thiochrome forms have spontaneously synthesized. Therefore, it is complicated to clearly identify the vibration bands on the IR spectra. However, the primer coordination via pyrimidin-N1 can be assumed based on the crystallographic data of similar soft metal ion-thiamine complexes [38–40]. Moreover, the dominant change of the intensities between 3500 and 3000 cm^{-1} was also observed thanks to the presence of the metallic surface [41,42].

We evaluated the stability of the prepared NCs as well. The pH-dependent DLS and fluorescence measurements (Figure S4) were carried out, which can be used to determine the stability region of the B_1-Au NCs. Note that the primer sizes of the cluster cores cannot be directly observed due to their small sizes. However, the cluster adducts in aqueous media are measurable with classical colloidal techniques. Based on the registered data, it can be concluded that the prepared NCs show a weak fluorescence under acidic conditions due to the large charge-shielding effect of the environment and form smaller aggregates based on the measured hydrodynamic diameters (d_H ~ 15 nm). In contrast, a dominant aggregation process can be observed at pH = 6.0 because the detected d_H is ca. 630 nm, and the ζ-potential is also close to zero mV. A possible explanation is that, at this pH value, the dominant form of the free thiamine is the pseudobase form [43]; thus, the sterically stabilizing molecules lost their dominant charge excess, and the formed NCs' structure becomes unstable. Nonetheless, the fluorescent intensity shows a growing tendency due aggregation-induced emissions (AIE), in which intramolecular rotations and vibration are inhibited due to the close contact of cluster cores [44]. The alkaline condition has no dominant effect on the sizes and the PL property; the detected d_H values are close to the lower limit of the nanometer range. The stability is also proven by the measured ζ-potential values ($|\zeta| > 20$ mV).

3.2. Antioxidant Studies

It is well known that the Vitamin B molecular family shows an excellent antioxidant effect [45]. In our previous study, it was shown that the Vitamin B_3 derivative niacinamide, after the synthesis of Au NCs, is still usable as an antioxidant agent (ORAC value for B_3 (amide) = 0.56 μM, for B_3 (amide)-Au NCs = 0.48 μM) [46]. Thiamine shows a larger preventive effect against ROS with a chain breaker mechanism [47], because the antioxidant can donate an electron and a proton to ROS at the same time, which annihilates the harmful effect of ROS on the chemical environment.

Apart from the surface ligand Vitamin B_1, gold-based nanomaterials can contribute to this mechanism due to their electron-rich surfaces [48]. For the determination of the potential antioxidant activity of the B_1-Au NCs, two different methods were selected, in which the concentration was related to the B_1 content (determined by spectrophotometry measurements) in the samples.

In the first case, the ABTS test was applied, in which the fading of the bluish-green color at 734 nm was registered with a spectrophotometer (Figure 2a). This method has several advantages; it can be used for both hydrophilic and lipophilic compounds, it can be applied in a wide pH range, it is cheap, and the total antioxidant capacity of a complex sample (e.g., nanoclusters, metal alloys, other nanohybrid systems) can be determined. For the measurement, the pure Vitamin B_1 served as a reference. As Figure 2b shows, the inhibition percent strongly depends on the applied concentration (In the case of the B_1-Au NCs, the concentration was related to the Vitamin B_1 content of the NCs suspension). In the case of the pure B_1, the IC_{50} value was determined to be 76.4 ± 3.7 μM. In contrast, the presence of the Au cores, as well as the oxidized thiochrome in the cluster surface, can facilitate scavenging activity, because the IC_{50} value is 36.9 ± 2.1 μM, which clearly demonstrates the better antioxidant activity of the prepared complex structure than that of the initial pure thiamine.

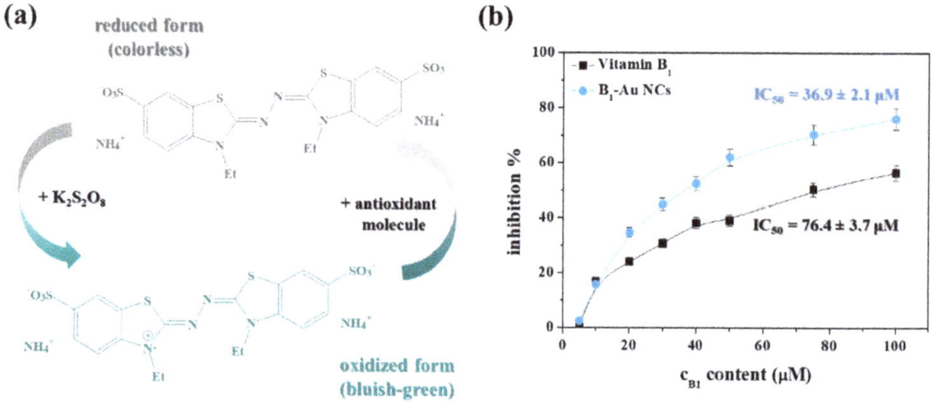

Figure 2. (**a**) The transformation of the ABTS molecule during the antioxidant measurement protocol from the reduced form to the oxidized form. (**b**) The radical scavenging activity curve (λ_{abs} = 734 nm, T = 25 °C) of the pure Vitamin B_1 (■) and the B_1-Au NCs (•) applying 5–100 μM B_1 content.

To investigate the radical chain reaction, an ORAC assay was applied, in which the inhibition of the oxidation of peroxyl radicals was studied. For the measurement in an aqueous medium, the hydrophilic 2,2′-azobis(2-amidinopropane) dihydrochloride was selected as the ROS generator for the oxidative degradation of the fluorescein molecule. As Figure 3 shows, the ORAC assay also demonstrates the better antioxidant activity of the newly prepared B_1-Au NCs. Based on the calculations, it can be estimated that the ORAC values are 0.36 ± 0.02 μM and 0.53 ± 0.01 μM in the case of Vitamin B_1 and B_1-Au NCs, respectively. As the calculated values demonstrate, both methods were suitable to determine the enhanced antioxidant behavior of the newly prepared blue-emitting Au NCs compared to that of the pure Vitamin B_1.

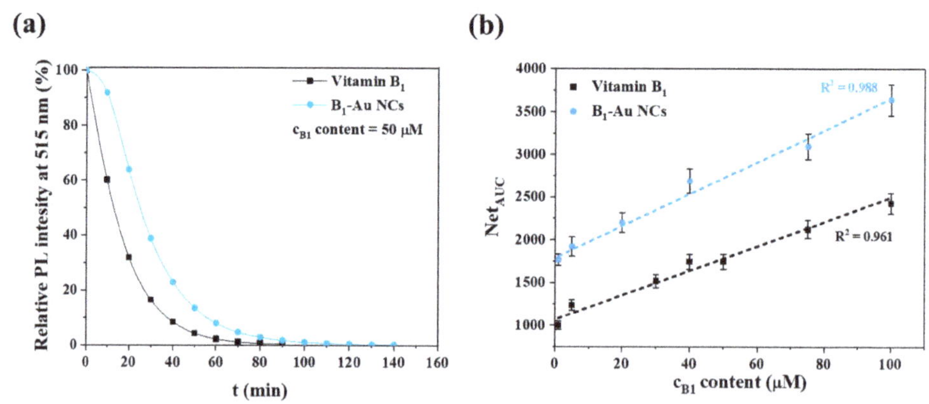

Figure 3. (**a**) The representative kinetic curves of fluorescence decay during the ORAC test in the presence of Vitamin B_1 (■) and B_1-Au NCs (•) (B_1 content of 50 μM, T = 25 °C, λ_{ex} = 485 nm). (**b**) The antioxidant dose-response curves between 1 and 100 μM of B_1 content.

3.3. Interaction of B_1-Au NCs with Bovine Serum Albumin

For future biomedical applications as in vitro or in vivo antioxidant agents, it is necessary to examine the interaction of the B_1-Au NCs with biologically important macromolecules. For this purpose, bovine serum albumin (BSA) was chosen as a model protein. Firstly, CD and PL measurements were carried out to analyze the optical characteristics of the interaction. During these measurements, the concentration of clusters was based on the metal content. The dispersion containing the NCs was prepared from their lyophilized powder form to obtain the exact metal concentration. During the registration of the CD spectra, the concentration of the BSA was constant (c_{BSA} = 0.05 mM), while the amount of the NCs varied between 0, 0.05, 0.01, 0.1, and 0.5 mM in the individual samples. The final samples were diluted 600-fold to reach the suitable optical signal. The spectra are presented in Figure S5, which show that the increasing cluster concentration had an increasing effect on the α-helix ratio from 54.3% to 73.2%. Therefore, it can be assumed that the binding process caused a contraction in the whole protein chain, which promoted the formation of an ordered structure.

To further investigate this binding process, PL measurements were carried out in two ways. In the first case, the quenching of the *Trp* amino acids of the protein chain in the 134th and 212th positions was examined. The fluorescence of this amino acid strongly depends on the chemical environment; thus, the conformation change of the protein chain also has a dominant impact on the extent of the intensity or the position of the maximum value. During these PL studies, the protein concentration was fixed at 0.5 mM. As it can be seen in Figure 4a, the intensity of the Trp emission decreases with the increase in the cluster's concentration. Based on the standard Stern–Volmer evaluation of the data (Figure S6), in which the relative fluorescence (F_0/F) is calculated depending on the applied Au concentration, it can be concluded that the binding causes a dominant quenching for the Trp emission. This decreasing tendency cannot be defined purely as static or dynamic quenching due to the upward curvature of the plot. Based on this phenomenon, the formation of a dark complex (static quenching) and an energy loss by collision (dynamic quenching) can also be present at the same time owing to the binding process. Moreover, the filling of the non-accessible binding sites, therefore the subsequent exposure of the Trp residues to the aqueous environment due to the change of the protein folding, can also cause similar differences from the linear Stern–Volmer-based dependence [49]. To further investigate the quenching process and the optical characteristics of the partners, the possibility of a resonance energy transfer (RET) between the BSA and B_1-Au NCs should also be considered due to the large overlap of the emission and excitation spectra of the Trp and B_1-Au NCs [50]. During this process, the energy excess can transfer from the donor (Trp in BSA) to an acceptor (Au NCs) via dipole–dipole coupling (Figure 4b), which can be facilitated by the bonding of the ultra-small cluster structures along the protein chain. This RET between the protein and NCs can also cause the nonlinearity of the quenching curves.

For this reason, the evaluation of the optical measurements was re-assessed based on the Scatchard plot (Equation (3)), which is a special methodology for protein/small molecule or protein/small particle interactions [51]:

$$\log\left(\frac{F_0}{F} - 1\right) = \log K_a + N \log[Q] \quad (3)$$

where the F_0 and F are the emission intensities at 350 nm before and after the addition of NCs, respectively, K_a is the binding constant, N is the number of binding sites of BSA to the cluster, and $[Q]$ is the applied NC concentration [52].

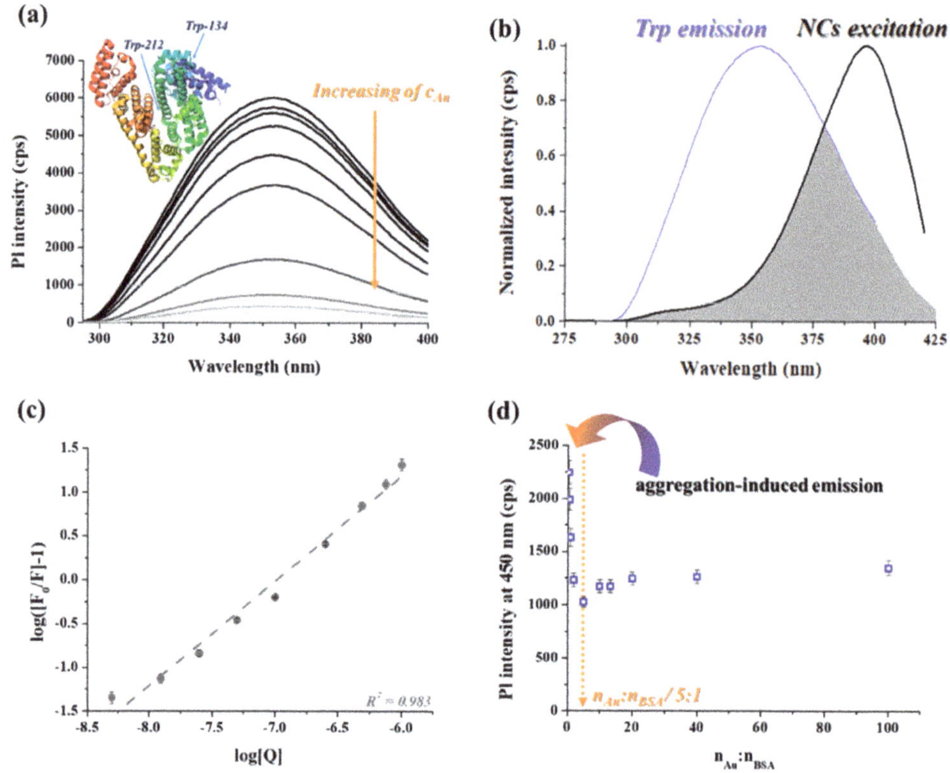

Figure 4. (**a**) The emission spectra of the BSA after addition of 0–1 mM Au NCs with the structure of BSA (PDB code: 3V03) (c_{BSA} = 0.5 mM; T = 25 °C; λ_{ex} = 280 nm). (**b**) The normalized emission spectrum of the Trp in BSA and the excitation spectrum of the B_1-Au NCs. (**c**) The Scatchard plot of the experienced quenching at 350 nm. (**d**) The change in the PL intensity of B_1-Au NCs depending on the amount of BSA (c_{Au} = 0.5 mM; λ_{ex} = 395 nm; λ_{em} = 450 nm; T = 25 °C).

By linear fitting (Figure 4c) the data points, the calculated K_a value is 2.34 × 108 ± 1.17 × 107 M^{-1}, which indicates a stronger interaction between the protein and NCs [53,54]. The determined N is 1.20 ± 0.05, which indicates a self-catalyzed binding; therefore, the affinity continually increases with the adsorption [53]. Based on the calculated N value, the presence of the metal core can slightly inhibit the attachment of thiamine in the binding pockets (Sudlow sites) of the BSA. Based on the $\Delta G = -RT \ln K_a$ equation, where R and T are the gas constant and the measurement temperature, respectively, the calculated Gibbs energy change of the interaction is -47.8 ± 2.3 kJ·mol^{-1}, which indicates a spontaneous, thermodynamic favorable binding process. Nonetheless, the internal and external surfaces of the protein molecule are also suitable to adsorb the clusters by hydrophobic and electrostatic interactions via surface ligands, as well as the emergence a strong Au–S bond via cysteine amino acids in contrast with the pure molecule. The possible H-bond and hydrophobic interactions between Vitamin B_1 and BSA are supported based on the work of R. Hosseinzadeh and K. Khorsandi, which included potentiometric and molecular docking studies [55]. Furthermore, in the work of M. Mallappa [56], spectroscopic and theoretical studies of similar bindings were also presented. Based on their measurements, it was concluded that the number of the binding sites is ca. 0.9, independently of the studied temperature, and the binding process is thermodynamically favorable ($\Delta G \sim -22$ kJ mol^{-1}). Additionally, the docking analysis showed that the binding is based on predominantly hydrophobic and H-bond interactions. Compared with the preciously published data, it can be clearly concluded that the presence of the ultra-small gold cores can facilitate the binding between the B_1 and BSA considering the determined number of binding sites, but the interaction is still spontaneous and predominantly driven by hydrophobicforces. However, this phenomenon should be further investigated by other techniques.

Besides the *Trp* quenching, the change in the NCs' emission by varying the BSA ratio was also investigated. Figure 4d shows that the intensity values interestingly reach a local minimum at a NCs:BSA/5:1 molar ratio. By applying a high cluster excess with large n_{Au}:n_{BSA} ratios, the detected reduced fluorescence intensities are almost constant. In contrast, the use of a large BSA concentration (at small n_{Au}:n_{BSA} ratios) can cause a dominant AIE effect due to the formation of dimers and tetramers of BSA [57], in which the bonded clusters in the folded proteins can repeatedly come close to each other, facilitating the energy transfer between the individual cluster cores. To verify the calculated K_a and ΔG values of the protein/cluster interaction, calorimetry measurements were carried out, in which the RET cannot influence the detected quenching process and it is not able to distort the calculated values.

The confirmation of the potential bioactivity was also investigated by comparisons with previously prepared antioxidant niacinamide-stabilized Au NCs (NAM-Au NCs) [46]. As can be seen on Figure 5, the interaction with the serum protein dramatically depends on the chemical structure of the stabilizing molecule of the metal surface. In the case of the NAM-Au NCs, the NAM molecule has only a few functional groups, which are mostly occupied by the Au NCs. The possible negligible binding by the BSA can be decisively facilitated by hydrophobic interactions via the aromatic ring of NAM. Moreover, the prepared metal cores are significantly smaller than in the case of the B_1-Au NCs. Based on the registered enthalpograms, it can be concluded that the NAM-Au NCs do not show any considerable interaction with BSA. In contrast, the characteristic K_a value of the B_1-Au NCs/BSA complex systems, as well as their thermodynamic nature and stoichiometry, can be determined by the application of a two-site binding model with best fitting.

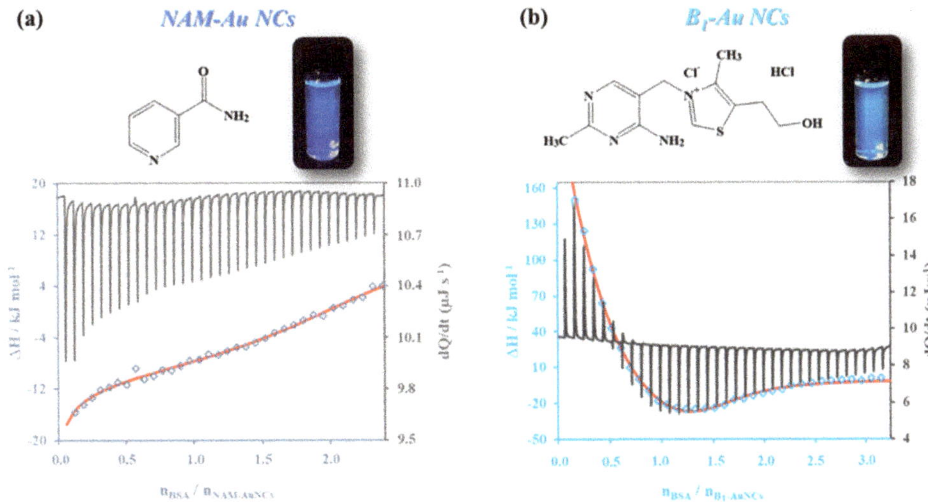

Figure 5. The calorimetric enthalpograms of the interaction between BSA and (**a**) NAM-Au NCs or (**b**) B_1-Au NCs' fitting by two-site binding model with the structural formula of the stabilizing ligands and the photos of the NC samples under UV lamp (λ_{max} = 365 nm).

As can be seen in Table 1, the assessed K_a values are significantly lower than in the case of the optical measurement. According to the reciprocal values of K_a, the dissociation constants are in the micromolar range, which are ca. 1.6 μM and ca. 6.2 μM in the case of the N_1 and N_2 sites, respectively. The magnitude of the dissociation constants refers to a medium-strength interaction between the protein and NCs. Furthermore, the binding is spontaneous and thermodynamically favorable ($\Delta G < 0$) in the case of both sites. Nevertheless, the determined data indicate very different behaviors for the two binding pockets. In the case of the second site, the calculated stoichiometry ($N_2 \sim 1.30$) is in good agreement with the evaluated fluorescence data ($N \sim 1.20$). The negative values of the ΔH and ΔS refer to the dominant presence of secondary forces, such as H-bonds and electrostatic interactions, during the formation of the BSA/NCs complex [58].

Table 1. The calculated binding constants (K_a), the Gibbs energy (ΔG), the enthalpy (ΔH), and entropy changes (ΔS) with the stoichiometry (N) of the binding between BSA and B_1-Au NCs based on the ITC measurement.

	First Binding Site	Second Binding Site
K_a (M^{-1})	$6.1 \times 10^5 \pm 8.4 \times 10^4$	$1.6 \times 10^5 \pm 2.4 \times 10^4$
ΔG ($kJ \cdot mol^{-1}$)	-32.99 ± 0.34	-29.73 ± 0.36
ΔH ($kJ \cdot mol^{-1}$)	779.90 ± 23.64	-97.36 ± 4.14
ΔS ($J \cdot mol^{-1} \cdot K^{-1}$)	2728 ± 0.00	-227 ± 0.00
N	0.20 ± 0.00	1.30 ± 0.00

In contrast, in the case of the first site, the binding is negligible based on the calculated N_1 value. Moreover, the binding is controlled by hydrophobic forces due to the positive values of ΔH and ΔS [59], which are in good agreement with the pure vitamin B_1 and BSA interaction studies. Therefore, it can be concluded that the binding process predominantly depends on the surface Vitamin B_1 molecules, but the presence of gold cores can facilitate this reaction.

4. Conclusions

In our article, the optical and structural characteristics of newly prepared B_1-Au NCs are presented. Based on their intensive blue emissions, the Au_8 cluster core presumably can utilize the excitation light with ca. 3%. The stabilization of the cluster cores is realized through the pyrimidine ring of the Vitamin B_1 molecule; moreover, the oxidized thiochrome form also takes part in the final structure stabilization presumably by $\pi \cdots \pi$ stacking with surface ligands. Based on the ABTS and ORAC assays, it was estimated that the presence of the metal cores having few atoms can enhance the antioxidant capacity compared with that of pure thiamine. For the investigation of further bioactivity, the interaction with the BSA protein was also measured with three different techniques. Based on the measurement data, it was concluded that the binding of the clusters along the protein chain is self-catalyzed, and the interaction is spontaneous and mostly controlled by hydrogen bonds and electrostatic interactions.

Supplementary Materials: The following supporting information can be downloaded at: https://www.mdpi.com/article/10.3390/antiox12040874/s1. Figure S1: The measured PL intensities of individual samples depending on the examined parameters (λ_{em} = 450 nm, λ_{ex} = 395 nm). The optimized parameters are as follows: (a) applied Vitamin B_1 concentration: c_{Au} = 1 mM; non-regulated pH; 20 °C; 1 day (b) the concentration of gold(III) salt: c_{B1} = 25 mM; pH = 3.5; 20 °C; 1 day (c) the pH of the reaction mixture: c_{B1} = 25 mM, c_{Au} = 1 mM; 20 °C; 1 day with the chemical structure of the thiamine forms (d) the temperature: c_{B1} = 25 mM; c_{Au} = 1 mM; pH = 3.5; 1 day (e) the time of the synthesis: c_{B1} = 25 mM; c_{Au} = 1 mM; pH = 3.5; 25 °C. Scheme S1: The schematic illustration of the B_1-Au NCs formation with a possible final cluster structure (unscaled). Figure S2: The XPS spectra of the (a) carbon (C), the (b) sulfur (S), the (c) nitrogen (N), the (d) chlorine (Cl), and the (e) oxygen (O) content in the B_1-Au NCs sample. Figure S3: The FT-IR spectra of Vitamin B_1 (black) and B_1-Au NCs (blue) in the range of 3500–1000 cm^{-1} (left) and 1000–500 cm^{-1} (right). Figure S4: The measured (a) hydrodynamic diameters (○) and the ζ-potential (■) values, as well as the (b) PL intensities of the B_1-Au NCs depending on the pH. Figure S5: The CD spectra of the BSA after addition of B_1-Au NCs in various concentrations (c_{BSA} = 0.083 µM). Figure S6: The Stern–Volmer plot of the *Trp* quenching in BSA by B_1-Au NCs (c_{BSA} = 0.05 mM). Theoretical background for the ITC measurements [60].

Author Contributions: Conceptualization, D.U.; methodology, D.U., G.G. and Á.J.; investigation, D.U., G.G., Á.J. and G.F.S.; writing—original draft preparation and editing, D.U.; writing—review, G.F.S. and E.C.; funding acquisition, D.U., Á.J. and E.C. All authors have read and agreed to the published version of the manuscript.

Funding: The research was supported by the National Research, Development, and Innovation Office-NKFIH through the PD137938 and FK131446 projects. Project no. TKP2021-EGA-32 was implemented with support provided by the Ministry of Innovation and Technology (MIT) of Hungary from the National Research, Development, and Innovation Fund (NRDIF), financed under the TKP2021-EGA funding scheme. Ditta Ungor is grateful for financial support from the János Bolyai Research Scholarship of the Hungarian Academy of Sciences. Á. Juhász was financially supported by the ÚNKP-22-4 -SZTE-497 New National Excellence Program of the Ministry for Innovation and Technology through the NRDIF.

Institutional Review Board Statement: Not applicable.

Informed Consent Statement: Not applicable.

Data Availability Statement: Data is contained within the article and supplementary material.

Acknowledgments: The authors would like to thank Samuel Coulburn (former undergraduate student at the University of Szeged) for his preliminary studies on the optimization process.

Conflicts of Interest: The authors declare no conflict of interest.

References

1. Ungor, D.; Csapó, E.; Kismárton, B.; Juhász, Á.; Dékány, I. Nucleotide-Directed Syntheses of Gold Nanohybrid Systems with Structure-Dependent Optical Features: Selective Fluorescence Sensing of Fe^{3+} Ions. *Colloids Surf. B Biointerfaces* **2017**, *155*, 135–141. [CrossRef] [PubMed]
2. Ungor, D.; Dékány, I.; Csapó, E. Reduction of Tetrachloroaurate(III) Ions With Bioligands: Role of the Thiol and Amine Functional Groups on the Structure and Optical Features of Gold Nanohybrid Systems. *Nanomaterials* **2019**, *9*, 1229. [CrossRef] [PubMed]
3. Leng, Y.; Fu, L.; Ye, L.; Li, B.; Xu, X.; Xing, X.; He, J.; Song, Y.; Leng, C.; Guo, Y.; et al. Protein-Directed Synthesis of Highly Monodispersed, Spherical Gold Nanoparticles and Their Applications in Multidimensional Sensing. *Sci. Rep.* **2016**, *6*, 28900. [CrossRef] [PubMed]
4. Xavier, P.L.; Chaudhari, K.; Baksi, A.; Pradeep, T. Protein-Protected Luminescent Noble Metal Quantum Clusters: An Emerging Trend in Atomic Cluster Nanoscience. *Nano Rev.* **2012**, *3*, 14767. [CrossRef] [PubMed]
5. Sarkar, P.; Nandi, N.; Barnwal, N.; Sahu, K. Mercaptopropionic Acid-Assisted Synthesis of Green and Blue Emissive Copper Nanoclusters for Multimodal Sensing, Logic Gate, and White Light Applications. *Mater. Today Chem.* **2023**, *27*, 101341. [CrossRef]
6. Chen, T.-H.; Tseng, W.-L. (Lysozyme Type VI)-Stabilized Au_8 Clusters: Synthesis Mechanism and Application for Sensing of Glutathione in a Single Drop of Blood. *Small* **2012**, *8*, 1912–1919. [CrossRef] [PubMed]
7. Zhou, T.; Su, Z.; Tu, Y.; Yan, J. Determination of Dopamine Based on Its Enhancement of Gold-Silver Nanocluster Fluorescence. *Spectrochim. Acta Part A Mol. Biomol. Spectrosc.* **2021**, *252*, 119519. [CrossRef] [PubMed]
8. Ungor, D.; Szilágyi, I.; Csapó, E. Yellow-Emitting Au/Ag Bimetallic Nanoclusters with High Photostability for Detection of Folic Acid. *J. Mol. Liq.* **2021**, *338*, 116695. [CrossRef]
9. Ungor, D.; Horváth, K.; Dékány, I.; Csapó, E. Red-Emitting Gold Nanoclusters for Rapid Fluorescence Sensing of Tryptophan Metabolites. *Sens. Actuators B Chem.* **2019**, *288*, 728–733. [CrossRef]
10. Luo, Y.; Miao, H.; Yang, X. Glutathione-Stabilized Cu Nanoclusters as Fluorescent Probes for Sensing pH and Vitamin B_1. *Talanta* **2015**, *144*, 488–495. [CrossRef]
11. Shang, L.; Stockmar, F.; Azadfar, N.; Nienhaus, G.U. Intracellular Thermometry by Using Fluorescent Gold Nanoclusters. *Angew. Chem. Int. Ed.* **2013**, *52*, 11154–11157. [CrossRef]
12. Zheng, K.; Setyawati, M.I.; Leong, D.T.; Xie, J. Surface Ligand Chemistry of Gold Nanoclusters Determines Their Antimicrobial Ability. *Chem. Mater.* **2018**, *30*, 2800–2808. [CrossRef]
13. Jindal, S.; Gopinath, P. Exploration of Connexin-43 Modulating, Multifunctional Silver Nanocluster-Hydrogel System for Theranostic Management of Cancer. *Mater. Today Chem.* **2022**, *26*, 101213. [CrossRef]
14. Li, D.; Wang, Z.; Kumari, B.; Mei, X.; Wang, Z.Y. Anti-Amyloid Nanoclusters for the Treatment of Brain Hazards Associated with Incurable Neurodegenerative Diseases. *Mater. Today Chem.* **2023**, *27*, 101256. [CrossRef]
15. Qi, F.; Huang, H.; Wang, M.; Rong, W.; Wang, J. Applications of Antioxidants in Dental Procedures. *Antioxidants* **2022**, *11*, 2492. [CrossRef]

16. Alam, M.W.; Al Qahtani, H.S.; Souayeh, B.; Ahmed, W.; Albalawi, H.; Farhan, M.; Abuzir, A.; Naeem, S. Novel Copper-Zinc-Manganese Ternary Metal Oxide Nanocomposite as Heterogeneous Catalyst for Glucose Sensor and Antibacterial Activity. *Antioxidants* **2022**, *11*, 1064. [CrossRef]
17. Cortesi, R.; Esposito, E.; Drechsler, M.; Pavoni, G.; Cacciatore, I.; Sguizzato, M.; Di Stefano, A. L-Dopa Co-Drugs in Nanostructured Lipid Carriers: A Comparative Study. *Mater. Sci. Eng. C* **2017**, *72*, 168–176. [CrossRef]
18. Hallan, S.; Sguizzato, M.; Drechsler, M.; Mariani, P.; Montesi, L.; Cortesi, R.; Björklund, S.; Ruzgas, T.; Esposito, E. The Potential of Caffeic Acid Lipid Nanoparticulate Systems for Skin Application: In Vitro Assays to Assess Delivery and Antioxidant Effect. *Nanomaterials* **2021**, *11*, 171. [CrossRef]
19. Sguizzato, M.; Pepe, A.; Baldisserotto, A.; Barbari, R.; Montesi, L.; Drechsler, M.; Mariani, P.; Cortesi, R. Niosomes for Topical Application of Antioxidant Molecules: Design and In Vitro Behavior. *Gels* **2023**, *9*, 107. [CrossRef]
20. Sicurella, M.; Sguizzato, M.; Cortesi, R.; Huang, N.; Simelière, F.; Montesi, L.; Marconi, P.; Esposito, E. Mangiferin-Loaded Smart Gels for HSV-1 Treatment. *Pharmaceutics* **2021**, *13*, 1323. [CrossRef]
21. Katana, B.; Kókai, K.P.; Sáringer, S.; Szerlauth, A.; Takács, D.; Szilágyi, I. The Influence of Solvents and Colloidal Particles on the Efficiency of Molecular Antioxidants. *Antioxidants* **2022**, *12*, 99. [CrossRef] [PubMed]
22. Alves, P.M.; Barrias, C.C.; Gomes, P.; Martins, M.C.L. Smart Biomaterial-Based Systems for Intrinsic Stimuli-Responsive Chronic Wound Management. *Mater. Today Chem.* **2021**, *22*, 100623. [CrossRef]
23. Xiao, F.; Xu, T.; Lu, B.; Liu, R. Guidelines for Antioxidant Assays for Food Components. *Food Front.* **2020**, *1*, 60–69. [CrossRef]
24. Zulueta, A.; Esteve, M.J.; Frígola, A. ORAC and TEAC Assays Comparison to Measure the Antioxidant Capacity of Food Products. *Food Chem.* **2009**, *114*, 310–316. [CrossRef]
25. Edwards, K.A.; Tu-Maung, N.; Cheng, K.; Wang, B.; Baeumner, A.J.; Kraft, C.E. Thiamine Assays—Advances, Challenges, and Caveats. *ChemistryOpen* **2017**, *6*, 178–191. [CrossRef]
26. Wood, D.M.; Ashcroft, N.W. Quantum Size Effects in the Optical Properties of Small Metallic Particles. *Phys. Rev. B* **1982**, *25*, 6255–6274. [CrossRef]
27. Rincon, L.; Hasmy, A.; Marquez, M.; Gonzalez, C. A Perturbatively Corrected Tight-Binding Method with Hybridization: Application to Gold Nanoparticles. *Chem. Phys. Lett.* **2011**, *503*, 171–175. [CrossRef]
28. Zheng, J.; Zhou, C.; Yu, M.; Liu, J. Different Sized Luminescent Gold Nanoparticles. *Nanoscale* **2012**, *4*, 4073. [CrossRef]
29. Yang, T.-Q.; Peng, B.; Shan, B.-Q.; Zong, Y.-X.; Jiang, J.-G.; Wu, P.; Zhang, K. Origin of the Photoluminescence of Metal Nanoclusters: From Metal-Centered Emission to Ligand-Centered Emission. *Nanomaterials* **2020**, *10*, 261. [CrossRef]
30. Bubeshko, N.N.; Stsiapura, V.I.; Stepuro, I.I. Fluorescent Properties of Thiochrome in Solvents of Different Polarity. *J. Appl. Spectrosc.* **2011**, *78*, 337–343. [CrossRef]
31. Yamabe, S.; Tsuchida, N.; Yamazaki, S. How Is Vitamin B_1 Oxidized to Thiochrome? Elementary Processes Revealed by a DFT Study. *Org. Biomol. Chem.* **2021**, *19*, 4529–4536. [CrossRef]
32. Wakchaure, P.D.; Ganguly, B. Unraveling the Role of π-Stacking Interactions in Ligand Binding to the Thiamine Pyrophosphate Riboswitch with High-Level Quantum Chemical Calculations and Docking Study. *J. Phys. Chem. B* **2022**, *126*, 1076–1084. [CrossRef]
33. Battistoni, C.; Mattogno, G.; Cariati, F.; Naldini, L.; Sgamellotti, A. XPS Photoelectron Spectra of Cluster Compounds of Gold. *Inorg. Chim. Acta* **1977**, *24*, 207–210. [CrossRef]
34. Shchukarev, A.; Korolkov, D. XPS Study of Group IA Carbonates. *Open Chem.* **2004**, *2*, 347–362. [CrossRef]
35. Jansen, R.J.J.; van Bekkum, H. XPS of Nitrogen-Containing Functional Groups on Activated Carbon. *Carbon* **1995**, *33*, 1021–1027. [CrossRef]
36. Butler, I.S.; Kawai, N.T.; Yining, H.; Louloudi, M.; Hadjiliadis, N. Effect of High Pressure on the Infrared Spectra of the Thiamine Enzyme 'Active Aldehyde' Intermediate 2-(α-Hydroxybenzyl)Thiamine Chloride (HBT) and the Mercury(II) Complex, Hg(HBT)Cl3. *Inorg. Chim. Acta* **1992**, *196*, 119–122. [CrossRef]
37. Sethiya, A.; Soni, J.; Manhas, A.; Jha, P.C.; Agarwal, S. Green and Highly Efficient MCR Strategy for the Synthesis of Pyrimidine Analogs in Water via C–C and C–N Bond Formation and Docking Studies. *Res. Chem. Intermed.* **2021**, *47*, 4477–4496. [CrossRef]
38. Adeyemo, A.; Kolawole, G.; Oderinde, R. A Cobalt(II) Complex of Vitamin B_1. *J. Coord. Chem.* **1986**, *15*, 181–184. [CrossRef]
39. Archibong, E.; Adeyemo, A.; Aoki, K.; Yamazaki, H. Thiamine-Metal Ion and Thiamine-Anion Interactions. Crystal Structure of Cu(Thiamine)Br_2. *Inorg. Chim. Acta* **1989**, *156*, 77–83. [CrossRef]
40. Hu, N.-H.; Aoki, K.; Adeyemo, A.O.; Williams, G.N. Metal Ion and Anion Coordination in the Thiamine–$[Pt^{II}(NO_2)_4]^{2-}$ System. Structures of a Metal Complex, Pt(Thiamine)$(NO_2)_3$, and Two Salts, (H-Thiamine)$[Pt(NO_2)_4]\cdot 2H_2O$ and (Thiamine Monophosphate)2$[Pt(NO_2)_4]\cdot 2H_2O$. *Inorg. Chim. Acta* **2001**, *325*, 9–19. [CrossRef]
41. Rajamanikandan, R.; Ilanchelian, M. Simple and Visual Approach for Highly Selective Biosensing of Vitamin B_1 Based on Glutathione Coated Silver Nanoparticles as a Colorimetric Probe. *Sens. Actuators B Chem.* **2017**, *244*, 380–386. [CrossRef]
42. Lin, L.; Wang, J.; Liu, W.; Luo, Y.; Xiao, Y.; Wang, Y. Rapid and Visual Readout of Vitamin B_1 Based on the Electrostatic Interaction Induced Aggregation of Gold Nanoparticles. *RSC Adv.* **2018**, *8*, 35850–35854. [CrossRef] [PubMed]
43. Maier, G.D.; Metzler, D.E. Structures of Thiamine in Basic Solution 1. *J. Am. Chem. Soc.* **1957**, *79*, 4386–4391. [CrossRef]
44. Bera, N.; Kiran Nandi, P.; Hazra, R.; Sarkar, N. Aggregation Induced Emission of Surface Ligand Controlled Gold Nanoclusters Employing Imidazolium Surface Active Ionic Liquid and PH Sensitivity. *J. Photochem. Photobiol. A Chem.* **2023**, *437*, 114471. [CrossRef]

45. Lukienko, P.I.; Mel'nichenko, N.G.; Zverinskii, I.V.; Zabrodskaya, S.V. Antioxidant Properties of Thiamine. *Bull. Exp. Biol. Med.* **2000**, *130*, 874–876. [CrossRef]
46. Gombár, G.; Ungor, D.; Samu, G.F.; Dömötör, O.; Csapó, E. Synthesis and Characterization of Novel Blue-Emitting Nicotinamide-Gold Nanoclusters with "Chain-Breaker" Antioxidant Property. *J. Mol. Liq.* **2022**, *359*, 119372. [CrossRef]
47. Higashi-Okai, K.; Nagino, H.; Yamada, K.; Okai, Y. Antioxidant and Prooxidant Activities of B Group Vitamins in Lipid Peroxidation. *J. UOEH* **2006**, *28*, 359–368. [CrossRef]
48. Valgimigli, L.; Baschieri, A.; Amorati, R. Antioxidant Activity of Nanomaterials. *J. Mater. Chem. B* **2018**, *6*, 2036–2051. [CrossRef]
49. Strambini, G.B.; Gabellieri, E. Phosphorescence Properties and Protein Structure Surrounding Tryptophan Residues in Yeast, Pig, and Rabbit Glyceraldehyde-3-Phosphate Dehydrogenase. *Biochemistry* **1989**, *28*, 160–166. [CrossRef]
50. Lakowicz, J.R. *Principles of Fluorescence Spectroscopy*, 3rd ed.; Lakowicz, J.R., Ed.; Springer: Boston, MA, USA, 2010; Volume 1961, ISBN 978-0-387-31278-1/978-0-387-46312-4.
51. Scatchard, G. The Attractions of Proteins for Small Molecules and Ions. *Ann. N. Y. Acad. Sci.* **1949**, *51*, 660–672. [CrossRef]
52. Sandu, N.; Chilom, C.G.; David, M.; Florescu, M. Evaluation of the Interaction of Levothyroxine with Bovine Serum Albumin Using Spectroscopic and Molecular Docking Studies. *J. Biomol. Struct. Dyn.* **2022**, *40*, 1139–1151. [CrossRef]
53. Shang, L.; Brandholt, S.; Stockmar, F.; Trouillet, V.; Bruns, M.; Nienhaus, G.U. Effect of Protein Adsorption on the Fluorescence of Ultrasmall Gold Nanoclusters. *Small* **2012**, *8*, 661–665. [CrossRef]
54. Shang, L.; Yang, L.; Seiter, J.; Heinle, M.; Brenner-Weiss, G.; Gerthsen, D.; Nienhaus, G.U. Nanoparticles Interacting with Proteins and Cells: A Systematic Study of Protein Surface Charge Effects. *Adv. Mater. Interfaces* **2014**, *1*, 1300079. [CrossRef]
55. Hosseinzadeh, R.; Khorsandi, K. Interaction of Vitamin B_1 with Bovine Serum Albumin Investigation Using Vitamin B_1-Selective Electrode: Potentiometric and Molecular Modeling Study. *J. Biomol. Struct. Dyn.* **2016**, *34*, 1903–1910. [CrossRef]
56. Mallappa, M.; Shivakumar, A.; Gowda, B.G.; Nageshbabu, R. Binding Study of Thiamine Hydrochloride to Bovine Serum Albumin: Spectroscopic and Molecular Modeling Methods. *J. Chem. Pharm. Res.* **2017**, *9*, 85–91.
57. Molodenskiy, D.; Shirshin, E.; Tikhonova, T.; Gruzinov, A.; Peters, G.; Spinozzi, F. Thermally Induced Conformational Changes and Protein–Protein Interactions of Bovine Serum Albumin in Aqueous Solution under Different PH and Ionic Strengths as Revealed by SAXS Measurements. *Phys. Chem. Chem. Phys.* **2017**, *19*, 17143–17155. [CrossRef]
58. Tian, Z.-Y.; Song, L.-N.; Zhao, Y.; Zang, F.-L.; Zhao, Z.-H.; Chen, N.-H.; Xu, X.-J.; Wang, C.-J. Spectroscopic Study on the Interaction between Naphthalimide-Polyamine Conjugates and Bovine Serum Albumin (BSA). *Molecules* **2015**, *20*, 16491–16523. [CrossRef]
59. Ross, P.D.; Subramanian, S. Thermodynamics of Protein Association Reactions: Forces Contributing to Stability. *Biochemistry* **1981**, *20*, 3096–3102. [CrossRef]
60. Wiseman, T.; Williston, S.; Brandts, J.F.; Lin, L.-N. Rapid measurement of binding constants and heats of binding using a new titration calorimeter. *Anal. Biochem.* **1989**, *179*, 131–137. [CrossRef]

antioxidants

MDPI

Article

Nanoemulsion Composed of α-Tocopherol Succinate and Dequalinium Shows Mitochondria-Targeting and Anticancer Effects

Le Thi Thuy [1], Seulgi Lee [2], Viet Dongquoc [3] and Joon Sig Choi [1,*]

[1] Department of Biochemistry, Chungnam National University, 99 Daehak-ro, Yuseong-gu, Daejeon 34134, Republic of Korea
[2] KM Science Research Division, Korea Institute of Oriental Medicine, Yuseong-daero 1672, Yuseong-gu, Daejeon 34054, Republic of Korea
[3] Department of Materials Science and Engineering, Chungnam National University, 99 Daehak-ro, Yuseong-gu, Daejeon 34134, Republic of Korea
* Correspondence: joonsig@cnu.ac.kr; Tel.: +82-42-821-7528; Fax: +82-42-822-7548

Abstract: Targeted drugs have been used to treat mitochondrial dysfunction-related diseases, including metabolic disorders and cancer; however, targeting and penetrating intracellular organelles remains a challenge. Dominant targeting approaches for therapeutic delivery are detailed in many nanoemulsion studies and show the tremendous potential of targeted delivery to inhibit cancer cell growth. Dequalinium (DQA) and α-tocopherol succinate (α-TOS) are good agents for targeting mitochondria. In this study, we aimed to develop a mitochondria-targeting emulsion, using DQA and α-TOS (DTOS), for cancer treatment. DTOS emulsions of 150–170 nm in diameter were formulated using homogenization. DQA and α-TOS were used as bifunctional agents (surfactants) to stabilize the nanoemulsion and anticancer drugs. Various molar ratios of DQA and α-TOS were tested to determine the optimal condition, and DTOS 5-5 was selected for further study. The DTOS emulsion showed improved stability, as evidenced by its ability to remain stable for three years at room temperature. This stability, combined with its effective targeting of mitochondria, led to inhibition of 71.5% of HeLa cells after 24 h. The DTOS emulsion effectively inhibited spheroid growth in the 3D model, as well as prevented the growth of HeLa cells grafted onto zebrafish larvae. These results highlight the DTOS emulsion's promising potential for mitochondria-targeting and cancer treatment.

Keywords: 3D spheroid; anticancer agent; dequalinium; nanoemulsion; tocopherol succinate

1. Introduction

Mitochondria are energy-generating machines of the cells. They play a critical role in metabolism, which involves various vital cell pathway processes [1–3]. Many of these processes relate to diseases, such as cancer; therefore, carriers or drugs that target the mitochondria may be an efficient therapy. The main impediment in mitochondria therapy for cancer treatment is the effective transport of the anticancer drug to the mitochondria because of the dependence on the physicochemical properties of the drug, such as size, solubility, and interaction with the plasma, to overcome the mitochondrial membrane [4]. Therefore, the development of utilitarian nanomaterials is crucial in the field of nanomedicine.

Nano-sized systems such as liposomes, micelles, and nanoemulsions have been explored to deliver drugs [5–8]. Nanoemulsion is the heterogeneous dispersion of two immiscible liquids (oil in water or water in oil) at the nanoscale. Surfactants, compounds with an amphiphilic profile, are used to reduce the interfacial tension between two immiscible phases and stabilize the system [9]. The stability of nanomedicine is one of the requirements of drug delivery [10]. Previous studies showed that emulsions can be stored for around 3–6 months at room temperature [11]. The emulsions do not have a sufficiently long shelf-life and they present destabilization mechanisms such as creaming, sedimentation, coalescence, and flocculation [12]. Using a polyelectrolyte nano-capsulate layer-by-layer around the solid template can protect the emulsion [13]. The secondary emulsions oil–water–oil (O/W/O) and water–oil–water (W/O/W) have been applied to improve the stability of the emulsion [14]. Another approach is using a high-pressure homogenizer to prepare emulsions together with a food-grade polymer to stabilize O/W nanoemulsions; however, the final colloidal systems presented a wide size distribution, predictably leading to fast destabilization [15]. The merger of relevant techniques and surfactants can provide a stable emulsion. Previous studies have also highlighted that emulsions are able to achieve an efficient therapeutic effect, and a poor-solubility anticancer agent can be loaded into the oil phase, which can cover the droplet for cell- or organ-targeting [16]. Ganta developed a folate nanoemulsion to deliver docetaxel to target ovarian cancer cells [17]. Moreover, lycopene emulsions have been used to treat human colon cancer cell lines (HT-29) [18], a taxoid prodrug in fish oil emulsion was found to be effective against prostate cancer [19], and methotrexate emulsion was more effective for leukemia than the free drug was [20]. In addition, emulsions have been used to treat breast cancer, melanoma, and lung cancer [21–23].

Dequalinium (DQA) is an amphiphilic component that has been explored as a mitochondrial moiety [24]. DQA can form a vesicular structure because of its amphiphilic structure and was reported to induce apoptosis in U373-MG and HeLa cells [25]. Therefore, drug delivery systems modified with DQA offer great promise in future cancer therapies. Recently, DQA was combined with other lipid components to form mitochondrial-targeted liposomes [26]. DQA liposomes easily transferred the drug to the mitochondria and improved the effectiveness of the drug. DQA can be modified directly to the polymer for polymersome formulation. Glycol chitosan–DQA was developed for curcumin delivery [27]. Therefore, DQA is a good candidate for an emulsion system targeted at the mitochondria. However, there are no studies about the use of DQA in emulsions.

Among the vitamin E derivatives, α-tocopherol succinate (α-TOS) shows the most attractiveness in cancer treatment. α-TOS is well-known as an antioxidant component. α-TOS can cause reactive oxygen species (ROS) and lead to cancer cell death [28]. Cancer cells express the antiapoptotic Bcl-2 and Bcl-xL. Bcl-2 can bind onto Bax, and this enables the survival of cancer cells by inhibiting cell apoptosis. Tocopherol succinate is able to block the BH3 domain of the Bcl-2 and Bcl-xl complex. Therefore, it decreases the binding of Bcl-2 on Bax protein. Depending on that mechanism, α-TOS is sensitive to cancer cells. In addition, α-TOS is a coenzyme Q10 inhibitor because it can bind to complex II in mitochondria [29]. Coenzyme Q10 is an electron carrier in mitochondria. However, this process is inhibited by α-TOS, which leads to the release of electrons in the cell. These unpaired electrons react with cellular oxygen to form various reactive oxygen species, causing cell death. Therefore, using α-TOS can improve the effectiveness of cancer treatment. Tocopherol succinate emulsion for paclitaxel has an effect on the human ovarian carcinoma cell line A2780/taxol. Guo et al. [30] reported that α-TOS is a nonionic surfactant with anticancer effects. Tocopherol succinate can inhibit the multidrug-resistant efflux pump P-glycoprotein [31]. Tocopherol succinate also supports vitamin K to produce apoptosis in cancer cells [32].

Harashima's group has demonstrated the potential of lipid-based formulations as a means of delivering poorly water-soluble drugs, with mitochondria-targeting being a promising therapeutic strategy [33–35]. To this end, we developed a novel nanoemulsion system using DQA and α-TOS as emulsifiers (DTOS emulsion) and anticancer agents. Figure 1 shows the representation of the DTOS emulsion's mechanism of cellular uptake and mitochondria-targeting. The high-pressure homogenization process was used to achieve mono-dispersion, and the combination of DQA and α-TOS was used to enhance stability. Various mole ratios of DQA and α-TOS were evaluated to determine the optimal conditions for encapsulation efficiency and stability. The DTOS 5-5 emulsion was selected for in-depth examination and its stability was found to be consistent for three years when stored at room temperature. The efficacy of its anticancer properties was also observed to be unchanged for three months. Treatment of HeLa cells with the DTOS emulsion resulted in increased cellular uptake and alteration of mitochondrial potential. This treatment led to over 70% inhibition of cell growth in cervical carcinoma (HeLa cells), breast cancer (MCF-7 cells), and murine melanoma (B16F10 cells). Furthermore, the DTOS emulsion demonstrated its anticancer potential in both 3D models (HeLa spheroid) and HeLa cells xenografted onto zebrafish larvae. These results suggest that the combination of DQA and α-TOS can be used to create a nanoemulsion for mitochondria-targeting in cancer therapy.

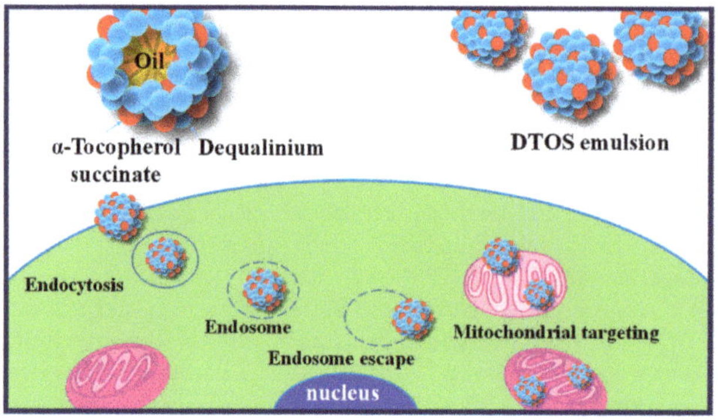

Figure 1. Illustration of the cellular uptake and mitochondria-targeting of the DTOS emulsion.

2. Materials and Methods

2.1. Materials

DQA chloride, castor oil, PEG-8 caprylic/capric glycerides, isopropyl myristate (IPM), lecithin, and N-(2-hydroxyethyl) piperazine-N′-2-ethanesulfonic acid (HEPES) were purchased from Sigma-Aldrich (St. Louis, MO, USA). Fetal bovine serum (FBS), 100× antibiotic-antimycotic agent and Dulbecco's modified Eagle's medium (DMEM) were purchased from GIBCO (Gaithersburg, MD, USA). HeLa, B16F10, and MCF-7 cell lines were obtained from the Korea Cell Line Bank (Seoul, Republic of Korea).

2.2. Control Emulsion

IPM, PEG-8 caprylic/capric glycerides, and lecithin were dissolved in a 20 mL bottle and sonicated for 15–20 min. Then, 10 mL of water was added, and the solution was sonicated again for 30 min to 1 h and homogenized for 2 h. Then, the solution was filtered with a 0.8 μm filter.

2.3. DQA Emulsion

DQA chloride 5 mM was dissolved in castor oil and sonicated for 15–20 min. Then, 10 mL of water was added, and the solution was sonicated again for 30 min to 1 h, and then the solution was homogenized. The solution was then filtered with a 0.8 μm filter.

2.4. DTOS Emulsion

DQA chloride and α-TOS were dissolved in castor oil and sonicated for 15–20 min. Then, 10 mL of water was added, and the solution was sonicated again for 30 min to 1 h, and then the solution was homogenized. The solution was then filtered with a 0.8 μm filter. The emulsion formulation process is shown in Figure 2.

2.5. Nile Red-Loaded Emulsion

DQA chloride, α-TOS, and Nile red were dissolved in castor oil and sonicated for 15–20 min. Then, 10 mL of water was added, and the solution was sonicated again for

30 min to 1 h, and then the solution was homogenized. The solution was then filtered with a 0.8 μm filter.

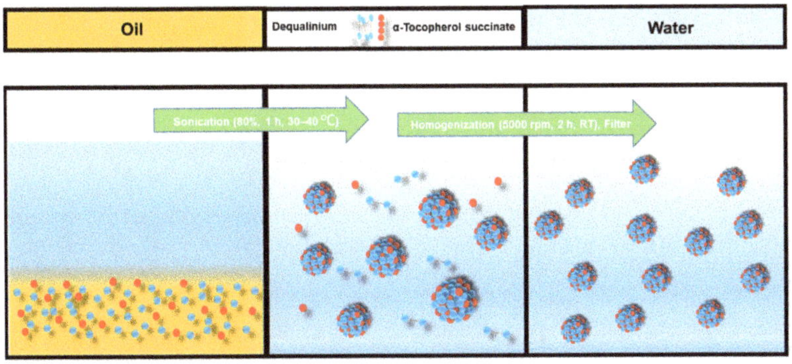

Figure 2. Emulsification process of DTOS emulsion.

2.6. Absorbance

Absorbance of the emulsion was detected using a UV-Vis spectrophotometer (Optizen POP; Mecasys, Daejeon, Republic of Korea). Methanol was used as a solvent for DQA, and the absorbance was found to be 330 nm for DQA and 290 nm for α-TOS.

2.7. Fourier Transform Infrared Spectrum (FTIR) Spectroscopy

The IR spectra of the DTOS emulsion, DQA, α-TOS, and their mixture were recorded using the FT-IR Nicolet™ iS™50 spectrometer. The spectra were acquired as an average of 64 spectra with a resolution of 4 cm^{-1}, and the dried state of the emulsion was placed into the holder for the analysis. The recording was performed in the spectral range of 600–4000 cm^{-1}.

2.8. Size and Zeta Potential

The size of the emulsion was measured using a Photal ELSZ particle size analyzer (Otsuka Electronics, Tokyo, Japan). Measurements were performed in triplicate and evaluated as the z-average (size). The surface charge of the emulsion was measured using a Zetasizer Nano ZS (Malvern Panalytical, Malvern, UK) at room temperature.

2.9. Stability of Emulsion over Time

The emulsions were kept at room temperature or in a refrigerator, and the size was measured using DLS at certain times.

2.10. Cell Uptake of Emulsion

HeLa cells (8×10^3 cells/well) were seeded in confocal dishes (μ-Slide 8 Well; ibidi, Fitchburg, WI, USA) and allowed to adhere in 270 μL of DMEM media (10% FBS and 1% (*w*/*v*) penicillin/streptomycin) at 37 °C in a humidified atmosphere of 5% CO_2 for 24 h. Then, cells were incubated with 30 μL of Nile red emulsion for 24 h. The medium was removed, cells were washed with Dulbecco's phosphate-buffered saline (DPBS) twice, and the nucleus was stained for 10 min with 200 μL of bisbenzimide (Hoechst 33342). The mitochondria were stained with 200 μL of MitoGreen (2 μM) for 20 min. Finally, cells were washed and observed using a Zeiss LSM 880 Live confocal laser microscope (Zeiss, Oberkochen, Germany).

2.11. Assessment of Mitochondrial Potential (ΔΨm) by JC-1 Staining

JC-1 (5, 59, 6, 69-tetrachloro-1, 19, 3, 39-tetraethylbenzimidazolcarbocyanine iodide) is a cationic dye used to target mitochondria. When a cell is healthy, JC-1 aggregated inside the mitochondria emit red fluorescence (590 ± 10 nm). However, when a cell is unhealthy, the mitochondrial potential is low, and the JC-1 monomers stay in the cytoplasm and emit green fluorescence (525 ± 10 nm). To assess the mitochondrial membrane potential of the DTOS emulsion, HeLa cells were seeded in confocal dishes (μ-Slide 8 Well; ibidi, Fitchburg, WI, USA) (8×10^3 cells/well) and allowed to adhere at 37 °C under 5% CO_2 for 24 h. Sample-treated (24 or 48 h) cells were then washed and incubated with 2 μM of JC-1 at 37 °C for 20 min. Cells were washed twice with DPBS, and analyzed using a Zeiss LSM 880 Live confocal laser microscope (Zeiss, Oberkochen, Germany).

2.12. Cell Viability

To determine the cell viability of the emulsions, a colorimetric WST-1 assay was performed. HeLa, B16F10, and MCF-7 cells were cultured in DMEM medium containing 10% (*v*/*v*) FBS and 1% (*w*/*v*) penicillin/streptomycin at 37 °C in a humidified atmosphere of 5% CO_2. Then, 1.3×10^4 cells/well were seeded in a 96-well plate and incubated in 90 μL of media for 24 h. Cells were then treated with 10 μL of DTOS emulsion along with the positive controls. After 24 h of incubation, 10 μL of EZ-Cytox reagent was added to each well (except for the negative control), incubated for 2 h, and the absorbance was measured at a 450 nm wavelength.

2.13. Anticancer Effect in 3D Spheroid Tumor Models

The anticancer effect of the DTOS emulsion was evaluated in 3D spheroid tumor models. The 3D spheroids were generated using a 1% agarose coating in a 96-well plate. Briefly, 0.2 g of agarose was dissolved in sterile distilled water and heated for 2 min in a microwave oven. Then, 100 μL of the homogenous agarose solution was quickly pipetted into the 96-well plate to coat a thin layer and left for 30 min to solidify. To form spheroids, 2×10^3 cells/well were seeded in agarose-coated 96-well plates and left undisturbed for 24 h at 37 °C under 5% CO_2. Spheroids were allowed to grow for 3 days, and samples were treated at different concentrations of DQA (0.6, 12.5, 25, 50, and 100 μM). The media in medium-containing samples were replaced every alternative day and spheroid growth was monitored. A spheroid without any treatment was used as a control.

2.14. Anticancer Effect in Zebrafish Models

Wildtype zebrafish were cultivated in a 28 °C incubator under a photoperiod of 10D/14L. Zebrafish eggs were maintained in salt water at 28 °C. After 48 hpf, dechorionated eggs were prepared in a Petri dish. To examine the toxicity of the DQA and DTOS emulsions, larvae were incubated with the samples, after which the number of surviving larvae were counted, and the morphology of the larvae was observed. We generated the zebrafish cancer models using the HeLa cell line for biodistribution and anticancer experiments. HeLa cells were stained using a cell fluorescence tracker (CellTracker™ Green CMFDA Dye, Invitrogen, Carlsbad, CA, USA) and injected into the yolk of larvae (48 hpf) using a microinjector (≈100 cells/larva for biodistribution and ≈150 cells/larva for anticancer). To determine the biodistribution, the xenografted larvae were incubated with 20 μM of Nile red-loaded DTOS 5-5 emulsion for 2 days. For the anticancer effect, the xenografted larvae were incubated with 30 μM of Nile red-loaded DTOS 5-5 emulsion for 3 days. After the incubation, the larvae were anesthetized using 0.04% tricaine and observed under a confocal microscope (Zeiss, Oberkochen, Germany).

2.15. Statistical Analysis

The results are expressed as mean ± SD. Statistical analysis (*p*-value) was performed using GraphPad Prism 5 (*t*-test and ANOVA). Differences between groups were considered statistically significant at $p < 0.001$ (***).

3. Results

3.1. Fabrication of DTOS Emulsion

Dequalinium and α-TOS formed an emulsion at different molar ratios (Table 1 and Figure 2). Based on the amount of the DQA and α-TOS, we prepared DTOS 1-9, DTOS 2-8, DTOS 3-7, DTOS 4-6, DTOS 5-5, DTOS 6-4, DTOS 7-3, DTOS 8-2, and DTOS 9-1 emulsions. The DTOS emulsions were obtained using a homogenizer, which is effective for generating emulsions with suspended droplets < 200 nm in diameter. All emulsions were formed at nano-size (around 150–170 nm) (Figure 3). The size distribution range was small, as demonstrated by the polydispersity index (PDI) value, where a PDI value < 0.2 represented a monodispersed droplet size distribution. The results implied that we successfully created a homogeneous nanoemulsion containing DQA, α-TOS, and castor oil using a homogenizer. The encapsulation efficiency of DQA and α-TOS was evaluated using a standard curve (Figure S1, Supplementary Materials). DTOS 5-5 was the best ratio for the emulsion formulation with a high DQA and α-TOS encapsulation efficiency (Table 1). The higher the DQA concentration, the higher the encapsulation efficiency of α-TOS. This may be due to the surfactant property of DQA.

Table 1. Encapsulation efficiency of DQA and α-TOS emulsions.

	DQA (mM):α-TOS (mM):Castor Oil (%)	DQA Encapsulation Efficiency (%)	α-TOS Encapsulation Efficiency (%)
DTOS 1-9	1:9:3	98.7	11.7
DTOS 2-8	2:8:3	89.1	36.8
DTOS 3-7	3:7:3	54.9	28.2
DTOS 4-6	4:6:3	58.8	43.3
DTOS 5-5	5:5:3	99.6	99.6
DTOS 6-4	6:4:3	75.2	91.9
DTOS 7-3	7:3:3	96.4	96.9
DTOS 8-2	8:2:3	83.8	99.9
DTOS 9-1	9:1:3	71.7	99.1

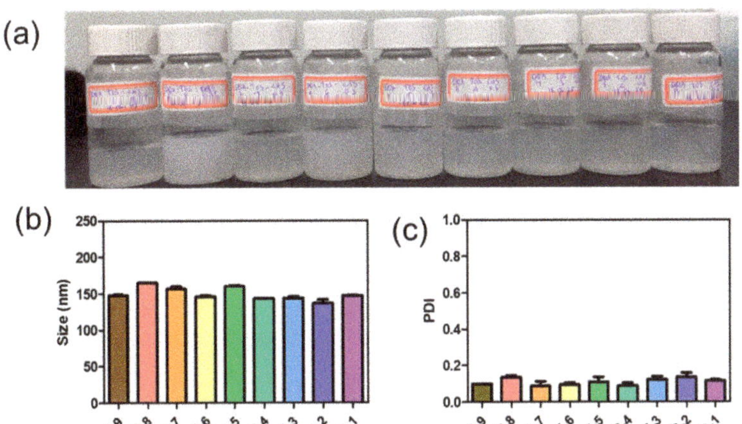

Figure 3. (**a**) Digital photograph of the dequalinium (DQA) and α-tocopherol succinate (α-TOS) (DTOS) emulsions after preparation. (**b**) Dynamic light scattering (DLS)-measured diameter of the DTOS emulsion after preparation. (**c**) Polydispersity index (PDI) of the DTOS emulsion after preparation. The data are presented as the mean value ± standard deviation of triplicate experiments.

3.2. Characterization of Emulsion

The confirmation of the emulsion component was evaluated using UV-Vis absorbance. DQA had an absorbance at 330 nm and α-TOS had an absorbance at 290 nm (Figure 4a). The DTOS 5-5 emulsion presented both peaks of α-TOS and DQA. The FTIR results showed the presence of DQA and α-TOS in the emulsion (Figure 4b), providing confirmation of the successful production of the DTOS emulsion. The shape, size, and surface charge of the nanoparticle are important factors for nanomedicine. The spherical nanoemulsion was detected using field emission scanning electron microscopy (Figure 4c). The DQA and DTOS 5-5 emulsion sizes were 208.4 ± 3.36 and 155.8 ± 0.9, which were smaller than the control IPM emulsion (435.67 ± 30.17 nm). The surface charges of the emulsions were determined: the control emulsion had a negative charge (−4.2 ± 0.4 mV), and the DQA and DTOS 5-5 emulsions had a positive charge (42.77 ± 3.34 and 34.4 ± 4.2) (Table 2). The positive charge of the emulsion may enhance its binding to cancer cells, facilitating intracellular targeted delivery [36]. These data are promising for cancer treatment. Nanoemulsions can easily target the tumor side due to the enhanced permeability and retention effect. The positive charge around the DTOS 5-5 emulsion facilitates interaction with the cell membrane.

Table 2. Size and zeta potential of dequalinium (DQA) emulsion and α-TOS/DQA 5-5 emulsion (DTOS 5-5).

	Zeta Potential (mV)	Size (nm)	PDI
Control emulsion	−4.23 ± 0.37	435.67 ± 30.17	0.39 ± 0.01
DQA	42.77 ± 3.34	208.40 ± 3.36	0.17 ± 0.01
DTOS 5-5	34.40 ± 4.22	155.83 ± 0.85	0.15 ± 0.01

3.3. Stability of Emulsion

The emulsions were stored at room temperature. The size was confirmed at a certain time using an ELS-Z particle size analyzer (Otsuka Electronics, Otsuka, Japan). Figure 5 shows the stability of the emulsions depending on the amount of the DQA and α-TOS. The emulsion containing only DQA and castor oil (DQA emulsion) was not stable, and its size changed after 2 weeks, and the PDI value also increased. This indicates that the DQA emulsion cannot avoid the aggregation of oil droplets after forming nanoparticles. α-TOS plays an important role of a co-surfactant in stabilizing the emulsion, which is a good indicator for the application of our emulsion. The sizes of DTOS 3-7, DTOS 4-6, DTOS 5-5, DTOS 6-4, and DTOS 7-3 emulsions were stable for over two years at room temperature (Figure 5a). However, the PDI value of DTOS 5-5 was the most stable (Figure 5b). Therefore, the DTOS 5-5 emulsion was selected for further experiments. The HeLa cells were tested for the anticancer effect of DTOS 5-5 when fresh and after storage at room temperature for 1 and 3 months. Figure S2 revealed that the bioactivity was consistently similar, implying the stability of the emulsion. However, the DTOS 5-5 emulsion was not stable at 4 °C (Figure 5c). The DQAsome has been demonstrated to be unstable under low temperatures. The mechanism of emulsion stability has been unclear until now. The combination of DQA and α-TOS increased the stability of the emulsion, leading to improved potential in nanomedicine applications.

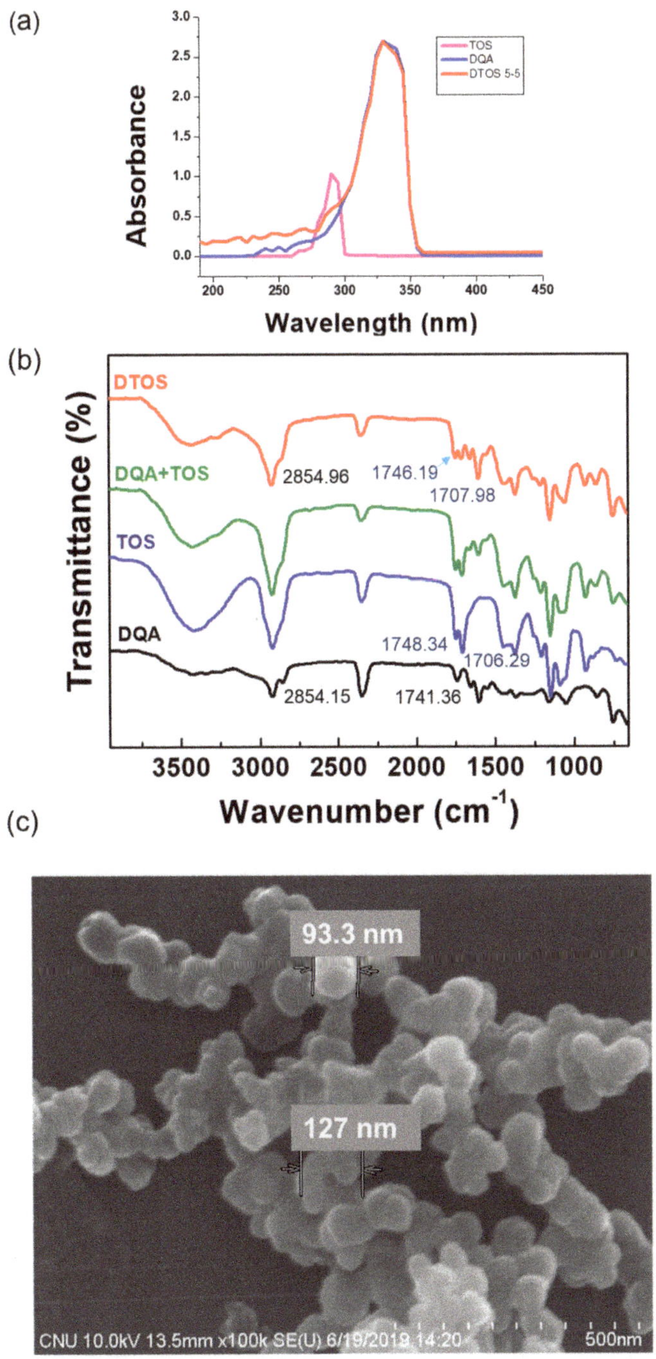

Figure 4. (**a**) UV-Vis absorption spectra of α-TOS, DQA, and DTOS emulsions. (**b**) FTIR spectra of α-TOS, DQA, the mixture of DQA and α-TOS, and DTOS emulsions. (**c**) Field emission scanning electron microscopy of DTOS 5-5.

3.4. Nile Red-Loaded Emulsion, Cell Uptake, and Mitochondria-Targeting

Nile red was used as a fluorescence model and was loaded into the emulsions and characterized. The Nile red emulsion was incubated with HeLa cells for 24 h. Mitochondria were stained with mitogen. The nucleus was stained with Hoechst dye and imaged using confocal laser scanning microscopy (Figure 6). The red fluorescence showed the location of the emulsion and the nanoemulsion produced a high-intensity red color, indicating that the emulsion can be taken up inside the cell membrane. The positive surface charge of nanoemulsion supports that it can effectively interact with the cell membrane, which is the first step of the endocytosis pathway. In addition, the Nile red emulsion can be localized at the mitochondria, where we can find the yellow color in the cells. The DQA and DTOS emulsions were both found to be able to efficiently target the mitochondria.

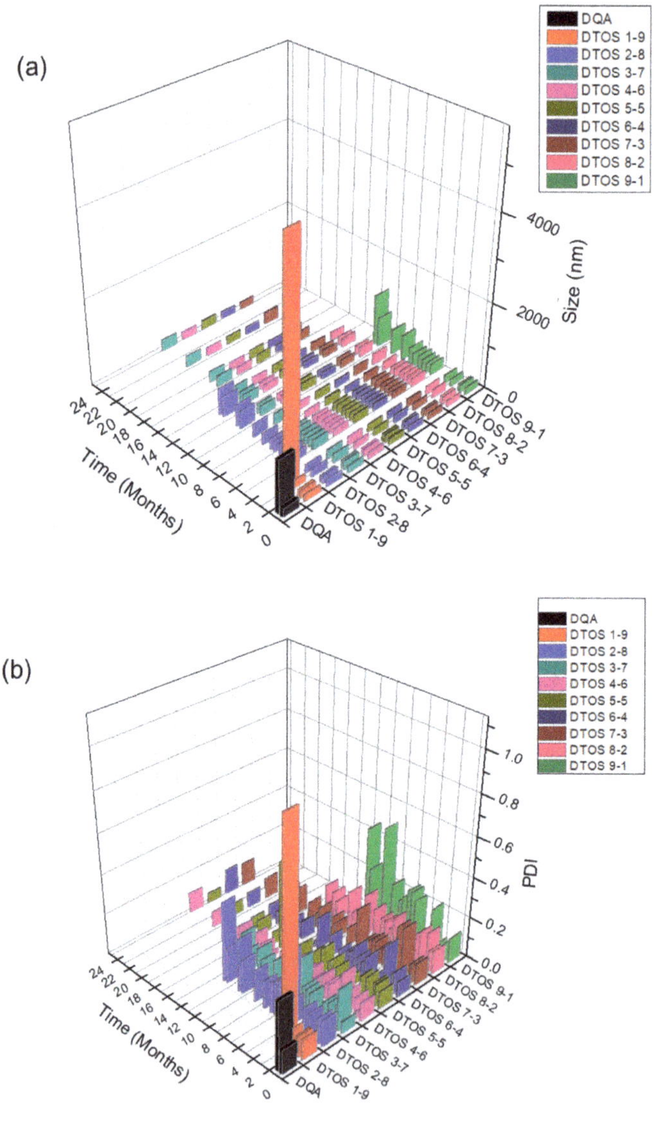

Figure 5. *Cont.*

(c)

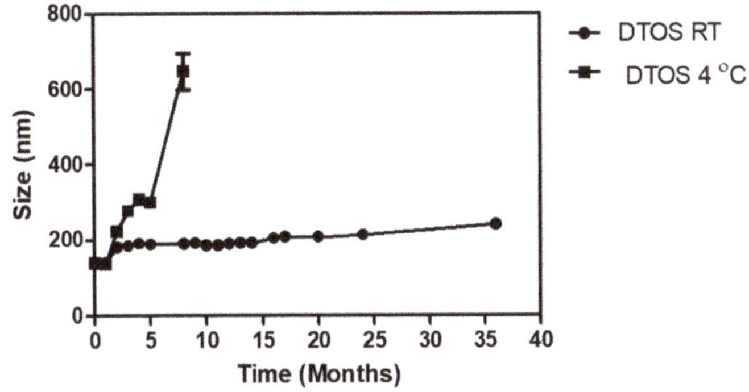

Figure 5. The stability of the DTOS emulsion. (**a**) Mean DLS diameter of the DTOS emulsion at a defined time. (**b**) Mean polydispersity index of the DTOS emulsion at a defined time. (**c**) DTOS emulsion stability under different temperatures at a specified time. The data are presented as the mean value ± standard deviation of triplicate experiments.

(a)

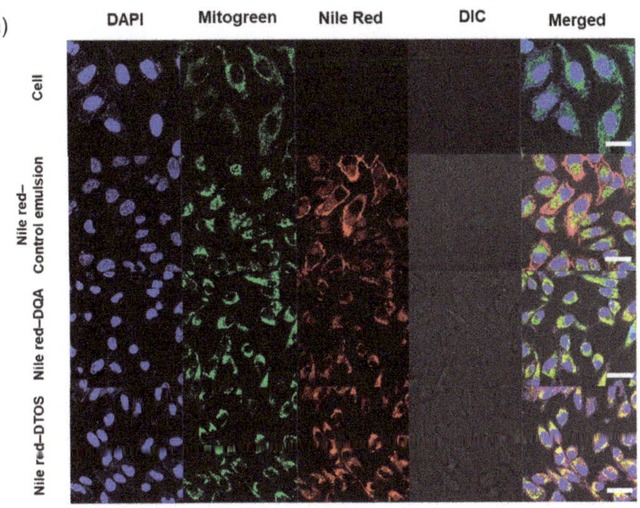

(b)

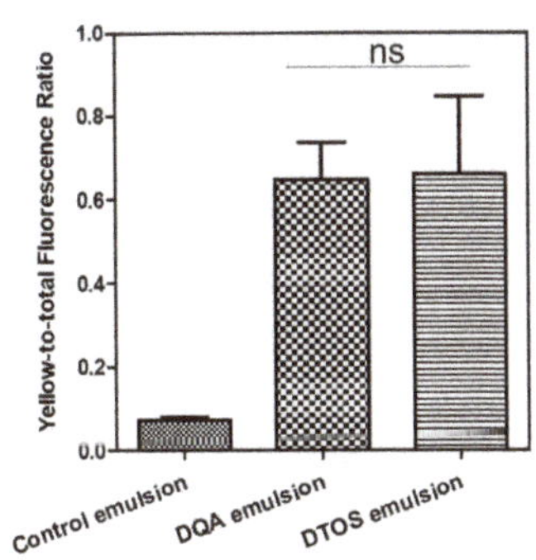

Figure 6. (**a**) Confocal laser scanning microscopy images of HeLa cells after 24 h of incubation with the Nile red emulsion. Labeled nanoparticles are shown in red (Nile red). The mitochondria are

stained with MitoGreen. The cell nucleus is stained blue by 4′,6-diamidino-2-phenylindole (DAPI). DIC, differential interference contrast; DQA, dequalinium emulsion; DTOS, DQA/α-TOS emulsion. The scale bar represents 30 μm. (**b**) The DTOS emulsion showed significant colocalization with mitochondria comparable to the DQA emulsion. Data points are represented as mean ± SD (n = 3 images for each group). Statistical analysis was conducted using *t*-test. ns: not significant. The scale bar represents 30 μm.

3.5. Mitochondrial Membrane Potential

HeLa cells were treated either with the DQA emulsion or the DTOS 5-5 emulsion. Mitochondrial oxidative phosphorylation uncoupler (CCCP), which has low potential, was used as a positive control. Then, the fluorescent probe JC-1 was added. The data showed a decreased red (~590 nm) to green (~529 nm) fluorescence intensity ratio in response to both DQA and DTOS emulsion exposure in relation to mitochondria depolarization, which is clearly observable in the fluorescence images. The results also showed that the impact of the DQA emulsion was less than that of the DTOS emulsion (Figure 7).

(a)

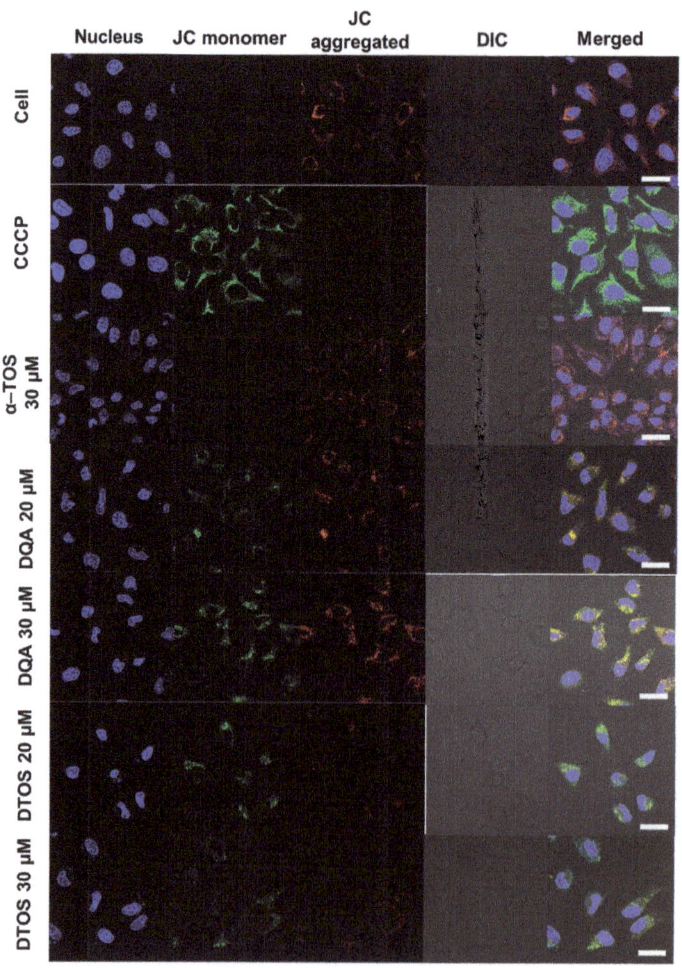

Figure 7. *Cont.*

(b)

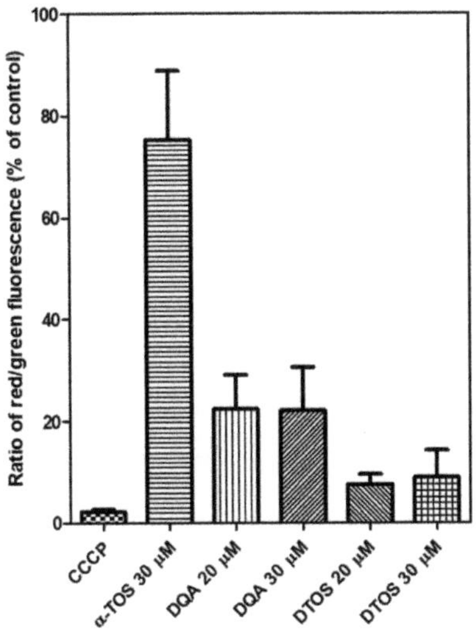

Figure 7. Assay of HeLa cell mitochondrial membrane potential with the JC-1 probe staining method. (**a**) Depolarization of mitochondrial membrane potential was observed after the cells were exposed to the emulsion, for 24 h, with CCCP as the positive control. (**b**) Quantitative analysis of the ratio of red/green fluorescence intensity. Results of the red and green fluorescence are overlapped and expressed as the mean ± standard deviation of triplicates. DIC, differential interference contrast; DQA, dequalinium emulsion; α-TOS, α-tocopherol succinate; DTOS, DQA/α-TOS emulsion. The scale bar represents 30 μm.

3.6. Cell Viability

The cytotoxicity effects of DTOS 5-5 were evaluated in HeLa cells using a WST-1 assay. Figure 8 shows that the DQA and DTOS 5-5 emulsions had an anticancer effect on the HeLa cells. Moreover, the DTOS emulsion caused toxicity in the B16F10 and MCF-7 cells (Figure S3). Previous studies have shown that DQA has the ability to inhibit cancer cell growth [25]. Dequalinium has a positive charge and hydrophobic head. It may cause a high interaction with the cell membrane and destroy the stability of the cell membrane. In other words, the accumulation of a high concentration of DQA inside the mitochondria can produce impaired mitochondria. In addition, the presence of α-TOS can improve the accumulation of DQA, increasing the impairment of the mitochondria and even causing cell death.

3.7. 3D Spheroid

A 3D spheroid model was formed by seeding HeLa cells in agarose-coated 96-well plates, and single spheroids were successfully grown for 3 days before sample treatment. The spheroids acquired a spheroid shape and became darker over time owing to the increase in the cell population. The morphology and size of the spheroids were monitored, followed by sample treatment. Interestingly, as shown in Figure 9, the DTOS 5-5-exposed spheroid showed peripheral cell damage. Compared to a 2D culture, where DTOS 5-5 effects are noticeable within 24 h of treatment, 3D models provide a closer insight into tumors where drug penetration and availability are limited due to their dense core and rigid extracellular matrix. These results suggest that 3D organization and tissue formation make tumors more resistant and predominantly complex compared to 2D culture models when therapeutic drugs are tested.

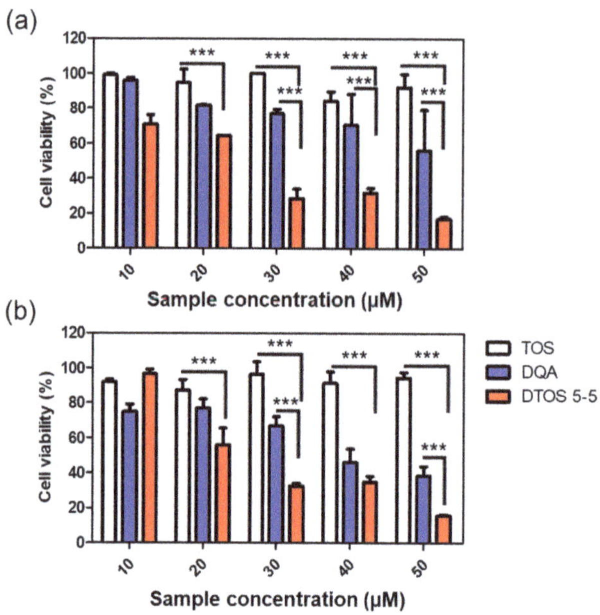

Figure 8. Cell viability of α-TOS, DQA, and DTOS 5-5 emulsions at different concentrations measured in HeLa cells at (**a**) 24 and (**b**) 48 h. Data points are represented as mean ± SD of four individual copies. Statistical analysis of data was conducted by one-way ANOVA with Tukey's post-hoc test. Differences between groups were considered statistically significant at $p < 0.001$ (***).

3.8. Zebrafish Animal Experiments

Human cancer cell xenografts in zebrafish larvae are a helpful preclinical tool in oncology research. Before evaluating the anticancer effect of the DTOS 5-5 emulsion, we examined its toxicity on the larvae. The larvae (48 h post-fertilization (hpf)) were incubated with various concentrations of the samples (10 μM to 50 μM) and observed at 72 and 96 h post-injection to record the number of alive larvae. α-TOS and DQA were used as the controls. Figure 10a showed that the α-TOS was safe for larvae even though they were treated at a high concentration. However, the DTOS 5-5 emulsion caused toxicity for larvae owing to the addition of DQA. The positive charge may interact with the fish, causing death. DTOS 5-5 doses of 10–30 μM were found to be safe for larvae. Moreover, DTOS 5-5 showed an anticancer effect at 30 μM in vitro. Therefore, we selected this concentration for further study. DTOS 5-5 at 30 μM was used to evaluate the toxicity of larvae for a certain time. The survival ratio of larvae was 80% at 96 dpi, while the DQA caused more toxicity. The morphology of the larvae was evaluated. We performed confocal laser scanning microscopy analysis to determine the biodistribution of the cancer cells and emulsion in the zebrafish larvae. We observed the HeLa cells as green and the emulsion as red. Figure 11a indicates that the cancer cell grew well on the larvae. The emulsion became distributed throughout the fish's body. The yellow color in the merged picture indicates the colocalization of cells and emulsions. The anticancer effect was then evaluated with DTOS 5-5, 30 μM. After the xenografted model was successfully prepared, the xenografted larvae were incubated with the DTOS 5-5 emulsion for 3 days. The local cancer cells were captured. Figure 11b shows that the DTOS 5-5 emulsion inhibited the growth of the HeLa cells on the larvae. The fluorescence intensity of the cell tracker-labeled HeLa cells in the zebrafish larvae was analyzed using Image J. Less fluorescence was found in the case of the DTOS 5-5 emulsion compared to that in the controls (Figure 11c), demonstrating the strong anticancer effect of the DTOS 5-5 emulsion.

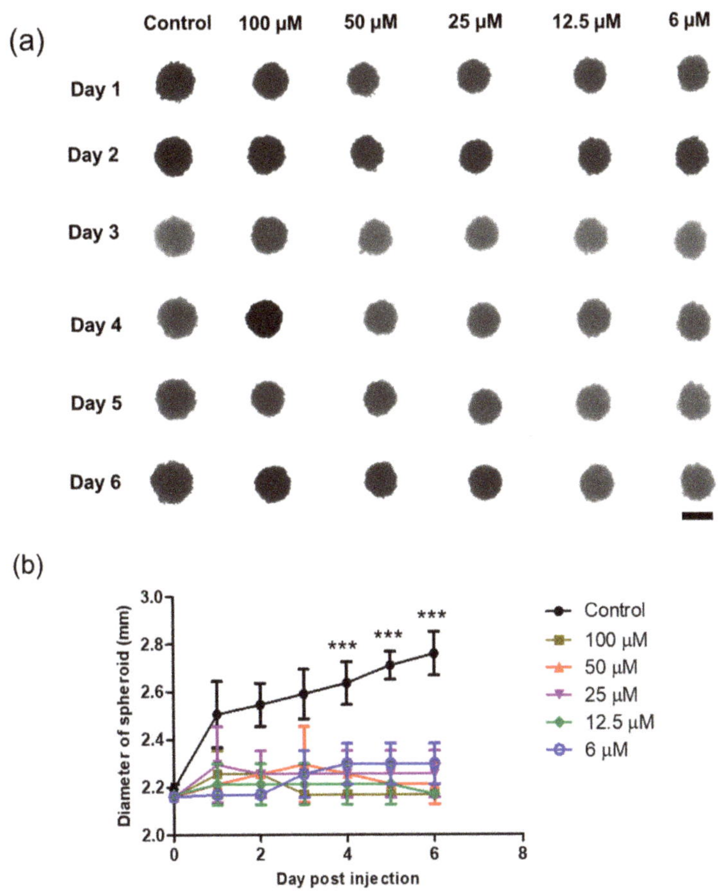

Figure 9. Three-dimensional spheroid study of the DTOS 5-5 emulsion. (**a**) Morphology and (**b**) diameter of spheroids. The scale bar represents 2.30 mm. A significant difference was observed between the emulsion treatment group (25 μM) and the control group. Data points are represented as mean ± SD of three individual copies. Statistical analysis of data was conducted using *t*-test (***, $p < 0.001$).

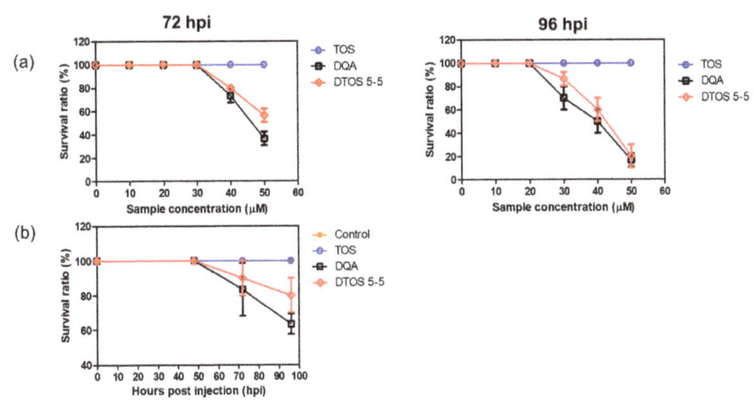

Figure 10. *Cont.*

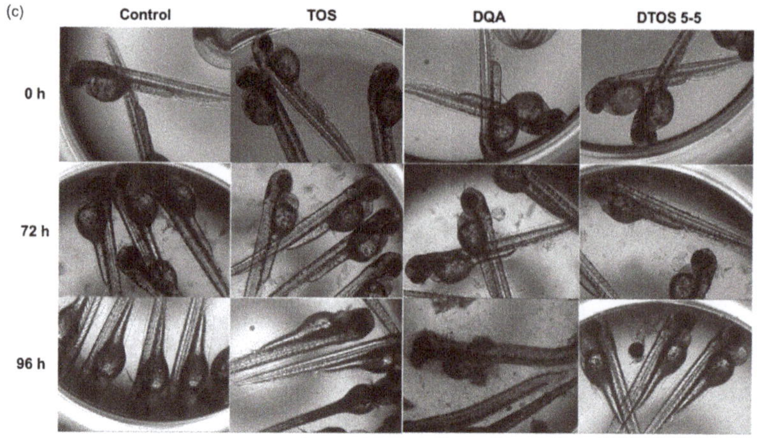

Figure 10. Evaluation of the in vivo toxicity of dequalinium (DQA) and α-tocopherol succinate (α-TOS) (DTOS) emulsions in zebrafish larvae. (**a**) The survival ratio of zebrafish larvae after treatment with various concentrations of samples at 72 and 96 hpi. Each value represents the average and standard deviation (n = 3). (**b**) The survival ratio of zebrafish larvae after treatment with 30 μM at a certain time. Each value represents the average and standard deviation (n = 3). (**c**) The morphology of the embryos after treatment with 30 μM of samples at a certain time. hpf, hours post-fertilization.

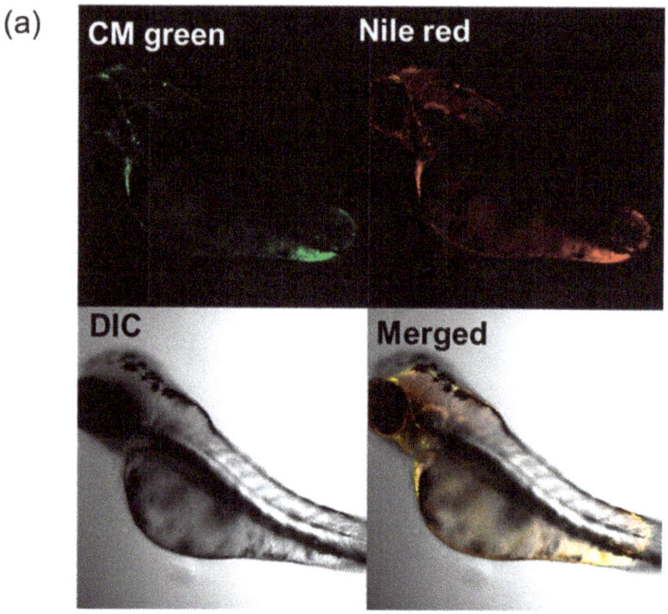

Figure 11. *Cont.*

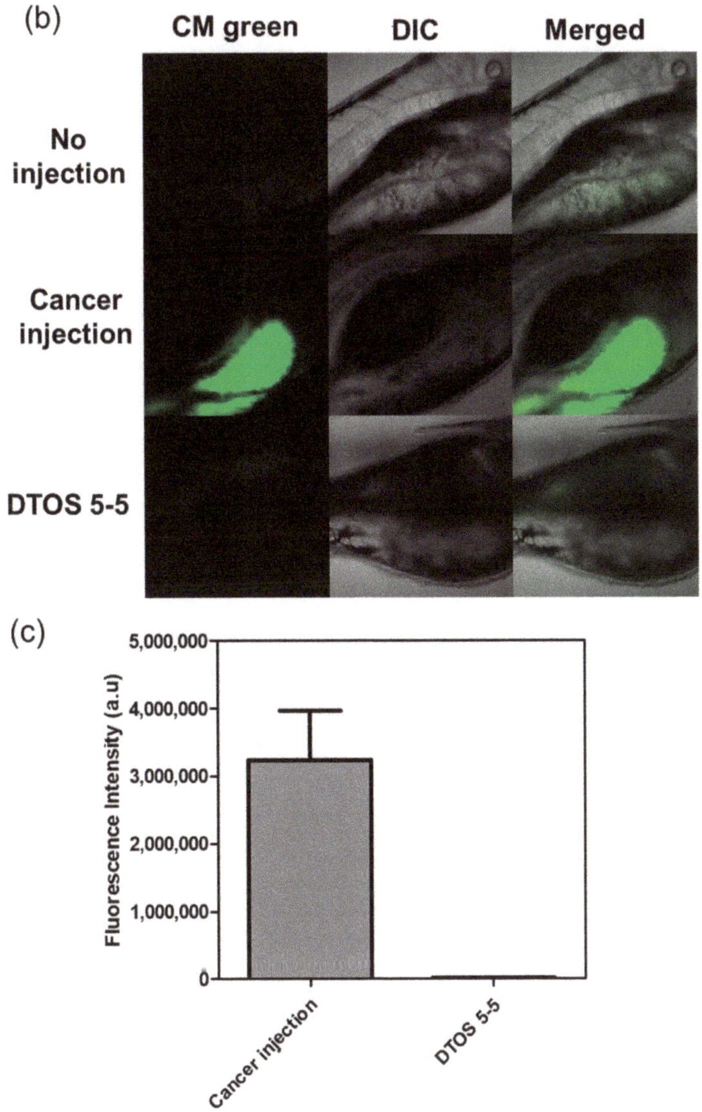

Figure 11. HeLa cells xenografted onto zebrafish larvae. (**a**) Colocalization of the emulsion and cancer cells. (**b**) Anticancer effect of the emulsion on the HeLa cells xenografted onto zebrafish larvae. (**c**) Fluorescence intensity of cell-tracker-labeled HeLa cells in zebrafish larvae. Each value presents the average and standard deviation (n = 3). DIC, differential interference contrast; hpf, hours post-fertilization; hpi, hours post-injection.

4. Discussion

Castor oil, which has been used as folk medicine since Ancient Egyptian times [37], was chosen as the oil phase. The castor oil is hydrolyzed in the small intestine by pancreatic enzymes, which results in the release of glycerol and ricinoleic acid, although 3,6-epoxyoctanedioic acid, 3,6-epoxydecanedioic acid, and 3,6-epoxydodecanedioic acid also appear as metabolites [38]. Castor oil and ricinoleic acid easily penetrate deep into the skin and enhance the transdermal penetration of other chemicals [39]. Among the different mitochondria-targeting moieties, DQA is suitable for emulsion emulsifiers due to its amphiphilic property. Moreover, α-TOS as a co-component can improve the effects of anticancer treatment. It has numerous important roles in the body and cells because of its antioxidant activity. Oxidants have been linked to numerous possible conditions and diseases, including cancer.

Herein, we explored whether the combination of castor oil, DQA, and α-TOS is suitable for anticancer effects. The stability of the emulsion is related to the concentration of DQA and α-TOS. We found that the range of each component from 3 mM to 7 mM is perfect for the stability of the DTOS emulsion at RT (Table 1 and Figure 5). α-TOS contributed to this characterization of the emulsion. The DQA emulsion was found unstable (data not shown). The stability mechanism is still ambiguous. We hypothesized that it is related to the surfactant ability of DQA. The size of the emulsion is small, which facilitates passing the enhanced permeability and retention (EPR) effect to reach the tumor site (Figure 3). The positive charge of the emulsion is good to interact with cell membranes (Table 2); however, it may be a disadvantage of our emulsion due to the interaction with plasma protein. The surface modification of the DTOS emulsion is needed in further studies. The cell uptake data showed that the DTOS emulsion can be located in the mitochondria (Figure 6). Moreover, mitochondria membrane potential has been considered the master signal between cell death and survival. Lipophilic cations can accumulate inside the inner membrane of the mitochondria and reduce the membrane potential. Previous reports have shown that anti-apoptotic signals from the cancer cell arise from the impairment of the mitochondrial membrane potential [40]. Therefore, to understand the mechanism of cell death related to mitochondria, the mitochondrial membrane potential needs to be confirmed. The JC-1 probe can be used to evaluate the mitochondrial potential. When the membrane potential is low, the JC-1 probe is not taken up by the mitochondria and is present in the cytoplasm as a fluorescent green monomer rather than being taken up and forming a fluorescent red aggregate when the mitochondrial membrane potential is intact. Our data showed that the mitochondrial membrane potential was low in the case of the DQA and DTOS emulsions (Figure 7). This may be a cause of cell death. In addition, the cell viability results demonstrated cell death after being treated with the DTOS emulsion (Figure 8).

The 3D tumor spheroids are universally used for drug screening and have recently obtained noticeable attention in cancer therapy for the study of cancer cell-to-cell communication, invasion, and drug resistance mechanisms [41]. Three-dimensional spheroid tumor models reportedly have better potential to mimic in vivo tumor environments than 2D culture models; therefore, we modeled the anticancer effects of DTOS 5-5 in a 3D tumor spheroid (Figure 9 and Figure S4). In 2D models, cancer cells are equally exposed to cytotoxic drugs, which do not sufficiently mimic the complexity of in vivo tumors. In contrast, 3D tumor models possess several features, such as drug penetration, hypoxia, and an extracellular matrix, that could shorten the gap between 2D testing and animal models. For the in vivo application, the zebrafish larvae were used as a model to evaluate the ability of the emulsion on anticancer effects. The cancer cells were xenografted on the larvae and then treated with the emulsion. The DTOS emulsion can enter and distribute inside the zebrafish larvae and inhibit cancer cell growth (Figure 11).

5. Conclusions

Here, we reported the fabrication of a mitochondria-targeting emulsion containing DQA and α-TOS. The resulting nanoemulsion, termed DTOS, was a homogenous emulsion shown to be 150–170 nm in diameter and stable for a long time at room temperature. After testing different ratios, the DTOS 5-5 emulsion was chosen as the agent for further study. The DTOS 5-5 emulsion can target mitochondria and reduce the mitochondrial membrane potential. It can inhibit the cell proliferation of cancer in both 2D and 3D models, as well as in cell xenografts on zebrafish larvae. Our results highlight that a straightforward combination of DQA and α-TOS is a beneficial combination for emulsion formulation that should be further researched for its positive potential in nanomedicine applications.

Supplementary Materials: The following supporting information can be downloaded at: https://www.mdpi.com/article/10.3390/antiox12020437/s1. DQA and α-Tos encapsulation efficiency. Figure S1: The standard curve of (a) DQA at 330 nm, (b) DQA at 290 nm and (c) α-TOS at 290 nm.; Figure S2: Measurement of HeLa cell viability after 24 hours of exposure to 30 μM DTOS 5-5 emulsion stored at room temperature for the specified period.; Figure S3: Cell viability of DTOS 5-5 emulsion at varying concentrations measured in MDA-MB-231, MCF-7, B16F10 cells at (a) 24 and (b) 48 h; Figure S4: The magnification of the spheroid after treatment with DTOS emulsion on day 6.

Author Contributions: Conceptualization, L.T.T. and J.S.C.; methodology, S.L. and V.D.; software, L.T.T. and S.L.; validation, L.T.T. and J.S.C.; formal analysis, S.L. and L.T.T.; investigation, S.L. and L.T.T.; resources, S.L., V.D. and L.T.T.; data curation, L.T.T. and V.D.; writing—original draft preparation, L.T.T., S.L. and V.D.; writing—review and editing, L.T.T. and J.S.C.; visualization, V.D. and L.T.T.; supervision, J.S.C.; project administration, J.S.C.; funding acquisition, J.S.C. All authors have read and agreed to the published version of the manuscript.

Funding: This research was supported by the Bio & Medical Technology Development Program of the National Research Foundation (NRF), funded by the Korean government (MSIT) (NRF-2018M3A9B5024060, NRF-2018M3A9B5024068, and 2022M3E5F1081315).

Institutional Review Board Statement: All zebrafish experiments were carried out in compliance with approved guidelines and regulations of the Animal Ethics Committee of Chungnam National University (CNU00160).

Informed Consent Statement: Not applicable.

Data Availability Statement: Data are contained within the article and the Supplementary Materials.

Acknowledgments: The authors sincerely thank Hye Won Park and Jeil Lee for their helpful discussion and assistance.

Conflicts of Interest: The authors declare no conflict of interest.

References

1. Yan, W.H.; Diao, S.; Fan, Z.P. The role and mechanism of mitochondrial functions and energy metabolism in the function regulation of the mesenchymal stem cells. *Stem Cell Res. Ther.* **2021**, *12*, 140. [CrossRef] [PubMed]
2. Abel, E.D. Mitochondrial Dynamics and Metabolic Regulation in Cardiac and Skeletal Muscle. *Trans. Am. Clin. Climatol. Assoc.* **2018**, *129*, 266–278.
3. Bhatti, J.S.; Bhatti, G.K.; Reddy, P.H. Mitochondrial dysfunction and oxidative stress in metabolic disorders—A step towards mitochondria based therapeutic strategies. *Biochim. Biophys. Acta (BBA)-Mol. Basis Dis.* **2017**, *1863*, 1066–1077. [CrossRef] [PubMed]
4. Dhanasekaran, S.; Venugopal, D.; Al-Dayan, N.; Ravinayagam, V.; Mohammed, A.A. Emerging insights into mitochondria-specific targeting and drug delivering strategies: Recent milestones and therapeutic implications. *Saudi J. Biol. Sci.* **2020**, *27*, 3581–3592. [CrossRef]
5. Patra, J.K.; Das, G.; Fraceto, L.F.; Campos, E.V.R.; Rodriguez-Torres, M.D.P.; Acosta-Torres, L.S.; Diaz-Torres, L.A.; Grillo, R.; Swamy, M.K.; Sharma, S.; et al. Nano based drug delivery systems: Recent developments and future prospects. *J. Nanobiotechnol.* **2018**, *16*, 71. [CrossRef]
6. Liu, Y.; Castro Bravo, K.M.; Liu, J. Targeted liposomal drug delivery: A nanoscience and biophysical perspective. *Nanoscale Horiz.* **2021**, *6*, 78–94. [CrossRef]
7. Bose, A.; Roy Burman, D.; Sikdar, B.; Patra, P. Nanomicelles: Types, properties and applications in drug delivery. *IET Nanobiotechnol.* **2021**, *15*, 19–27. [CrossRef]
8. Anwer, M.K.; Aldawsari, M.F.; Iqbal, M.; Almutairy, B.K.; Soliman, G.A.; Aboudzadeh, M.A. Diosmin-Loaded Nanoemulsion-Based Gel Formulation: Development, Optimization, Wound Healing and Anti-Inflammatory Studies. *Gels* **2023**, *9*, 95. [CrossRef]
9. Patel, M.R.; Patel, R.B.; Thakore, S.D. *Applications of Nanocomposite Materials in Drug Delivery*, 1st ed.; Woodhead Publishing: Cambridge, UK, 2018; pp. 667–700. ISBN 9780128137413. [CrossRef]
10. Dordevic, S.; Gonzalez, M.M.; Conejos-Sanchez, I.; Carreira, B.; Pozzi, S.; Acurcio, R.C.; Satchi-Fainaro, R.; Florindo, H.F.; Vicent, M.J. Current hurdles to the translation of nanomedicines from bench to the clinic. *Drug Deliv. Transl. Res.* **2022**, *12*, 500–525. [CrossRef]

11. Ostbring, K.; Matos, M.; Marefati, A.; Ahlstrom, C.; Gutierrez, G. The Effect of pH and Storage Temperature on the Stability of Emulsions Stabilized by Rapeseed Proteins. *Foods* **2021**, *18*, 1657. [CrossRef]
12. Ravera, F.; Dziza, K.; Santini, E.; Cristofolini, L.; Liggieri, L. Emulsification and emulsion stability: The role of the interfacial properties. *Adv. Colloid Interface Sci.* **2021**, *288*, 102344. [CrossRef] [PubMed]
13. Mateos-Maroto, A.; Abelenda-Nunez, I.; Ortega, F.; Rubio, R.G.; Guzman, E. Polyelectrolyte Multilayers on Soft Colloidal Nanosurfaces: A New Life for the Layer-By-Layer Method. *Polymers* **2021**, *13*, 1221. [CrossRef]
14. Tenorio-Garcia, E.; Araiza-Calahorra, A.; Simone, E.; Sarkar, A. Recent advances in design and stability of double emulsions: Trends in Pickering stabilization. *Food Hydrocoll.* **2022**, *128*, 107601. [CrossRef]
15. Procopio, A.; Lagreca, E.; Jamaledin, R.; La Manna, S.; Corrado, B.; Di Natale, C.; Onesto, V. Recent Fabrication Methods to Produce Polymer-Based Drug Delivery Matrices (Experimental and In Silico Approaches). *Pharmaceutics* **2022**, *15*, 872. [CrossRef] [PubMed]
16. Kalepu, S.; Nekkanti, V. Insoluble drug delivery strategies: Review of recent advances and business prospects. *Acta Pharm. Sin. B* **2015**, *5*, 442–453. [CrossRef] [PubMed]
17. Ganta, S.; Singh, A.; Rawal, Y.; Cacaccio, J.; Patel, N.R.; Kulkarni, P.; Ferris, C.F.; Amiji, M.M.; Coleman, T.P. Formulation development of a novel targeted theranostic nanoemulsion of docetaxel to overcome multidrug resistance in ovarian cancer. *Drug Deliv.* **2016**, *23*, 968–980. [CrossRef]
18. Huang, R.F.S.; Wei, Y.J.; Inbaraj, B.S.; Chen, B.H. Inhibition of colon cancer cell growth by nanoemulsion carrying gold nanoparticles and lycopene. *Int. J. Nanomedicine.* **2015**, *10*, 2823–2846. [CrossRef]
19. Ahmad, G.; El Sadda, R.; Botchkina, G.; Ojima, I.; Egan, J.; Amiji, M. Nanoemulsion formulation of a novel taxoid DHA-SBT-1214 inhibits prostate cancer stem cell-induced tumor growth. *Cancer Lett.* **2017**, *406*, 71–80. [CrossRef]
20. Karasulu, H.Y.; Karabulut, B.; Goker, E.; Guneri, T.; Gabor, F. Controlled release of methotrexate from w/o microemulsion and its in vitro antitumor activity. *Drug Deliv.* **2007**, *14*, 225–233. [CrossRef]
21. Zhang, T.; Li, M.; Yang, R.Y.; Zhang, D.; Guan, J.B.; Yu, J.; Yang, B.; Zhang, H.C.; Zhang, S.W.; Liu, D.; et al. Therapeutic efficacy of lipid emulsions of docetaxel-linoleic acid conjugate in breast cancer. *Int. J. Pharm.* **2018**, *546*, 61–69. [CrossRef]
22. Forouz, F.; Dabbaghi, M.; Namjoshi, S.; Mohammed, Y.; Roberts, M.S.; Grice, J.E. Development of an Oil-in-Water Self-Emulsifying Microemulsion for Cutaneous Delivery of Rose Bengal: Investigation of Anti-Melanoma Properties. *Pharmaceutics* **2020**, *12*, 947. [CrossRef] [PubMed]
23. Nie, Y.L.; Liu, K.X.; Mao, X.Y.; Li, Y.L.; Li, J.; Zhang, M.M. Effect of injection of brucea javanica oil emulsion plus chemoradiotherapy for lung cancer: A review of clinical evidence. *J. Evid.-Based Med.* **2012**, *5*, 216–225. [CrossRef] [PubMed]
24. Pawar, A.; Korake, S.; Gajbhiye, K.R. Dequalinium-Derived Nanoconstructs: A Promising Vehicle for Mitochondrial Targeting, Curr. *Drug Deliv.* **2021**, *18*, 1056–1063. [CrossRef] [PubMed]
25. Bae, Y.; Jung, M.K.; Lee, S.; Song, S.J.; Mun, J.Y.; Green, E.S.; Han, J.; Ko, K.S.; Choi, J.S. Dequalinium-based functional nanosomes show increased mitochondria targeting and anticancer effect. *Eur. J. Pharm. Biopharm.* **2018**, *124*, 104–115. [CrossRef] [PubMed]
26. Bae, Y.; Jung, M.K.; Song, S.J.; Green, E.S.; Lee, S.; Park, H.S.; Jeong, S.H.; Han, J.; Mun, J.Y.; Ko, K.S.; et al. Functional nanosome for enhanced mitochondria-targeted gene delivery and expression. *Mitochondrion* **2017**, *37*, 27–40. [CrossRef]
27. Mallick, S.; Song, S.J.; Bae, Y.; Choi, J.S. Self-assembled nanoparticles composed of glycol chitosan-dequalinium for mitochondria-targeted drug delivery. *Int. J. Biol. Macromol.* **2019**, *132*, 451–460. [CrossRef]
28. Pekmez, M.; Onay-Ucar, E.; Arda, N. Effect of alpha-tocopheryl succinate on the molecular damage induced by indomethacin in C6 glioma cells. *Exp. Ther. Med.* **2015**, *9*, 585–590. [CrossRef]
29. Ralph, S.J.; Moreno-Sanchez, R.; Neuzil, J.; Rodriguez-Enriquez, S. Inhibitors of succinate: Quinone reductase/Complex II regulate production of mitochondrial reactive oxygen species and protect normal cells from ischemic damage but induce specific cancer cell death. *Pharm. Res.* **2011**, *28*, 2695–2730. [CrossRef]
30. Guo, Y.; Luo, J.; Tan, S.; Otieno, B.O.; Zhang, Z. The applications of Vitamin E TPGS in drug delivery. *Eur. J. Pharm. Sci.* **2013**, *49*, 175–186. [CrossRef]
31. Liang, L.; Peng, Y.; Qiu, L. Mitochondria-targeted vitamin E succinate delivery for reversal of multidrug resistance. *J. Control. Release* **2021**, *337*, 117–131. [CrossRef]
32. Tomasetti, M.; Nocchi, L.; Neuzil, J.; Goodwin, J.; Nguyen, M.; Dong, L.; Manzella, N.; Staffolani, S.; Milanese, C.; Garrone, B.; et al. Alpha-tocopheryl succinate inhibits autophagic survival of prostate cancer cells induced by vitamin K3 and ascorbate to trigger cell death. *PLoS ONE* **2012**, *7*, e52263. [CrossRef] [PubMed]
33. Abbasi, S.; Higashino, H.; Sato, Y.; Minami, K.; Kataoka, M.; Yamashita, S.; Harashima, H. Maximizing the Oral Bioavailability of Poorly Water-Soluble Drugs Using Novel Oil-Like Materials in Lipid-Based Formulations. *Mol. Pharm.* **2021**, *18*, 3281–3289. [CrossRef] [PubMed]
34. Tsujioka, T.; Sasaki, D.; Takeda, A.; Harashima, H.; Yamada, Y. Resveratrol-Encapsulated Mitochondria-Targeting Liposome Enhances Mitochondrial Respiratory Capacity in Myocardial Cells. *Int. J. Mol. Sci.* **2022**, *23*, 112. [CrossRef]
35. Satrialdi; Takano, Y.; Hirata, E.; Ushijima, N.; Harashima, H.; Yamada, Y. An effective in vivo mitochondria-targeting nanocarrier combined with a pi-extended porphyrin-type photosensitizer. *Nanoscale Adv.* **2021**, *3*, 5919–5927. [CrossRef] [PubMed]
36. Forest, V.; Pourchez, J. Preferential binding of positive nanoparticles on cell membranes is due to electrostatic interactions: A too simplistic explanation that does not take into account the nanoparticle protein corona. *Mater. Sci. Eng. C* **2017**, *70*, 889–896. [CrossRef]

37. Metwaly, A.M.; Ghoneim, M.M.; Eissa, I.H.; Elsehemy, I.A.; Mostafa, A.E.; Hegazy, M.M.; Afifi, W.M.; Dou, D. Traditional ancient Egyptian medicine: A review. *Saudi J. Biol. Sci.* **2021**, *28*, 5823–5832. [CrossRef]
38. Johnson, W. Final report on the safety assessment of Ricinus Communis (Castor) Seed Oil, Hydrogenated Castor Oil, Glyceryl Ricinoleate, Glyceryl Ricinoleate SE, Ricinoleic Acid, Potassium Ricinoleate, Sodium Ricinoleate, Zinc Ricinoleate, Cetyl Ricinoleate, Ethyl Ricinoleate, Glycol Ricinoleate, Isopropyl Ricinoleate, Methyl Ricinoleate, and Octyldodecyl Ricinoleate. *Int. J. Toxicol.* **2007**, *26*, 31–77. [CrossRef]
39. Mein, E.A.; Richards, D.G.; McMillin, D.L.; Nelson, C.D. Transdermal Absorption of Castor Oil. *Evid.-Based Integr. Med.* **2005**, *2*, 239–244. [CrossRef]
40. Klein, K.; He, K.; Younes, A.I.; Barsoumian, H.B.; Chen, D.; Ozgen, T.; Mosaffa, S.; Patel, R.R.; Gu, M.; Novaes, J.; et al. Role of Mitochondria in Cancer Immune Evasion and Potential Therapeutic Approaches. *Front. Immunol.* **2020**, *11*, 573326. [CrossRef]
41. Lee, K.H.; Kim, T.H. Recent Advances in Multicellular Tumor Spheroid Generation for Drug Screening. *Biosensors* **2021**, *11*, 445. [CrossRef]

antioxidants

MDPI

Article

Bio-Based Nano-Enabled Cosmetic Formulations for the Treatment of *Cutibacterium acnes*-Associated Skin Infections

Kristina Ivanova [1,†], Eva Ramon [1,†], Aleksandra Ivanova [1], Susana Sanchez-Gomez [2] and Tzanko Tzanov [1,*]

1 Grup de Biotecnologia Molecular i Industrial, Department of Chemical Engineering, Universitat Politècnica de Catalunya, Rambla Sant Nebridi 22, 08222 Terrassa, Spain
2 Bionanoplus S.L., Pol. Mocholi, Plaza Cein 5, Nave B14, 31110 Noain, Spain
* Correspondence: tzanko.tzanov@upc.edu
† These authors contributed equally to this work.

Abstract: Acne is a common chronic skin condition with serious physical and psychosocial consequences. In some cases, the appearance of pimples, whiteheads, or blackheads on the face, neck, and back may lead to scarring, disfiguring, depression, frustration, and anxiety in patients. Current treatments rely on antibiotics to eradicate *Cutibacterium acnes* (*C. acnes*), the bacterium responsible for this skin condition. However, these approaches do not scavenge the reactive oxidative species (ROS) generated during disease development and raise concerns about the increase in antimicrobial resistance. In this study, an environmentally friendly and cost-effective self-assembly nanoencapsulation technology based on zein, a bio-based hydrophobic protein, was employed to produce multifunctional essential oil (EO)-loaded nanocapsules (NCs) with superior antioxidant and bactericidal activity toward *C. acnes*. The NCs displayed "smart" release of the active cargo only under the conditions that were conducive to acne proliferation on skin. Once incorporated into creams, the EO-loaded NCs led to a complete inhibition of *C. acnes* and demonstrated the capacity to scavenge ROS, thus preventing damage to human skin cells. The in vitro permeation studies revealed that the nanoformulated EO was able to penetrate through the epidermis, indicating its potential for the treatment of skin diseases, such as acne.

Keywords: oregano oil; zein nanocapsules; pH-controlled cargo release; cosmetic formulations; antibacterial and antioxidant nanocapsules; *Acne vulgaris* treatment

1. Introduction

Acne vulgaris, or acne, is a chronic skin disorder affecting 95% of the global population, and it is considered the eighth prevalent health condition worldwide [1,2]. This disease starts as soon as age nine and continues into adulthood, and it has huge psychosocial impact on individuals. Affected patients exhibit comedones, nodules, pustules, and scarring on the face and the upper part of the body, frequently associated with psychological issues, such as dissatisfaction with one's appearance, lack of self-confidence, lower self-estimation, and social dysfunction. The psychological sequelae of acne also include increased risk of insomnia, anxiety, depression, suicidal thoughts, and even suicide [3,4].

Acne is a multifactorial disorder caused by sebum over-production in skin cells, hormonal changes, and microbiome imbalance [5,6]. This disease is triggered by an overlapping of several events in the pilosebaceous follicles, such as hyperproliferation of the Gram-positive anaerobic bacterium *Cutibacterium acnes* (*C. acnes*) and the presence of reactive oxidative species (ROS), e.g., nitrous oxide, hydroxyl, and superoxide, that are generated as the side products of the host immune response and sebum oxidation by *C. acnes* [7].

Current topical treatments, which are based on comedolytic agents (e.g., retinoids, benzoyl peroxide, and salicylic acid) or antibiotics (e.g., clindamycin and erythromycin)

for controlling the colonization of *C. acnes*, frequently aggravate skin irritation and inflammation. These approaches are not effective because they (i) do not present antioxidant properties that are able to reduce ROS harmful effects; (ii) do not pass through the skin epidermis; (iii) cause side effects, such as toxicity and skin drying; and (iv) over long periods, with the use of antibiotics in particular, can lead to the appearance of resistance strains, jeopardizing not only *acne vulgaris* treatment outcomes, but also other *C. acnes*-associated diseases, e.g., infective endocarditis [8,9]. Natural extracts from plants' leaves, flowers, roots, or stems have been introduced as alternative and more effective solutions for managing *acne vulgaris*. Aloe, tea tree oil, propolis, rosemary, and chamomile are largely employed as they feature strong antioxidant properties and bactericidal activity towards *C. acnes*, thus implying less selective pressure for antimicrobial resistance (AMR) appearance [10–12]. Despite their prominent anti-*C. acnes* potential, these bio-actives show uncontrolled biodegradability and induce toxicity and inflammation.

Advances in nanotechnology have allowed the redesigning of natural actives, potentiating their activity and stability [13]. Nanocarriers, including liposomes, niosomes, solid lipid nanoparticles, and micro-emulsions, provide protection for the encapsulated hydrophilic and lipophilic actives, target and control delivery while minimizing their toxicity toward other tissues, and allow higher skin penetration and time residence. Nanoformulation changes the chemical and physical properties of natural actives, endowing them with superior antibacterial performance and long-term stability when compared to their free form. The surface area-to-volume ratio increases the interaction with bacterial cells, causing cellular damage at lower dosages in contrast to non-encapsulated actives [14–16].

In this study, we developed novel anti-acne formulations comprising multifunctional zein-based nanocapsules (NCs) loaded with plant-derived antibacterial and antioxidant essential oil (EO) for efficient *acne vulgaris* treatment, targeting simultaneously the inhibition of ROS production and *C. acnes* overgrowth. Stable oregano oil NCs (EO-loaded NCs) were generated using a proprietary self-assembling encapsulation technology based on zein, a hydrophobic protein found in corn seed, which is included in the US FDA (Food and Drug Administration) Inactive Ingredients Database and classified as GRAS (Generally Recognized as Safe). This environmentally friendly, scalable, and cost-effective self-assembling encapsulation method yielded EO-loaded nano-delivery vehicles without the need for additional downstream processes, such as purification or drying steps. The use of a highly lipophilic and biodegradable zein protein is anticipated to enhance stability and impart controlled release of poorly water-soluble EO actives [17]. Nano-transformation will additionally boost the anti-acne performance of EO due to improved interaction and disruption of bacterial cells at a lower non-toxic concentration [14,18]. Incorporating EO-loaded NCs into cosmetic formulation will outperform conventional anti-acne products in terms of skin permeation and enhanced antibacterial efficacy. The innovative nano-cosmeceuticals were validated for their potential to inhibit *C. acnes* and to scavenge free radicals in vitro. The biocompatibility and antioxidant activity of the nano-enabled formulations were assessed with human skin cells. The release profile and transdermal delivery of the NCs upon a specific trigger of acne infection, such as pH 7, were evaluated using Franz cells.

2. Materials and Methods

2.1. Materials

Zein, a protein extracted from maize, was purchased from Flo Chemical Corporation (Ashburnham, MA, USA) and employed for NC generation. Oregano oil from Thymbra capitata (100% pure) was kindly provided by the TELIC S.A. (Barcelona, Spain). *Cutibacterium acnes* CECT 5684 was obtained from the Spanish Type Culture Collection (CECT, Valencia, Spain). A reinforced clostridial medium, obtained from Sigma-Aldrich (Madrid, Spain), was used for *C. acnes* cultivation in all antimicrobial tests. Brain Heart Infusion (BHI) agar for bacterial culturing and viable cell counting was also purchased from Sigma-Aldrich (Madrid, Spain). Dulbecco's Modified Eagle Medium (DMEM) media; Hank's Balanced Salt Solution (HBBS); Fetal Serum Bovine (FBS); mixture of 5000 Units penicillin (Pen), 5 mg mL^{-1} streptomycin (Strp), 200 mM of glutamin (Gln), and 10 mM of phosphate buffer at a pH of 7 (PBS) were provided by Sigma-Aldrich (Madrid, Spain). Human keratinocytes cells (HaCaT) were purchased from the American Type Culture Collection (Manassas, VA, USA). The AlamarBlue Cell Viability Reagent and GasPak^{TM} EZ to induce a microaerophilic/CO_2-enriched environment were supplied by Thermo Fisher Scientific (Barcelona, Spain). HCl, oleic acid, and Tween 20 were provided by Panreac Applichem (Barcelona, Spain). All other reagents were purchased from Sigma-Aldrich if not specified otherwise.

2.2. Preparation of EO NCs

NCs containing oregano oil were prepared as described previously [19]. Briefly, 0.2% (*w/w*) zein and 9.8% (*w/w*) propylene glycol were mixed until complete dissolution and further incorporated into a homogeneous mixture of 6% (*w/w*) propanediol (DuPont Tate & Lyle Bioproducts, Loudon. TN, USA), 6% (*w/w*) denatured alcohol (Barcelona, Spain), 6% (*w/w*) Tween 20, 0.8% (*w/w*) oleic acid, 0.01% (*w/w*) HCl, and 0.5% (*w/w*) oregano oil. The resultant surfactant–EO–zein mixture (29 g) was added dropwise under continuous agitation into water (71 g) to generate the NCs [20].

2.3. Characterization of EO-Loaded NCs

The NCs were characterized in terms of their macroscopic appearance, e.g., absence of aggregates and precipitates. The NCs' surface charge, size, and polydispersity were determined using a Zetasizer Nano ZS (Malvern Instruments Inc., Malvern, Worcestershire, UK). The number of NCs per milliliter were assessed by Nanoparticles Tracking Analysis using the NanoSight NS 300 (Malvern Instruments Inc., UK) in the flow mode and the software NTA 3.2 to capture several frames of the NC suspension. The size and the morphology of the NCs were also studied using a Transmission Electron Microscopy, TEM (Tecnai G2 F20, FEI company, Hillsboro, OR, USA), at 80 kV acceleration voltage. Prior to observation, 10 µL of the samples were placed on ultrathin carbon on holey carbon grids and air dried.

The amount of EO encapsulated in the NCs was assessed by carvacrol quantification using high performance liquid chromatography (HPLC). The HPLC experiments were performed using an Agilent 1260 Infinity system equipped with a quaternary pump, an auto-sampler with a high-sensitivity cell, a thermostatted column compartment, and a diode array detector. The ultraviolet (UV) spectra were collected at 220 and 278 nm. The Agilent OpenLab CDS software version 2.2 was used for instrument control, data collection, and data processing. The column used was a Zorbax SB-C18 (250 × 4.6 mm, 5 µm). The mobile phase was an isocratic combination of acetonitrile:water (50:50) with a flow rate of 2 mL min^{-1}. The injection volume for all samples and standard solutions was 10 µL. The encapsulation efficiency (EE) was calculated as follows:

$$EE\ (\%) = (C_{total} - C_{non\text{-}encapsulated})/C_{total} \times 100, \quad (1)$$

where C_{total} is the total carvacrol concentration in the suspension, and $C_{non\text{-}encapsulated}$ is the concentration of the "non-encapsulated" active—the filtrate collected after NC centrifugation for 30 min at 4000× *g* using Amicon® centrifugal filters (100 kDa cut-off, Millipore, Madrid, Spain).

The EO release from the NCs was assessed in PBS at a pH of 5.5 and at a pH of 7 for 4 h at 32 °C (the temperature of the skin). A total of 0.2 g of the NCs was redispersed in 10 mL of PBS, at a pH of 5.5 or 7, and incubated at 32 °C with shaking (30 rpm). At defined time intervals, 500 µL of each sample was collected and replaced with fresh PBS. The collected samples were centrifugated for 30 min at 4000× *g* using Amicon® centrifugal filters (100 kDa cut-off, Millipore, Madrid, Spain), and the filtrates were subjected to HPLC analysis to quantify the amount of EO released.

2.4. Antibacterial Activity of EO-Loaded NCs

Broth Microdilution Test. The minimal inhibitory concentration (MIC) of the NCs and the bulk EO was determined by the standardized broth microdilution method. *C. acnes* was grown in the reinforced clostridial medium under anaerobic conditions using an anaerobic container system at 37 °C for 3 days. For the antibacterial tests, the turbidity of the bacterial suspension was adjusted to an optical density of 0.01 at 600 nm in the reinforced clostridial medium, corresponding to 1×10^6 colony-forming units (CFU mL^{-1}). A total of 50 μL of the *C. acnes* suspension was mixed with 50 μL of the EO-loaded NCs and the bulk EO at different concentrations (0.0125–0.2 EO % (*v/v*)) in a sterile 96-round-bottom-well plate and incubated in an anaerobic environment at 37 °C for 24 h. The reinforced clostridial medium served as a negative control. The lowest concentration required to inhibit *C. acnes* growth was defined as the MIC. Each sample was tested in a triplicate.

Time-kill kinetic assay. The minimal time necessary for the NCs to completely eradicate *C. acnes* was determined using a time-kill kinetic assay. The *C. acnes* suspension was diluted in a sterile phosphate-buffered saline at a pH of 7 (PBS) to an OD = 0.01 at λ = 600 nm (~10^6 CFU mL^{-1}). For the assay, 250 μL of the bacterial inoculum was mixed with 250 μL of the samples and incubated at 37 °C under anaerobic conditions. At different time points, 15 μL of the samples was taken, and the survived bacteria were enumerated on a BHI agar using the drop plate method. *C. acnes* in the PBS was used as a negative control (no bactericidal activity).

2.5. Formulation of Anti-Acne Cosmetics Containing EO-Loaded NCs

Anti-acne cosmetic formulation was prepared by incorporating the encapsulated EO (0.02%) into a cosmetic facial cream base containing water, glycerin, and dimethicone. The antimicrobial activity of the nano-enabled anti-acne cream was assessed and compared to the cream with the bulk EO. The creams were prepared using a standard reverse emulsification method. An aqueous phase containing 5 g of triethanolamine was added dropwise into an oil phase containing 30 g of stearic acid, 5 g of liquid paraffin, 3 g of white beeswax, and 2 g of the NCs, while the mixture was stirred at 400 rpm. The temperature of the aqueous phase and the oil phase was adjusted to 70 and 65 °C, respectively. The mixture was stirred at 200 rpm (C-MAG HS7, IKA®, Staufen, Germany) and allowed to cool down to room temperature to form the creams.

2.6. Antibacterial Activity of the Nano-Enabled Cosmetic Formulations

The antibacterial activity of the creams was evaluated by using an agar diffusion test. *C. acnes* was grown in the reinforced clostridial broth for 3 days under anaerobic conditions at 37 °C. Afterwards, a BHI agar was inoculated with *C. acnes* (~10^8 CFU mL^{-1}), and 25 mL was poured into sterile plastic petri dishes. The agar was allowed to solidify, and 3 holes with a diameter of 7 mm were punched aseptically with a sterile cork borer. Then, 0.1 g of the samples were placed into the wells, and the plates were incubated at 37 °C under anaerobic conditions for 24–48 h. Then, the antimicrobial activity of the creams was assessed by measuring the diameter of the zones of inhibition that appeared as clear zones. All diffusion tests were performed in two independent experiments, and antibacterial activity was expressed as mean ± standard deviation.

2.7. Radical Scavenging Activity of the Anti-Acne Creams

The antioxidant activity of the NC-containing cream was determined based on their scavenging activity over ROS using 1 diphenyl-2-picryl hydrazyl (DPPH) free radical in a methanol solution. A total of 0.1 mL of the sample solution was added to 3.9 mL of 60 μM of the DPPH free radical solution. After 1 h in the dark, the absorbance of the preparations was measured at 517 nm (Abs_{517}) and compared to the corresponding absorbance of the blank (DPPH without the sample). Ascorbic acid at 0.5 mg mL^{-1} was used as a positive control. The % of inhibition was calculated as follows:

$$\text{Radical scavenging activity (\%)} = ((\text{Abs}_{517\,\text{blank}} - \text{Abs}_{517\,\text{scavenging activity sample}})/(\text{Abs}_{517\,\text{blank}})) \times 100 \quad (2)$$

2.8. Biocompatibility of the Anti-Acne Creams

The cells were seeded at a density of 6 × 10^4 cells per well on a 96-well tissue culture-treated polystyrene plate. On the next day, the cells were exposed to 3% creams diluted in a DMEM media containing 10% FBS, 2 mM of Gln, 50 Units of Pen, and 50 mg of Strp per mL at a pH of 7.5 (complete DMEM media) and incubated at 37 °C in a humidified atmosphere with 5% CO_2 for 2 h. After the indicated time of incubation, the NCs were removed, and the cells were washed with 200 μL of PBS and covered with 100 μL of 10% (*v/v*) AlamarBlue® reagent diluted in the complete DMEM media. After 4 h at 37 °C, the absorbance at 570 nm was measured, using 600 nm as a reference wavelength, in a TECAN infinite M200 (Tecan Group, Switzerland). Resazurin, the active ingredient of AlamarBlue® reagent, is non-toxic, cell-permeable compound that is blue in color, and when it is reduced to resorufin by viable cells, it becomes red. The quantity of the resorufin formed is directly proportional to the number of viable cells. The relative viability (%) of HaCaT cells was determined for each concentration of the creams with EO-loaded NCs and compared with the cells incubated with only a cell culture medium. All tests were performed in triplicate. Additionally, the cells were also subjected to a cytotoxicity assessment using the Live/Dead Viability/Cytotoxicity Kit for mammalian cells (Molecular Probes, ThermoFisher Scientific, Madrid, Spain). This kit includes two fluorescent probes, calcein and ethidium homodimer-1, that provide simultaneous determination of live (green fluorescence) and dead cells (red fluorescence) [19]. The cells were stained with a mixture of both stains in a ratio of calcein:ethidium homodimer of (4:1) in PBS for 15 min in the dark and were visualized using a fluorescence microscopy at 480/500 nm for calcein and at 490/635 nm for ethidium homodimer.

2.9. Intracellular ROS Measurement

This method uses HaCaT cells and allows for a more realistic screening of antioxidant activity against ROS than other methods using stable free-radical molecules, such as ABTS or DPPH [21]. Briefly, the cells were seeded at a density of 6 × 10^4 cells in 100 μL of complete DMEM media per well on a black, clear-bottom, 96-well microplate. Next day, the growth medium was removed, and the cells were washed with 200 μL of PBS. The cells were treated per triplicate for 2 h with 100 μL of 3% of cream formulations diluted in HBSS at a pH of 7 and 25 μM of 2′,7′-dichlorofluorescein diacetate. Ascorbic acid (150 μg mL^{-1}) was used as a positive control for antioxidant activity. The cells were further washed with 200 μL of PBS, and, subsequently, oxidative stress was induced by the addition of 600 μM of 2,2′-azobis(2-methylpropionamidine) dihydrochloride in 100 μL of HBSS. Immediately, the 96-well microplate was placed into a TECAN infinite M200 (Tecan Group, Männedorf, Switzerland). Emission at 535 nm was measured after excitation at 485 nm for 1 h every 5 min. After the subtraction of the initial fluorescence values, the area under the curve for fluorescence versus time was integrated to calculate the CAA value as follows:

$$CAA\,(\%) = 1 - \left(\frac{\int SA}{\int CA}\right) \quad (3)$$

where $\int SA$ is the integrated area under the curve of the sample fluorescence versus time, and $\int CA$ is the integrated area from the control curve. The CAA values (%) are presented as mean ± SD for the triplicate data from one experiment.

2.10. EO Permeation Studies

Dermatomized porcine skin (400 μm thickness) was used for the permeation studies using Franz diffusion cells. At first, the integrity of the skin was confirmed by its visual inspection and transepidermal water loss measurements (Tewameter® TM 300). Then, the dermatomized skin was mounted on the Franz diffusion cells with a 1.767 cm^2 cross-sectional area and 7 mL receptor volume. The anti-acne formulations ($n = 5$) were applied onto the skin in the donor compartment, and the system was maintained at 32 ± 1 °C with the help of a thermo-regulated outer water jacket, while the diffusion medium (PBS, pH 7) was stirred continuously using a magnetic stirrer. Finally, the system was disassembled, and the concentration of EO in the skin was quantified by HPLC.

2.11. Statistical Analysis

All data are presented as mean ± standard deviation. For multiple comparisons, statistical analysis was performed using a one-way analysis of variance (ANOVA), with p values less than 0.05 considered as statistically significant.

3. Results and Discussion

In this work, EO was nanoformulated using a proprietary self-assembling technology based on zein and non-volatile solvent propylene glycol [20]. Zein is a water-insoluble maize protein with amphiphilic characteristics, which is able to self-assemble into nano- and micro-structures. This protein has been used as a platform for encapsulating a range of hydrophobic and hydrophilic actives, including heparin, curcumin, α-tocopherol, and EO, achieving high loading capacity coupled with enhanced stability, sustained release, photoprotection, and bioavailability [22–25].

3.1. NP Characterization

The obtained EO-loaded NC suspension appears opalescent-transparent and yellowish, due to the zein, containing a high concentration of the yellow pigment xanthophyll (Figure 1A) [26]. The NCs are spherical in shape with an average size of 164 ± 5 nm and a narrow particle size distribution (0.4 ± 0.004). The NCs' concentration, as determined by NTA, is 3×10^9 NCs mL^{-1}. The EO-loaded NCs possess relatively high positive ζ-potential of 21 ± 2 mV, indicating good colloidal stability. Visible aggregate formation and phase separation due to NC precipitation were not observed even after 12 months of storage at room temperature. The size and ζ-potential values of the NCs did not change, further confirming the long-term storage stability of the NCs (Figure 1). This is explained by the use of the non-ionic surfactant Tween 20 in the NC formulation, enhancing the electrostatic and steric repulsion against aggregation. Since carvacrol represents 73.8% of the EO composition, this was used as a standard to determine the EE [27]. The HPLC analysis determined a 86 ± 1% EO encapsulation yield.

3.2. In Vitro EO Release

Maintaining a pH between 5–6 is vital for normal skin functioning and homeostasis. Higher pHs cause changes in healthy skin's microbiome balance and promote *C. acnes* proliferation and occurrence of *acne vulgaris* [28]. The release behavior of the NCs was assessed at a pH of 5.5 and a pH of 7, mimicking the physiological conditions in healthy and conditioned skin, respectively. At defined time intervals, the percentage of EO released from the NCs was quantified by HPLC (Figure 2). At a pH of 5.5, the NCs did not show any EO leakage, indicating good stability and retention of actives. Increasing the pH to 7, however, triggered the release, and approximately 45% of the encapsulated EO was liberated from the NCs within 4 h of incubation, which was attributed to pH-induced destabilization and rearrangement of the zein's secondary structure [28–30].

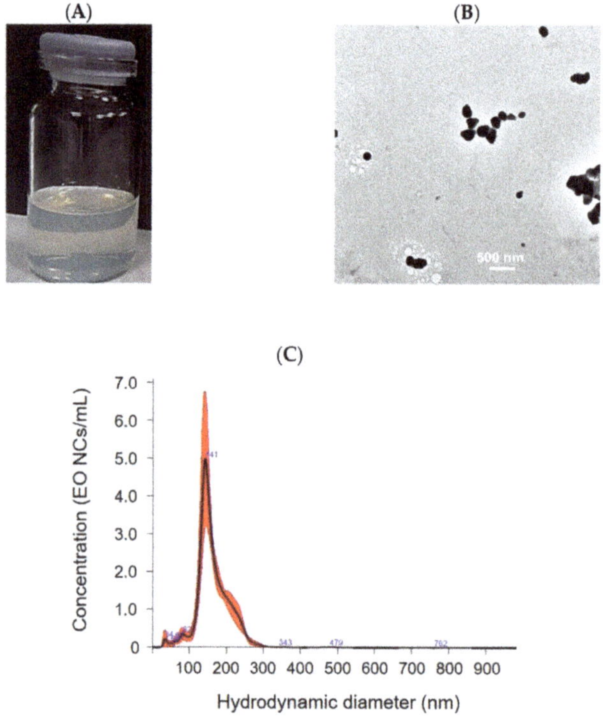

Figure 1. Characterization of EO-loaded NCs: (**A**) macroscopic appearance, (**B**) TEM images, and (**C**) size distribution.

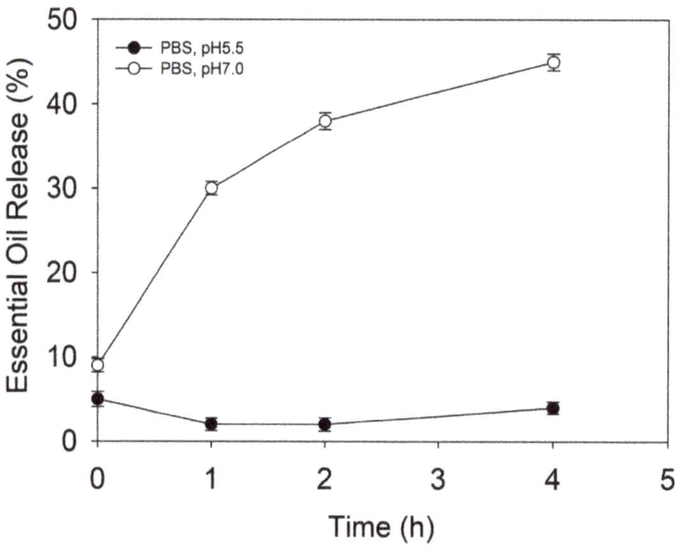

Figure 2. EO release from the NCs under conditions mimicking healthy skin (pH 5.5) and conditioned skin (pH 7) promoting *acne vulgaris* occurrence.

3.3. Antimicrobial Activity of EO-Loaded NCs against C. acnes

Plant-derived antimicrobials have gained significant attention as being more efficient against both susceptible and resistant bacteria than other antibiotic alternatives, with lower potential for resistance development. Although the strong anti-*C. acnes* activity of natural oils, such as cloves, cactus, and tea tree, has been previously described, their enhanced bactericidal effect due to the nano-size transformation has not yet been reported [31]. Our results demonstrated up to 8-fold increase in the antimicrobial activity of oregano oil against *C. acnes* upon nanoformulation ($p < 0.05$). A complete inhibition (100%) of bacterial growth was observed for the EO-loaded NCs at 0.025% (*v/v*) of the oil, while 0.2% of the bulk active was needed to achieve the same effect (Figure 3A). It is noteworthy that the antibacterial effect of the empty NCs, without the EO, was also evaluated, but any activity against *C. acnes* was not observed. These results are in agreement with our previous works validating nano-scale transformation as an innovative approach potentiating the antibacterial performance of different actives, including biopolymers, EO, enzymes, and metals, mainly due to improved interaction and disturbance of bacterial membrane [19,32,33].

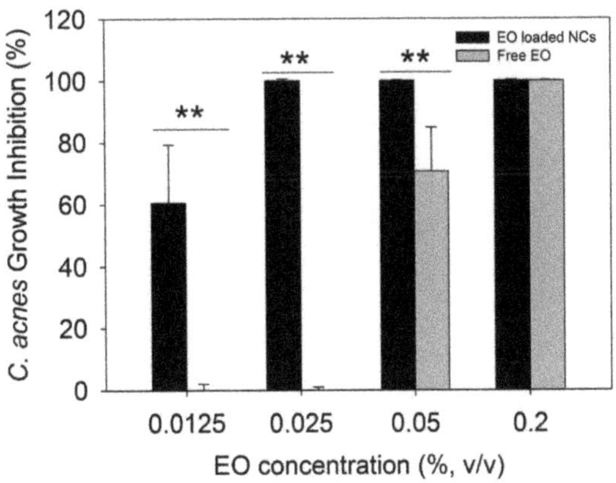

(A)

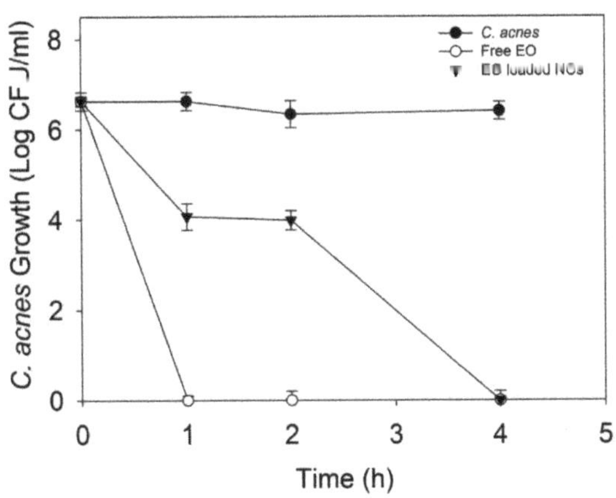

(B)

Figure 3. *Cont.*

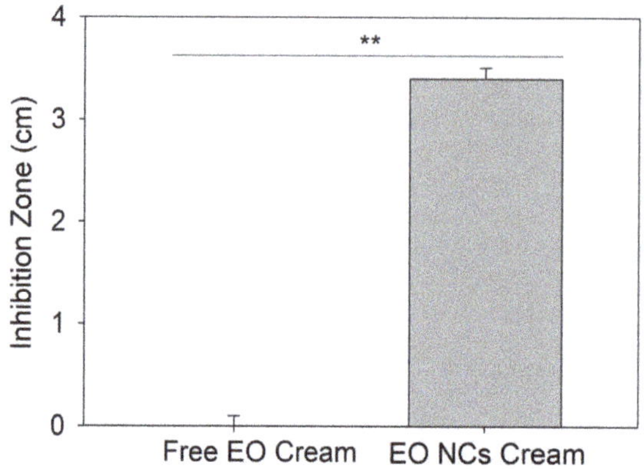

(C)

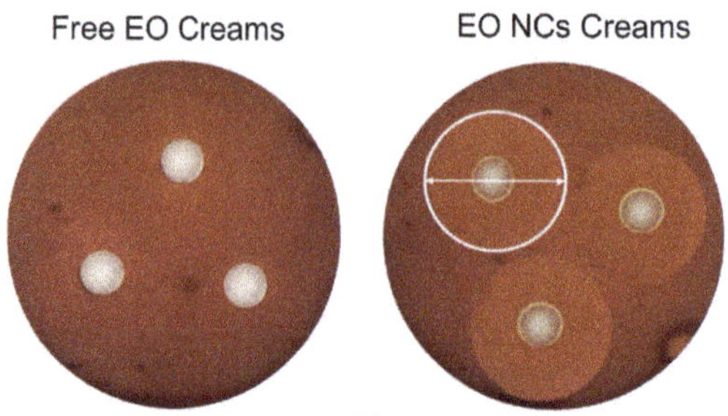

(D)

Figure 3. (**A**) Antibacterial activity of non-encapsulated and encapsulated EO against *C. acnes*. (**B**) Time-kill curves, (**C**) zone of inhibition (cm) of *C. acnes* growth by the free EO or EO-loaded NC anti-acne creams, and (**D**) agar plates inoculated with *C. acnes* and the free EO or EO-loaded NC anti-acne creams. All experiments were performed in triplicate, and the data are expressed as the mean ± standard deviation. ** stands for $p < 0.05$, considered statistically significant.

A time-kill kinetic assay was further performed at the MIC of the free EO and EO-loaded NCs to assess the kinetics of their bactericidal activity toward the target pathogen overtime. At the MIC, the bulk EO completely eradicated *C. acnes* within the first hour of incubation, while the EO-loaded NCs demonstrated a slower killing rate. A decrease in the live cell count by 2.6 $\log_{10}$ and 2.3 $\log_{10}$ (CFU·mL^{-1}) was achieved within the first and second hours, respectively, while complete bacterial removal was reached at the fourth hour of incubation (Figure 3B). These results confirm the bactericidal effect of the developed NCs and are in agreement with the sustained release of antibacterial EO from the zein matrix as a function of specific skin condition, e.g., *C. acnes* infection (Figure 2).

The anti-*C. acnes* EO-loaded NCs were further incorporated into a commercial cream's base formulation, and its bactericidal performance was assessed in vitro using a zone of inhibition assay. The EO-loaded NC-containing creams showed superior antibacterial efficiency against the target bacterium compared to the control, i.e., anti-acne formulation with the free active ($p < 0.05$). No zones of inhibition were observed for the cream with the bulk EO, while the nano-enabled anti-acne formulation reached an inhibition zone of 3 cm (Figure 3C).

Carvacrol, a phenolic compound present at high percentage in oil, is considered the principal active responsible for the strong antibacterial activity against *C. acnes*. The intrinsic hydrophobicity of this compound is thought to facilitate its interaction with bacterial cell through the direct binding with proteins, causing changes in the cells' morphology and disintegration of the membrane, which lead to cellular dysfunction and death. Inactivation of essential enzymes implicated in the synthesis of structural cell components is also likely to occur. Furthermore, the improved membrane-disturbing capacity due to the nanoform potentiates the antibacterial effect of this active at lower concentrations and results in higher anti-acne performance in regard to the cream loaded with the bulk active [34].

3.4. *Antioxidant Activity Using DPPH and Cellular Antioxidant Activity*

Recently, several studies have demonstrated the importance of antioxidant actives in the treatment of *acne vulgaris*. Apart from the oxidative species produced by *C. acnes* creating a favorable microenvironment for bacteria growth, neutrophils' defensive mechanisms for controlling the infection also generate reactive species [35]. This excessive amount of ROS overwhelms the natural antioxidant defense of the body, damaging the epithelium and the pilosebaceous area, and worsening the acne condition of affected individuals [12,36,37]. In addition to the enhanced antibacterial effect, higher antioxidant activity was observed for the nanoformulated EO when compared to the bulk material at the same amounts. Up to 60% of DPPH reduction was achieved by 0.0125% of encapsulated EO, while the same amount of the bulk oil did not demonstrate antioxidant properties ($p < 0.05$). The enhancement of the EO's intrinsic radical scavenging potential upon its nanoformulation can be explained by the large surface area-to-mass ratio of the NCs and the improved absorption of the free DPPH radicals. The control zein NCs without EO possess negligible antioxidant activity (15%), further demonstrating the advantage of using nanoformulated actives. Previous studies that focused on the nanoformulation of different bio-actives already reported similar behavior [38,39]. To this end, we assessed the antioxidant activity of the developed EO-loaded NC creams. The hydrogen-donating ability was assessed using a method based on the reduction of a methanol solution of the free radical DPPH (purple color) to its non-radical form (yellow color) [40]. The results showed the increased ability of the EO-loaded NC creams to scavenge free DPPH ($p < 0.05$) due to the intrinsic antioxidant properties of the oil (Figure 4A,B) [41].

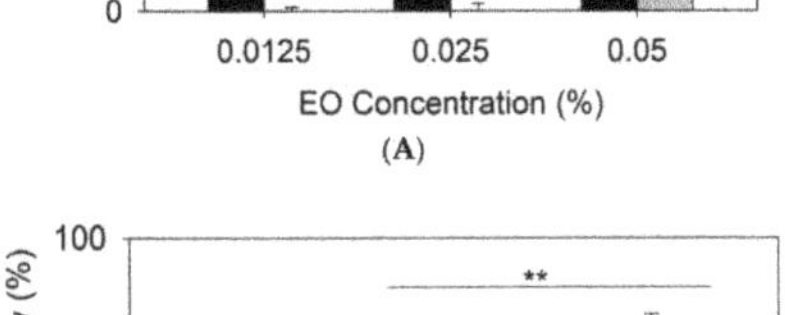

(A)

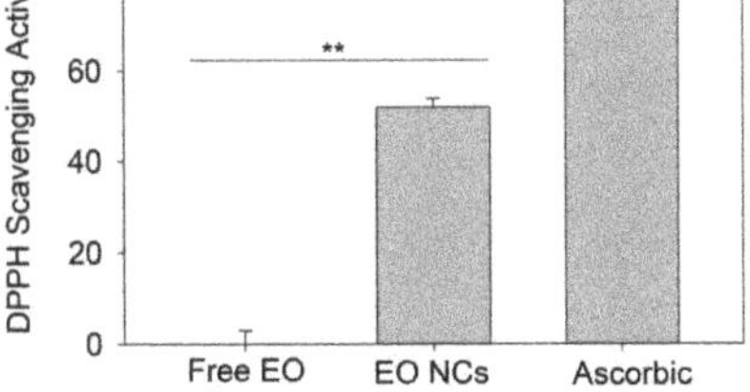

(B)

Figure 4. *Cont.*

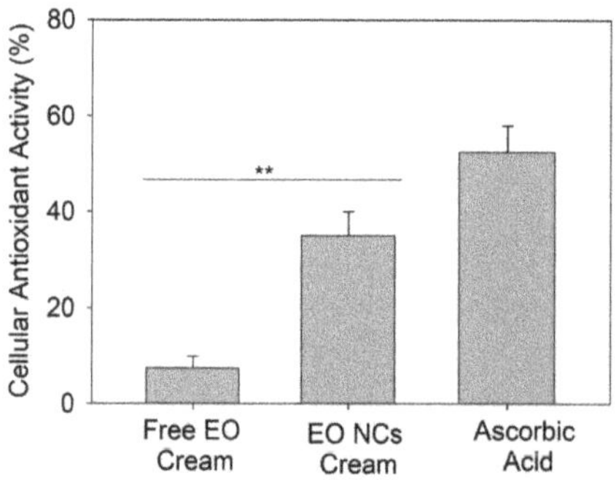

(C)

Figure 4. (**A**) Antioxidant activity of bulk EO and EO-loaded NCs, (**B**) free DPPH radical scavenging by the free EO and EO-loaded NC creams, and (**C**) cellular antioxidant activity of the free EO and EO-loaded NC creams. All experiments were performed in triplicate, and the data are expressed as the mean ± standard deviation. ** stands for $p < 0.05$, considered statistically significant.

Additionally, the antioxidant activity of the NC creams was assessed in HaCaT cells as a more realistic way than the currently used "test tube" DPPH method [21]. An accumulation of ROS due to cellular oxidative metabolism or external factors can cause molecular damage, leading to cell apoptosis [42]. This assay determines the ability of compounds to penetrate the membrane and act intracellularly as antioxidants [21]. The cellular antioxidant activity assay demonstrated that the EO-loaded NC formulations displayed higher free radical scavenging potential than the control cream with the non-encapsulated active ($p < 0.05$), which is attributed to the potentiating effect of the nano-form (Figure 4A,C) [43]. The antioxidant capacity of oregano oil is associated with the phenolic compound carvacrol, which is able to reduce free radicals [21,44,45].

3.5. EO Permeation Studies

Percutaneous absorption studies using Franz diffusion cells were conducted with porcine skin to evaluate the degree of EO penetration through the skin. Porcine skin was employed due to its resemblance to human skin physiological and anatomical properties and the lack of concern about ethical issues arising from its use [46]. In epidermis, the outermost layer is structured in a similar keratinizing stratified organization, and the thickness ratio between the dermis and the epidermis is identical between human and pork. This ratio is important for maintaining the viscoelastic properties of the skin, which are responsible for (i) protecting the body against external microbial infection, (ii) wound healing, and (iii) recovering skin shape after a force has been applied [47].

The dermatomized porcine skin was placed in the Franz diffusion cells, and the amount of active released from the EO-loaded NC creams and from the EO-loaded NCs into the skin were determined. The results revealed that about 1.5 ± 0.2% and 2.6 ± 0.3% of EO of the total applied dose of NCs and NC creams, respectively, were delivered into the skin (Figure 5). The higher EO penetration for the NC-containing cosmetics than the EO-loaded NCs alone ($p < 0.05$) is attributed to the presence of permeation enhancers, such as water, alcohols, and non-ionic surfactants in both the NCs and the cream matrix. These enhancers for transdermal delivery of antibacterial and antioxidant EO diminished the barrier properties of skin and boosted the NCs to reach deeper regions of the epidermis [48].

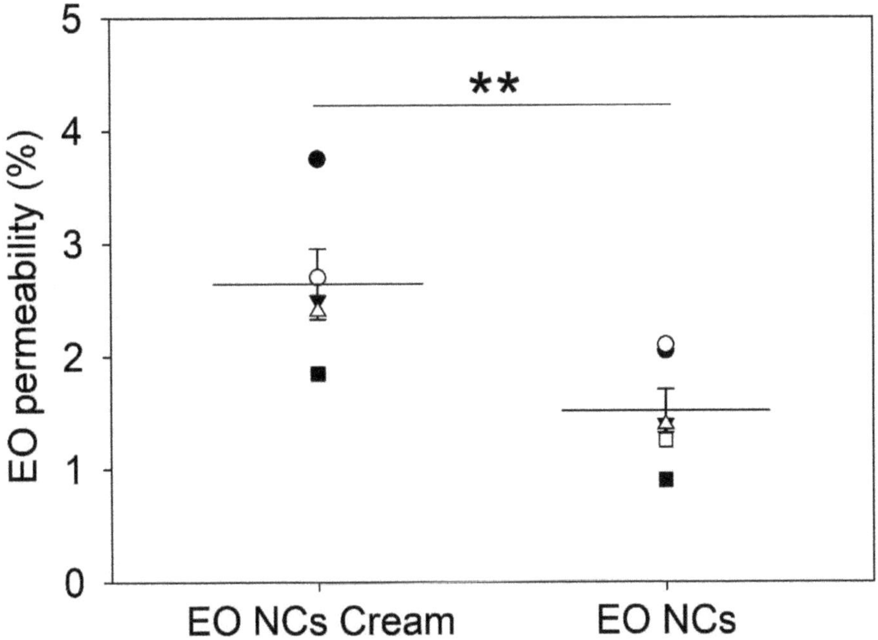

Figure 5. Percentage of EO permeation through the skin after 2 h of administering the EO-loaded NCs and the EO-loaded NC creams. Data are expressed as the mean of five replicates ± standard deviation. ** stands for $p < 0.05$, considered statistically significant.

3.6. Nanosafety of Anti-Acne EO-Loaded NC-Containing Cosmetic Formulations

The inclusion of nanomaterials in cosmetic products has raised some discussion about their toxicity due to size, safe dosage administration, and material composition. The high surface/volume ratio of these materials makes them more reactive than their pristine forms [49]. The nano-size allows them to easily pass through cell membranes and potentially interact with molecules that are important for cell viability (e.g., DNA and proteins) [50]. Therefore, it is critical to assess whether the developed anti-acne creams are safe toward skin cells. An in vitro viability test using keratinocytes (HaCaT cell line) was carried out to confirm the biocompatibility of the nano-enabled cosmetic products. Keratinocytes are the major cell type of the protective thin outer layer of skin epidermis, where the creams are intended to be applied [51].

The results showed that the anti-acne formulation did not cause significant side effects on the human HaCaT cells, confirming that the EO-loaded zein-based NCs and the compounds employed for the preparation of the cosmetic base formulation are safe for use (Figure 6A). After 24 h of exposure, the cells exhibited intact membranes, allowing the intracellular retention of the green dye calcein and showing a similar behavior as the control creams with the non-encapsulated active (Figure 6B).

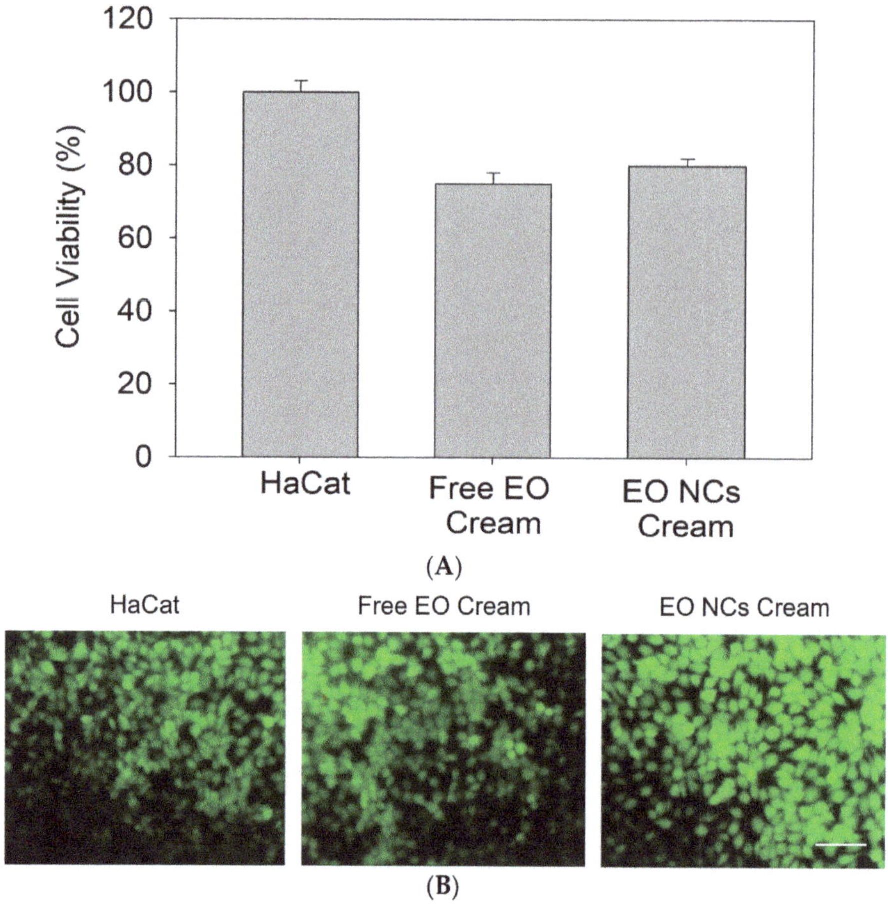

Figure 6. Biocompatibility of the free EO and EO-loaded NC anti-acne creams assessed by (**A**) Alamar Blue and (**B**) Live/Dead assay in HaCaT cells. All experiments were performed in triplicate, and the data are expressed as the mean ± standard deviation.

4. Conclusions

Despite the large number of marketed anti-acne products intended to reduce inflammation or *C. acnes* overgrowth, these products do not scavenge ROS produced by the host immune system's defense mechanism against infection. In this work, we developed innovative bio-based cosmetic formulations containing EO-loaded NCs to simultaneously decrease ROS generation and eradicate *C. acnes*, which is responsible for the severity of acne disease. Taking advantage of the intrinsic EO bio-activities and zein self-assembling capability and biocompatibility, stable EO-loaded NCs with superior antioxidant and antibacterial performance than the bulk EO were synthesized. The novel multifunctional delivery nanosystems released the encapsulated actives upon a pH typical for acne skin infection and completely eradicated the pathogen within 4 h. The cosmetic cream formulations containing the bio-based anti-acne nano-actives showed higher ROS scavenging potential and enhanced bactericidal effect toward *C. acnes* than the bulk oil at concentrations that are safe to human skin cells. The compounding of EO nano-actives in cosmetic formulations increased the EO's transdermal permeation into the skin, indicating its capability to reach inflamed areas that are colonized by *C. acnes*. The use of nanoformulated EO with improved antimicrobial capacity is an innovative approach for effective acne treatment, which is expected to impart less pressure for the selection of AMR.

Author Contributions: Conceptualization, methodology, investigation, formal analysis, writing—original draft, and writing—review and editing, K.I.; Conceptualization, methodology, investigation, formal analysis, writing—original draft, and writing—review and editing, E.R.; Methodology, investigation, formal analysis, and writing—review and editing, A.I.; Methodology, investigation, formal analysis, and writing—review and editing, S.S.-G.; Conceptualization, methodology, formal analysis, resources, writing—review and editing, and supervision, T.T. All authors have read and agreed to the published version of the manuscript.

Funding: This research was funded by the MCIN/AEI/10.13039/501100011033 and the EU "NextGenerationEU"/PRTR", under the framework of the Project TARDIS- PCI2022-13292.

Institutional Review Board Statement: Not applicable.

Informed Consent Statement: Not applicable.

Data Availability Statement: All data generated or analyzed during this study are included in this manuscript.

Conflicts of Interest: The authors declare no conflict of interest.

References

1. Tan, J.K.L.; Bhate, K. A Global Perspective on the Epidemiology of Acne. *Br. J. Dermatol.* **2015**, *172*, 3–12. [CrossRef] [PubMed]
2. Skroza, N.; Tolino, E.; Mambrin, A.; Zuber, S.; Balduzzi, V.; Marchesiello, A.; Bernardini, N.T.; Proietti, I.; Potenza, C. Adult Acne versus Adolescent Acne: A Retrospective Study of 1,167 Patients. *J. Clin. Aesthet. Dermatol.* **2018**, *11*, 21–25.
3. Trivedi, M.K.; Bosanac, S.S.; Sivamani, R.K.; Larsen, L.N. Emerging Therapies for Acne Vulgaris. *Am. J. Clin. Dermatol.* **2018**, *19*, 505–516. [CrossRef] [PubMed]
4. Xu, S.; Zhu, Y.; Hu, H.; Liu, X.; Li, L.; Yang, B.; Wu, W.; Liang, Z.; Deng, D. The Analysis of Acne Increasing Suicide Risk. *Medicine* **2021**, *100*, e26035. [CrossRef] [PubMed]
5. Kumar, B.; Pathak, R.; Mary, P.B.; Jha, D.; Sardana, K.; Gautam, H.K. New Insights into Acne Pathogenesis: Exploring the Role of Acne-Associated Microbial Populations. *Dermatologica Sin.* **2016**, *34*, 67–73. [CrossRef]
6. Lee, Y.B.; Byun, E.J.; Kim, H.S. Potential Role of the Microbiome in Acne: A Comprehensive Review. *J. Clin. Med.* **2019**, *8*, 987. [CrossRef] [PubMed]
7. Bowe, W.P.; Logan, A.C. Clinical Implications of Lipid Peroxidation in Acne Vulgaris: Old Wine in New Bottles. *Lipids Health Dis.* **2010**, *9*, 141. [CrossRef]
8. Kurokawa, I.; Layton, A.M.; Ogawa, R. Updated Treatment for Acne: Targeted Therapy Based on Pathogenesis. *Dermatol. Ther.* **2021**, *11*, 1129–1139. [CrossRef]
9. Platsidaki, C. Recent Advances in Understanding Propionibacterium Acnes (*Cutibacterium acnes*) in Acne. *F1000Research* **2018**, *7*, 1–12. [CrossRef]
10. Mazzarello, V.; Donadu, M.G.; Ferrari, M.; Piga, G.; Usai, D.; Zanetti, S.; Sotgiu, M.A. Treatment of Acne with a Combination of Propolis, Tea Tree Oil, and Aloe Vera Compared to Erythromycin Cream: Two Double-Blind Investigations. *Clin. Pharmacol. Adv. Appl.* **2018**, *10*, 175–181. [CrossRef] [PubMed]
11. Dessinioti, C.; Katsambas, A. Propionibacterium Acnes and Antimicrobial Resistance in Acne. *Clin. Dermatol.* **2017**, *35*, 163–167. [CrossRef]
12. Vora, J.; Srivastava, A.; Modi, H. Antibacterial and Antioxidant Strategies for Acne Treatment through Plant Extracts. *Inform. Med. Unlocked* **2018**, *13*, 128–132. [CrossRef]
13. Kaul, S.; Gulati, N.; Verma, D.; Mukherjee, S.; Nagaich, U. Role of Nanotechnology in Cosmeceuticals: A Review of Recent Advances. *J. Pharm.* **2018**, *2018*, 3420204. [CrossRef]
14. Fernandes, M.M.; Ivanova, K.; Hoyo, J.; Pérez-Rafael, S.; Francesko, A.; Tzanov, T. Nanotransformation of Vancomycin Overcomes the Intrinsic Resistance of Gram-Negative Bacteria. *ACS Appl. Mater. Interfaces* **2017**, *9*, 15022–15030. [CrossRef]
15. Ferreres, G.; Bassegoda, A.; Hoyo, J.; Torrent-burgue, J.; Tzanov, T. Metal—Enzyme Nanoaggregates Eradicate Both Gram-Positive and Gram-Negative Bacteria and Their Bio Fi Lms. *ACS Appl. Mater. Interfaces* **2018**, *10*, 40434–40442. [CrossRef] [PubMed]
16. Wang, L.; Hu, C.; Shao, L. The Antimicrobial Activity of Nanoparticles: Present Situation and Prospects for the Future. *Int. J. Nanomed.* **2017**, *12*, 1227–1249. [CrossRef]
17. Hadavi, M.; Hasannia, S.; Faghihi, S.; Mashayekhi, F.; Homazadeh, H.; Mostofi, S.B. Zein Nanoparticle as a Novel BMP6 Derived Peptide Carrier for Enhanced Osteogenic Differentiation of C2C12 Cells. *Artif. Cells Nanomed. Biotechnol.* **2018**, *46*, 559–567. [CrossRef] [PubMed]

18. Ivanova, A.; Ivanova, K.; Hoyo, J.; Heinze, T.; Sanchez-Gomez, S.; Tzanov, T. Layer-By-Layer Decorated Nanoparticles with Tunable Antibacterial and Antibiofilm Properties Against Both Gram-Positive and Gram-Negative Bacteria. *ACS Appl. Mater. Interfaces* **2018**, *10*, 3314–3323. [CrossRef]
19. Ivanova, K.; Ivanova, A.; Ramon, E.; Hoyo, J.; Sanchez-Gomez, S.; Tzanov, T. Antibody-Enabled Antimicrobial Nanocapsules for Selective Elimination of Staphylococcus Aureus. *ACS Appl. Mater. Interfaces* **2020**, *12*, 35918–35927. [CrossRef]
20. Salman, H.H.A.; Azcarate, I.G.; Catalan, I.E. Nanoparticles Comprising a Vegetable Hydrophobic Protein and a Water Miscible Non-Volatile Organic Solvent and Uses Thereof. U.S. Patent 9,974,753, 22 May 2018.
21. Wolfe, K.L.; Rui, H.L. Cellular Antioxidant Activity (CAA) Assay for Assessing Antioxidants, Foods, and Dietary Supplements. *J. Agric. Food Chem.* **2007**, *55*, 8896–8907. [CrossRef] [PubMed]
22. De Marco, I. Zein Microparticles and Nanoparticles as Drug Delivery Systems. *Polymers* **2022**, *14*, 2172. [CrossRef]
23. Hashem, F.M.; Al-Sawahli, M.M.; Nasr, M.; Ahmed, O.A.A. Optimized Zein Nanospheres for Improved Oral Bioavailability of Atorvastatin. *Int. J. Nanomed.* **2015**, *10*, 4059–4069. [CrossRef]
24. Zhang, H.; Van Os, W.L.; Tian, X.; Zu, G.; Ribovski, L.; Bron, R.; Bussmann, J.; Kros, A.; Liu, Y.; Zuhorn, I.S. Development of Curcumin-Loaded Zein Nanoparticles for Transport across the Blood-Brain Barrier and Inhibition of Glioblastoma Cell Growth. *Biomater. Sci.* **2021**, *9*, 7092–7103. [CrossRef] [PubMed]
25. Zou, L.; Zheng, B.; Zhang, R.; Zhang, Z.; Liu, W.; Liu, C.; Xiao, H.; McClements, D.J. Enhancing the Bioaccessibility of Hydrophobic Bioactive Agents Using Mixed Colloidal Dispersions: Curcumin-Loaded Zein Nanoparticles plus Digestible Lipid Nanoparticles. *Food Res. Int.* **2016**, *81*, 74–82. [CrossRef]
26. Sessa, D.J.; Eller, F.J.; Palmquist, D.E.; Lawton, J.W. Improved Methods for Decolorizing Corn Zein. *Ind. Crops Prod.* **2003**, *18*, 55–65. [CrossRef]
27. Merino, N.; Berdejo, D.; Bento, R.; Salman, H.; Lanz, M.; Maggi, F.; Sánchez-Gómez, S.; García-Gonzalo, D.; Pagán, R. Antimicrobial Efficacy of *Thymbra Capitata* (L.) Cav. Essential Oil Loaded in Self-Assembled Zein Nanoparticles in Combination with Heat. *Ind. Crops Prod.* **2019**, *133*, 98–104. [CrossRef]
28. Prakash, C.; Bhargave, P.; Tiwari, S.; Majumdar, B.; Bhargava, R.K. Skin Surface PH in Acne. *J. Clin. Aesthet. Dermatol.* **2017**, *10*, 33–39.
29. Kuo, S.H.; Shen, C.J.; Shen, C.F.; Cheng, C.M. Role of PH Value in Clinically Relevant Diagnosis. *Diagnostics* **2020**, *10*, 107. [CrossRef]
30. Cabra, V.; Arreguin, R.; Vazquez-Duhalt, R.; Farres, A. Effect of Temperature and PH on the Secondary Structure and Processes of Oligomerization of 19 KDa Alpha-Zein. *Biochim. Biophys. Acta Proteins Proteom.* **2006**, *1764*, 1110–1118. [CrossRef]
31. Taleb, M.H.; Abdeltawab, N.F.; Shamma, R.N.; Abdelgayed, S.S.; Mohamed, S.S.; Farag, M.A.; Ramadan, M.A.; Origanum Vulgare, L. Essential Oil as a Potential Anti-Acne Topical Nanoemulsion—In Vitro and in Vivo Study. *Molecules* **2018**, *23*, 2164. [CrossRef]
32. Ivanova, K.; Ivanova, A.; Hoyo, J.; Pérez-Rafael, S.; Tzanov, T. Nano-Formulation Endows Quorum Quenching Enzyme-Antibiotic Hybrids with Improved Antibacterial and Antibiofilm Activities against Pseudomonas Aeruginosa. *Int. J. Mol. Sci.* **2022**, *23*, 7632. [CrossRef]
33. Ivanova, A.; Ivanova, K.; Fiandra, L.; Mantecca, P.; Catelani, T.; Natan, M.; Banin, E.; Jacobi, G.; Tzanov, T. Antibacterial, Antibiofilm, and Antiviral Farnesol-Containing Nanoparticles Prevent Staphylococcus Aureus from Drug Resistance Development. *Int. J. Mol. Sci.* **2022**, *23*, 7527. [CrossRef]
34. Folle, C.; Marqués, A.M.; Díaz-Garrido, N.; Espina, M.; Sánchez-López, E.; Badia, J.; Baldoma, L.; Calpena, A.C.; García, M.L. Thymol-Loaded PLGA Nanoparticles: An Efficient Approach for Acne Treatment. *J. Nanobiotechnol.* **2021**, *19*, 359. [CrossRef]
35. Sahib, A.; AlAnbari, H.; Raghif, A. Oxidative Stress in Acne Vulgaris: An Important Therapeutic Target. *J. Mol. Pathophysiol.* **2013**, *2*, 27. [CrossRef]
36. Arican, O.; Kurutas, E.B.; Sasmaz, S. Oxidative Stress in Patients with Acne Vulgaris. *Mediat. Inflamm.* **2005**, *2005*, 380–384. [CrossRef] [PubMed]
37. Mills, O.H.; Criscito, M.C.; Schlesinger, T.E.; Verdicchio, R.; Szoke, E. Addressing Free Radical Oxidation in Acne Vulgaris. *J. Clin. Aesthet. Dermatol.* **2016**, *9*, 25–30.
38. Shi, Q.; Wang, X.; Tang, X.; Zhen, N.; Wang, Y.; Luo, Z.; Zhang, H.; Liu, J.; Zhou, D.; Huang, K. In Vitro Antioxidant and Antitumor Study of Zein/SHA Nanoparticles Loaded with Resveratrol. *Food Sci. Nutr.* **2021**, *9*, 3530–3537. [CrossRef]
39. Fernandes, M.M.; Rivera, D.; Francesko, A.; Šližytė, R.; Mozuraityte, R.; Rommi, K.; Lantto, R.; Tzanov, T. Bio/Sonochemical Conversion of Fish Backbones into Bioactive Nanospheres. *Process Biochem.* **2015**, *50*, 1843–1851. [CrossRef]
40. Kedare, S.B.; Singh, R.P. Genesis and Development of DPPH Method of Antioxidant Assay. *J. Food Sci. Technol.* **2011**, *48*, 412–422. [CrossRef]
41. Kozics, K.; Bučková, M.; Puškárová, A.; Kalászová, V.; Cabicarová, T.; Pangallo, D. The Effect of Ten Essential Oils on Several Cutaneous Drug-Resistant Microorganisms and Their Cyto/Genotoxic and Antioxidant Properties. *Molecules* **2019**, *24*, 4570. [CrossRef]
42. Redza-Dutordoir, M.; Averill-Bates, D.A. Activation of Apoptosis Signalling Pathways by Reactive Oxygen Species. *Biochim. Biophys. Acta Mol. Cell Res.* **2016**, *1863*, 2977–2992. [CrossRef]
43. Ma, J.J.; Yu, Y.G.; Yin, S.W.; Tang, C.H.; Yang, X.Q. Cellular Uptake and Intracellular Antioxidant Activity of Zein/Chitosan Nanoparticles Incorporated with Quercetin. *J. Agric. Food Chem.* **2018**, *66*, 12783–12793. [CrossRef] [PubMed]

44. Carpena, M.; Nuñez-Estevez, B.; Soria-Lopez, A.; Garcia-Oliveira, P.; Prieto, M.A. Essential Oils and Their Application on Active Packaging Systems: A Review. *Resources* **2021**, *10*, 7. [CrossRef]
45. Fernandes, M.M.; Ivanova, K.; Francesko, A.; Rivera, D.; Torrent-Burgués, J.; Gedanken, A.; Mendonza, E.; Tzanov, T. Escherichia Coli and Pseudomonas Aeruginosa Eradication by Nano-Penicillin G. *Nanomed. Nanotechnol. Biol. Med.* **2016**, *12*, 2061–2069. [CrossRef] [PubMed]
46. Neupane, R.; Boddu, S.H.S.; Renukuntla, J.; Babu, R.J.; Tiwari, A.K. Alternatives to Biological Skin in Permeation Studies: Current Trends and Possibilities. *Pharmaceutics* **2020**, *12*, 152. [CrossRef]
47. Wang, Y.; Marshall, K.L.; Baba, Y.; Lumpkin, E.A.; Gerling, G.J. Compressive Viscoelasticity of Freshly Excised Mouse Skin Is Dependent on Specimen Thickness, Strain Level and Rate. *PLoS ONE* **2015**, *10*, e0120897. [CrossRef]
48. Kim, B.; Cho, H.-E.; Moon, S.H.; Ahn, H.-J.; Bae, S.; Cho, H.-D.; An, S. Transdermal Delivery Systems in Cosmetics. *Biomed. Dermatol.* **2020**, *4*, 10. [CrossRef]
49. Gatoo, M.A.; Naseem, S.; Arfat, M.Y.; Mahmood Dar, A.; Qasim, K.; Zubair, S. Physicochemical Properties of Nanomaterials: Implication in Associated Toxic Manifestations. *BioMed Res. Int.* **2014**, *2014*, 498420. [CrossRef] [PubMed]
50. Lebre, F.; Chatterjee, N.; Costa, S.; Fernández-De-gortari, E.; Lopes, C.; Meneses, J.; Ortiz, L.; Ribeiro, A.R.; Vilas-Boas, V.; Alfaro-Moreno, E. Nanosafety: An Evolving Concept to Bring the Safest Possible Nanomaterials to Society and Environment. *Nanomaterials* **2022**, *12*, 1810. [CrossRef]
51. Keppel Hesselink, J.M.; Kopsky, D.J.; Bhaskar, A.K. Skin Matters! The Role of Keratinocytes in Nociception: A Rational Argument for the Development of Topical Analgesics. *J. Pain Res.* **2017**, *10*, 1–8. [CrossRef]

antioxidants

MDPI

Article

Facile Fabrication of α-Bisabolol Nanoparticles with Improved Antioxidant and Antibacterial Effects

Sangwoo Kim [1,2], Sohyeon Yu [1,3], Jisu Kim [1,2], Nisar Ul Khaliq [4], Won Il Choi [1], Hyungjun Kim [4,*] and Daekyung Sung [1,*]

[1] Center for Bio-Healthcare Materials, Bio-Convergence Materials R&D Division, Korea Institute of Ceramic Engineering and Technology, 202 Osongsaengmyeong 1-ro, Osong-eup, Heungdeok-gu, Cheongju 28160, Republic of Korea

[2] Department of Chemical and Biomolecular Engineering, Yonsei University, 50 Yonsei-ro, Seodaemun-gu, Seoul 03722, Republic of Korea

[3] Department of Chemical Engineering, Hanyang University, 222 Wangsimni-ro, Seongdong-gu, Seoul 04763, Republic of Korea

[4] Department of Chemistry and Bioscience, Kumoh National Institute of Technology, 61 Daehak-ro, Gumi 39177, Republic of Korea

* Correspondence: hyungjun@kumoh.ac.kr (H.K.); dksung@kicet.re.kr (D.S.); Tel.: +82-54-478-7830 (H.K.); +82-43-913-1511 (D.S.); Fax: +82-54-478-7859 (H.K.); +82-43-913-1597 (D.S.)

Abstract: Bioactive compounds are widely used in the bio-industry because of their antioxidant and antibacterial activities. Because of excessive oxidative stress, which causes various diseases in humans, and because preservatives used in bioproducts cause allergies and contact dermatitis, it is important to use natural bioactive compounds in bioproducts to minimize oxidative stress. α-bisabolol (ABS) is a natural compound with both antioxidant and antibacterial properties. However, its water-insolubility makes its utilization in bioproducts difficult. In this study, ABS-loaded polyglyceryl-4 caprate nanoparticles (ABS@NPs) with improved aqueous stability and ABS loading were fabricated using an encapsulation method. The long-term stability of the ABS@NPs was analyzed with dynamic light scattering and methylene blue-staining to determine the optimized ABS concentration in ABS@NPs (10 wt%). The ABS@NPs exhibited excellent antioxidant activity, according to the 2,2-diphenyl-1-picrylhydrazyl assay and in vitro reactive oxygen species generation in NIH-3T3 fibroblast cells, and an outstanding antibacterial effect, as determined using the *Staphylococcus aureus* colony-counting method. Furthermore, we evaluated the biocompatibility of the ABS@NPs in vitro. This study suggests that ABS@NPs with improved antioxidant and antibacterial properties can be used to treat diseases related to various oxidative stresses and can be applied in many fields, such as pharmaceuticals, cosmetics, and foods.

Keywords: bioactive compound; α-bisabolol; polyglyceryl-4 caprate; nanoparticle; solubilization; encapsulation; antioxidant; antibacterial

1. Introduction

Bioactive compounds have various properties, such as antioxidant and antibacterial activities, and they are widely used in the pharmaceutical, cosmetic, and food industries [1–3]. Terpenoid, a representative bioactive compound, is a natural organic compound composed of isoprene units that is produced by isopentenyl diphosphate, which is a precursor to isoprene, and its isomer, dimethylallyl diphosphate (DMAPP). It is known for its excellent ability to scavenge reactive oxygen species (ROS), that is, antioxidant ability, owing to which it has been a subject of many studies [4–6]. ROS, which are highly reactive forms of intermediates, include hydrogen peroxide (H_2O_2), superoxide radical (O_2^-), and hydroxyl radical (OH^-). They cause extreme damage to biomolecules in cells and mitochondria, thereby inducing inflammation and excessive oxidative stress in the body resulting in various diseases, such as cancer and Alzheimer's disease (AD), in humans [7–12]. Therefore, compounds with antioxidant properties that have the ability to remove these free radicals have garnered considerable interest in relation to the development of various bioproducts in the modern urbanized society, where many factors, such as ultraviolet rays, fine dust, and blue light, induce the formation of active oxygen species [13–15].

Antibacterial activity is an important property for bioproduct development [16]. Compared to chemical and plastic products, bioproducts are more susceptible to contamination and denaturation, which makes it difficult to maintain the product quality [16–19]. As bioproducts are in an aqueous environment, where microorganisms, such as bacteria, can easily grow, it is essential to add preservatives to prevent their degradation [19–21]. In the bio-industry, preservatives are added to decrease the bacteria purity during manufacturing, packaging, and storage [21]. However, preservatives such as formaldehyde, iodopropynyl butylcarbamate, and triclosan cause allergies and contact dermatitis in users, even when used in small amounts; therefore, their use is being reduced gradually [22–24]. One way to minimize this issue is to use natural substances with antibacterial effects in bioproducts [25–27].

In this study, we focused on α-bisabolol (ABS), a natural bioactive compound with antioxidant and antibacterial properties. ABS is a naturally occurring sesquiterpene alcohol that is widely present in plant sources, such as *Matricaria chamomilla*, and several studies have indicated that it has useful pharmacological and cosmetic activities, including anti-inflammatory, anti-irritant, anti-tumor, antioxidant, antibacterial, and anti-allergic properties [28–33]. However, owing to the insolubility of ABS in water, its bioavailability is low, and it is difficult to develop a bioproduct based on ABS due to its lipophilicity [28,34–37]. To overcome these disadvantages, nanocapsule techniques using amphiphilic polymers or solubilizers have been developed to enhance the bioavailability and solubility of hydrophobic substances, such as ABS [7,28–30,36,37]. However, the ABS loading and physicochemical stability of the previously developed systems are low, the manufacturing process is complicated, and the fabrication requires temperature-controlled environmental conditions [29–31,37]. Therefore, the development of an ideal nanocarrier for ABS requires an optimization technology that can enhance both the loading and the physicochemical stability of ABS in a simple and convenient manner.

In this study, we developed a nanoprecipitation technique using amphiphilic polyglyceryl-4 caprate, which contains a hydrophilic carboxyl group segment and a hydrophobic hydrocarbon chain segment, to fabricate ABS-loaded nanoparticles (ABS@NPs) with higher loading and stability of ABS than previously achieved. The objective of this study was to improve the long-term stability and effectiveness of ABS as an antioxidant and antibacterial material in an aqueous environment (Figure 1). To evaluate the stability of ABS@NPs, many physicochemical properties, such as the particle diameter, surface charge, and polydispersity index (PDI), were analyzed via dynamic light scattering (DLS). The stability of the nanoparticle system was also confirmed visually using a methylene blue staining test. The ROS-scavenging activity of ABS@NPs was analyzed in situ using the 2,2-diphenyl-1-picrylhydrazyl (DPPH) assay and through in vitro studies using mouse embryonic fibroblast cells (NIH 3T3). Furthermore, the antibacterial activity of ABS@NPs was confirmed using the colony-counting method. Finally, we confirmed the biocompatibility of ABS@NPs with an in vitro experiment using NIH 3T3 cells. The improved antioxidant and antibacterial properties of ABS@NPs make them suitable candidates for treating diseases related to oxidative stress, and they are expected to have applications in various fields, such as pharmaceuticals, cosmetics, and foods.

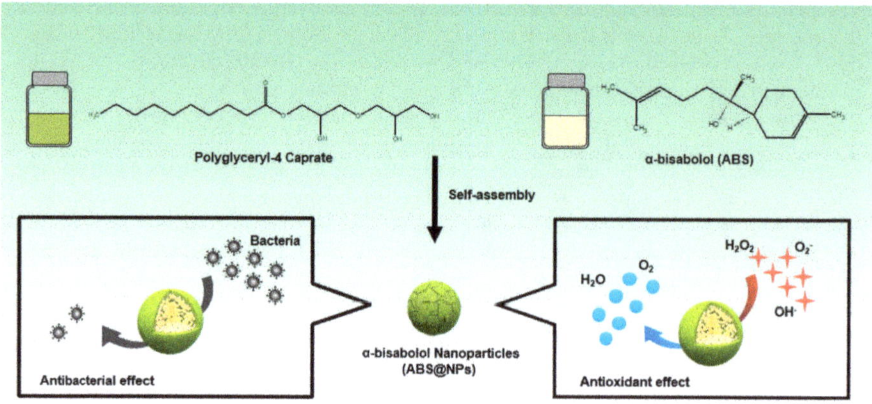

Figure 1. Schematic illustration of the preparation of α -bisabolol-loaded nanoparticles (ABS@NPs) and improved antioxidant and antibacterial effects.

2. Materials and Methods

2.1. Materials

ABS and tetrahydrofuran (THF; anhydrous, 99.9%) were purchased from Sigma-Aldrich (St. Louis, MO, USA), polyglyceryl-4 caprate was purchased from Special Chemical Co. (Paris, France), and deionized water (DIW) were obtained from HyClone (Logan, UT, USA) for fabricating ABS nanoparticles. For high-performance liquid chromatography (HPLC), deionized water (DIW) was purchased from Milli-Q® (Molsheim, France), and acetonitrile (HPLC grade) and phosphoric acid were obtained from Merck® (Darmstadt, Germany). For the dye solubility method, methylene blue was obtained from Sigma-Aldrich (St. Louis, MO, USA). For the in situ antioxidants experiment, the reagents 2,2-diphenyl-1-picrylhydrazyl (DPPH) and ascorbic acid (AA) were obtained from Sigma-Aldrich (St. Louis, MO, USA). For in vitro cell incubation, penicillin–streptomycin, trypsin (0.25%), fetal bovine serum (FBS), and dulbecco's modified Eagle's medium (DMEM) were purchased from Gibco (Grand Island, NY, USA). For in vitro experiments, reagents such as 2,7-dichlorodihydrofluorescein diacetate (H2DCFDA) and 3-(4,5-dimethylthiazol-2-yl)-2,5-diphenyltetrazolium bromide (MTT) were obtained from Invitrogen (Carlsbad, CA, USA), hydrogen peroxide (H_2O_2, 30%) was purchased from Junsei Chemical Co. (Tokyo, Japan), dimethyl sulfoxide-d6 (DMSO-d6, 99.8%) was obtained from Sigma-Aldrich (St. Louis, MO, USA), and phosphate-buffered saline (PBS, pH 7.4) was purchased from HyClone (Logan, UT, USA). For the Gram-positive bacterium, *Staphylococcus aureus* ATCC 6538, culture, Luria–Bertani (LB) agar and Luria–Bertani (LB) broth were obtained from BD Difco (Sparks, MD, USA). For the antibacterial assay, the Gram-positive bacterium, *Staphylococcus aureus* ATCC 6538 was obtained from the American Type Culture Collection (ATCC; Manassas, VA, USA). All solvents were used as received without additional purification.

2.2. Preparation of ABS@NPs

ABS@NPs were fabricated through self-assembly in the aqueous phase after mixing hydrophobic ABS with amphiphilic polyglyceryl-4 caprate, which contains a hydrophilic carboxyl group segment and a hydrophobic hydrocarbon chain segment. First, ABS (1, 2, 4, or 8 mg) and polyglyceryl-4 caprate (20 mg) were dissolved in THF (1 mL) in 4 mL vial under magnetic stirring at room temperature for 2 h. Then, utilizing a syringe pump (LEGATO100, KD Scientific, Korea), the THF solution with ABS and polyglyceryl-4 caprate was added dropwise to 5 mL of DIW with stirring at 530 rpm. The ABS@NPs (ABS loading of 5, 10, 20, and 40 wt% with respect to polyglyceryl-4 caprate) were stabilized by mild stirring (530 rpm) for 1 h. Finally, the solvent was completely evaporated via vacuum evaporation for 2 h and the remaining was diluted with DIW to 5 mL. The resulting products are denoted as ABS@NP × wt%, where × wt% represents the ABS loading respect to polyglyceryl-4 caprate. The same method was used to prepare empty nanoparticles (NPs) of polyglyceryl-4 caprate without the addition of ABS (denoted as ABS@NP 0 wt%) [7]. The zeta potential, PDI, and particle size of ABS@NPs were estimated through DLS using an electrophoretic light-scattering spectrophotometer (ELS-Z2, Otsuka Electronics Co., Tokyo, Japan). The loading content and loading efficiency of ABS in nanoparticles were analyzed via HPLC of unloaded ABS. Utilizing Amicon Ultra-15 centrifugal filters (molecular weight cutoff: 100 kDa), unloaded ABS was purified through ultrafiltration at 2000 rpm for 15 min [36] The chromatographic conditions used for the HPLC experiment are as follows: the injection volume was 20 µL, the detection wavelength was 200 nm, and the mobile phases were a mixture of (A) acetonitrile and (B) water. In addition, acetonitrile and phosphoric acid were used at 80:19:1 by volume in a linear gradient elution program from A:B (50:50) to 100% A in 25 min, returning to A:B (50:50) in 5 min. The eluent flow rate was 0.8 mL/min. All HPLC experiments were performed at room temperature. After this, the loading content and loading efficiency were calculated as follows [34–36]:

$$Loading\ content\ (\%) = \left[\frac{(weight\ of\ fed\ ABS - weight\ of\ unloaded\ ABS)}{weight\ of\ NPs}\right] \times 100 \quad (1)$$

$$Loading\ efficiency\ (\%) = \left[\frac{(weight\ of\ fed\ ABS - weight\ of\ unloaded\ ABS)}{weight\ of\ fed\ ABS}\right] \times 100 \quad (2)$$

2.3. *Methylene Blue Staining of ABS@NPs*

To visually confirm the encapsulation, stability, and transparency of the dispersed phase of the fabricated ABS@NPs with various ABS concentrations (0 wt%, 5 wt%, 10 wt%, 20 wt%, and 40 wt%), a dye solubility method was carried out utilizing methylene blue, a hydrophilic dye. First, methylene blue was dissolved in DIW at 120 nM concentration. Next, 2 mL of the dye solution was added to 2 mL of the ABS@NPs suspension and mixed in a 4 mL vial. Finally, the solution was visually examined to confirm the precipitation or dispersion of ABS@NPs [7,38].

2.4. *Assessment of the Stability of ABS@NPs*

The stability of ABS@NPs was analyzed over 112 days via DLS. The PDI and particle size of ABS@NPs were estimated at ABS concentrations of 0, 5, and 10 wt% in DIW on days 0, 1, 3, 7, 14, 28, 56, and 112.

2.5. *In Situ Antioxidant Activity of ABS@NPs by the DPPH Assay*

The antioxidant activity of ABS@NPs was evaluated utilizing a DPPH assay [39]. As control groups, solutions of AA and ABS in DIW were prepared at two concentrations each (5 and 10 wt%). The ABS@NPs were prepared at three ABS concentrations (0, 5, and 10 wt%). Then, a 0.1 mM DPPH solution was diluted with ethanol and stored in dark conditions at 4 °C. Subsequently, the prepared DPPH solution 50 µL was added with each ABS@NP suspension of 150 µL. The negative control group was 50 µL of DPPH solution added to 150 µL of DIW, which hardly showed any antioxidant activity. As a positive control, AA was used and ABS in DIW and ABS@NP 0 wt% were used as negative control groups for comparison with ABS@NPs. All mixtures were stored in dark condition at 25 °C for 24 h. Using a microplate reader (VICTOR X5, PerkinElmer, Singapore, Republic of Singapore), the absorbance of each mixture was analyzed at a wavelength of 515 nm. The antioxidant activity was calculated utilizing the following equation: [40,41]

$$Antioxidant\ activity\ (\%) = \left[\frac{\Delta A_{515}\ of\ control - \Delta A_{515}\ of\ sample}{\Delta A_{515}\ of\ control}\right] \times 100 \quad (3)$$

2.6. In Vitro Antioxidant Activity of ABS@NPs

To estimate the intracellular antioxidant effect of the ABS@NPs with ABS concentrations of 5 and 10 wt%, mouse embryonic fibroblast cells (NIH 3T3) were cultured in 96-well plates at a density of 10,000 cells/well and incubated for 24 h. ROS were induced in NIH 3T3 fibroblast cells via stimulation with H_2O_2, as an oxidative stress agent. After sample treatment, changes in the ROS levels were estimated using the following steps: first, suspensions of ABS@NP 10 wt% with various ABS concentrations (1–1000 nM) and 5 μM hydrogen peroxide (H_2O_2) were added to fibroblast cells and cultured for 8 h. For comparison, a negative control group without H_2O_2 and a positive control group with H_2O_2 were used. Then, after washing with PBS (200 μL to each 96-well plate) to eliminate the remaining sample solution, the NIH 3T3 cells were treated with a 10 μM H2DCFDA solution, which is an ROS fluorescence indicator, and seeded for 90 min in the dark. Finally, the in vitro antioxidant activity of the samples was estimated by measuring the fluorescence intensity of dichlorofluorescein (DCF), which was oxidized by ROS, at the emission wavelength of 535 nm (excitation wavelength: 485 nm) and using a microplate reader [7,31].

2.7. Antibacterial Activity of ABS@NPs

To estimate the antibacterial activity of ABS@NPs, a colony-counting method using *Staphylococcus aureus* ATCC 6538 (*S. aureus* ATCC 6538) was used. The bacteria were incubated in Luria–Bertani (LB) agar plates (BD Difco, Sparks, MD, USA) containing 1.5% agar at 37 °C. Before utilization, a single colony was inoculated in the LB broth and incubated overnight at 37 °C. This culture was subsequently diluted in the LB broth until the optical density (OD600) reached 0.1. Next, ABS@NPs (with 0 and 10 wt% ABS) were added to each culture to estimate the inhibition of bacterial growth over 24 h in an incubator. PBS and the ABS solution in DIW were used as negative control groups. Finally, after incubation, the suspensions were diluted to a factor of 10^7, and 100 μL of each suspension was spread over an agar plate using glass beads. After overnight incubation, the number of colonies was counted to determine the antibacterial activity against *S. aureus* ATCC 6538 [42,43].

2.8. In Vitro Cytotoxicity of ABS@NPs

The biocompatibility of ABS@NPs was evaluated utilizing NIH 3T3 cells, which were incubated in the DMEM solution including 1% penicillin–streptomycin and 10% FBS. Cell viability analysis was performed using the 3-(4,5-dimethylthiazol-2-yl)-2,5-diphenyltetrazolium bromide (MTT) assay 24 h after the addition of ABS@NPs. First, the cells were cultured at a density of 10,000 cells/well in 96-well plates. After 24 h of culture, the cells were incubated with different concentrations of ABS@NPs (1–10 μM) and cultured at 37 °C for 24 h. Thereafter, a 1 mg/mL MTT solution was added to the medium, and DMEM solution (containing 1% penicillin–streptomycin and 10% FBS) was added to each well of the plate and incubated for 3 h. Finally, the medium was washed with PBS and DMSO-d6 was used to dissolve the purple formazan dye crystals. Using a microplate reader (BioTek, Winooski, VT, USA), the absorbance of the formazan generated by live cells was estimated at 570 nm. The percentage of viable cells was estimated using the following equation: [7,29,36,44]

$$\text{Cell viability } (\%) = \left(\frac{\Delta A_{570} of\ test\ group}{\Delta A_{570} of\ control\ group}\right) \times 100 \quad (4)$$

2.9. Statistical Analysis

The resulting data are presented as mean ± standard deviation values, and every experiment was performed in triplicate. Using Student's t-test method, differences between experimental groups were compared. Statistical significance in all evaluations was confirmed at $p < 0.05$.

3. Results and Discussion

3.1. Characterization of ABS@NPs

ABS, a sesquiterpene alcohol, is a natural hydrophobic bioactive compound with various effects, including antioxidant and antibacterial activities [28–30,32,33]. However, its application in the bio-industry, such as in functional foods, pharmaceuticals, and cosmetics, is difficult owing to its low solubility and stability in the aqueous phase [28–31,37]. Therefore, it is necessary to develop a carrier that improves the stability and solubility of lipophilic ABS. In this study, polyglyceryl-4 caprate NPs with various ABS concentrations (ranging from 0 to 40 wt%) were produced by an encapsulation method. Polyglyceryl-4 caprate self-assembles in water to form stable NPs consisting of a hydrophilic shell and a hydrophobic core in which hydrophobic compounds can be encapsulated (Figure 1). The physicochemical properties, including PDI and size, of ABS@NPs did not differ significantly as the ABS concentration was varied (0–40 wt%) (Figure 2A,B). The ABS@NP 0 wt% (without ABS) exhibited a negative zeta potential of approximately -14.48 ± 0.92 mV, and the value tended to be the same as the concentration of ABS in the ABS@NPs was increased up to 10 wt%. However, in the ABS concentration range of 20 to 40 wt%, the surface zeta potential became increasingly negative as the loading content of ABS increased (Figure 2C). The encapsulation of ABS in the ABS@NPs was estimated using staining with a hydrophilic dye, methylene blue. Because ABS is colorless, the non-encapsulated part of the ABS@NPs cannot be observed well visually. With methylene blue added, the suspensions of ABS@NPs with up to 10 wt% ABS were clearly transparent, indicating that ABS was successfully encapsulated in the NPs up to a concentration of 10 wt%. However, at ABS concentrations above 10 wt.%, the suspensions became opaque, indicating the presence of unencapsulated ABS (Figure 2D). To quantify the encapsulation of ABS in the ABS@NPs, the ABS loading contents and efficiencies of ABS@NPs were analyzed via HPLC at different ABS concentrations, and the results are as follows: 5 wt% ABS@NPs: L.C. = 4.10, L.E. = 82.07, 10 wt% ABS@NPs: L.C. = 8.13, L.E. = 81.34, 20 wt% ABS@NPs: L.C. = 13.52, L.E. = 67.60, and 40 wt% ABS@NPs: L.C. = 15.17, L.E. = 37.92. Based on the experimental data, we concluded that 10 wt% is the optimal loading of ABS in ABS@NPs.

3.2. Long-Term Stability of The ABS@NPs

Particles of an oil phase in water are metastable, that is, they are thermodynamically unstable owing to their high energy level. Therefore, suspensions of oil particles dispersed in water using surfactants easily phase-separate through destabilization processes, such as precipitation, flocculation, and coalescence. Therefore, the long-term stability of ABS@NPs in DIW was analyzed at 25 °C by evaluating the changes in the NP size and PDI using DLS. The initial particle size (Figure 3A) and PDI (Figure 3B) of ABS@NPs indicated stability for a prolonged period, up to 112 days, without any notable change at ABS concentrations ranging from 0 to 10 wt%. In addition, all samples had a particle size of 300 nm or less and a PDI value of 0.3 or less. Thus, the results indicated that the fabricated ABS@NPs have remarkable long-term stability, and the system can be used as a successful platform for developing stable drug delivery systems.

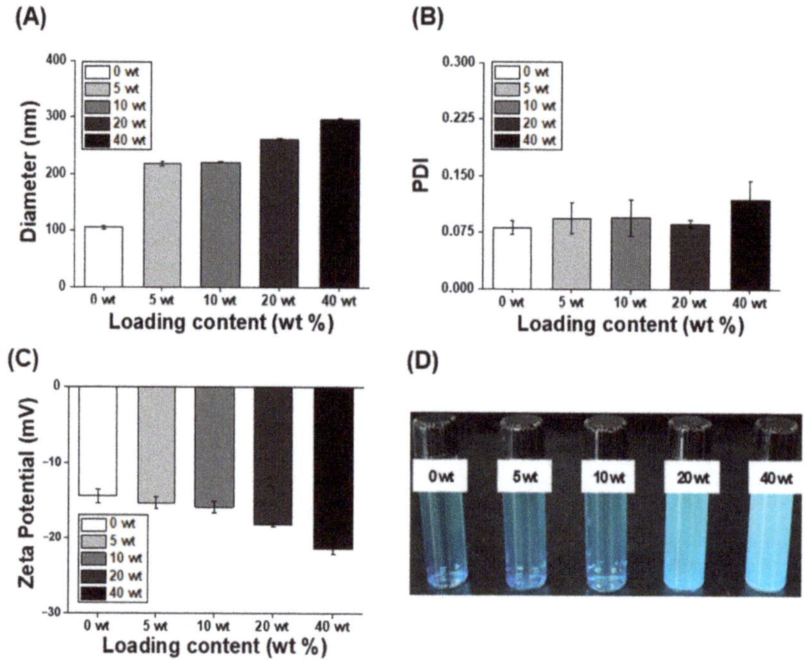

Figure 2. (**A**) Particle size, (**B**) polydispersity index (PDI), and (**C**) zeta potential of ABS@NPs with different ABS loadings in the range of 0 to 40 wt%. (**D**) Methylene blue staining test of the ABS@NPs with different ABS loadings.

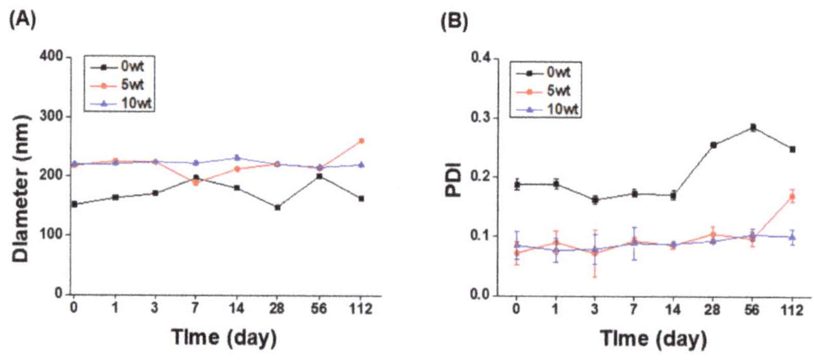

Figure 3. Long-term stability of ABS@NPs at ABS concentrations ranging from 0 to 40 wt%. Variation of the (**A**) particle size and (**B**) polydispersity index (PDI) of ABS@NPs over 112 days.

3.3. In Situ DPPH Radical-Scavenging Activity and In Vitro Antioxidant Activity of the ABS @NPs

ABS is a stronger antioxidant than garlic [45]. However, maximizing the antioxidant activity of ABS in the aqueous phase is challenging because of its hydrophobic properties. Therefore, we fabricated ABS@NPs to maximize the ABS activity in an aqueous solution. To measure the antioxidant activity of ABS@NPs, an in situ DPPH antioxidant activity assay and an in vitro radical-scavenging activity assay were performed. First, using the DPPH radical-scavenging assay, the antioxidant activities of ABS@NPs and various control groups were evaluated (Figure 4A). DPPH, which is an organic nitrogen radical, absorbs at the wavelength of 515 nm in the visible range. When a solution of DPPH radicals reacts with an antioxidant, the color of the resulting solution shifts from violet to yellow because the DPPH receives electrons or hydrogen atoms from the radical scavenger, and its absorbance at 515 nm decreases. Thus, the percentage of scavenged DPPH radicals were determined based on the absorbance of the samples at 515 nm. ABS in DIW had little effect in scavenging DPPH radicals in comparison with the positive control of AA in DIW. In other words, this experiment showed that bio-applications are limited if alpha-bisabolol is not water-soluble through encapsulation. However, ABS@NPs exhibited more effective DPPH radical-scavenging activity than that of AA, and the antioxidant effect increased with the increase in the ABS concentration in the ABS@NPs from 5 to 10 wt%. In addition, in the case of ABS@NP 0 wt% (without ABS), there was little scavenging of DPPH radicals, suggesting that the solubilizer, polyglyceryl-4 caprate, had little effect on the antioxidant activity (Figure 4A). H2DCFDA, which is an ROS fluorescence indicator, diffuses through the cell membrane and is oxidized very quickly to highly fluorescent DCF, which fluoresces green in the presence of intracellular ROS, and its fluorescence intensity at the emission wavelength of 535 nm (excitation wavelength: 485 nm) increases [10]. Hence the in vitro antioxidant activity assay was conducted by analyzing H2DCFDA fluorescence after the addition of H_2O_2 in mouse NIH 3T3 fibroblast cells. H_2O_2, which is an oxidative stress agent, spontaneously formed a cellular environment, leading to the generation of ROS. The NIH 3T3 cells treated with H_2O_2 alone were used as the negative control group. As expected, the ROS levels of the cells treated with ABS@NP 10 wt% decreased considerably to approximately 15% as the ABS concentration increased from 1 to 1000 nM. However, the ROS levels of the cells treated with ABS in DIW and ABS@NP 0 wt% were reduced up to 49% and 56%, respectively. Therefore, we consider that these two samples have little effect on the ROS-scavenging activity in vitro (Figure 4B). These results indicate that the encapsulation of ABS enhances its antioxidant activity.

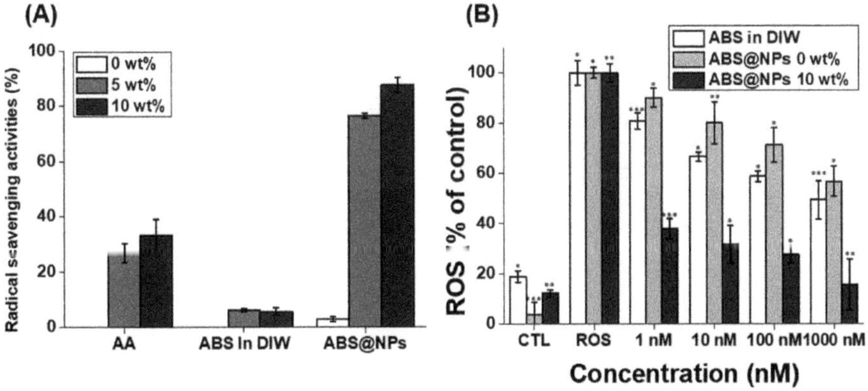

Figure 4. (**A**) Antioxidation activity of ABS@NPs with 0, 5, and 10 wt% ABS, compared to that of ascorbic acid (AA) in deionized water (DIW), assessed using the 2,2-diphenyl-1-picrylhydrazyl (DPPH) radical-scavenging assay. (**B**) Results of in vitro assays using the H2DCFDA assay kit. Antioxidation activity of ABS@NP 10 wt% at ABS concentrations ranging from 1 to 1000 nM; reactive oxygen species (ROS) and the control (CTL) groups represent the highest and lowest levels of ROS, respectively (* $p < 0.05$, ** $p < 0.01$, *** $p < 0.005$).

3.4. Antibacterial Activity of ABS@NPs

ABS has previously been reported to exhibit antibacterial activity [31,32]. However, owing to its hydrophobic properties, its antibacterial properties are not effectively manifested in the aqueous phase. In this study, we used a colony-counting method to analyze the antibacterial activity of ABS@NPs against *S. aureus* ATCC 6538. It was visually observed that the ABS@NPs significantly inhibited the growth of *S. aureus* compared to the control groups of PBS and ABS@NP 0 wt% (Figure 5A). The viability of *S. aureus* ATCC 6538 was reduced to 1 and 30% after treatment with ABS@NPs and ABS in DIW, respectively. Notably, these results show that the antibacterial effect of ABS increased considerably after encapsulation (Figure 5B), indicating that even a small amount of ABS exhibits considerably enhanced antibacterial activity.

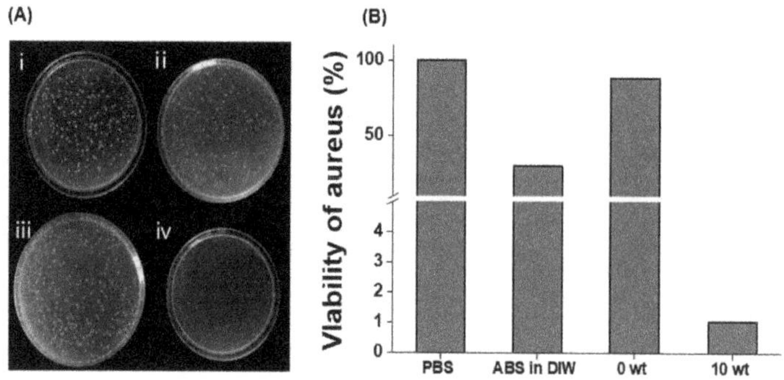

Figure 5. Antibacterial activity of ABS@NPs. (**A**) Photographs of staphylococcus aureus ATCC 6538 colonies in (i) phosphate-buffered saline, (ii) ABS in deionized water (DIW), (iii) ABS@NP 0 wt% in DIW, and (iv) ABS@NP 10 wt% in DIW. (**B**) Viability of S. aureus after treatment with phosphate-buffered saline (PBS), ABS in DIW, ABS@NP 0 wt% in DIW, and ABS@NP 10 wt% in DIW.

3.5. In Vitro Cytotoxicity Activity of ABS @NPs

To assess the biocompatibility of ABS@NPs in NIH 3T3 fibroblast cells, an MTT assay was performed after treatment with ABS@NPs. There was almost no reduction in the viability of the NIH 3T3 cells. No toxic effects were observed in cells treated with ABS at concentrations ranging from 1 to 10 μM (Figure 6). We found that ABS@NPs did not show cytotoxic effects up to a concentration of 10 μM, and did not induce toxic effects in cells.

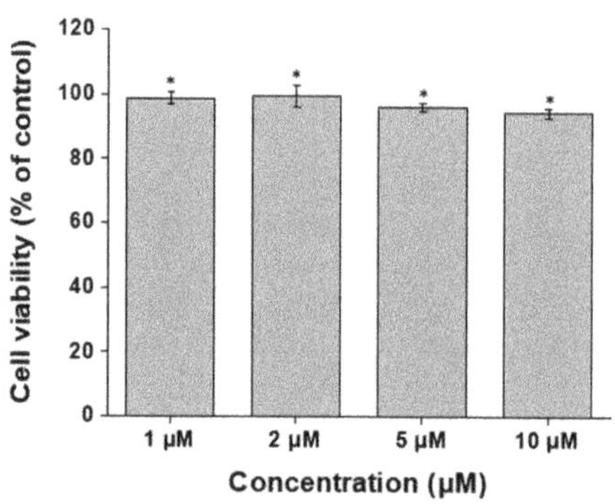

Figure 6. Cytotoxicity analysis of 10 wt% ABS@NPs at ABS concentrations in the range of 1 to 10 μM (* $p < 0.05$).

4. Conclusions

Bioactive compounds have various properties, such as antioxidant and antibacterial activities, and are widely used in the pharmaceutical, cosmetic, and food industries. ROS, which are highly reactive forms of intermediates, include H_2O_2, a superoxide radical (O_2^-), and a hydroxyl radical (OH^-). They cause extreme damage to biomolecules in cells and mitochondria, thereby inducing inflammation and excessive oxidative stress in the body, resulting in various diseases, such as cancer and AD in humans. Therefore, compounds with antioxidant properties have become of great interest for the development of various bioproducts in modern urbanized society, where many factors, such as ultraviolet rays, fine dust, and blue light, induce the formation of active oxygen species. The antibacterial activity of natural substances is an important property for bioproduct development as it minimizes preservatives, such as formaldehyde, iodopropynyl butylcarbamate, and triclosan, which induce issues such as allergies and contact dermatitis in users. ABS, a sesquiterpene alcohol, is a natural hydrophobic bioactive compound with various effects, including antioxidant and antibacterial activities. However, its application in the bio-industry is difficult owing to its low solubility and stability in the aqueous phase. In this study, we demonstrated the successful and facile fabrication of ABS@NPs, which have potential antioxidant and antibacterial effects, using an emulsification method. The optimized ABS@NPs were thermodynamically stable and exhibited excellent stability for up to 112 days. Moreover, the improved aqueous solubility of ABS@NPs led to a remarkable increase in the bioavailability of ABS and induced improved effects of ABS compared to those of non-encapsulated ABS. We confirmed that ABS@NPs successfully scavenge ROS and kill bacteria without toxicity. The ABS@NPs are expected to be used as drug carriers with outstanding stability in various fields, including foods, cosmetics, and pharmaceuticals.

Author Contributions: Conceptualization, D.S., H.K. and W.I.C.; methodology, S.K. and S.Y.; software, S.K. and J.K.; validation, S.K., N.U.K. and J.K.; formal analysis, S.K. and S.Y.; investigation, S.K.; resources, J.K.; data curation, S.K.; writing—original draft preparation, S.K.; writing—review and editing, D.S., H.K. and W.I.C.; visualization, S.K.; supervision, D.S.; project administration, W.I.C.; funding acquisition, D.S. All authors have read and agreed to the published version of the manuscript.

Funding: This work was supported by the National Research Foundation of Korea (NRF) grant funded by the Korea government (MSIT) (2021M3C1C3097647, 2021R1F1A1061145, 2021R1F1A1063492). This research was supported by Brain Pool program funded by the Ministry of Science and ICT through the National Research Foundation of Korea (2022H1D3A2A02053125), and a grant from the Korea Institute of Ceramic Engineering and Technology (KICET) (1415181794).

Institutional Review Board Statement: Not applicable.

Informed Consent Statement: Not applicable.

Data Availability Statement: Not applicable.

Conflicts of Interest: The authors declare no conflict of interest.

References

1. Apone, F.; Barbulova, A.; Colucci, M.G. Plant and Microalgae Derived Peptides Are Advantageously Employed as Bioactive Compounds in Cosmetics. *Front. Plant Sci.* **2019**, *10*, 756. [CrossRef]
2. Borowitzka, M.A. Microalgae as sources of pharmaceuticals and other biologically active compounds. *J. Appl. Phycol.* **1995**, *7*, 3–15. [CrossRef]
3. Kaur, S.; Das, M. Functional foods: An overview. *Food Sci. Biotechnol.* **2011**, *20*, 861–875. [CrossRef]
4. Dubey, V.S.; Bhalla, R.; Luthra, R. An overview of the non-mevalonate pathway for terpenoid biosynthesis in plants. *J. Biosci.* **2003**, *28*, 637–646. [CrossRef]
5. Joshi, S.; Chanotiya, C.S.; Agarwal, G.; Prakash, O.; Pant, A.K.; Mathela, C.S. Terpenoid Compositions, and Antioxidant and Antimicrobial Properties of the Rhizome Essential Oils of Different Hedychium Species. *Chem. Biodivers.* **2008**, *5*, 299–309. [CrossRef]
6. Pichersky, E.; Raguso, R.A. Why do plants produce so many terpenoid compounds? *New Phytol.* **2018**, *220*, 692–702. [CrossRef]
7. Yang, H.; Yu, S.; Kim, J.; Baek, K.; Lee, Y.R.; Lee, H.S.; Choi, W.I.; Sung, D. Facile Solvent-Free Preparation of Antioxidant Idebenone-Loaded Nanoparticles for Efficient Wound Healing. *Pharmaceutics* **2022**, *14*, 521. [CrossRef]
8. Saravanakumar, G.; Kim, J.; Kim, W.J. Reactive-Oxygen-Species-Responsive Drug Delivery Systems: Promises and Challenges. *Adv. Sci.* **2017**, *4*, 1600124. [CrossRef]
9. Ye, H.; Zhou, Y.; Liu, X.; Chen, Y.; Duan, S.; Zhu, R.; Liu, Y.; Yin, L. Recent Advances on Reactive Oxygen Species-Responsive Delivery and Diagnosis System. *Biomacromolecules* **2019**, *20*, 2441–2463. [CrossRef]
10. Choi, S.-I.; Lee, J.S.; Lee, S.; Lee, H.J.; Kim, B.-J.; Yeo, J.; Jung, T.-D.; Cho, B.-Y.; Choi, S.-H.; Lee, J.-H. Antioxidant and anti-aging effects of extracts from leaves of Castanea crenata Siebold & Zucc. in human dermal fibroblast. *J. Food Hyg. Saf.* **2017**, *32*, 243–248.
11. Liu, Y.e.; Chen, C.; Wang, X.; Sun, Y.; Zhang, J.; Chen, J.; Shi, Y. An epigenetic role of mitochondria in cancer. *Cells* **2022**, *11*, 2518. [CrossRef] [PubMed]

12. Fang, X.; Zhang, J.; Roman, R.J.; Fan, F. From 1901 to 2022, how far are we from truly understanding the pathogenesis of age-related dementia? *GeroScience* **2022**, *44*, 1879–1883. [CrossRef] [PubMed]
13. Godic, A.; Poljsak, B.; Adamic, M.; Dahmane, R. The role of antioxidants in skin cancer prevention and treatment. *Oxidative Med. Cell. Longev.* **2014**, *2014*, 860479. [CrossRef] [PubMed]
14. Yoshitomi, T.; Nagasaki, Y. Reactive oxygen species-scavenging nanomedicines for the treatment of oxidative stress injuries. *Adv. Healthc. Mater.* **2014**, *3*, 1149–1161. [CrossRef] [PubMed]
15. Zhu, Y.; Matsumura, Y.; Velayutham, M.; Foley, L.M.; Hitchens, T.K.; Wagner, W.R. Reactive oxygen species scavenging with a biodegradable, thermally responsive hydrogel compatible with soft tissue injection. *Biomaterials* **2018**, *177*, 98–112. [CrossRef] [PubMed]
16. Mu, H.; Tang, J.; Liu, Q.; Sun, C.; Wang, T.; Duan, J. Potent Antibacterial Nanoparticles against Biofilm and Intracellular Bacteria. *Sci. Rep.* **2016**, *6*, 18877. [CrossRef]
17. Hillyer, C.D.; Josephson, C.D.; Blajchman, M.A.; Vostal, J.G.; Epstein, J.S.; Goodman, J.L. Bacterial contamination of blood components: Risks, strategies, and regulation: Joint ASH and AABB educational session in transfusion medicine. *Hematol. Am. Soc. Hematol. Educ. Program* **2003**, *2003*, 575–589. [CrossRef]
18. Hussain, M.A. Food Contamination: Major Challenges of the Future. *Foods* **2016**, *5*, 21. [CrossRef]
19. Jimenez, L. Molecular diagnosis of microbial contamination in cosmetic and pharmaceutical products: A review. *J. AOAC Int.* **2001**, *84*, 671–675. [CrossRef]
20. Astray, G.; Gonzalez-Barreiro, C.; Mejuto, J.C.; Rial-Otero, R.; Simal-Gándara, J. A review on the use of cyclodextrins in foods. *Food Hydrocoll.* **2009**, *23*, 1631–1640. [CrossRef]
21. Sheng, Z.; Liu, Y. Potential impacts of silver nanoparticles on bacteria in the aquatic environment. *J. Environ. Manag.* **2017**, *191*, 290–296. [CrossRef] [PubMed]
22. Hughes, O.B.; Maderal, A.D.; Tosti, A. Preservative Sensitization—Safety With and Safety Without. *Curr. Treat. Options Allergy* **2016**, *3*, 345–358. [CrossRef]
23. Magos, L. Review on the toxicity of ethylmercury including its presence as a preservative in biological and pharmaceutical products. *J. Appl. Toxicol.* **2001**, *21*, 1–5. [CrossRef]
24. Herman, A. Antimicrobial Ingredients as Preservative Booster and Components of Self-Preserving Cosmetic Products. *Curr. Microbiol.* **2019**, *76*, 744–754. [CrossRef]
25. Yang, S.C.; Lin, C.H.; Sung, C.T.; Fang, J.Y. Antibacterial activities of bacteriocins: Application in foods and pharmaceuticals. *Front. Microbiol.* **2014**, *5*, 241. [CrossRef] [PubMed]
26. Bondi, M.; Lauková, A.; de Niederhausern, S.; Messi, P.; Papadopoulou, C. Natural Preservatives to Improve Food Quality and Safety. *J. Food Qual.* **2017**, *2017*, 1090932. [CrossRef]
27. Dreger, M.; Wielgus, K. Application of essential oils as natural cosmetic preservatives. *Herba Pol.* **2013**, *59*, 142–156. [CrossRef]
28. De Marchi, J.G.B.; Jornada, D.S.; Silva, F.K.; Freitas, A.L.; Fuentefria, A.M.; Pohlmann, A.R.; Guterres, S.S. Triclosan resistance reversion by encapsulation in chitosan-coated-nanocapsule containing alpha-bisabolol as core: Development of wound dressing. *Int. J. Nanomed.* **2017**, *12*, 7855–7868. [CrossRef]
29. Marongiu, L.; Donini, M.; Bovi, M.; Perduca, M.; Vivian, F.; Romeo, A.; Mariotto, S.; Monaco, H.L.; Dusi, S. The inclusion into PLGA nanoparticles enables α-bisabolol to efficiently inhibit the human dendritic cell pro-inflammatory activity. *J. Nanopart. Res.* **2014**, *16*, 2554. [CrossRef]
30. Terroso, T.F.; Condotta, K.B.; da Fonseca, F.N.; Jornada, D.S.; Ferreira, G.O.; Ellwanger, J.H.; Schmidt, J.A.; Pohlmann, A.R.; Guterres, S.S. In vivo prophylactic gastroprotection using α-bisabolol encapsulated in lipid-core nanocapsules and in cocoa-theospheres. *J. Drug Deliv. Sci. Technol.* **2016**, *36*, 99–109. [CrossRef]
31. Sathya, S.; Shanmuganathan, B.; Devi, K.P. Deciphering the anti-apoptotic potential of alpha-bisabolol loaded solid lipid nanoparticles against Abeta induced neurotoxicity in Neuro-2a cells. *Colloids Sur. B Biointerfaces* **2020**, *190*, 110948. [CrossRef] [PubMed]
32. Ramazani, E.; Akaberi, M.; Emami, S.A.; Tayarani-Najaran, Z. Pharmacological and biological effects of alpha-bisabolol: An updated review of the molecular mechanisms. *Life Sci.* **2022**, *304*, 120728. [CrossRef] [PubMed]
33. Eddin, L.B.; Jha, N.K.; Goyal, S.N.; Agrawal, Y.O.; Subramanya, S.B.; Bastaki, S.M.A.; Ojha, S. Health Benefits, Pharmacological Effects, Molecular Mechanisms, and Therapeutic Potential of alpha-Bisabolol. *Nutrients* **2022**, *14*, 1370. [CrossRef]
34. Na, Y.; Lee, J.S.; Woo, J.; Ahn, S.; Lee, E.; Il Choi, W.; Sung, D. Reactive oxygen species (ROS)-responsive ferrocene-polymer-based nanoparticles for controlled release of drugs. *J. Mater. Chem. B* **2020**, *8*, 1906–1913. [CrossRef]
35. Sao Pedro, A.; Detoni, C.; Ferreira, D.; Cabral-Albuquerque, E.; Sarmento, B. Validation of a high-performance liquid chromatography method for the determination of (−)-alpha-bisabolol from particulate systems. *Biomed. Chromatogr.* **2009**, *23*, 966–972. [CrossRef] [PubMed]
36. Na, Y.; Woo, J.; Choi, W.I.; Lee, J.H.; Hong, J.; Sung, D. alpha-Tocopherol-loaded reactive oxygen species-scavenging ferrocene nanocapsules with high antioxidant efficacy for wound healing. *Int. J. Pharm.* **2021**, *596*, 120205. [CrossRef] [PubMed]
37. D'Almeida, A.P.L.; Pacheco de Oliveira, M.T.; de Souza, E.T.; de Sa Coutinho, D.; Ciambarella, B.T.; Gomes, C.R.; Terroso, T.; Guterres, S.S.; Pohlmann, A.R.; Silva, P.M.; et al. alpha-bisabolol-loaded lipid-core nanocapsules reduce lipopolysaccharide-induced pulmonary inflammation in mice. *Int. J. Nanomed.* **2017**, *12*, 4479–4491. [CrossRef]

38. Hosseinpour, M.; Mobini-Dehkordi, M.; Saffar, B.; Teimori, H. Antiproliferative effects of Matricaria chamomilla on Saccharomyces cerevisiae. *J. HerbMed Pharmacol.* **2013**, *2*, 49–51.
39. Kim, K.W.; Thomas, R. Antioxidative activity of chitosans with varying molecular weights. *Food Chem.* **2007**, *101*, 308–313. [CrossRef]
40. Apak, R.; Gorinstein, S.; Böhm, V.; Schaich, K.M.; Özyürek, M.; Güçlü, K. Methods of measurement and evaluation of natural antioxidant capacity/activity (IUPAC Technical Report). *Pure Appl. Chem.* **2013**, *85*, 957–998. [CrossRef]
41. Oh, H.; Lee, J.S.; Sung, D.; Lim, J.-M.; Choi, W.I. <p>Potential Antioxidant and Wound Healing Effect of Nano-Liposol with High Loading Amount of Astaxanthin. *Int. J. Nanomed.* **2020**, *15*, 9231–9240. [CrossRef] [PubMed]
42. Oliveira, F.S.; Freitas, T.S.; Cruz, R.P.D.; Costa, M.D.S.; Pereira, R.L.S.; Quintans-Junior, L.J.; Andrade, T.A.; Menezes, P.D.P.; Sousa, B.M.H.; Nunes, P.S.; et al. Evaluation of the antibacterial and modulatory potential of alpha-bisabolol, beta-cyclodextrin and alpha-bisabolol/beta-cyclodextrin complex. *Biomed. Pharm.* **2017**, *92*, 1111–1118. [CrossRef] [PubMed]
43. Oh, H.; Lee, J.S.; Lee, H.S.; Sung, D.; Choi, W.I. A Novel Polyvinylpyrrolidone-Stabilized Illite Microparticle with Enhanced Antioxidant and Antibacterial Effect. *Polymers* **2021**, *13*, 4275. [CrossRef] [PubMed]
44. Sathya, S.; Shanmuganathan, B.; Manirathinam, G.; Ruckmani, K.; Devi, K.P. α-Bisabolol loaded solid lipid nanoparticles attenuates Aβ aggregation and protects Neuro-2a cells from Aβ induced neurotoxicity. *J. Mol. Liq.* **2018**, *264*, 431–441. [CrossRef]
45. Herrera-Calderon, O.; Chacaltana-Ramos, L.J.; Huayanca-Gutierrez, I.C.; Algarni, M.A.; Alqarni, M.; Batiha, G.E. Chemical Constituents, In Vitro Antioxidant Activity and In Silico Study on NADPH Oxidase of *Allium sativum* L. (Garlic) Essential Oil. *Antioxidants* **2021**, *10*, 1844. [CrossRef]

antioxidants

MDPI

Article

A Study of the Interface of Gold Nanoparticles Conjugated to Cowpea Fe-Superoxide Dismutase

Edurne Tellechea [1,*], Aaron C. Asensio [1,†], Paula Ciaurriz [1,‡], Javier Buezo [2,§], Pedro López-Gómez [2], Marina Urra [2] and Jose F. Moran [2,*]

1 NAITEC-Technological Center of Automotive and Mechatronics, C/Tajonar 20, 31006 Pamplona, Spain
2 Institute for Multidisciplinary Research in Applied Biology (IMAB), Department of Sciences, Public University of Navarre (UPNA); Avda. de Pamplona 123, 31192 Mutilva, Spain
* Correspondence: eteiletxea@naitec.es (E.T.); jose.moran@unavarra.es (J.F.M.); Tel.: +34-948-292900 (E.T.); Tel.: +34-948-168018 (J.F.M.)
† Current address: Centro Stirling, Carretera de Tafalla 10, 31132 Villatuerta, Spain.
‡ Current address: CENER, National Renewable Energy Center of Spain, Polígono Industrial Rocaforte, Parcela G2-H1, 31400 Sangüesa, Spain.
§ Current address: Department of Forest Engineering, Forest Management Planning and Terrestrial Measurements, University of Transilvania, 1, Ludwig van Beethoven Str., 500123 Brașov, Romania.

Abstract: The iron superoxide dismutase (FeSOD) is a first barrier to defend photosynthetic organisms from superoxide radicals. Although it is broadly present in plants and bacteria, FeSODs are absent in animals. They belong to the same phylogenic family as Mn-containing SODs, which are also highly efficient at detoxifying superoxide radicals. In addition, SODs can react with peroxynitrite, and FeSOD enzyme has already been used to evaluate the anti-nitrative capacity of plant antioxidants. Gold nanoparticles (AuNPs) have been shown to significantly improve the functionality and the efficiency of ligands, providing they are properly assembled. In this work, the characteristics of the recombinant cowpea (*Vigna unguiculata*) FeSOD (r*Vu*FeSOD) immobilized onto AuNPs were investigated as a function of (1) NP surface chemistry and (2) biofunctionalization methods, either physical adsorption or covalent bonding. The NP surface chemistry was studied by varying the concentration of the ligand molecule 11-mercaptoundecanoic acid (MUA) on the NP surface. The coverage and activity of the protein on AuNPs was determined and correlated to the surface chemistry and the two biofunctionalization methods. rVuFeSOD–AuNPs conjugate stability was monitored through absorption measurements, agarose gel electrophoresis and DLS, enzymatic activity by a colorimetric assay and by in-gel activity assay, and coverage was measured by colorimetric assay. When using physical adsorption, the NP is the most perturbing agent for the activity of the enzyme. In contrast, only the NP coverage was affected by MUA ligand concentration. However, during covalent attachment, both the NP and the concentration of MUA on the surface influenced the enzyme activity, while the coverage of the NP remained constant. The results evidence the importance of the biomolecule and AuNP interaction for the functionality of the hybrid. These strategies can be used to develop electrochemical biosensors for $O_2^{\bullet -}$ and for peroxynitrite in biomedical applications.

Keywords: biofunctionalization; gold nanoparticle; superoxide dismutase; SOD

1. Introduction

Superoxide dismutases (SODs; superoxide:superoxide oxidoreductase, EC 1.15.1.1) are an essential group of metalloenzymes that have been crucial for the evolution and maintenance of oxygenic life. They represent a first line of defense against free radical production from oxygen by specifically catalyzing the dismutation of superoxide radicals ($O_2^{\bullet -}$). SODs catalyze two-step reactions in which two superoxide anions dismutate to hydrogen peroxide and water, while a metal cofactor cycles between its reduced and oxidized forms [1]. Superoxide dismutation by SODs is among the fastest enzyme reactions known [2], and is only limited by diffusion velocity. SODs are found in all three domains of life, and may well have been present in LUCA (the last universal common ancestor of life), long before the existence of an oxygenic atmosphere on earth, to break the $O_2^{\bullet-}$ produced from the UV-radiation-derived splitting of water. Virtually all organisms that spend any time in the presence of oxygen possess copies of this enzyme. Three major families of superoxide dismutase are currently known, and these families depend on the metal cofactor: the Cu/Zn type, the Ni type and the Fe and Mn type [2].

In every living organism, the regulation of $O_2^{\bullet-}$ production and elimination is very important. The excess $O_2^{\bullet-}$ are involved in many physiological and pathological processes. $O_2^{\bullet-}$ is strongly correlated with tissue injury and associated inflammation, and certain cancers and aged–related disease, such amyotrophic lateral sclerosis, Parkinson's disease, Alzheimer's disease, cataracts and various neurological disorders [2]. Therefore, the monitorization of superoxide anions in biological systems, both in vivo and in vitro, is of great importance to reveal and counteract $O_2^{\bullet-}$ physiological functions. Superoxide radicals are highly reactive and short-lived, and therefore difficult to detect in complex biological matrices. In recent years, different detection techniques have been developed, i.e., electron paramagnetic resonance (EPR) [3], surface-enhanced Raman spectroscopy (SERS), fluorescence imaging, photoprotein-based bioluminescence, and electrochemical biosensors [4]. Considerable attention has been paid to the direct electrochemistry of SOD and related $O_2^{\bullet-}$ detection [5] as a non-damaging, low-cost, and effective selective technique, but it requires the immobilization of SOD onto the electrode surface. Several strategies have been employed to improve electron transfer between SOD redox enzyme and electrodes, and it appears a promising way to use nanomaterials as the protein carriers. These hybrid electrodes can be built on a nanometric scale at low cost, and with strong analytical response. The electrode surfaces are chemically and physically diverse, and they include CeO_2 nanoparticles [6], Pt–Pd multiwalled carbon nanotubes [6] (MWCNTs), ZnO nanoparticles [7], and gold nanoparticles (AuNPs) [8–11], AuNPs being one of the most studied nanomaterials. Another interesting application of SOD–AuNP complexes is the development of highly sensitive colorimetric detection of the temporal evolution of SOD1 aggregates implicated in the pathology of amyotrophic lateral sclerosis (ALS) [12]. Additionally, AuNPs have been described as a new class of surface immobilized pH-stimulus-responsive hybrid material based on tethered SOD1 [13], and as SOD carriers for possible therapeutic applications [14].

Many immobilization methods have been developed for SOD and AuNPs, such as direct binding, encapsulation, and crosslinking, although the most popular biofuction-alization method is noncovalent immobilization [5–7,10]. CuZnSOD (SOD1) is the most frequently used SOD [8–10,12,13]), while FeSOD, is the least studied group of the main SOD families [15,16]. Generally, these studies focus on the effect of whole conjugates (SOD–AuNPs) on the application (i.e., electrochemical measurements). While some enzymes retain their activity once they are localized upon the AuNPs [14,17], others are strongly affected [15]. In some cases, the NPs can improve enzyme activity and stability [18]. Moreover, it has been observed that the ligand used to passivate nanoparticles also plays an important role in enzyme activity [15]. Thus, the characterization of the VuFeSOD enzyme interaction with AuNPs, and the stability of the resulting particle complexes, is of critical importance to many functional applications.

Here we investigate the characteristics of a recombinant (r*Vu*FeSOD) protein from the legume cowpea (*Vigna unguiculata*) immobilized on 9.6 nm AuNPs. Cowpea is an important legume crop originating from tropical and subtropical areas. It is of increasing agronomic interest due to its ability to tolerate drought. Cowpea FeSOD has been shown to participate in the response to drought stress by eliminating superoxide radicals [19]. Within eukaryotes, the FeSOD family is typically found in chloroplasts, with few exceptions, the most important being the FeSOD of the legume plants. Thus, VuFeSOD belongs to a second family of FeSODs localized in the cytosol, and they are more important than the chloroplastic family in terms of biological activity within the cells [19,20]. VuFeSOD has been crystallized [21], its 3D structure has been solved, and the model refined to 1.97 Å resolution [22]. FeSOD is a homodimer enzyme with one binding site for superoxide anions per subunit, which is located at a cleft close to the dimer interface. The dimer interface also shows that some amino acids are considered to play an important role in the catalysis due to subunit cooperation [22]. rVuFeSOD plays a role in symbiotic nodules during biological fixation of atmospheric nitrogen, where it can protect the cytosolic symbiotic hemoglobin from oxidation with superoxide. The *Vu*FeSOD contents in the plant cells increase with the age of the plant, and VuFeSOD also participates in the plant response to abiotic stresses such us drought, salt, high irradiance, and others, which limits field agronomic production. This protein has a high affinity for the superoxide anion, and it is possible to overexpress and purify it in very high concentrations [23].

In addition, VuFeSOD has been used as a sensor of the harmful peroxynitrite anion, since peroxynitrite targets important metalloproteins, as superoxide dismutases, with high affinity [24–26]. In this respect, VuFeSOD has been used to test, in vitro, the anti-nitrative and protective capacity of different antioxidants from plants [26,27]. Peroxynitrite also targets hemoproteins and other metalloproteins with high affinity [27]. Hence, VuFeSOD bound to AuNPs can be useful as an affordable and specific sensor to detect either superoxide or peroxynitrite radicals, or to protect hemoglobins and other proteins from oxidation. There is a broad array of biomedical applications that can benefit from this technology, including different medical situations, such as inflammation, cardiovascular diseases, or hypoxia–reperfusion injury.

Here we show that the r*Vu*FeSOD enzyme can conjugate to AuNPs covalently and noncovalently, using mercaptoundecanoic acid as a ligand. The effect of ligand concentration on protein activity and coverage was determined to ascertain its correlation with surface chemistry. Our results show that both the surface chemistry and how the enzyme interacts with the NP, either covalently or by physical adsorption, affects the activity and coverage. These results improve the FeSOD utility and efficiency in its range of applications, potentially enhancing, for example, the capabilities of electrochemical nanosensors for SOD detection or even biomedics, with nanodeposition of Au particles via FeSOD in tissues where pathologic SOD production is typically detected, e.g., in anoxia–reperfusion injuries.

2. Materials and Methods

2.1. Chemicals and Biological Material

All chemicals were purchased from Sigma-Aldrich Co. (St. Louis, MO, USA), except when indicated. HisTrap HP 5 mL chromatography columns were supplied by GE Healthcare (Uppsala, Sweden). The buffer used with the protein contained 10 mM sodium phosphate (NaP) and was adjusted to pH 7.4. MilliQ Water (Millipore, Bedford, MA, USA) was used throughout this study.

2.2. Methods

2.2.1. Overexpression, Purification and Activity of Recombinant VuFeSOD

The *Vu*FeSOD was recombinantly engineered into pET28a+ as described previously [19]. Overexpression and purification of the recombinant *Vu*FeSOD was established by the optimized method, as reported previously. Protein purification was assessed by gel electrophoresis (10% PAGE, *w*/*v*), and purified protein aliquots were pooled and stored at −20 °C until used. In order to quantify total protein, Bradford dye binding assay was used with bovine serum albumin (BSA) as a standard. Enzymatic activity of SOD was assayed on 12.5% (*w*/*v*) native acrylamide gel [28].

2.2.2. Gold Nanoparticles Synthesis (AuNPs)

Water-soluble, citrate-stabilized AuNPs (d = 9.6 ± 2.2 nm) were synthesized according to literature methods [29]. Briefly, 80 mL of 1% tetrachloroauric acid ($HAuCl_4$) was reduced by adding a mixture of 4 mL of 1% sodium citrate (*w*/*v*), 0.1 mL of 1% tannic acid (*w*/*v*), 1 mL of 25 mM sodium carbonate, and 14.9 mL of H_2O at 60 °C under vigorous stirring.

At the beginning, the color of the solution was purple, but changed to red as the reaction continued. After 10 min at stable temperature, the colloidal solution was cooled down at room temperature.

After the synthesis was completed, transmission electron microscopy (TEM) images were captured to evaluate size distribution of the particles. The average size of the particles was obtained by analysis of TEM images JEOL 2011 (JEOL, Inc., Peabody, MA, USA) with ImageJ software (https://imagej.net, accessed on 16 May 2022) [30].

The concentration of the AuNP solution was calculated by absorption spectrophotometry. The AuNPs (9.6 nm) showed an absorption peak at 517.5 nm. Gold nanoparticles were assumed to possess the bulk structure of gold, and a population of atoms per volume unit (~5.9×10^{28} m^{-3}) was reported previously [31]. Accordingly, the 9.6 nm AuNPs in our study were composed of approximately 27,332 atoms with an extinction coefficient of about 9.1×10^7 $cm^{-1} \times M^{-1}$ [32]. The concentrations of certain AuNP solutions were then calculated via the Lambert–Beer law, where absorbance at 800 nm is subtracted from the peak absorbance as a baseline value (Equation (1)).

$$C = \frac{Abs_{517.5\text{nm}} - Abs_{800\text{nm}}}{\varepsilon_{abs}} \quad (1)$$

2.2.3. Surface Modification of AuNPs

The surfaces of the NPs were modified with mercaptoundecanoic acid (MUA) using different NP:ligand stoichiometry: 1:100, 1:250, 1:500, 1:750, and 1:1000. MUA contains a thiol group in one side of the chain that facilitates a covalent bond to Au and a carboxyl group on the other side. Gel electrophoresis, size, and UV–Vis spectra were used to assay the surface chemistry. Agarose gel electrophoresis (0.5%) was performed in Tris-acetate (TA) buffer at E = 80 mA/cm for 60 min.

2.2.4. Conjugation of SOD to AuNPs

Two different approaches were used to conjugate the protein to nanoparticles. The first approach used physical adsorption between the particle and protein to generate supramolecular assemblies; the second used covalent linkage of the protein to the particle by means of stable amide bond formation between the carboxylic group of MUA and protein.

Protein adsorption: NP–r*Vu*FeSOD conjugation was achieved by incubating r*Vu*FeSOD with the NPs in solution at room temperature for 1 h. The incubation ratio was 1:500 NP:r*Vu*FeSOD, which was chosen based on the titration method. This ratio most likely represents a large excess of protein; thus, it helps to ensure conjugation. NP–r*Vu*FeSOD conjugates were purified by centrifugation at 4 °C.

Covalent linkage: an initial activation of the carboxylic groups of MUA was accomplished by loading the NPs with freshly prepare activation solution EDC/sulfo-NHS (ratio 2:1). EDC (1-ethyl-3-(3-dimethylaminopropyl) carbodiimide hydrochloride) is a water-soluble zero-length carbodiimide crosslinker that activates carboxyl groups for spontaneous reaction with primary amines, enabling protein conjugation. The addition of sulfo-NHS (*N*-hydroxy sulfosuccinimide) to reactions increases the efficiency and enables the carboxylic group to be activated for longer period of time [32]. The activation solution contained different concentrations of EDC/sulfo-NHS for every NP:MUA stoichiometry, and it depended on the concentration of carboxylic groups on the nanoparticle surface. The ratio COOH:EDC was always 1:10. After 1 h of incubation, the nanoparticles were washed with coupling buffer using centrifugation and resuspended using a sonic probe. The proteins were introduced in the solution to produce the covalent attachment via ester linkage. After 2 h of incubation, NP–r*Vu*FeSOD conjugates were purified by centrifugation at 4 °C. The purified conjugates were finally dispersed in buffer and storage at 4 °C. Surface chemistry was assay by agarose gel electrophoresis (0.5%) in TA at E = 80 mA/cm for 60 min. Enzyme coverage was quantified by the Bradford protein assay using BSA as standard. The number of r*Vu*FeSOD per NP was obtained from the difference between the initial and final protein concentrations in solution, divided by the initial NP concentration.

2.2.5. Superoxide Dismutase In-Gel Activity Assays for the Conjugates

In-gel SOD activity assays for AuNP–r*Vu*FeSOD conjugates were performed by electrophoresis on agarose gels (0.5%) in 0.5× Tris-acetate buffer pH 8 at 75 V for 90 min. After the electrophoresis, the gels were stained according to [28], with the following modifications. Agarose gels were kept in the buffer (50 mM sodium phosphate, pH 7.8) for 30 min. Secondly, the gel was transferred to 0.5 mM nitroblue tetrazolium-containing buffer, and it was further incubated for 20 min. Finally, they were incubated in the reaction buffer supplemented with 0.03 mM riboflavin and 0.2% tetramethylethylenediamine (TEMED) (v/v) for 20 min. All incubations were performed in darkness. Gels were then exposed to white light for 2–5 min to visualize SOD activity bands.

2.2.6. Spectrophotometric Activity Assay

The enzymatic activity of r*Vu*FeSOD was spectrophotometrically quantified, based on the ability of SODs to inhibit NBT reduction by the xanthine + xanthine oxidase (XOD) system [33]. Reduction in NBT was monitored at 25 °C by following the increase in absorbance at 560 nm for 5 min. The reaction cocktail contained reaction buffer (10 mM potassium phosphate, 0.1 mM Na_2EDTA, pH 7.4), 0.1 mM xanthine, and 0.25 mM NBT. The reaction was started by the addition of 40 µL of 1:1600 diluted XOD. Sample volumes of NP–r*Vu*FeSOD conjugates were adjusted to reduce activity rate to around 50%. Subsequently, 10–20 µg of r*Vu*FeSOD was finally employed. A sample without XOD was used as a blank (negative control). Data from different syntheses and experimental replicates were collected to calculate the average (minimum n = 3).

2.2.7. Dynamic Light Scattering

Size measurements were performed by dynamic light scattering (DLS) with a Zetasizer Nano series instrument (Malvern Instruments, Worcestershire, UK). Nanoparticle average hydrodynamic diameter (intensity) as well as the polydispersity index (PdI) were measured before and after conjugation. DLS measurements were performed using the following settings: laser wavelength of 633 nm (He–Ne) and scattering angle 90°; measurement temperature 25 °C, medium viscosity 0.8872 mPa·s, and medium refractive index 1.330. All the samples were sonicated before measurement and standard 1 mL disposable polystyrene cuvettes were used.

3. Results and Discussion

3.1. Engineering the NP Surface Chemistry

r*Vu*FeSOD is a homodimeric enzyme with one noncovalently bound iron atom cofactor per monomer (Figure 1A). The r*Vu*FeSOD monomer has 245 amino acid residues, seven α-helices, and three β-sheet structures. Its overall size is ~45 × 31 × 36 Å, the isoelectric point is 5.31, and the molecular weight is 27,467 Da, including one atom of Fe per monomer. Additionally, the 3D model obtained by X-ray diffraction is available [21,22]. The r*Vu*FeSOD was produced and purified according to the protocol described in the Materials and Methods of [23]. The protein was produced in a soluble state, with little or no inclusion bodies. The purification steps of r*Vu*FeSOD are shown in Figure 1B. Activity of r*Vu*FeSOD was checked using gel stained for SOD activity assay. After electrophoresis on native polyacrylamide gels and staining, the negative banding corresponding to the SOD activity was visualized (Figure 1C).

Citrate-stabilized AuNPs were synthesized (Figure 2A—red solution). AuNP present the localized surface plasmon resonance (LSPR), which refers to the collective oscillation of electrons within the material when they are excited by light [34], giving rise to a characteristic absorption peak (Figure 2C) that varies depending on the AuNPs size, form, and surrounding medium [35]. Transmission electron microscopy (TEM) images showed spherical shaped particles with an average diameter of 9.6 ± 2.2 nm, while dynamic light scattering (DLS) measurements revealed an average hydrodynamic diameter (intensity) of 11.3 ± 0.6 nm (Figure 2). As expected, the DLS size was slightly larger than in

TEM, since the latter corresponds to a dry particles size. NP surfaces were modified with 11-mercaptoundecanoic acid (MUA, SH-$(CH_2)_{11}$-COOH). MUA is well known to bind to the gold atoms by the -SH group, and the carboxylic terminal group is relatively easy to bind covalently to the protein. Different amounts of surface coating MUA ligand were used so that the effect of NP surface chemistry on r*Vu*FeSOD behavior could be studied. We used NP−citrate as the starting material, and then modified it with different concentrations of MUA. Under these conditions, MUA is well known to bind to gold atoms by the -SH group.

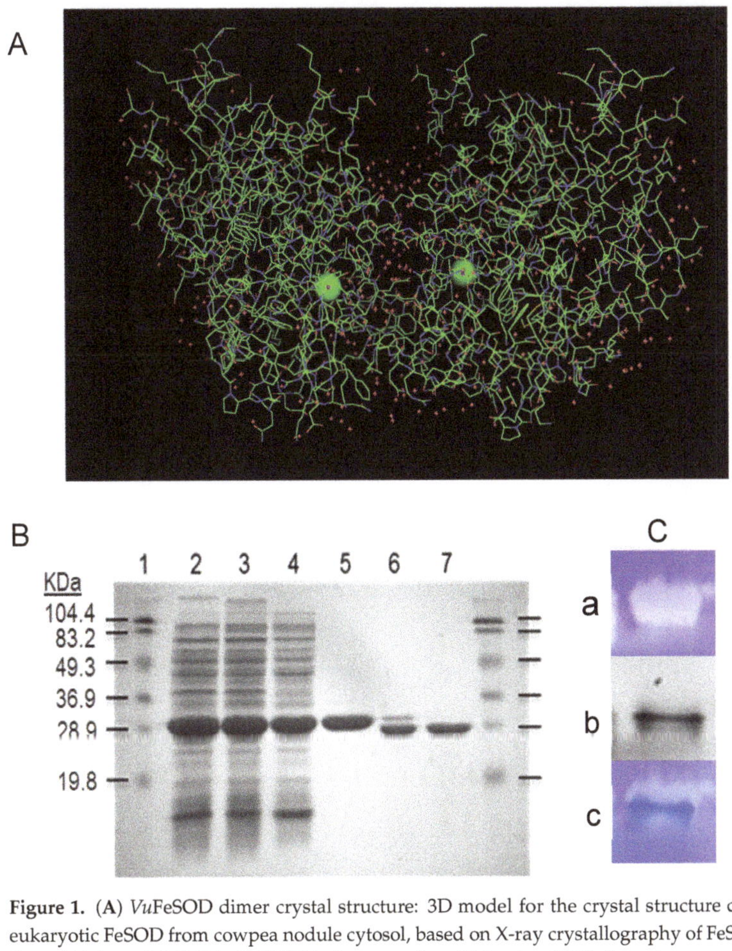

Figure 1. (**A**) *Vu*FeSOD dimer crystal structure: 3D model for the crystal structure dimer of the eukaryotic FeSOD from cowpea nodule cytosol, based on X-ray crystallography of FeSOD crystals (http://doi.org/10.2210/pdb1UNF/pdb accessed on 16 October 2022). Iron atoms are presented as green circles. (**B**) SDS-PAGE gel of the r*Vu*FeSOD purification steps: samples were electrophoresed in a 12.5% SDS-PAGE gel and stained with Coomassie Blue. Line 1: Molecular mass markers (KDa); Line 2: Crude extract, Cell disruption; Line 3: Crude extract, pellet; Line 4: Crude extract, supernatant; Line 5: Pure r*Vu*FeSOD; Line 6: Pure r*Vu*FeSOD partially digested with thrombin; and Line 7: Pure r*Vu*FeSOD digested with thrombin. (**C**) r*Vu*FeSOD gel activity: (a) Gel stained for SOD activity assay (~2 μg of protein), (b) replica gel stained with Coomassie blue brilliant, and (c) superposition of gel stained with Coomassie and gel stained for SOD activity.

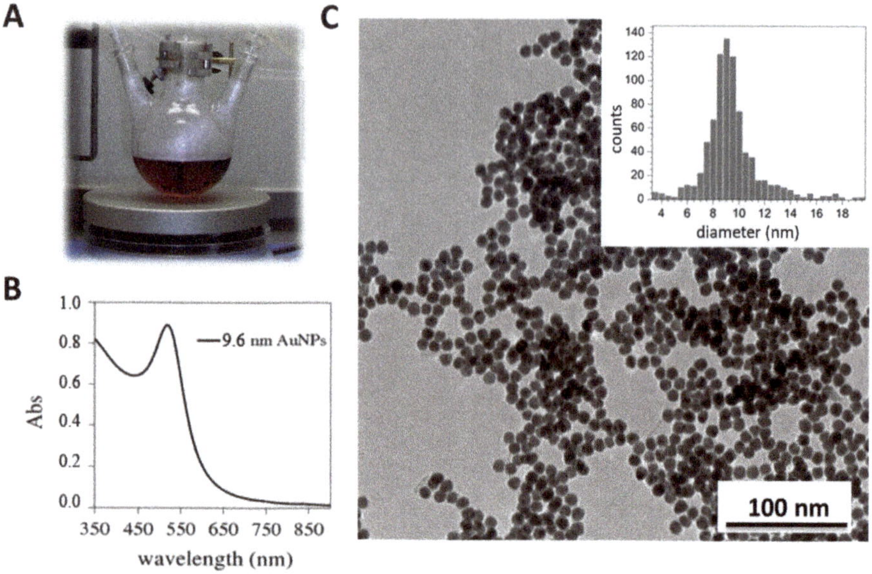

Figure 2. Synthesis of 9.6 nm gold nanoparticle: (**A**) reduction in tetrachloroauric acid in the presence of a reducing agent (citrate) to form colloid AuNPs (red solution); (**B**) UV–Vis absorption spectra of AuNPs with an absorption peak at 517.5 nm; and (**C**) TEM images of AuNPs and their respective size distribution histograms.

We probed the following NP:MUA stoichiometries: 1:100, 1:250, 1:500, 1:750, and 1:1000 to assess the density of the packing. The packing density of MUA onto spherical gold nanoparticles has been measured previously. Thus, it was determined that the packing density for AuNPs modified with a MUA was 4.97 ± 0.01 ligand molecules·nm-2 [36], while other investigators previously reported a value of 5.7 ± 0.13 [37]. Since the packing density of MUA is nanoparticle-size-independent, the highest possible packing on the 9.6 nm AuNPs modified with MUA is in the range of 1450–1650 molecules per nanoparticle. Therefore, our particles are not totally covered by the SAM.

NPs with different surface ligand coatings presented slight differences in hydrodynamic diameter. The hydrodynamic diameter increased from 11.30 to 13.94 nm (Figure 3A). Gel electrophoresis also showed mobility shifts that varied with surface chemistry (Figure 3B). NP−citrate was not stable enough in the buffer to run in the gel (lane 1), which has been observed previously [38]. MUA functionalization increased the NP mobility in gel electrophoresis (from lane 2 to line 6), which may be due to the negative charge from MUA. As we increased the concentration of MUA on the NPs surface, the NPs began to gradually become more stable in the gel [39], run more homogeneously, and shifted to lower mobility, most likely due to the increase in size.

3.2. Gold Nanoparticle Protein Conjugation

NPs with different surface chemistries were then conjugated to r*Vu*FeSOD. Two different approaches were used to conjugate the protein to nanoparticles. The first approach used physical adsorption of the protein to the particle surface. For this purpose, conjugation was achieved by simple incubation for 1 h at a ratio of AuNPs to r*Vu*FeSOD of 1:500. Determination of the optimal NP:r*Vu*FeSOD ratio was achieved using the titration method [40] (Figure 4). Unbound r*Vu*FeSOD was separated by spin centrifugation. The second method used direct covalent linkage of the protein to the particle surface. The covalent attachment involves a series of consecutive steps. First, activation of the MUA's carboxylic groups was accomplished by loading the nanoparticles with activation solution EDC/sulfo-NHS [41].

In order to avoid the aggregation of NPs, we determined the activation conditions for each NP:MUA sample, to ensure the protein–AuNP linkage. Several ratios of EDC were revealed with each NP:MUA ratio. Finally, a 1:10 MUA:EDC ratio was chosen. AuNPs were activated for 1 h, and then the protein (1:500 NP: protein ratio) was loaded in the solution to produce the covalent attachment via active ester methods. After 2 h of incubation, AuNP–r*Vu*FeSOD conjugates were purified by centrifugation at 4 °C. r*Vu*FeSOD contains 18 lysine (-NH_2) susceptible to form the covalent bond. They were distributed across the surface of the protein (Figure 5). We assumed that the junction between the MUA and protein will be random, having higher probability those residues located at the surface.

A

	Diameter (nm)	
NP: MUA	Intensity	sd
1:0	11.3	0.6
1:100	11.7	0.7
1:250	12.0	0.7
1:500	12.6	0.9
1:750	13.5	0.4
1:1000	13.9	0.4

B

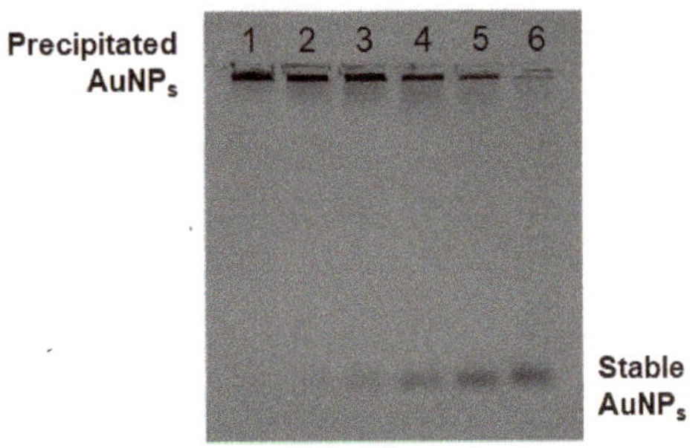

Figure 3. AuNPs surface modification with different concentrations of MUA. (**A**) AuNPs hydrodynamic size measured by Zetasizer in water. The diameter (intensity) increases linearly with MUA concentration on the surface. (**B**) Gel electrophoresis mobility shift of NP–citrate modified with MUA: Lanes: (1) NP–citrate, (2) 1:100 NP:MUA ratio, (3) 1:250 NP:MUA ratio, (4) 1:500 NP:MUA ratio, (5) 1:750 NP:MUA ratio, and (6) 1:1000 NP:MUA ratio.

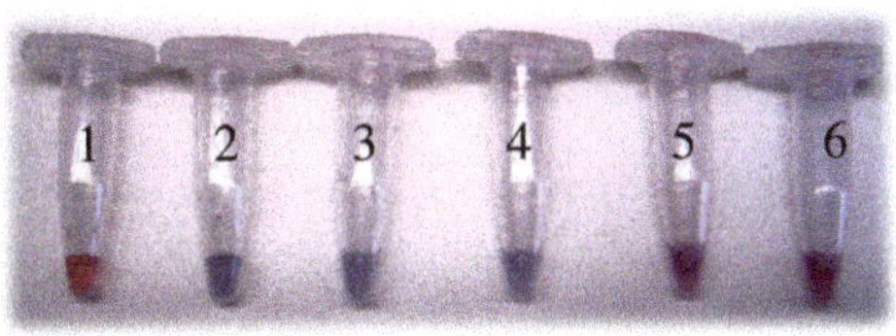

Figure 4. Determination of the optimal NP:r*Vu*FeSOD ratio: Lines (1) Citrate AuNPs, (2) 1:1 Citrate AuNP:r*Vu*FeSOD, (3) 1:10 Citrate AuNP:r*Vu*FeSOD, (4) 1:100 Citrate AuNP:r*Vu*FeSOD, (5) 1:500 Citrate AuNP:r*Vu*FeSOD, and (6) 1:1,000 Citrate AuNP:r*Vu*FeSOD. The lowest amount of protein that maintained a stable colloidal solution after addition of NaCl was selected, corresponding to 1:500 AuNP:r*Vu*FeSOD (tube #5).

Gel electrophoresis showed mobility shifts that varied with surface chemistry. The mobility shift is more pronounced for physical adsorption, rather than for covalent attachment. In physical adsorption, all the conjugates ran in the positive direction, indicating successful NPs stabilization and a net negative charge (Figure 6A). In addition, the narrow band indicated a uniform charge distribution, and thus uniform protein functionalization. The mobility of the conjugates increased with the concentration of MUA on the NP surface. The different mobilities can be explained by the protein coverage and by MUA concentration on the NPs surface. As we increase the negative charge of the nanoparticles with MUA, fewer proteins bind to the NPs, probably because r*Vu*FeSOD has a net negative charge at neutral pH, and the interaction between the negative particles and the protein becomes weaker.

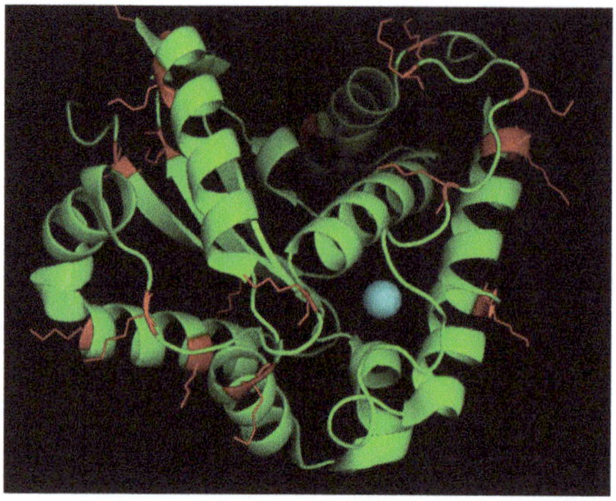

Figure 5. 3D model for a monomer of *Vu*FeSOD: Lysine residues are presented in red.

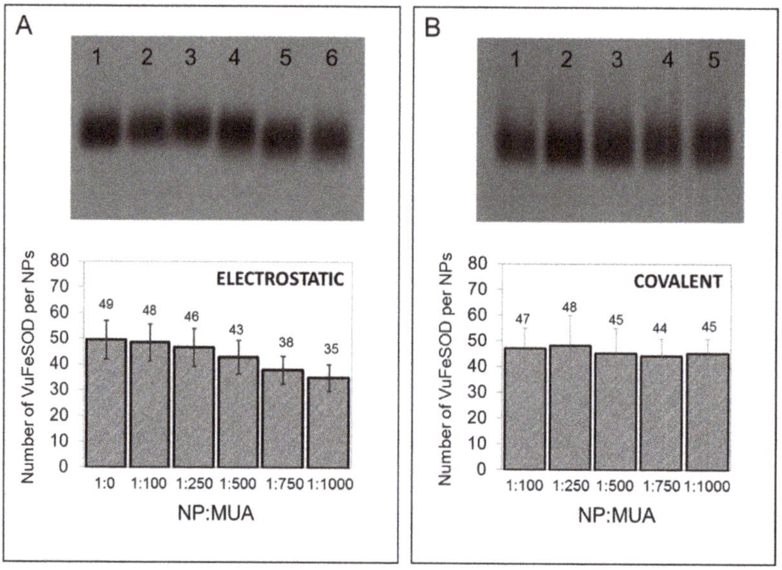

Figure 6. Effect of surface chemistry of AuNP-linked r*Vu*FeSOD on native gel electrophoresis and coverage: (**A**) Physical adsorption: Lanes: (1) NPs–r*Vu*FeSOD, (2) 1:100 NP:MUA–r*Vu*FeSOD, (3) 1:250 NP:MUA–r*Vu*FeSOD, (4) 1:500 NP:MUA–r*Vu*FeSOD, (5) 1:750 NP:MUA–r*Vu*FeSOD, and (6) 1:1,000 NP:MUA–r*Vu*FeSOD. (**B**) Covalent: Lanes: (1) 1:100 NP:MUA–r*Vu*FeSOD, (2) 1:250 NP:MUA–r*Vu*FeSOD, (3) 1:500 NP:MUA–r*Vu*FeSOD, (4) 1:750 NP:MUA–r*Vu*FeSOD, and (5) 1:1,000 NP:MUA–r*Vu*FeSOD.

In covalent bonding, all the conjugates also ran in the positive direction, indicating a net negative charge (Figure 6B). They presented a similar narrow band. The mobility of conjugates was very similar for all samples, although it seems that the mobility slightly increases on the gel with MUA. Although covalent attachment of proteins to NPs provides conjugates that are stable toward dissociation, in our case, covalently binding nanoparticles presented a light trail of nanoparticles in the gel, which did not appear upon physical adsorption, indicating a greater heterogeneity of the samples.

For physical adsorption, the coverage was determined as 49 r*Vu*FeSOD per NPs—citrate. NPs—citrate modified with MUA progressively resulted in lower coverage 48 (1:100

NP:MUA), 46 (1:250 NP:MUA), 43 (1:500 NP:MUA), 38 (1:750 NP:MUA), and 35 (1:1000 NP:MUA), indicating that MUA inhibited conjugation (Figure 6). AuNPs modified with MUA are negatively charged particles; therefore, as we increase the MUA concentration on the nanoparticle, the nanoparticles surface become more negatively charged. All the bioconjugation assays were performed at the pH 7.4, at which r*Vu*FeSOD is also negatively charged (pI. 5.31). The repulsion tendency between negatively charged nanoparticles and negatively charged proteins starts to be more important as the negative charge on the NPs surface increases. These results correlate with those obtained in the gel electrophoresis.

For the covalent attachment, there were not significant differences on the sample to sample coverage: 47 (1:100 NP:MUA), 48 (1:250 NP:MUA), 45 (1:500 NP:MUA), 44 (1:750 NP:MUA), and 45 (1:1000 NP:MUA). The number of active carboxyl groups on the surface that we observed did not have any significant effect on coverage. These results also correlate with those obtained in the gel electrophoresis analysis.

We also checked the size of the conjugates with DLS (Table 1). We measured the size of the protein, and of the nanoparticles before and after conjugation. For physical adsorption, the size of the conjugates decreased as there was more MUA (carboxyl group) on the NP surface, which agrees with the gel electrophoresis and coverage results. For covalent bonding, the sizes slightly decreased with the number of carboxyl groups on the NPs surface. All the resulting conjugates presented a monolayer of protein lower than protein dimer hydrodynamic size (7.8 nm) indicating that our conjugates form a monolayer and not a multilayer. This result also agrees with the gel electrophoresis and coverage results.

Table 1. Protein layer thickness and LSPR shift (nm) of AuNP–VuFeSOD conjugates (physical adsorption and covalent linkage).

NP:MUA		1:0	1:100	1:250	1:500	1:750	1:1000	**r*Vu*FeSOD (Dimer Size)**
Protein layer thickness *	Physical adsorption	6.1	5.4	4.7	4.3	3.5	3.1	7.8
	Covalent	-	5.6	6.0	4.8	4.7	4.9	
$\Delta\ \lambda_{LSPR}$ (nm)	Physical adsorption	7.0	6.8	6.5	5.6	5.0	4.3	-
	Covalent	-	7.2	7.1	7.2	7.0	6.0	

* Protein layer thickness (DLS, intensity, nm).

Conjugated stability was monitored via absorption measurements of the particles. Binding of the SOD on the AuNPs surface causes a small shift in the LSPR peak of the AuNPs. Absorption spectra for all conjugates showed that the LSPR peak underwent red shifts between 7 and 4 nm, accompanied by an increase in the intensity, indicating a proper bioconjugation. These results correlate with the DLS measurements.

Considering the previous results, the coverage values obtained were slightly higher than expected in the monolayer. We have estimated between 20–21 monomer proteins (10 full protein dimers, Figure 7A) per AuNPs as the maximum theoretical surface coverage for a 9.6 nm AuNP using crystallographic overall size of *Vu*FeSOD [21]. Depending on the protein arrangement, the theoretical number of proteins could be duplicated to 40 proteins (20 dimers) per AuNP, providing that one of the monomers binds to the NPs and the other does not (Figure 7B); however, it remains below the values obtained. The third possibility would be something intermediate between A and B. It is important to note that we calculated the concentration of r*Vu*FeSOD as a function of BSA calibration curve, therefore, these numbers probably are not the real coverage, but an estimate. Thus, NP surface chemistry was found to influence the coverage only when the protein was conjugated by physical adsorption.

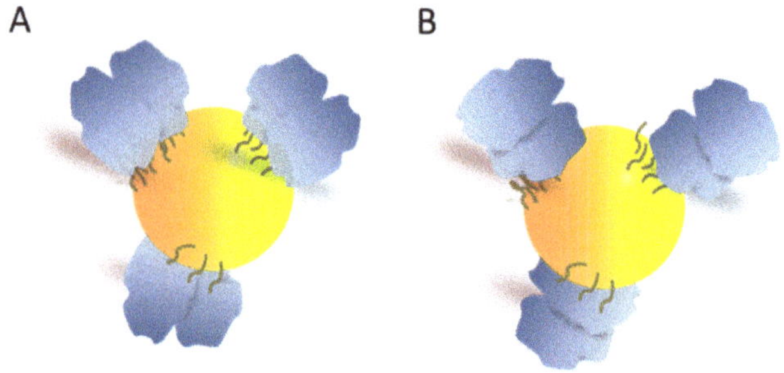

Figure 7. Different conformations of conjugates. (**A**) Both VuFeSOD monomers bind to the nanoparticles (**B**) one of the monomers binds to the NPs and the other does not.

To understand how MUA ligands impacted SOD function, the enzymatic activity of r*Vu*FeSOD on the different NPs was measured. First, SOD activity was measured in gels. Agarose gel was used to separate the NP–protein conjugates (Figure 8). During the physical adsorption process, a decrease in the activity in gel was observed as we increased the MUA concentration on the surface. Apparently, this may be related to the decrease in the coverage observed, and it would indicate that the −COOH groups did not necessarily affect the activity of the protein (Figure 8A). However, MUA caused a clear reduction in r*Vu*FeSOD activity onto AuNPs with covalent attachment (Figure 8B).

A

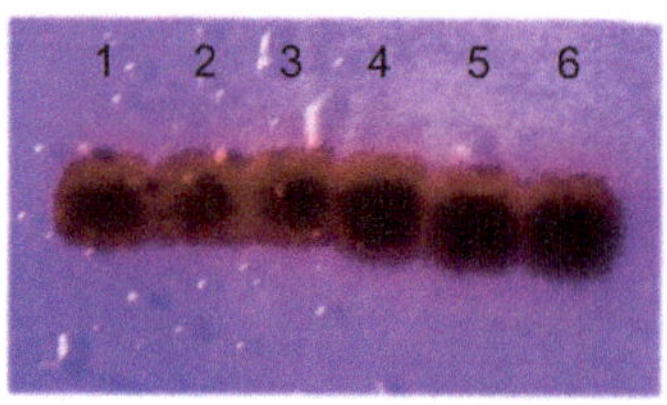

PHYSICAL ADSORPTION

NP:MUA	Coverage	% Actives protein	# of active protein
1:0	49	31	16
1:100	48	37	18
1:250	47	31	15
1:500	43	31	13
1:750	38	36	14
1:1000	35	38	13

B

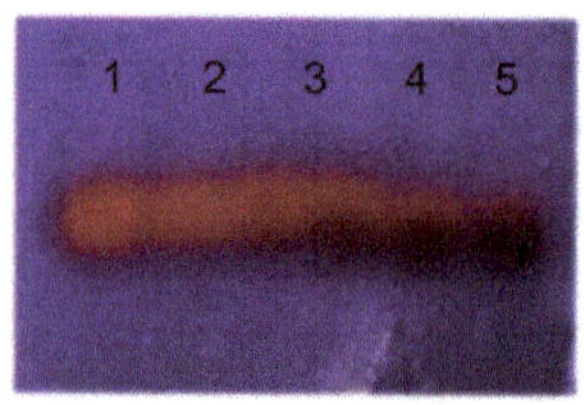

COVALENT

NP:MUA	Coverage	% Actives protein	# of active protein
1:0	--	--	--
1:100	47	31	15
1:250	48	27	13
1:500	45	25	11
1:750	44	21	9
1:1000	45	9	4

Figure 8. Effect of surface chemistry of AuNP-linked r*Vu*FeSOD on the superoxide dismutase activity assay outcome. (**A**) Physical adsorption: AuNP–*Vu*FeSOD activity gel for different NP:MUA stoichiometry and in the table, data of coverage, percentage of remaining superoxide dismutase activity, and number (#) of active proteins on the NPs. (**B**) Covalent attachment: NP–*Vu*FeSOD activity gel for different NP:MUA stoichiometry and in the table, data of coverage, percentage of remaining superoxide dismutase activity, and number of active proteins on the NPs.

Secondly, an activity assay method was performed on the AuNP–*Vu*FeSOD solutions to assess the loss of activity after binding. For physical adsorption, the remaining active r*Vu*FeSOD on the NPs was in the range of 30–40%, indicating that r*Vu*FeSOD activity was compromised when bound to NPs. The activity measurements show that modifying citrate-stabilized NPs with MUA did not significantly influence r*Vu*FeSOD enzymatic activity, which indicates how strong a perturbing agent NPs are. Therefore, we can consider that the MUA molecule has not an effect on enzymatic activity of the protein, just on the coverage, and consequently, the coverage has no significant effect on the activity.

Given that the retained activity of the r*Vu*FeSOD is lower than expected, we hypothesize that the protein behavior, which is based on a cooperative mechanism between the two monomers of the protein, is affected by the interaction of critical amino acids involved in the cooperative mechanism and the NPs [22]. In addition, at a physiological pH, SOD has a net negative charge. However, the deep and narrow active channel above the catalytic active site exhibits a highly positive charge that electrostatically attracts and guides the negatively charged $O_2^{\bullet-}$ anions to the catalytic Fe metal at the bottom of the active channel [42]. This positive channel may be electrostatically attracted by the negative AuNPs surface, interfering or even blocking the access of $O_2^{\bullet-}$ to the catalytic metal, and possibly exposing internal amino acids to enable binding to the NP.

The r*Vu*FeSOD has only one Cys108 in each monomer. It is not on the surface of the protein, but relatively close to it (Figure 9); therefore, it may potentially bind to the nanoparticles, destabilizing the protein structure, similar to what it has been observed for yeast cytochrome *c* from *Saccharomyces cerevisiae* [43]. It is noteworthy that the cysteine molecule is neither at the interface of two proteins or near the active center (the FeCys distance is 12.93 Å), but quite near to His102, which is one of the four catalytic residues. Moreover, the cysteine molecule connects a loop with an alpha helix and is near two lysines ($-NH_2$ containing), Lys110 and Lys226, which may interact with the carboxyl groups of the surface. Thus, it may be that the thiol from one monomer of r*Vu*FeSOD links to the NPs, forcing them to destabilize the folding of this monomer and disturb the dimer. In this situation, the protein involved may well lose an important part of its activity. It has been observed in *Escherichia coli* MnSOD (*Ec*MnSOD) that the disruption of the interaction between Tyr202 from one monomer with the neighboring monomer, His47, reduces the SOD activity to 30% to 40% [44]. In our case, the activity reduction is between 60–70%, indicating that a major form of disruption is taking place. It has been also indicated for FeSODs that have a cooperativity mechanism between the two monomers during catalysis. Indeed, in nature, FeSODs, and also MnSOD, are never monomers, they are always found as dimers or tetramers, but in the latter case they behave as a pair of dimers [22]. All these interactions may well explain the loss of 60–70% of the protein activity. In addition, the monolayer formed by the protein at its maximum coverage (DLS, 7.0 nm) is very close to the 7.8 nm of the protein diameter, supporting this hypothesis.

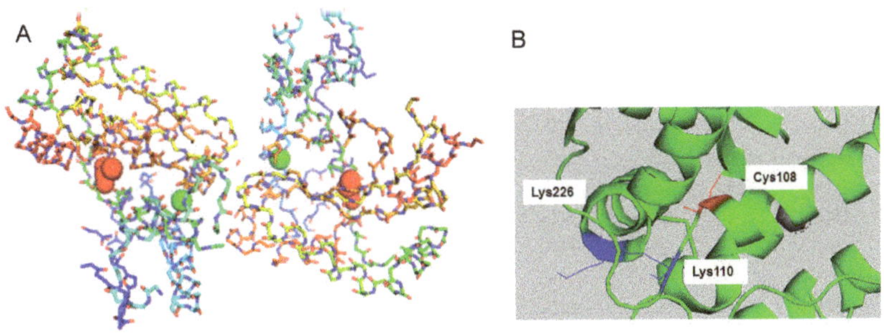

Figure 9. (**A**) VuFeSOD dimer crystal structure: 3D model for the monomer of the eukaryotic FeSOD from cowpea nodule cytosol, based on X-ray crystallography of FeSOD crystals. Iron atom presented as green circles and cysteine in red. The distance between the two Fe atoms is 18.01 Å and between the Fe atom and Cys from the same monomer 12.93 Å. (**B**) In red are the cysteine molecule (Cys108) of one monomer, and in blue are the two lysines that are near the Cys108: Lys110 and Lys226.

For covalent bonding, the proportion of active r*Vu*FeSOD still present on the AuNPs was lower than 31%, indicating that r*Vu*FeSOD activity was especially compromised when covalently bound to NPs. This result points to the activation of carboxylic groups in MUA, as its interaction with Lys–NH_2 residues is essentially implicated in the binding and loss of activity. Thus, the change in the MUA and NP surface chemistry induced a higher loss in protein activity. At this point, active r*Vu*FeSOD decreased when MUA concentration increased at the surface down to 9% at 1:1,000 NP:MUA, although the coverage was very similar in all conjugates. This suggests that increasing the probability of covalent linkage with highest MUA concentration reduces the stability of the r*Vu*FeSOD protein dimer. Similarly, it has been found that the covalent linkage of the CuZnSOD to a flat surface reduced SOD activity nearly 50% relative to the adsorbed state [16]. The coverage was very similar in all samples, but the monolayer size measured by DLS decreased slightly with MUA, suggesting that the surface caused the protein to change conformation without the possibility of a possible rearrangement of the protein. This conformational change has a direct impact on the activity.

4. Conclusions

In summary, a recombinant iron-superoxide dismutase from *Vigna unguiculata* (r*Vu*FeSOD) was conjugated to 9.6 nm AuNPs using either physical adsorption or covalent bonding. r*Vu*FeSOD was produced and purified to homogeneity in high yields using a self-induction overexpression system. In addition, 9.6 nm AuNPs with a high degree of control were synthesized, and their surfaces were modified with different concentrations of 11-mercaptoundecanoic acid ligand very easily.

Interactions with NPs can significantly alter the coverage and function of r*Vu*FeSOD. The NPs are generally a strongly perturbing agent for r*Vu*FeSOD, and the interactions between r*Vu*FeSOD and the NPs and NP ligands resulted in the significant inactivation of the protein activity.

Different bioconjugation strategies produced different effects on the interaction between r*Vu*FeSOD and NPs. For physical adsorption, the impact of MUA concentration on the surface was more important in terms of coverage than activity. The MUA ligand acted more as a steric barrier that was also enhanced by the electrostatic repulsion, producing a reduction in coverage. However, the amount of MUA on the surface did not affect the activity, indicating that the strongly perturbing agent is the NPs itself. Evaluation of functional properties of the conjugate indicated that upon conjugation, proteins retained 31–39% of activity.

For covalent attachment, however, the opposite effect was observed. The impact of MUA concentration was more important in terms of activity than coverage. As the concentration of MUA increased on the surface, the inactivation of the protein was higher; protein can lose 90% of its activity. This suggests that as well as the NP, the covalent linkage also destabilized the protein activity, probably due to an excess of attachment points to the surface. Overall, we have reported some remarkable results. The binding method, either physical adsorption or covalent linkage can help to improve or worsen the activity. For our system, physical adsorption has resulted in a better strategy. These results suggest that more optimization is needed for a better understanding of the interaction between r*Vu*FeSOD and AuNPs. Nevertheless, these strategies can be useful for applications, which require tethering the r*Vu*FeSOD and other enzymes to a surface.

Author Contributions: Conceptualization, E.T., A.C.A. and J.F.M..; methodology, E.T. and P.C.; validation, E.T., A.C.A. and P.C.; investigation, E.T., J.B. and P.L.-G.; formal analysis, M.U.; data curation, M.U.; writing—original draft preparation, E.T. and J.B.; writing—review and editing, E.T. and P.L.-G.; supervision, A.C.A. and J.F.M.; funding acquisition, E.T. and J.F.M. All authors have read and agreed to the published version of the manuscript.

Funding: This research was funded by the Government of Navarra, Department of Innovation, Business and Employment for financial support within the project SABioD. E.T., P.C. and A.C. were funded by SABioD grant. The authors also acknowledge a grant from the Public University of Navarre (Res 309/2022) to J.F.M. M.U. is a recipient of a pre-doctoral fellowship from the Government of Navarre, Spain. J.B. and P.L. have received pre-doctoral fellowships from the Public University of Navarre, Spain. J.B. is supported by the Romanian Ministry of Education and research, grant CNCS-UEFISCDI, project number PN-III-P4-ID-PCE-2020-2696, within PNCDI III.

Institutional Review Board Statement: Not applicable.

Informed Consent Statement: Not applicable.

Data Availability Statement: Data is contained within the article.

Conflicts of Interest: The authors declare no conflict of interest.

References

1. Abreu, I.A.; Cabelli, D.E. Superoxide dismutases—A review of the metal-associated mechanistic variations. *Biochim. Biophys. Acta Proteins Proteom.* **2010**, *1804*, 263–274. [CrossRef] [PubMed]
2. Halliwell, B.; Gutteridge, J.M.C. Free Radicals in Biology and Medicine. *Free Radic. Biol. Med.* **2015**, *5*, 961. [CrossRef]
3. Gopalakrishnan, B.; Nash, K.M.; Velayutham, M.; Villamena, F.A. Detection of nitric oxide and superoxide radical anion by electron paramagnetic resonance spectroscopy from cells using spin traps. *J. Vis. Exp.* **2012**, *66*, e2810. [CrossRef]
4. Jie, Z.; Liu, J.; Shu, M.; Ying, Y.; Yang, H. Detection strategies for superoxide anion: A review. *Talanta* **2022**, *236*, 122892. [CrossRef] [PubMed]
5. Zhu, X.; Niu, X.; Zhao, H.; Tang, J.; Lan, M. Immobilization of superoxide dismutase on Pt-Pd/MWCNTs hybrid modified electrode surface for superoxide anion detection. *Biosens. Bioelectron.* **2015**, *67*, 79–85. [CrossRef] [PubMed]
6. Zhu, A.; Sun, K.; Petty, H.R. Titanium doping reduces superoxide dismutase activity, but not oxidase activity, of catalytic CeO_2 nanoparticles. *Inorg. Chem. Commun.* **2012**, *15*, 235–237. [CrossRef] [PubMed]
7. Deng, Z.; Tian, Y.; Yin, X.; Rui, Q.; Liu, H.; Luo, Y. Physical vapor deposited zinc oxide nanoparticles for direct electron transfer of superoxide dismutase. *Electrochem. Commun.* **2008**, *10*, 818–820. [CrossRef]
8. Wang, L.; Mao, W.; Ni, D.; Di, J.; Wu, Y.; Tu, Y. Direct electrodeposition of gold nanoparticles onto indium/tin oxide film coated glass and its application for electrochemical biosensor. *Electrochem. Commun.* **2008**, *10*, 673–676. [CrossRef]
9. Wang, Y.; Wu, Y.; Wang, J.; Di, J. Disposable superoxide anion biosensor based on superoxide dismutase entrapped in silica sol-gel matrix at gold nanoparticles modified ITO electrode. *Bioprocess Biosyst. Eng.* **2009**, *32*, 531–536. [CrossRef]
10. Wang, L.; Wen, W.; Xiong, H.; Zhang, X.; Gu, H.; Wang, S. A novel amperometric biosensor for superoxide anion based on superoxide dismutase immobilized on gold nanoparticle-chitosan-ionic liquid biocomposite film. *Anal. Chim. Acta* **2013**, *758*, 66–71. [CrossRef]
11. El-Deab, M.S.; Ohsaka, T. Direct electron transfer of copper-zinc superoxide dismutase (SOD) on crystallographically oriented Au nanoparticles. *Electrochem. Commun.* **2007**, *9*, 651–656. [CrossRef]
12. Hong, S.; Choi, I.; Lee, S.; Yang, Y.I.; Kang, T.; Yi, J. Sensitive and colorimetric detection of the structural evolution of superoxide dismutase with gold nanoparticles. *Anal. Chem.* **2009**, *81*, 1378–1382. [CrossRef] [PubMed]
13. Kang, T.; Hong, S.; Choi, I.; Sung, J.J.; Kim, Y.; Hahn, J.S.; Yi, J. Reversible pH-driven conformational switching of tethered superoxide dismutase with gold nanoparticle enhanced surface plasmon resonance spectroscopy. *J. Am. Chem. Soc.* **2006**, *128*, 12870–12878. [CrossRef] [PubMed]
14. Pudlarz, A.M.; Ranoszek-Soliwoda, K.; Czechowska, E.; Tomaszewska, E.; Celichowski, G.; Grobelny, J.; Szemraj, J. A Study of the Activity of Recombinant Mn-Superoxide Dismutase in the Presence of Gold and Silver Nanoparticles. *Appl. Biochem. Biotechnol.* **2019**, *187*, 1551–1568. [CrossRef] [PubMed]
15. Tellechea, E.; Cornago, I.; Ciaurriz, P.; Moran, J.F.; Asensio, A.C. Conjugation of active iron superoxide dismutase to nanopatterned surfaces. *IEEE Trans. Nanobioscience* **2012**, *11*, 176–180. [CrossRef]
16. Ge, B.; Scheller, F.W.; Lisdat, F. Electrochemistry of immobilized CuZnSOD and FeSOD and their interaction with superoxide radicals. *Biosens. Bioelectron.* **2002**, *18*, 295–302. [CrossRef]
17. Asuri, P.; Karajanagi, S.S.; Vertegel, A.A.; Dordick, J.S.; Kane, R.S. Enhanced stability of enzymes adsorbed onto nanoparticles. *J. Nanosci. Nanotechnol.* **2007**, *7*, 1675–1678. [CrossRef]
18. Lv, M.; Zhu, E.; Su, Y.; Li, Q.; Li, W.; Zhao, Y.; Huang, Q. Trypsin-gold nanoparticle conjugates: Binding, enzymatic activity, and stability. *Prep. Biochem. Biotechnol.* **2009**, *39*, 429–438. [CrossRef]
19. Moran, J.F.; James, E.K.; Rubio, M.C.; Sarath, G.; Klucas, R.V.; Becana, M. Functional Characterization and Expression of a Cytosolic Iron-Superoxide Dismutase from Cowpea Root Nodules. *Plant Physiol.* **2003**, *133*, 773–782. [CrossRef]
20. Asensio, A.C.; Gil-Monreal, M.; Pires, L.; Gogorcena, Y.; Aparicio-Tejo, P.M.; Moran, J.F. Two Fe-superoxide dismutase families respond differently to stress and senescence in legumes. *J. Plant Physiol.* **2012**, *169*, 1253–1260. [CrossRef]
21. Muñoz, I.G.; Moran, J.F.; Becana, M.; Montoya, G. Crystallization and preliminary X-ray diffraction studies of the eukaryotic iron superoxide dismutase (FeSOD) from Vigna unguiculata. *Acta Cryst.* **2003**, *D59*, 1070–1072. [CrossRef]

22. Muñoz, I.G.; Moran, J.F.; Becana, M.; Montoya, G. The crystal structure of an eukaryotic iron superoxide dismutase suggests intersubunit cooperation during catalysis. *Protein Sci.* **2005**, *14*, 387–394. [CrossRef] [PubMed]
23. Urarte, E.; Auzmendi, I.; Rol, S.; Ariz, I.; Aparicio-Tejo, P.; Arredondo-Peter, R.; Moran, J.F. A Self-Induction Method to Produce High Quantities of Recombinant Functional Flavo-Leghemoglobin Reductase. *Methods Enzymol.* **2008**, *436*, 411–423. [CrossRef]
24. Ischiropoulos, H.; Zhu, L.; Chen, J.; Tsai, M.; Martin, J.C.; Smith, C.D.; Beckman, J.S. Peroxynitrite-mediated tyrosine nitration catalyzed by superoxide dismutase. *Arch. Biochem. Biophys.* **1992**, *298*, 431–437. [CrossRef]
25. Ischiropoulos, H.; Zhu, L.; Beckman, J.S. Peroxynitrite formation from macrophage-derived nitric oxide. *Arch. Biochem. Biophys.* **1992**, *298*, 446–451. [CrossRef]
26. Larrainzar, E.; Urarte, E.; Auzmendi, I.; Ariz, I.; Arrese-Igor, C.; González, E.M.; Moran, J.F. Use of Recombinant Iron-Superoxide Dismutase as A Marker of Nitrative Stress. *Methods Enzymol.* **2008**, *437*, 605–618. [PubMed]
27. Urarte, E.; Asensio, A.C.; Tellechea, E.; Pires, L.; Moran, J.F. Evaluation of the anti-nitrative effect of plant antioxidants using a cowpea Fe-superoxide dismutase as a target. *Plant Physiol. Biochem.* **2014**, *83*, 356–364. [CrossRef]
28. Beauchamp, C.; Fridovich, I. Superoxide dismutase: Improved assays and an assay applicable to acrylamide gels. *Anal. Biochem.* **1971**, *44*, 276–287. [CrossRef]
29. Beesley, J.E. Colloidal gold: A new perspective for cytochemical marking. *Trends Biochem. Sci.* **1989**, *14*, 392. [CrossRef]
30. Abràmoff, M.D.; Magalhães, P.J.; Ram, S.J. Image processing with ImageJ Part II. *Biophotonics Int.* **2005**, *11*, 36–43.
31. Park, S.; Brown, K.A.; Hamad-Schifferli, K. Changes in oligonucleotide conformation on nanoparticle surfaces by modification with mercaptohexanol. *Nano Lett.* **2004**, *4*, 1925–1929. [CrossRef]
32. Brown, K.A. Noncovalent Adsorption of Nucleotides in Gold Nanoparticle DNA Conjugates: Bioavailability at the Bio-Nano Interface. 2008. Available online: https://dspace.mit.edu/handle/1721.1/44866 (accessed on 11 October 2022).
33. Sun, Y.; Oberley, L.W.; Li, Y. A simple method for clinical assay of superoxide dismutase. *Clin. Chem.* **1988**, *34*, 497–500. [CrossRef] [PubMed]
34. Mie, G. Contributions to the optics of turbid media, particularly of colloidal metal solutions. *Ann. Phys.* **1976**, *25*, 377–445.
35. Haynes, C.L.; van Duyne, R.P. Nanosphere lithography: A versatile nanofabrication tool for studies of size-dependent nanoparticle optics. *J. Phys. Chem. B* **2001**, *105*, 5599–5611. [CrossRef]
36. Ivanov, M.R.; Haes, A.J. Anionic functionalized gold nanoparticle continuous full filling separations: Importance of sample concentration. *Anal. Chem.* **2012**, *84*, 1320–1326. [CrossRef]
37. Hinterwirth, H.; Kappel, S.; Waitz, T.; Prohaska, T.; Lindner, W.; Lämmerhofer, M. Quantifying thiol ligand density of self-assembled monolayers on gold nanoparticles by inductively coupled plasma-mass spectrometry. *ACS Nano* **2013**, *7*, 1129–1136. [CrossRef]
38. Reed, A.M.W.; Metallo, S.J. Oriented protein adsorption to gold nanoparticles through a genetically encodable binding motif. *Langmuir* **2010**, *26*, 18945–18950. [CrossRef]
39. Sperling, R.A.; Parak, W.J. Surface modification, functionalization and bioconjugation of colloidal inorganic nanoparticles. *Philos. Trans. R. Soc. A Math. Phys. Eng. Sci.* **2010**, *368*, 1333–1383. [CrossRef]
40. Pissuwan, D.; Cortie, C.H.; Valenzuela, S.M.; Cortie, M.B. Gold nanosphere-antibody conjugates for hyperthermal therapeutic applications. *Gold Bull.* **2007**, *40*, 121–129. [CrossRef]
41. Hermanson, G.T. Chapter 4. Zero-Length Crosslinkers. In *Bioconjugate Techniques*, 3rd ed.; Academic Press: Cambridge, MA, USA, 2013; pp. 259–273, ISBN 9780123822390. [CrossRef]
42. Getzoff, E.D.; Tainer, J.A.; Weiner, P.K.; Kollman, P.A.; Richardson, J.S.; Richardson, D.C. Electrostatic recognition between superoxide and copper, zinc superoxide dismutase. *Nature* **1983**, *306*, 287–290. [CrossRef]
43. Aubin-Tam, M.E.; Hamad-Schifferli, K. Gold nanoparticle-cytochrome C complexes: The effect of nanoparticle ligand charge on protein structure. *Langmuir* **2005**, *21*, 12080–12084. [CrossRef] [PubMed]
44. Edwards, R.A.; Whittaker, M.M.; Whittaker, J.W.; Baker, E.N.; Jameson, G.B. Removing a Hydrogen Bond in the Dimer Interface of Escherichia coli Manganese Superoxide Dismutase Alters Structure and Reactivity. *Biochemistry* **2001**, *40*, 4622–4632. [CrossRef] [PubMed]

antioxidants

MDPI

Article

Zinc Oxide Nanoparticles (ZnO-NPs) Suppress Fertility by Activating Autophagy, Apoptosis, and Oxidative Stress in the Developing Oocytes of Female Zebrafish

Suzan Attia Mawed [1], Carlotta Marini [2], Mahmoud Alagawany [3], Mayada R. Farag [4,*], Rasha M. Reda [5], Mohamed T. El-Saadony [6], Walaa M. Elhady [4], Gian E. Magi [2], Alessandro Di Cerbo [2,*] and Wafaa G. El-Nagar [1]

1 Zoology Department, Faculty of Science, Zagazig University, Zagazig 44519, Egypt
2 School of Biosciences and Veterinary Medicine, University of Camerino, 62024 Matelica, Italy
3 Poultry Department, Agriculture Faculty, Zagazig University, Zagazig 44519, Egypt
4 Forensic Medicine and Toxicology Department, Faculty of Veterinary Medicine, Zagazig University, Zagazig 44519, Egypt
5 Department of Fish Diseases and Management, Faculty of Veterinary Medicine, Zagazig University, Zagazig 44511, Egypt
6 Department of Agricultural Microbiology, Faculty of Agriculture, Zagazig University, Zagazig 44511, Egypt
* Correspondence: dr.mayadarf@gmail.com (M.R.F.); alessandro.dicerbo@unicam.it (A.D.C.)

Abstract: In vertebrates, the core mechanisms that control gametogenesis are largely multiple, complex, successive, and orchestrated by intrinsic and extrinsic factors. However, age, health status, and hormonal activity are important factors for good fertility; other intangible intracellular molecular mechanisms that manage oocyte development are still unclear. The present study was designed to elucidate the ultrastructure changes in the ovary in response to its exposure to zinc oxide nanoparticles (ZnO-NPs) and to explore the role of autophagy and apoptosis during egg maturation and ovulation on the fertility of female zebrafish. In our study, ZnO-NPs could induce cytotoxicity in the maturing oocyte by activating autophagy and apoptosis in a caspase-dependent manner and could induce oxidative stress by generating reactive oxygen species (ROS) that elevated the mutated ovarian tP53 protein. Simultaneously, necroptosis developed, mimicking the features of apoptosis and necrosis. Collectively, ZnO-NPs created a suitable necrotic environment that led to follicular developmental retardation that altered oocyte ovulation and reduced fecundity of female zebrafish.

Keywords: zinc oxide nanoparticles; autophagy; apoptosis; oxidative stress; ovary; zebrafish

1. Introduction

Recently, nanoparticles (NPs) have attracted a lot of attention in the research community because they have greater chemical, physical, and biological properties than their bulky counterparts [1–3]. Zinc oxide nanoparticles (ZnO-NPs), as one of the ionic metal oxide nanoparticles, have attracted interest because of their diverse physical and chemical properties, as well as their antibacterial properties against a wide spectrum of pathogenic bacteria [4]. Therefore, ZnO-NPs have been widely used in the industrial sector in optoelectronics, catalysts, cosmetics, pigments, and ceramics due to their unique characteristics and their ability to create various nanostructures [4,5]. ZnO-NPs are also used in biological and biomedical sectors because of their anti-inflammatory, wound-healing, antiseptic, and anti-cancer characteristics [6,7].

However, increasing the use of ZnO-NPs has unavoidably resulted in higher human and environmental exposures, as well as toxicological impacts on environmental species. Nano-ZnO particles, on the other hand, are easily bioaccumulated by aquatic creatures, where they cause harmful consequences [8,9]. Of these harmful consequences, ZnO-NPs have toxic effects on the female reproductive system (oocytes), as well as the developing embryos [10,11].

Normal female reproduction and fetal development are required for the survival of all species, including humans and animals. In the female ovary, two essential processes are independently induced and cooperate before fertilization: oocyte maturation and ovulation.

Successful maturation requires the combination of intrinsic and extrinsic factors and passes through different developmental stages that were described earlier in the zebrafish [12]. The first stage of oocyte development is named the primary oocyte or previtellogenic oocyte, followed by the vitellogenic oocyte where the oocytes become more enlarged and reached their maximum size, followed by the third step named the post-ovulatory follicle, which occurs after ovulation [13,14]. In the vertebrate ovary, granulosa cells (GCs) and theca cells formed the follicular cell (FCs) mass around the developing oocyte and they can provide it with essential amino acids, cholesterol, and other nutrients before the ovulation [15,16].

In the developing oocyte and follicular cells cytoplasm, macrophagy (here, named autophagy) is one of the most-programmed regular intrinsic factors that maintain cellular homeostasis and energy production during germ cell starvation and manages the oogenesis process [17,18]. Autophagy is a bulk subcellular degradation process that helps in recycling the unused cytosolic components for cell survival, differentiation, growth, and development [19,20].

For further clarification, increasing evidence declared that autophagy played an essential role in the proliferation and survival of granulosa cells [21–23], suggesting its crucial role during the oogenesis to embryogenesis transition of both invertebrates and vertebrates [18,24–26].

Recent works have investigated different mechanisms for the relationship between ZnO-NP toxicity and female reproductive performance. For example, some authors reported that ZnO-NPs have cytotoxic effects in mouse ovarian germ cells (OGCs); even at low concentrations, ZnO-NPs impeded meiosis and developing abilities in OGCs [11].

Furthermore, ZnO-NPs caused oxidative stress, developmental toxicity, and DNA damage to zebrafish embryos, resulting in significant embryo hatching delays and increased deformity after a 96-h exposure [8].

The adult female zebrafish has asynchronous ovaries, containing ova in different developmental stages, making it a suitable model for studying all the concepts related to ovarian development [27–29]. In our study, we used the female zebrafish as a model to study the effects of ZnO-NPs on cytotoxicity, apoptosis, and autophagy in the developing oocytes in vivo.

To achieve this objective, we investigated the histological findings of the ovarian oocytes under a light and transmission electron microscope as well as the changes in gene expression in nano-ZnO-treated zebrafish ovarian tissue by Reverse transcription-quantitative polymerase chain reaction (RT-qPCR) and Western blot analysis.

2. Materials and Methods

2.1. ZnO-NPs Preparation and Characterization

The chemical Zn-NPs (Che-Zn-NPs) were prepared as follows; 12 g of Zn $(NO_3)_2 \cdot 6H_2O$ was dissolved in 1 L of distilled water then was stirred with NaOH (10%) solution on a hot plate magnetic stirrer for 25 min, then for 2 h at 70 °C. The mixed solution was cooled and filtrated [30].

The synthesized ZnO-NPs were characterized using several techniques. To determine the optical absorption spectra of ZnO-NPs, ultraviolet-visible spectroscopy (UV-vis) (LaxcoTM dual-beam spectrophotometer) was used. In addition, transmission electron microscope analysis (TEM, JEOL 1010, Shimadzu, Japan) was used to determine the morphological characteristics of ZnO-NPs, particularly their size and form. Dynamic light scattering analysis was used to measure the particle size in the colloidal solution of produced ZnO-NPs (DLS, Malvern Hills, UK). Zeta potential analysis was conducted to determine the surface charge of ZnO-NPs and their relative stability. The LC_{50} of ZnO-NPs was estimated in our laboratory and found to be 3.48 mg/L.

2.2. Animal Husbandry and Experiment Design

Adult female zebrafish (*Danio rerio*) (n = 180) were bought from a local fish supplier (Cairo, Egypt) and acclimatized for two weeks before the experiment. During the acclimatization and throughout the experiment, the females were kept in aerated water at 27.5 ± 1 °C in glass aquaria ($80 \times 40 \times 30$ cm, water capacity 60 L), 14 h light: 10 h dark, pH 6.7 ± 0.2 and dissolved oxygen 6.3 ± 0.5 mg/L. The fish were fed twice a day on *Artemia nauplii* (hatched shrimp's eggs) [31]. Acclimatized females were randomly divided into three experimental groups (n = 60/group), each in triplicate (20 fish) in separate tanks. The first group was used as the control group (receiving no treatment), the second group, termed the T1 group, was exposed to $1/5^{th}$ of the estimated LC_{50} of ZnO-NPs (0.69 mg/L) in water daily for two weeks (15 days), while the third group termed the T2 group was exposed to 1/5th of the estimated LC_{50} of ZnO-NPs daily for one month (30 days). The experimental procedures were carried out at the Zoology Department, Faculty of Science, Zagazig University, Zagazig, Egypt.

2.3. Fertility, Fecundity, and Gonad Somatic Index Calculations

Fertility refers to females that can lay ovulated eggs when crossed with adult males, whereas fecundity measures the reproductive potential through the number of fertilized spawned eggs after mating [32]. Herein, tracing fertility and fecundity assessment was conducted with 10 fish from each group, one-to-one paired with untreated males every 5 days. The spawning ratio for fertility was calculated [33]. In addition, to detect fecundity after mating between the females and males, spawned eggs were collected and counted after one hour of light in the morning. Data on fertility and fecundity was obtained from triplicate readings. The gonad somatic index (GSI) was calculated every five days. GSI is an indicator of reproductive capacity, commonly used to quantify the reproductive condition in fish (GSI = Gonad weight/Bodyweight $\times$100).

2.4. Determination of Zinc Residues in the Whole Fish Body

The bodies of female zebrafish (6 females/sample) were digested using acids [34]. In a clean screw-capped glass bottle, one gram of each sample was digested with 4 mL of digestion solution (perchloric/nitric acid, 1:1). Initial digestion was carried out at room temperature for 24 h, followed by heating for 2 h at 110 °C.

After cooling, deionized water was added, and the solution was warmed to expel nitrous gases for one hour in a water bath. Then, the digests were filtered using Whatman No. 1 filter and diluted to 25 mL with deionized water [35]. The resultant solution was then analyzed by a flame atomic absorption spectrophotometer (FAAS).

2.5. Histological Assessments and Transmission Electron Microscope (TEM) Preparations

For histological observations, the females were anesthetized in ice water and fixed as a whole-mount for 24 h at room temperature in Bouin's solution to preserve the ovary oocytes before dissection. Dissected fixed tissues were dehydrated and embedded in paraffin wax and sectioned transversely at 5 μm thicknesses (Leica Model, RM2125 RTS, Biosystems, Deer Park, USA). Sections were stained with hematoxylin and eosin [36]. The average number of oocytes at different stages was calculated to detect the percentage for each type per slide in triplicate.

For TEM observations, dissected ovaries from the three experimental groups were fixed in a mixture of 2.5% glutaraldehyde and 2.5% paraformaldehyde in 0.1 M Na-cacodylate buffer (pH = 7.3) for 24 h at 4 °C. After rinsing in 0.1 M Na-cacodylate buffer, the fixed samples were post-fixed at room temperature in 1% osmium tetroxide. After that, graded series of ethanol were used for the dehydration of samples. Finally, the tissues were embedded in an Epon-Araldite mixture. Semi-thin sections (1.5 mm thickness) were cut using a Reichert ultra-microtome. Ultrathin sections were stained with toluidine blue contrasted in 50% alcohol-uranyl acetate solution and lead citrate, then examined with a Philips EM 400 electron microscope (Philips, INCAEDX, Oxford, UK) at the Faculty of Science, Alexandria, Egypt.

2.6. RNA Isolation and Quantitative Real-Time PCR (qRT-PCR)

Total RNA was extracted from six ovaries of each group with TRIzol reagent according to the manufacturer's instructions (Life Technologies, Carlsbad, CA, USA). Total RNA concentration was evaluated by gel electrophoresis and spectrophotometer (METTLER, TOLEDO, Canada), respectively. Total RNA was used as a template for reverse transcription to produce cDNAs with the Prime Script TM RT reagent Kit with gDNA Eraser (Stratagene, Takara, San Jose, CA, USA).

qRT-PCR was conducted on the MSLPCR30 Thermal Cycler system (Biobase Biozone Co., Ltd., Guangdong, China) and β-actin was used to normalize the expression values. The specific primers used in this study are listed in Table 1.

Table 1. Target genes, accession number, and primer sequences for quantitative real-time PCR (qRT-PCR).

Target Gene	Accession Number in NCBI	Primer Sequences
	Reference Gene	
βactin	NM_131031	F: 5′ ATGGATGAGGAAATCGCTGC 3′ R:5′CTTTCTGTCCCATGCCAACC 3′
	Antioxidant enzymes	
Superoxide dismutase1 (*sod1*)	NM_131294	F: 5′ CGCACTTCAACCCTCATGAC 3′ R: 5′ TGAATCACCATGGTCCTCCC 3′
Superoxide dismutase2 (*sod2*)	NM_199976	F:5′CCTCCAGACAGAAGCA 3′ R:5′CTGAAATGAGCCAAAGT 3′
Glutathione peroxidase 1a (*gpx1a*)	NM_001007281	F:5′GCACAACAGTCAGGGAT 3′ R:5′TCAGGAACGCAAACAG 3′
Glutathione S-transferase pi 1.2 (*gstp1.2*)	NM_131734	F:5′CCAACCACCTCAAATGCT 3′ R:5′ACGGGAAAGAGTCCAGACAG 3′
Catalase (*cat*)	NM_130912	F:5′TGTGGAAGGAGGGTCG 3′ R:5′CTTTGGCTTTGGAGTAG 3′
	Autophagy-related genes	
Autophagy-related gene-7 homolog (*atg7*)	XM 021479676	F:5′ACGGTGATGCTGTTGGTCTG 3′ R: 5′ TTTGTCGGTGGATTTGAAGG 3′
Autophagy-related gene-5 homolog (*atg5*)	NM_205618	F: 5′ TGGAGTATCCCACCGAAGA3′ R:5′ CACTGGTCGGAAGAGC3′
Autophagy-related gene-12 homolog (*atg12*)	NM_001246200	F: 5′ TCATCTCACGCTTCCTCAA 3′ R: 5′ TCACTTCCGAAACACTCAAA 3′
Sequestosome 1 (sqstm1) (*p62*)	NM_001312913	F: 5′ TGGTGCTACTGCCTCTTCTCA 3′ R: 5′ GGGTTACTTTGGTCCGCTTT 3′
	Apoptosis-related genes	
Apoptosis-inducing factor (*siva1*)	NM_001327928	F: 5′ CCGCTACCGACAGGAGATCTACGA 3′ R: 5′ GGTGTGGAGCGCGCTCTGTGCAGT 3′
BCL2 associated X, apoptosis regulator (*baxa*)	NM_131562	F: 5′ GACAGGGATGCTGAAGTGA 3′ R: 5′ TGAGTCGGCTGAAGATTAGA 3′
Caspase a (*caspa*)	NM_131505	F: 5′ GACGGTGAGCCTGATGAGCCAA 3′ R: 5′ CCTGAACAGTTCCTCGATGTGA 3′

Table 1. *Cont.*

Target Gene	Accession Number in NCBI	Primer Sequences
	Oocyte maturation genes	
Methyltransferase like 3 (*mettl3*)	NM_212780	F: 5′ CCTAGAGCTGCTGAATACCAGT 3′ R: 5′ GATGATTCGCCTGAAGTGC 3′
Progesterone receptor membrane component-1 (*pgrmc1*)	NM_001007392	F: 5′ CAGACTATGGCCCGGTTGAGGAG 3′ R: 5′ CTGCATGGCATTGAGATCGG 3′
Zygote arrest 1 (*zar1*)	NM_194381	F: 5′ CAACCCGAAGACCGAC 3′ R: 5′ CACCACCGCTGCTGAC 3′
Gonadal soma-derived factor variant 2 (*gsdf*)	NM_001114668	F: 5′ GCTCCATCCGTCACCT 3′ R: 5′ TCACCGTAGACAGAACCAG 3′
SRY-box transcription factor 3 (*sox3*)	NM_001001811	F: 5′ ATTCCGCAGTCCAACA 3′ R: 5′ TTCTCCTGAGCCATCTTC 3′
	Ovulation-related genes	
Metallopeptidase with thrombospondin type 1 motif, 15a (*adamts15a*)	NM_001126429	F:5′GAGAGCAAAGATAACAAGGCACAAA3′ R: 5′TTTTCCACCTTTATTGACTCCACCT3′
Luteinizing hormone/choriogonadotropin receptor (*lhcgr*)	NM_205625	F: 5′ CGCTCTGATCAACTGGGACA 3′ R: 5′ GGCGCTGTTGGCATAAATCC 3′
Progesterone receptor (*pgr*)	NM_001166335	F: 5′ ACAGACAGCATACACCGC3′ R: 5′TCCACAGGTCAGAACTCC3′
Follicle-stimulating hormone receptor (fshr)	NM_001001812	F: 5′ CAAATGCGTCTACGCCATGC3′ R: 5′AAAGCGGGATTACGGACGGT3′
Follistatin a (*fsta*)	NM_131037	F: 5′ CATCAAGGCCAAGTCATGCG3′ R: 5′GCCTGCTTCATGGCACACTC3′

2.7. Protein Extraction and Western Blot Analysis

Total protein was obtained from the homogenates of 6 ovaries from each group by lysing in 800 μL of lysis buffer (7 M urea, 2 M thiourea, 2% DDT, 4% CHAPS, 20 mM Tris base, 1% protease inhibitor cocktail, 0.5 μL benzonase, and 20 μL/mL Bio-Lytes3/10, Fudebio-Tech, China). After centrifugation at 12,000× *g* round per minute (RPM) for 20 min at 4 °C, the supernatant was collected carefully. The procedure was managed according to previous reports [37]. After electrophoresis and electrotransfer, Nylon Fluoride (PVDF) membranes (Millipore, Burlington, MA, USA) were cut, blocked against Bovine Serum Albumin (5% BSA, AUG pharma, Giza, Egypt), resolved in Tris Buffered Saline with Tween (TBST) before one hour and then blotted with primary antibodies all night.

Procedures for all antibodies were performed following the manufacturer's instructions; recombinant anti-mutant P53 antibody (1:1000 dilution, Abcam, ab32049, Cambridge, UK), anti-VASA/VAS antibody (1:500 dilution, Abcam, ab209710, Cambridge, UK), anti-progesterone receptor Pgr (1:1000 dilution, Abcam, ab75857, Cambridge, UK), recombinant anti-Caspase-3 p12 antibody Caspase-3 (EPR16888) (1:1000 dilution, Abcam, ab179517, Cambridge, UK), and anti-β-actin antibody -N- terminal (1:500 dilution, Abcam, ab209869, Cambridge, UK), separately. Membranes were then incubated with horseradish peroxidase (HRP)-linked secondary antibody (1:5000) and visualized using enhanced Western blotting detection reagents (Amersham Pharmacia Biotech, London, UK).

Image J software (Version number (1.51K), National Institutes of Health, Rockville, MD, USA) was used for protein quantifications and blot scanning. These procedures were conducted in the Faculty of Medicine, Mansoura University, Mansoura, Egypt.

2.8. Statistical Analysis and Graph Preparation

Data were analyzed using GraphPad Prism8 software (8.00, GraphPad Software, Inc., La Jolla, CA, USA) and reported as the mean ± standard error of the mean (SEM). Differences in ovarian anomaly and ZnO-NPs residue accumulation were analyzed using a one-way analysis of variance (ANOVA), followed by Tukey's multiple comparisons test. A value of * $p < 0.05$ was considered significant.

3. Results

3.1. Zinc Oxide Nanoparticles (ZnO-NPs) Characterization

The UV-visible absorption spectra of ZnO-NPs are shown in Figure 1A. The samples of ZnO-NPs have a strong absorption maximum at 340 nm.

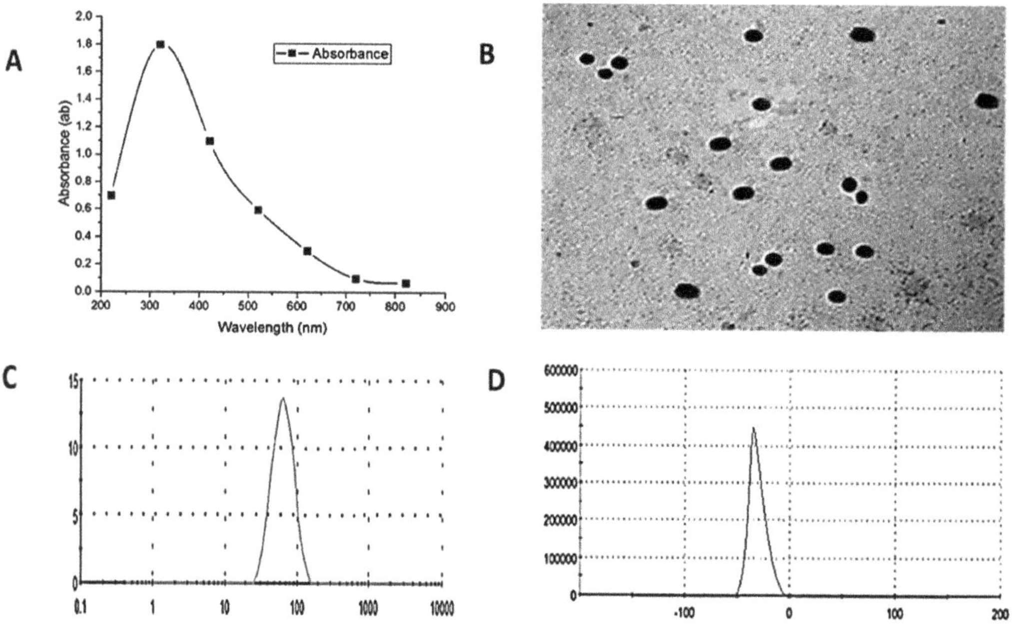

Figure 1. ZnO-NPs characterization: (**A**) shows the UV–VIS spectroscopy analysis of ZnO-NPs to estimate their optical properties; the maximum peak was 340 nm. (**B**) The size and shape of the ZnO-NPs were spherical with an average size of 108 nm by TEM. (**C**) DLS analysis showed that the exact size was 89 nm. (**D**) Zeta potential analysis showed that the net surface charge of ZnO-NPs was −33 mV.

Moreover, TEM measurements showed good distribution of ZnO-NPs, which had a spherical shape, an average size of 108 nm, and presented no agglomeration (Figure 1B).

DLS analysis of particle size distribution revealed an average particle size of around 89 nm (based on intensity distribution) (Figure 1C). The ZnO-NPs had a mean zeta potential of −33 mV, indicating moderate stability (Figure 1D).

3.2. ZnO-NPs Affect Ovarian Morphology and Alter Female Fertility and Fecundity

Females of the control group grew normally and did not manifest any ovarian abnormalities (Figure 2A(a,d)), whereas 50% of T1 females showed mild differences from the control upon dissection (Figure 2A(b,e)). On the other hand, 90% of the dissected treated females from T2 had diffused empty ovaries with confocal macro-necrosis compared with the matched control and T1 (Figure 2A(c,f)). At the experimental end, the percentage of females with ovarian malignancy was recorded (Figure 2B).

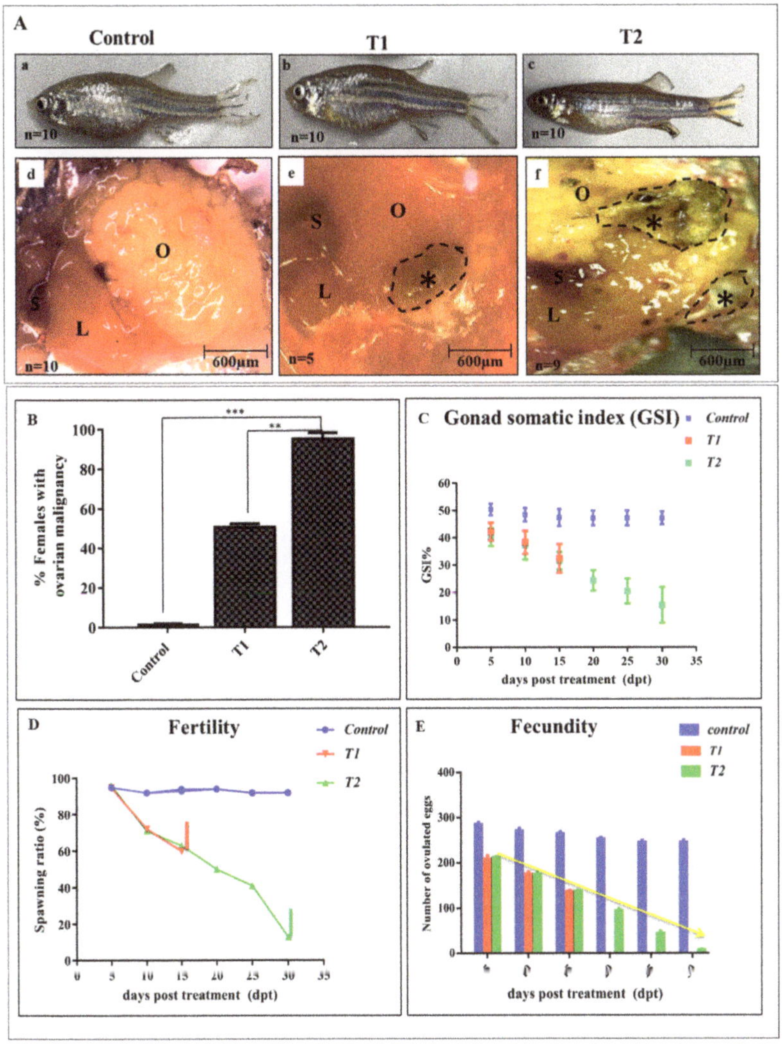

Figure 2. Effects of ZnO-NPs on Gonadosomatic index, fertility, and fecundity: (**A**) Representative pictures of the control, T1, and T2 females with normal ovaries in the control fish (**a**,**d**), transition state of malignancy in T1 (**b**,**e**), and ovarian necrosis in T2 (**c**,**f**) (Black asterisks). (**B**) Percentage of females with macroscopic ovarian malignancy for each experimental group ($n = 10$). (**C**) Distribution of gonad somatic index (GSI); notice the weight reduction of T2 females compared with the control. (**D**) Fertility assessment of the control, T1, and T2 groups declined at 30 dpt in T2 into 10%. (**E**) Tracing assessment of fecundity in the control, T1, and T2 with a significant reduction in T2 at 30 dpt. L: liver, O: ovary, S: spleen. The results are shown as the mean ± SEM. ** $p < 0.01$, *** $p < 0.001$. T1 = group was exposed to 1/5th of estimated LC_{50} of ZnO-NPs in water daily for two weeks (15 days). T2 = group was exposed to 1/5th of estimated LC_{50} of ZnO-NPs in water daily for one month (30 days).

During the exposure period, it was noticed that ZnO-NPs affected the females' body weight; accordingly, the GSI was reduced significantly after one-month post-ZnO-NPs exposure rather than two weeks (Figure 2C).

Moreover, fertility and fecundity assessments were conducted every five days and the spawned eggs were calculated after mating with the males. After one month of ZnO-NPs exposure, the females' fertility declined and nearly all of the treated females were infertile by 30 dpt compared with the control females (Figure 2D). Furthermore, the number of spawned eggs declined sharply after one month in the T2 females compared with the control (Figure 2E).

3.3. Zn Residues in the Female's Body

The tissue analysis of Zn residues in the whole body of the fish is represented in Table 2.

Table 2. Accumulation of ZnO-NPs residues in the whole body of treated female zebrafish (μg/g wet weight).

Groups	Zn Residues (μg/g Wet Weight)
control	15.83 ± 1.57^{c}
T1	32.10 ± 4.01^{b}
T2	57.85 ± 1.78^{a}
SEM	6.26
p-value	<0.001

Means within columns carrying different superscripts are significant at ($p < 0.05$). T1 = group was exposed to 1/5th of estimated LC_{50} of ZnO-NPs in water daily for two weeks (15 days). T2 = group was exposed to 1/5th of estimated LC_{50} of ZnO-NPs in water daily for one month (30 days).

Herein, the highest concentration of Zn was detected in the body tissue of females that were exposed to ZnO-NPs for one month, followed by fish exposed to ZnO-NPs for two weeks, then the control group that showed the lowest value of Zn residues.

3.4. Effect of ZnO-NPs on Histological Findings of Oocyte Maturation Levels

After one month, the ovaries of the control females had normal histological architecture and contained different stages of oocytes development, including primary oocytes or the primary growth stage (PGS), cortical alveolar stage I (CAS I), predominantly vitellogenic stage (VS), mature stage (MS), and atretic oocytes. In the primary oocytes stage, the oocyte was small, and spherical, with a central large nucleus containing deeply stained nucleoli at the peripheral zone, and the ooplasm was more intense compared with other stages (Figure 3A). The cortical alveolar stage I (CAS I) was characterized by the presence of cortical alveoli cells that gradually grew and began to fill the ooplasm around the central nucleus to differentiate into the cortical alveolar stage II (CASII) (Figure 3B,C).

The nucleoli at the CASII stage-oriented periphery migrated to the center of the nucleus, and at the same time, the zona radiata became well-developed (Figure 3C). As a consequence, the number of yolk granules increased in the ooplasm to give rise to the vitellogenic stage (VS) (Figure 3D).

At this stage, the nucleus was difficult to observe and the oocytes enlarged gradually and entered into the mature stage (MS), in which the oocyte was filled with large vitellus yolk granules. In this stage, the nucleus completely disappeared due to the intense diffusion of yolk granules (Figure 3E). Normally, ovarian follicles can either grow to mature oocytes or breakdown by a process of follicular atresia (a form of normal apoptosis to control the oocyte number in the ovarian pool); at this stage, the atretic oocytes (AS) were determined by the hypertrophy of granulosa and theca cells with irregularity in the zona radiata (Figure 3F).

Compared with the control ovaries (Figure 4A,B), the T1 females revealed a significant reduction in the number of mature oocytes, however cortical and vitellogenic stages were still present (Figure 4C,D). Contrarily, females of the T2 group exhibited abnormal ovarian structure with a significant tissue degeneration and a dominant distribution of primary oocytes. Here, cortical, vitellogenic, and mature stages were rarely observed and nearly absent in some sections (Figure 4E,F). Statistical analysis of the histological sections confirmed the previous observations and revealed the adverse consequences of ZnO-NPs on the developing granulosa cells around the nucleus of the oocytes that affected oocyte maturation and differentiation (Figure 4G).

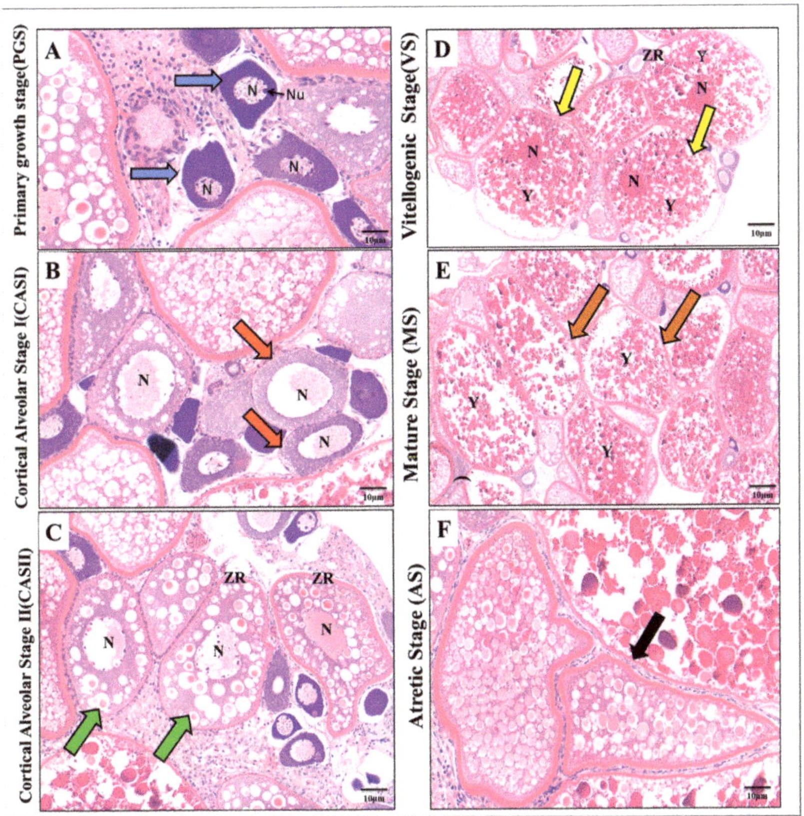

Figure 3. Histological structure showing the different stages of oocyte development in the control zebrafish ovary: (**A**) Primary growth stage (PGS) (blue arrow). (**B**) Cortical Alveolar Stage I (CASI) (red arrow). (**C**) Cortical Alveolar Stage II (CASII) (green arrow). (**D**) Vitellogenic Stage (VS) (yellow arrow). (**E**) Mature Stage (MS) (orange arrow). (**F**) Atretic Stage (AS) (black arrow). N: nucleus, Nu: nucleolus, Y: yolk, ZR: Zona radiata (H&E, 10 µm).

3.5. ZnO-NPs Induce Cytotoxicity and Autophagosome Formation at the Ultrastructural Level

The control-group oocyte's TEM analysis is displayed in Figure 5A–D. There were three main layers in the contact wall; zona theca (ZT) contained theca cells, zona granulosa (ZG), which included the granulosa cells, and zona radiata (ZR) that appeared as a complex perforated layer crossed by pores or canals contain oocyte microvilli. Zona radiata (ZR) was the main feature of the previtellogenic oocyte (Figure 5A). The ooplasm of the previtellogenic oocyte was rich with large yolk granules and mitochondria that had quite regular cisternae (Figure 5B,C). The nucleus had an intact regular nuclear envelope and many small nucleoli arranged in the peripheral zone at the nuclear membrane (Figure 5D).

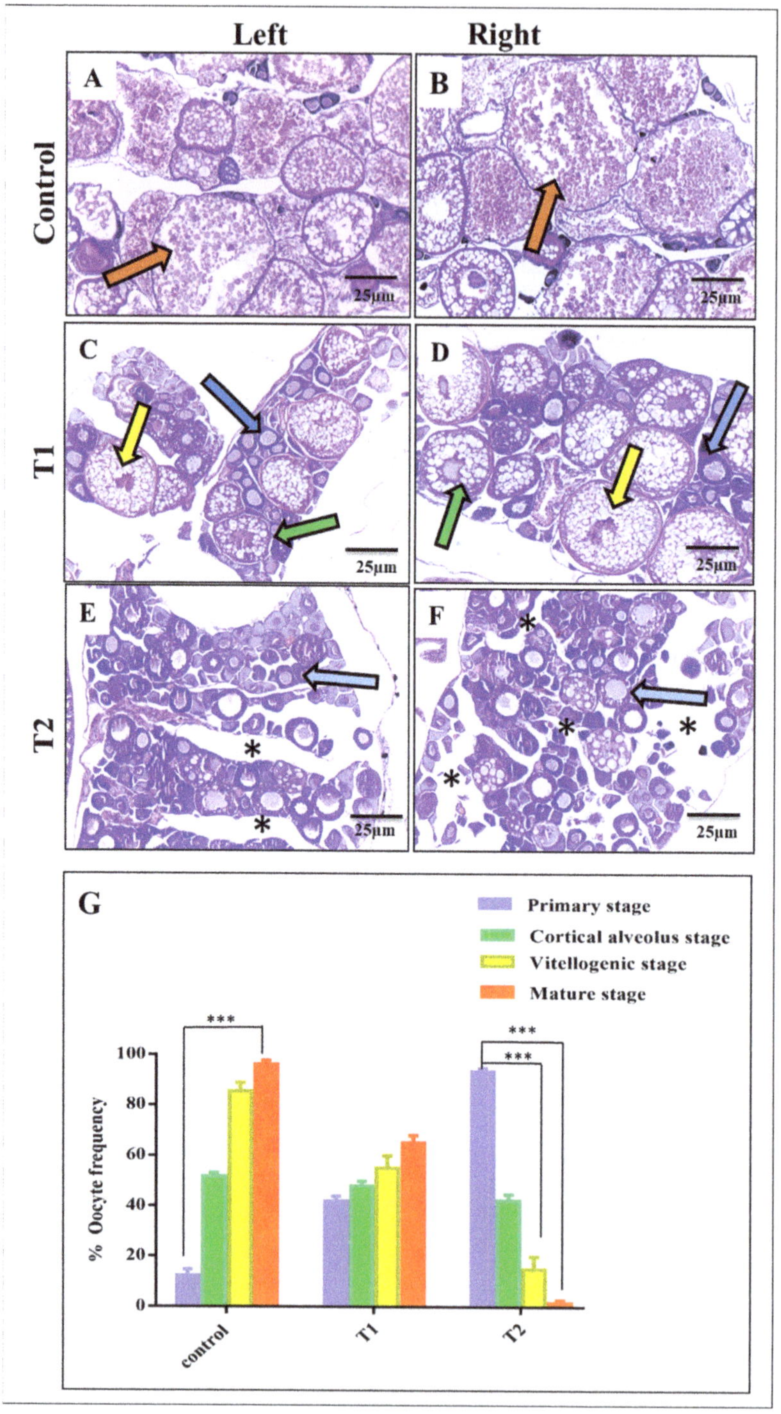

Figure 4. Comparative histological observations of the control, T1, and T2 left and right ovaries (H&E, 25 μm): (**A**,**B**) Photomicrographs showing the left and right ovaries of the control; notice the

presence of numerous mature oocytes (orange arrow). (**C,D**) Photomicrographs showing the left and right ovaries of T1; notice the presence of the primary growth stage (blue arrow), cortical alveolar stage II (green arrow), vitellogenic stage (yellow arrow), and the absence of the mature stage. (**E,F**) Photomicrographs showing the left and right ovaries of T2; notice the tissue degeneration (black asterisk) and the prominent distribution of primary oocytes (blue arrows). (**G**) Statistical analysis of ovary sections in the three experimental groups. Data are shown as the mean ± SEM. *** $p < 0.001$. T1 = group was exposed to 1/5th of estimated LC_{50} of ZnO-NPs in water daily for two weeks (15 days). T2 = group was exposed to 1/5th of estimated LC_{50} of ZnO-NPs in water daily for one month (30 days).

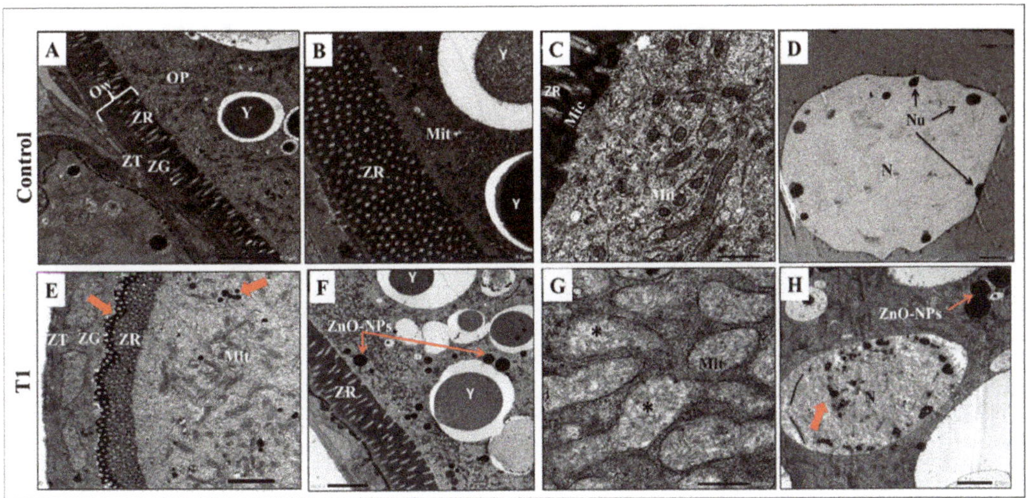

Figure 5. Transmission Electron Microscopy observation of the control and T1 ovaries: (**A–D**) Transmission electron micrographs of the control vitellogenic oocyte showing the intact oocyte membrane with distinct cell layers of theca cells (ZT), granulosa cells (ZG), and zona radiata (ZR), large yolk granules, plenty of normal mitochondria, and a normal nucleus. (**E–H**) Transmission electron micrographs of the T1 ovary showing diffusion of ZnO-NPs to the ooplasm through the cell membrane (red arrows); notice the mild alteration of the cell membrane, mitochondrial degeneration, and chromatin condensation. OW: oocyte wall, ZT: Zona theca, ZG: Zona granulosa, ZR: Zona radiata, OP: ooplasm, Y: yolk, Mit: Mitochondria, Mic: microvilli, N: nucleus, Nu: nucleolus. T1 = group was exposed to 1/5th of the estimated LC50 of ZnO-NPs in water daily for two weeks (15 days).

Contrarily, oocytes revealed mild alterations to the cell wall, ooplasm, and nucleus after two weeks of ZnO-NPs exposure in the T1 group. Herein, the zona radiata (ZR) manifested an irregular appearance with diffused ZnO-NPs that appeared as black droplets penetrating the zona radiata to the ooplasm (Figure 5E,F). In the ooplasm, there were signs of ruptured mitochondrial cisternae (Figure 5G). In addition, the nucleus had a state of chromatin condensation and diffused nuclear material (Figure 5H).

On the other hand, the long exposure to ZnO-NPs for 30 days had significant cytotoxic effects on the developing oocytes. The primary oocyte had a large, indented nucleus with an irregular envelope and separate nuclear components (Figure 6A). The observed vitellogenic oocyte manifested apoptotic features with a winding oocyte wall (Figure 6B). Moreover, the long ZnO-NPs exposure led to ooplasm vacuolization with organelle degeneration due to the high diffusion of the nanoparticles (Figure 6C,E). The nucleus appeared with an irregular tortuous membrane (Figure 6F), and the mitochondria had fragmented cisternae and a swollen appearance (Figure 6G). Interestingly, long exposure to ZnO-NPs activated macroautophagy (also termed autophagy) and altered the intracellular degradation system in the cytoplasm (Figure 6H,I). Here, the ooplasm of T2 contained numerous autophagosomes that were double-membrane vesicles that contained degenerated cellular organelles (Figure 6J). The process of macroautophagy was completed when the autophagosomes fused with the lysosomes to form autolysosomes where the inner cellular cargo degraded (Figure 6K,L).

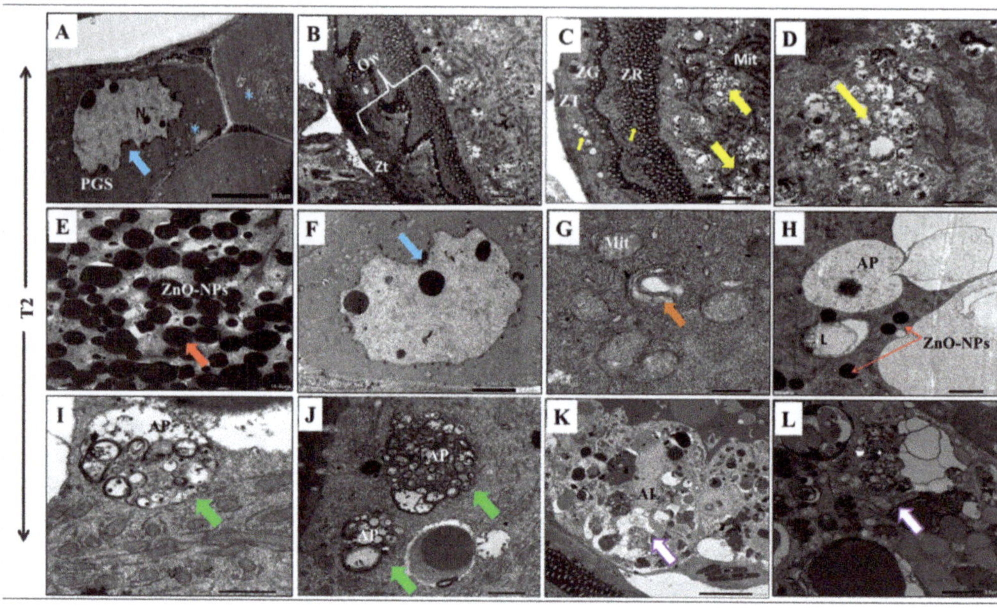

Figure 6. Transmission Electron Microscopy observation of T2 ovary: (**A**) Transmission electron micrographs of a primary oocyte (PGS) showing abnormal winding nuclear membrane (blue arrow) and cytoplasmic vocalizations (blue asterisks). (**B–G**) Micrographs of vitellogenic oocytes in abnormal conditions exhibited irregular cell walls with some vacuolization in the granulosa cell layer and the ooplasm (yellow arrow) with complete organelle degeneration (yellow arrow) due to the enormous diffusion of ZnO-NPs (red arrow). The nucleus appeared with a winding nuclear membrane (blue arrow) and the mitochondria exhibited atrophic cisternae and a swollen appearance (orange arrow). (**H–L**) Transmission electron micrographs showing the steps of autophagy; notice the presence of numerous autophagosomes (green arrow) and autolysosomes (white arrow). OW: oocyte wall, ZT: Zona theca, ZG: Zona granulosa, ZR: Zona radiata, N: nucleus, Mit: Mitochondria, PGS: primary growth stage, AP: autophagosome, AL: autolysosome.

3.6. Effect of ZnO-NPs on the Expression of Specific Genes (Antioxidant, Autophagy, Apoptosis, Oocyte Maturation, and Ovulation-Related Genes) in Zebrafish Ovarian Cells

TEM observations were supported by epigenetic expression evaluated by qRT-PCR. Herein, in T2, signals from the damaged mitochondria increased the ROS from the endoplasmic reticulum which led to high oxidative stress (OS). ROS activated DNA damage and autophagy pathways capable of inducing cell death (apoptosis). Accordingly, mRNA expression of antioxidant genes (*sod1*, *sod2*, *gpx1a*, *gstp1.2*, and *cat*) declined in the T2 group compared with the control and T1 groups (Figure 7A).

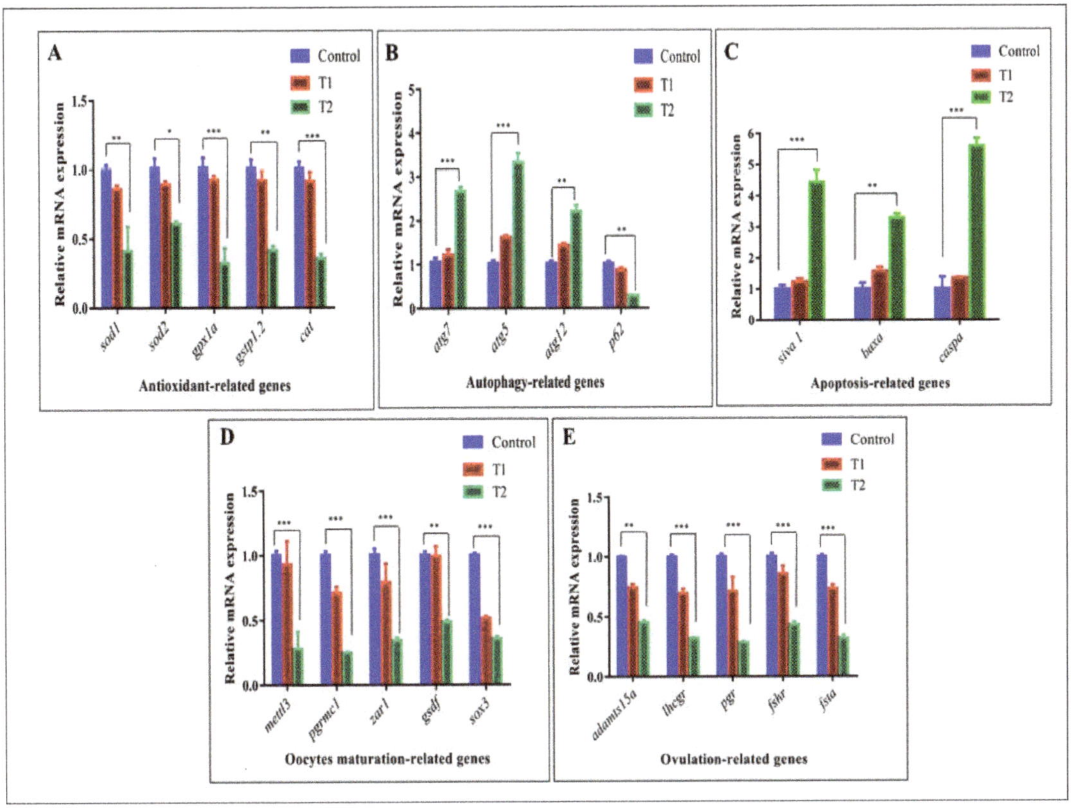

Figure 7. Effect of ZnO-NPs on oocyte maturation and ovulation via the induction of oxidative stress and the apoptotic pathway at the genetic level. (**A–C**) Expressions of mRNA evaluated by qRT-PCR indicate the downregulation of antioxidant-related genes in T2 (**A**), the upregulation of autophagy-related genes in T2 (**B**), and the induction of apoptosis-related genes in T2 (**C**). (**D**,**E**) mRNA expression shows the downregulation of oocyte maturation-related genes in T2 (**D**) and ovulation genes in T2 (**E**). The results from three dependent experiments are shown as the mean ± SEM. * $p < 0.05$, ** $p < 0.01$, *** $p < 0.001$. T1 = group was exposed to 1/5th of the estimated LC50 of ZnO-NPs in water daily for two weeks (15 days). T2 = group was exposed to 1/5th of the estimated LC_{50} of ZnO-NPs in water daily for one month (30 days).

On the contrary, mRNA expression of autophagy genes (*atg7*, *atg5*, and *atg12*) was gradually increased in the T2 group and involved in the autophagosome formation, whereas *p62*, the autophagic cargo receptor, gradually declined, thus indicating the actual autophagy activation (Figure 7B).

In addition, mRNA expression of apoptosis-related genes was elevated in the T2 group compared with the control and T1 siblings via a higher expression of *siva*, *bax*, and *caspa* (Figure 7C).

Most likely, oxidative stress, autophagy, and apoptosis induction were responsible for the oocyte ovulation and maturation suppression in the T2 ovary indicated by the downregulation of mRNA expression of oocyte maturation-related genes including *mettl3*, *pgrmc1*, *zar1*, *gsdf*, and *sox3*, that in turn affected the ovulation process via the suppression of ovulation-related genes (*adamts15a*, *ihcgr*, *pgr*, *fshr*, and *fsta*) (Figure 7D,E).

3.7. Effect of ZnO-NPs on the Expression of Proteins Related to Apoptosis Genes

To confirm the relationship between ZnO-NPs aggregation and necrotic tissue formation in the T2 ovary, a Western blot was performed on the ovaries of the control, T1, and T2 groups that revealed a higher accumulation of mutated **tP53** protein in the T2 group relative to the control and T1 siblings (Figure 8A,C). Mutated tP53 protein marked the damaged DNA and favored cancer cell survival. Furthermore, the T2 group exhibited a higher expression of the **Vasa** protein that was specific for germ cells and primordial gametocytes, indicating that ZnO-NPs did not affect germ cell differentiation, ensuring the presence of many primary oocytes in the T2 ovaries rather than the control and T1 groups (Figure 8A,D). On the other hand, the T2 group exhibited a significant reduction of the progesterone receptor protein **Pgr**, which plays an important role in the ovulation process (Figure 8A,E).

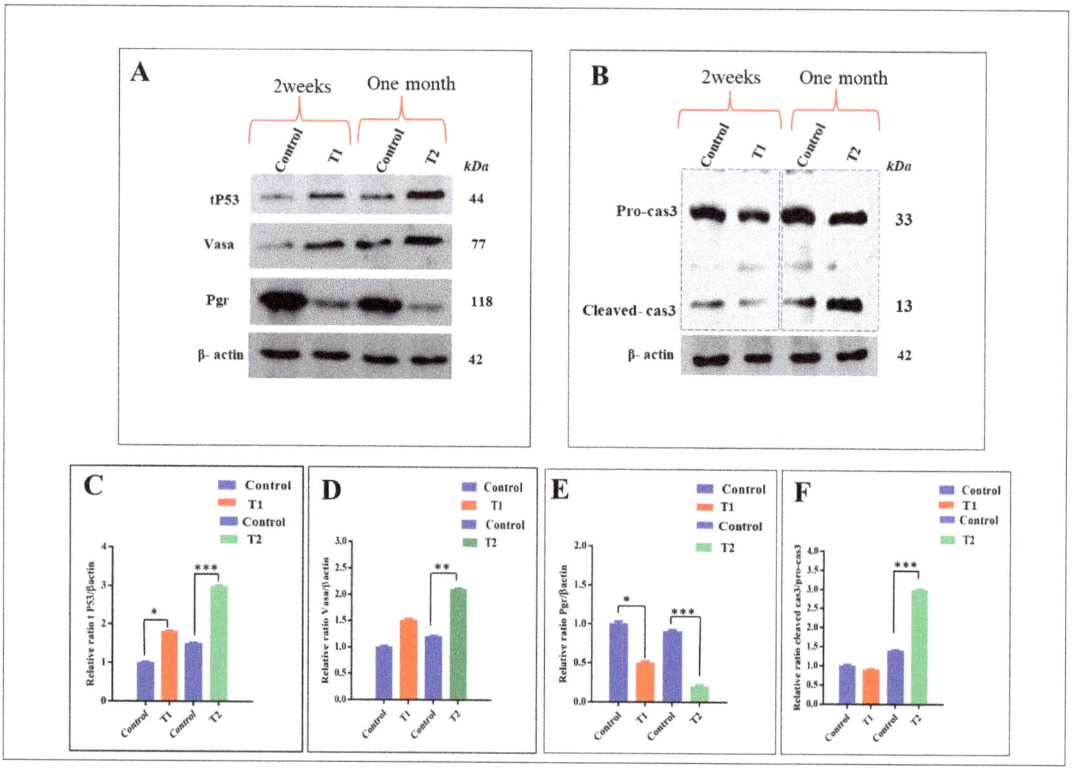

Figure 8. Effect of ZnO-NPs on necroptosis via mutated tP53 formation: (**A**) Western blot analysis of the tP53 protein, Vasa protein, and Pgr protein normalized to β-actin in control, T1, and T2 groups. (**B**) Western blot analysis of procaspase-3 and cleaved caspase-3 in the control, T1, and T2 groups revealed the overexpression of cleaved caspase-3 in T2 compared with the control and T1 groups. (**C–F**) Quantified protein expression revealed the ratio analysis of tP53/β-actin, Vasa/β-actin, Pgr/β-actin, and cleaved -cas3/pro-cas3, respectively quantified by the Image J software. Data expressed as mean ± SEM. * $p < 0.05$, ** $p < 0.01$, and *** $p < 0.001$. T1 = group was exposed to 1/5th of the estimated LC_{50} of ZnO-NPs in water daily for two weeks (15 days). T2 = group was exposed to 1/5th of the estimated LC_{50} of ZnO-NPs in water daily for one month (30 days).

In addition, ZnO-NPs induced the apoptosis of oocytes via the caspase pathway, revealed by the higher expressions of the **Cleaved-cas3** protein in the T2 group compared with the control and T1 (Figure 8B,F).

4. Discussion

In relation to the characterization of ZnO-NPs, their strong absorption at 340 nm was firstly confirmed by Dulta *et al.*, who reported that the maximum absorption of ZnO-NPs was in the range of 300–360 nm, with a very high peak at 340 nm [38]. The absorption spectra of produced nanoparticles are influenced by a variety of factors, including synthesis technique, temperature, size, and shape [39]. This strong absorption refers to the spherical shape of the NPs as well as the monodispersed nature of their distribution, which is confirmed by the results of the TEM measurements [40,41]. Because of the electrostatic repulsions between the individual particles, a large negative or positive value of zeta potential suggests a higher physical colloidal stability [42].

During the exposure period to ZnO-NPs, the ZnO-NPs affected the females' body weight; in fact, the resulting GSI significantly reduced after one month rather than after two weeks. Kime attributed the decrease in GSI to vitellogenesis suppression [43]. Vitellogenesis is the production and secretion of vitellogenins (Vtgs) from the liver as primary precursors of yolk proteins in response to the estrogen stimulation [44]. ZnO-NPs have been shown in studies to produce intracellular reactive oxygen species (ROS) [45,46], which damage biomolecules, such as DNA, lipids, and proteins in the liver and ovaries, as well as other organs, and hence hinder the vitellogenesis process [43,45,47].

Collectively, over time, ZnO-NPs alter female fertility and fecundity. The ZnO-NPs hampered the growth of the zebrafish embryo and larva and reduced their survivability and hatching rate, where the 84 h half-maximum effective concentration (EC_{50}) of ZnO-NPs on the hatching rate of zebrafish embryo was 2.065 mg/L [48]. ZnO-NPs reduced the hatching rate and caused pericardial edema of zebrafish embryos and larvae possibly by increasing ROS and altering the cellular response to oxidative stress [9]. ZnO-NPs delayed zebrafish embryo and larva development, decreased their survival and hatching rates, and caused serious tissue damage and ulcerations [10].

The current results agree with those of Tavabe et al., who found that ZnO-NPs have a dose-dependent effect on *Macrobrachium rosenbergii* egg weight, viable egg rate, and broodstock inter-spawning period [49]. Wang, et al. also noted that chronic exposure (13 weeks) to zebrafish of 0.1 mg L-1 titanium dioxide nanoparticles ($nTiO_2$) led to a reduction of 29.5% in the total egg number [50]. The NPs can overcome biological barriers and directly alter primary ovarian follicles, as well as subsequently affect the zebrafish vitellogenesis [50]. Tang et al. demonstrated that ZnO-NPs' detrimental effect on reproductive organs was generated by apoptosis and signaling in the endoplasmic reticulum [51], while Bacchetta, et al. attributed the reduced reproduction in *Daphnia magna* to a direct injury to the mitochondria, resulting in poor energy availability [52].

The detection of Zn residues in the female's body agrees with a previous work that found the accumulation of Zn resulting from waterborne exposure to ZnO-NPs to be 7 to 12 times higher in blackfish than in the control group [53]. Kaya, et al. found that 14 days of waterborne exposure by *Oreochromis niloticus* to small (30 nm) and large (100 nm) ZnO-NPs led to a significant accumulation of ZnO-NPs in the tissues [54]. On the contrary, the tissues of zebrafish exposed to ZnO-NPs at 500 μg/L or 5000 μg/L via the water revealed no significant uptake of zinc in the studied tissues evaluated (liver, gill, kidney, and brain) [55]. The physicochemical properties of NPs, as well as the exposure method and fish species, alter tissue distribution patterns and accumulation, which could explain the disparity in results [56].

For instance, Suganthi, et al. observed ovary histopathological abnormalities in *Oreochromis mossambicus* after exposure to ZnO-NPs for 4 days [57]. The histopathological abnormalities of *O. mossambicus* ovaries differed depending on the concentration of ZnO-NPs, where degenerated late vitellogenic oocytes (DLV) and the development of vacuolation (V) in the cytoplasm were seen in 30 ppm-exposed fish. Oocyte necrosis and vitellogenic fluid (Vf) in the ovarian parenchyma were seen at 50 ppm. Degenerated late vitellogenic oocytes (DLV) and vacuolation (V) production in the cytoplasm were detected at 70 ppm. In addition, it has been observed that the ZnO–NPs (50 mg/L) could induce more substantial histological damages to adult zebrafish ovaries than perfluorooctane sulfonate (PFOS) alone [58]. According to Liu et al., ZnO NPs have a detrimental effect on ovarian development because of their effects on neuronal factors, neuroendocrine cells, or the contents of essential elements found in the ovary [59]. On the other hand, mitotic catastrophe, vacuolization in the ooplasm, enlargement of the mitochondria, and degradation of the pore and microvilli structures of the zona radiata were recorded in zebrafish that were exposed to titanium dioxide nanoparticles (TiO_2-NPs) for 5 days [60]. Numerous studies support the histological impact of TiO_2-NPs on ovarian anomalies in zebrafish [50,61].

The most significant of several hypotheses suggests that TiO_2-NPs have a degenerative effect on folliculogenesis, alter sex hormone levels and decrease the fertility [50,61]. Moreover, the TEM study of mouse OGCs subjected to ZnO-NPs revealed a reduction of cell viability in a concentration- and time-dependent manner.

Treatment with 10 g/mL ZnO-NPs for one day was non-toxic, while the structures of the cells treated with 30 g/m ZnO-NPs for a day were disrupted [11]. Interestingly, a study performed in testicular cells revealed that ZnO-NPs increased the numbers of autophagosomes and caused an aberrant enlargement of the nuclear membrane intermembrane gap [62].

Moreover, a quantitative transcriptomics (RNA-seq) study on gene expressions in ovarian samples showed that a total of 222 genes were altered following the ZnO-NP treatments [59].

Numerous studies link ZnO-NPs' cytotoxic effects to oxidative stress development and the increase of ROS levels in the cells, which disrupts the cellular redox balance and can seriously harm biological macromolecules and cause genetic instability [63–65].

In mouse OGCs subjected to 20 and 30 g/mL ZnO-NPs, it was detected that ROS production caused a decrease in the viability of the OGCs [12]. Similarly, Chen et al. recorded that gene expressions associated with oxidative stress (Gclc) levels in the placentas of pregnant mice were downregulated after exposure to ZnO-NPs [66].

This downregulation resulted in impairing the ability of the body to effectively eliminate ROS, particularly H_2O_2, which led to an increase in oxidants and oxidative stress causing fetus damage and fetal abortions.

According to several studies, ZnO-NPs can trigger the autophagy process in cells by releasing zinc ions that harm lysosomes and disrupt autophagic flux and mitochondria [67,68]. The autophagy signaling system is controlled by a crucial molecular signal called mTOR.

More than 20 genes, including the Atg5, Atg7, and atg12 genes, can encode the proteins necessary for the autophagy field execution [69]. Numerous works have shown that ZnO-NPs can increase the expression of atg genes, particularly atg5 and atg7, and the proteins involved in the production of the autophagosome [68,70,71].

Similarly, in cultured primary astrocytes, it was discovered that ZnO-NPs activated caspase-3 and caused the production of the bax gene [72].

This was supported by Ahamed et al., who demonstrated that ZnO-NPs triggered apoptotic cell death by inducing p53 and caspase pathways through the action of the oxidative stress [73].

Additionally, Chen et al. reported that the silver nanoparticles (Ag-NPs) can trigger the maturation of zebrafish oocytes by inducing apoptosis in ovarian follicle cells as a result of oxidative stress [74]. While, according to Applerot et al., the lysosomal cells initially absorbed the nano-ZnO and then released Zn^{2+} [75].

This is consistent with Mishra et al. who stated that ZnO-NPs triggered apoptosis and the production of ROS [76].

Our results suggested that long exposure to ZnO-NPs maintains primary oocyte dormancy and the few growing oocytes died before complete maturation, hence ceasing the ovulation process. Within the normal female ovary, hormonal action has a key role in controlling oocyte maturation and ovulation, however, it depends on the cross-talk between other cellular and molecular mechanisms including autophagy, apoptosis, and necroptosis that also determine the fate of the oocytes [77,78].

Accordingly, as long as the autophagy process is stable, the other two pathways are controlled to maintain fertility for zebrafish females [23,79]. In addition, progesterone receptor membrane component 1 (Pgrmcl) plays an essential role in promoting the survival of both the normal and cancerous ovarian [80,81]. Pgrmcl expression has been correlated with tumor growth, angiogenesis, and infertility [82,83]. Oocyte maturation is essential for the ovulation step and any disturbance will affect the fertility [84]. Furthermore, incomplete maturation alters ovulation and follicular-stimulating genes [85].

As for the effects of ZnO-NPs on the expressions of proteins related to apoptosis-related genes, the Western blot revealed a higher accumulation of mutated tP53 protein in the T2 group relative to the control and T1 siblings. Mutated tP53 protein marked the damaged DNA favoring cancer cell survival. Furthermore, the T2 group exhibited a higher expression of the Vasa protein that is specific for germ cells and primordial gametocytes, indicating that ZnO-NPs did not affect germ cell differentiation, ensuring the presence of many primary oocytes in T2 ovaries rather than in the control and T1 groups.

On the other hand, the T2 group exhibited a significant reduction of progesterone receptor protein Pgr, which has an essential function in the ovulation process. In addition, ZnO-NPs induced oocyte apoptosis via the caspase pathway, which was revealed by the higher expression of cleaved -cas3 protein in the T2 group compared with the control and T1.

Moreover, the ovaries of the T2 females harboring high levels of the tP53-mutated protein that has been reported to be increased in half of the solid tumors, induced cancer cells to survive [86,87].

In zebrafish, the Vasa protein is involved in germ cell formation and is stable throughout early development [88], however, its relation to ovarian necrosis is still poorly understood. Here, we found that the expression of the Vasa protein is upregulated in T2 females compared with the control, supporting the previous results observed in other ovarian cancers [89–91].

5. Conclusions

In conclusion, our results revealed that ZnO-NPs can impair the fertility of female zebrafish in a time-dependent manner. Exposing zebrafish to 1/5th of the estimated LC_{50} of ZnO-NPs (0.69 mg/L) daily for one month caused cytotoxicity in the maturing oocyte by activating autophagy and apoptosis in a caspase-dependent manner and induced oxidative stress by generating ROS that elevated the mutated ovarian tP53 protein. These effects could be implicated in delaying the development of embryos and inducing embryonic abnormalities.

Author Contributions: Conceptualization, S.A.M., M.R.F. and M.A.; methodology, M.R.F., M.A., M.T.E.-S., S.A.M., R.M.R. and W.M.E.; software, M.T.E.-S.; validation, M.R.F., M.A., S.A.M. and A.D.C.; formal analysis, S.A.M. and M.R.F.; investigation, S.A.M. and M.R.F. and M.A.; resources, M.R.F. and W.G.E.-N.; data curation, M.R.F.; writing—original draft preparation, M.R.F., M.A., S.A.M., M.T.E.-S., W.M.E. and A.D.C.; writing—review and editing, M.A., M.R.F., W.M.E., G.E.M. and A.D.C.; visualization, M.A.; project administration, A.D.C., M.A. and M.R.F.; funding acquisition, A.D.C. and C.M. All authors have read and agreed to the published version of the manuscript.

Funding: This research received no external funding.

Institutional Review Board Statement: The animal study was reviewed and approved by the institutional Ethics Committee of Zagazig University, Egypt (Approval number: ZUIACUC/2/F/56/2021).

Informed Consent Statement: Not applicable.

Data Availability Statement: The data are contained within this article.

Conflicts of Interest: The authors declare no conflict of interest.

References

1. Heiligtag, F.J.; Niederberger, M. The fascinating world of nanoparticle research. *Mater. Today* **2013**, *16*, 262–271. [CrossRef]
2. Di Cerbo, A.; Pezzuto, F.; Scarano, A. Cytotoxic and Bacteriostatic Activity of Nanostructured TiO_2 Coatings. *Pol. J. Microbiol.* **2016**, *65*, 225–229. [CrossRef] [PubMed]
3. Guildford, A.L.; Poletti, T.; Osbourne, L.H.; Di Cerbo, A.; Gatti, A.M.; Santin, M. Nanoparticles of a different source induce different patterns of activation in key biochemical and cellular components of the host response. *J. R. Soc. Interf.* **2009**, *6*, 1213–1221. [CrossRef] [PubMed]
4. Mirzaei, H.; Darroudi, M. Zinc oxide nanoparticles: Biological synthesis and biomedical applications. *Ceram. Int.* **2017**, *43*, 907–914. [CrossRef]
5. Islam, F.; Shohag, S.; Uddin, M.J.; Islam, M.R.; Nafady, M.H.; Akter, A.; Mitra, S.; Roy, A.; Emran, T.B.; Cavalu, S. Exploring the Journey of Zinc Oxide Nanoparticles (ZnO-NPs) toward Biomedical Applications. *Materials* **2022**, *15*, 2160. [CrossRef]
6. Jiang, J.; Pi, J.; Cai, J. The Advancing of Zinc Oxide Nanoparticles for Biomedical Applications. *Bioinorg. Chem. Appl.* **2018**, *2018*, 1062562. [CrossRef]
7. Scarano, A.; Murmura, G.; Vantaggiato, G.; Lauritano, D.; Silvestre-Rangil, J.; Di Cerbo, A.; Lorusso, F. Delayed expansion of atrophic mandible (deam): A case report. *Oral Implantol. (Rome)* **2017**, *10*, 190–196. [CrossRef]
8. Zhao, X.; Wang, S.; Wu, Y.; You, H.; Lv, L. Acute ZnO nanoparticles exposure induces developmental toxicity, oxidative stress and DNA damage in embryo-larval zebrafish. *Aquat. Toxicol.* **2013**, *136*, 49–59. [CrossRef]
9. Zhu, X.; Wang, J.; Zhang, X.; Chang, Y.; Chen, Y. The impact of ZnO nanoparticle aggregates on the embryonic development of zebrafish (Danio rerio). *Nanotechnology* **2009**, *20*, 195103. [CrossRef]
10. Liu, J.; Zhao, Y.; Ge, W.; Zhang, P.; Liu, X.; Zhang, W.; Hao, Y.; Yu, S.; Li, L.; Chu, M.; et al. Oocyte exposure to ZnO nanoparticles inhibits early embryonic development through the gamma-H2AX and NF-kappaB signaling pathways. *Oncotarget* **2017**, *8*, 42673–42692. [CrossRef]
11. Saber, M.; Hayaei-Tehrani, R.S.; Mokhtari, S.; Hoorzad, P.; Esfandiari, F. In vitro cytotoxicity of zinc oxide nanoparticles in mouse ovarian germ cells. *Toxicol. Vitr.* **2021**, *70*, 105032. [CrossRef] [PubMed]
12. Selman, K.; Wallace, R.A.; Sarka, A.; Qi, X. Stages of oocyte development in the zebrafish, Brachydanio rerio. *J. Morphol.* **1993**, *218*, 203–224. [CrossRef] [PubMed]
13. Cakici, O.; İsisag Ucuncu, S. Oocyte Development In Zebrafish, Danio rerio (Teleostei: Cyprinidae). *J. Fish.Aqua. Sci.* **2007**, *24*, 137–141.
14. Lessman, C.A. Oocyte maturation: Converting the zebrafish oocyte to the fertilizable egg. *Gen. Comp. Endocrinol.* **2009**, *161*, 53–57. [CrossRef]
15. Eppig, J.J. Oocyte control of ovarian follicular development and function in mammals. *Reproduction* **2001**, *122*, 829–838. [CrossRef] [PubMed]
16. Su, Y.Q.; Sugiura, K.; Eppig, J.J. Mouse oocyte control of granulosa cell development and function: Paracrine regulation of cumulus cell metabolism. *Semin. Reprod. Med.* **2009**, *27*, 32–42. [CrossRef] [PubMed]
17. Gawriluk, T.R.; Hale, A.N.; Flaws, J.A.; Dillon, C.P.; Green, D.R.; Rucker, E.B., 3rd. Autophagy is a cell survival program for female germ cells in the murine ovary. *Reproduction* **2011**, *141*, 759–765. [CrossRef]
18. Agnello, M.; Chiarelli, R.; Martino, C.; Bosco, L.; Roccheri, M.C. Autophagy is required for sea urchin oogenesis and early development. *Zygote* **2016**, *24*, 918–926. [CrossRef]
19. Klionsky, D.J.; Emr, S.D. Autophagy as a regulated pathway of cellular degradation. *Science* **2000**, *290*, 1717–1721. [CrossRef]
20. Yoshimori, T. Autophagy: Paying Charon's toll. *Cell* **2007**, *128*, 833–836. [CrossRef]
21. D'Herde, K.; De Prest, B.; Roels, F. Subtypes of active cell death in the granulosa of ovarian atretic follicles in the quail (Coturnix coturnix japonica). *Reprod. Nutr. Dev.* **1996**, *36*, 175–189. [CrossRef] [PubMed]
22. Choi, J.Y.; Jo, M.W.; Lee, E.Y.; Yoon, B.K.; Choi, D.S. The role of autophagy in follicular development and atresia in rat granulosa cells. *Fertil. Steril.* **2010**, *93*, 2532–2537. [CrossRef]
23. Gioacchini, G.; Dalla Valle, L.; Benato, F.; Fimia, G.M.; Nardacci, R.; Ciccosanti, F.; Piacentini, M.; Borini, A.; Carnevali, O. Interplay between autophagy and apoptosis in the development of Danio rerio follicles and the effects of a probiotic. *Reprod. Fertil. Dev.* **2013**, *25*, 1115–1125. [CrossRef] [PubMed]
24. Thome, R.G.; Santos, H.B.; Arantes, F.P.; Domingos, F.F.; Bazzoli, N.; Rizzo, E. Dual roles for autophagy during follicular atresia in fish ovary. *Autophagy* **2009**, *5*, 117–119. [CrossRef] [PubMed]
25. Tsukamoto, S.; Kuma, A.; Mizushima, N. The role of autophagy during the oocyte-to-embryo transition. *Autophagy* **2008**, *4*, 1076–1078. [CrossRef] [PubMed]
26. Nakashima, A.; Aoki, A.; Kusabiraki, T.; Shima, T.; Yoshino, O.; Cheng, S.B.; Sharma, S.; Saito, S. Role of autophagy in oocytogenesis, embryogenesis, implantation, and pathophysiology of pre-eclampsia. *J Obstet Gynaecol. Res.* **2017**, *43*, 633–643. [CrossRef]
27. Ge, W. Intrafollicular paracrine communication in the zebrafish ovary: The state of the art of an emerging model for the study of vertebrate folliculogenesis. *Mol. Cell. Endocrinol.* **2005**, *237*, 1–10. [CrossRef]
28. Clelland, E.; Peng, C. Endocrine/paracrine control of zebrafish ovarian development. *Mol. Cell Endocrinol.* **2009**, *312*, 42–52. [CrossRef]

29. Elkouby, Y.M. All in one - integrating cell polarity, meiosis, mitosis and mechanical forces in early oocyte differentiation in vertebrates. *Int. J. Dev. Biol.* **2017**, *61*, 179–193. [CrossRef]
30. El-Saadony, M.T.; Alkhatib, F.M.; Alzahrani, S.O.; Shafi, M.E.; El Abdel-Hamid, S.; Taha, T.F.; Aboelenin, S.M.; Soliman, M.M.; Ahmed, N.H. Impact of mycogenic zinc nanoparticles on performance, behavior, immune response, and microbial load in Oreochromis niloticus. *Saudi J. Biol. Sci.* **2021**, *28*, 4592–4604. [CrossRef]
31. Westerfield, M. *The Zebrafish Book: A Guide for the Laboratory Use of Zebrafish (Danio Rerio)*; University of Oregon Press: Eugene, OR, USA, 2000.
32. Tang, H.; Liu, Y.; Luo, D.; Ogawa, S.; Yin, Y.; Li, S.; Zhang, Y.; Hu, W.; Parhar, I.S.; Lin, H.; et al. The kiss/kissr systems are dispensable for zebrafish reproduction: Evidence from gene knockout studies. *Endocrinology* **2015**, *156*, 589–599. [CrossRef] [PubMed]
33. Chen, Y.; Tang, H.; Wang, L.; He, J.; Guo, Y.; Liu, Y.; Liu, X.; Lin, H. Fertility Enhancement but Premature Ovarian Failure in esr1-Deficient Female Zebrafish. *Front. Endocrinol. (Lausanne)* **2018**, *9*, 567. [CrossRef] [PubMed]
34. Mahaffey, K.R.; Capar, S.G.; Gladen, B.C.; Fowler, B.A. Concurrent exposure to lead, cadmium, and arsenic. Effects on toxicity and tissue metal concentrations in the rat. *J. Lab. Clin. Med.* **1981**, *98*, 463–481. [PubMed]
35. Julshman, K. Analysis of Major and Minor Elements in Mollusks from Norway. Ph.D. Thesis, Institute of Nutrition Direction of Bergen Nygardsangen, Bergen University, Bergen, Norway, 1983.
36. Suvarna, K.; Layton, C. The Hematoxylin and eosin, Connective and mesenchymal tissues with their stains, Immunohistochemical techniques and Transmission electron microscopy. In *Bancroft's Theory and Practice of Histological Technique*; Livingstone, C., Ed.; Elsevier: Oxford, UK, 2013.
37. Mawed, S.A.; He, Y.; Zhang, J.; Mei, J. Strategy of Hepatic Metabolic Defects Induced by beclin1 Heterozygosity in Adult Zebrafish. *Int. J. Mol. Sci.* **2020**, *21*, 1533. [CrossRef]
38. Dulta, K.; Koşarsoy Ağçeli, G.; Chauhan, P.; Jasrotia, R.; Chauhan, P.K. A Novel Approach of Synthesis Zinc Oxide Nanoparticles by Bergenia ciliata Rhizome Extract: Antibacterial and Anticancer Potential. *J. Inorg. Organomet. Polym. Mater.* **2021**, *31*, 180–190. [CrossRef]
39. Iravani, S.; Korbekandi, H.; Mirmohammadi, S.V.; Zolfaghari, B. Synthesis of silver nanoparticles: Chemical, physical and biological methods. *Res. Pharm. Sci.* **2014**, *9*, 385–406.
40. Ezealisiji, K.M.; Siwe-Noundou, X.; Maduelosi, B.; Nwachukwu, N.; Krause, R.W.M. Green synthesis of zinc oxide nanoparticles using Solanum torvum (L) leaf extract and evaluation of the toxicological profile of the ZnO nanoparticles–hydrogel composite in Wistar albino rats. *Intern. Nano Lett.* **2019**, *9*, 99–107. [CrossRef]
41. Talam, S.; Karumuri, S.R.; Gunnam, N. Synthesis, Characterization, and Spectroscopic Properties of ZnO Nanoparticles. *ISRN Nanotec.* **2012**, *2012*, 372505. [CrossRef]
42. Agarwal, H.; Nakara, A.; Menon, S.; Shanmugam, V. Eco-friendly synthesis of zinc oxide nanoparticles using Cinnamomum Tamala leaf extract and its promising effect towards the antibacterial activity. *J. Drug Deliv. Sci. Technol.* **2019**, *53*, 101212. [CrossRef]
43. Kime, D.E. The effects of pollution on reproduction in fish. *Rev. Fish Biol. Fish.* **1995**, *5*, 52–95. [CrossRef]
44. Reading, B.; Sullivan, C. The Reproductive Organs and Processes: Vitellogenesis in Fishes. *Encyclopedia of Fish Physiology* **2011**, *1*, 635–646. [CrossRef]
45. Sharma, V.; Anderson, D.; Dhawan, A. Zinc oxide nanoparticles induce oxidative DNA damage and ROS-triggered mitochondria mediated apoptosis in human liver cells (HepG2). *Apoptosis* **2012**, *17*, 852–870. [CrossRef] [PubMed]
46. Shahzad, K.; Khan, M.N.; Jabeen, F.; Kosour, N.; Chaudhry, A.S.; Sohail, M.; Ahmad, N. Toxicity of zinc oxide nanoparticles (ZnO-NPs) in tilapia (Oreochromis mossambicus): Tissue accumulation, oxidative stress, histopathology and genotoxicity. *Int. J. Environ. Sci. Technol.* **2019**, *16*, 1973–1984. [CrossRef]
47. Yao, Y.; Zang, Y.; Qu, J.; Tang, M.; Zhang, T. The Toxicity Of Metallic Nanoparticles On Liver: The Subcellular Damages, Mechanisms, And Outcomes. *Int. J. Nanomed.* **2019**, *14*, 8787–8804. [CrossRef] [PubMed]
48. Zhu, X.; Zhu, L.; Duan, Z.; Qi, R.; Li, Y.; Lang, Y. Comparative toxicity of several metal oxide nanoparticle aqueous suspensions to Zebrafish (Danio rerio) early developmental stage. *J. Environ. Sci. Health Part A Toxic/Hazard. Subst. Environ. Eng.* **2008**, *43*, 278–284. [CrossRef]
49. Tavabe, K.R.; Kuchaksaraei, B.S.; Javanmardi, S. Effects of ZnO nanoparticles on the Giant freshwater prawn (Macrobrachium rosenbergii, de Man, 1879): Reproductive performance, larvae development, CHH concentrations and anti-oxidative enzymes activity. *Anim. Reprod. Sci.* **2020**, *221*, 106603. [CrossRef] [PubMed]
50. Wang, J.; Zhu, X.; Zhang, X.; Zhao, Z.; Liu, H.; George, R.; Wilson-Rawls, J.; Chang, Y.; Chen, Y. Disruption of zebrafish (Danio rerio) reproduction upon chronic exposure to TiO_2 nanoparticles. *Chemosphere* **2011**, *83*, 461–467. [CrossRef]
51. Tang, Y.; Chen, B.; Hong, W.; Chen, L.; Yao, L.; Zhao, Y.; Aguilar, Z.P.; Xu, H. ZnO Nanoparticles Induced Male Reproductive Toxicity Based on the Effects on the Endoplasmic Reticulum Stress Signaling Pathway. *Int. J. Nanomed.* **2019**, *14*, 9563–9576. [CrossRef]
52. Bacchetta, R.; Santo, N.; Marelli, M.; Nosengo, G.; Tremolada, P. Chronic toxicity effects of $ZnSO_4$ and ZnO nanoparticles in Daphnia magna. *Environ. Res.* **2017**, *152*, 128–140. [CrossRef]

53. Sayadi, M.H.; Pavlaki, M.D.; Martins, R.; Mansouri, B.; Tyler, C.R.; Kharkan, J.; Shekari, H. Bioaccumulation and toxicokinetics of zinc oxide nanoparticles (ZnO NPs) co-exposed with graphene nanosheets (GNs) in the blackfish (Capoeta fusca). *Chemosphere* **2021**, *269*, 128689. [CrossRef]
54. Kaya, H.; Aydın, F.; Gürkan, M.; Yılmaz, S.; Ates, M.; Demir, V.; Arslan, Z. Effects of zinc oxide nanoparticles on bioaccumulation and oxidative stress in different organs of tilapia (Oreochromis niloticus). *Environ. Toxicol. Pharmacol.* **2015**, *40*, 936–947. [CrossRef] [PubMed]
55. Johnston, B.D.; Scown, T.M.; Moger, J.; Cumberland, S.A.; Baalousha, M.; Linge, K.; van Aerle, R.; Jarvis, K.; Lead, J.R.; Tyler, C.R. Bioavailability of Nanoscale Metal Oxides TiO_2, CeO_2, and ZnO to Fish. *Environ. Sci. Technol.* **2010**, *44*, 1144–1151. [CrossRef] [PubMed]
56. Choi, S.J.; Choy, J.H. Biokinetics of zinc oxide nanoparticles: Toxicokinetics, biological fates, and protein interaction. *Int. J. Nanomed.* **2014**, *9 Suppl 2*, 261–269. [CrossRef]
57. Suganthi, P.; Murali, M.; Athif, P.; Sadiq Bukhari, A.; Syed Mohamed, H.E.; Basu, H.; Singhal, R.K. Haemato-immunological studies in ZnO and TiO_2 nanoparticles exposed euryhaline fish, Oreochromis mossambicus. *Environ. Toxicol. Pharmacol.* **2019**, *66*, 55–61. [CrossRef] [PubMed]
58. Du, J.; Wang, S.; You, H.; Jiang, R.; Zhuang, C.; Zhang, X. Developmental toxicity and DNA damage to zebrafish induced by perfluorooctane sulfonate in the presence of ZnO nanoparticles. *Environ. Toxicol.* **2016**, *31*, 360–371. [CrossRef]
59. Liu, X.Q.; Zhang, H.F.; Zhang, W.D.; Zhang, P.F.; Hao, Y.N.; Song, R.; Li, L.; Feng, Y.N.; Hao, Z.H.; Shen, W.; et al. Regulation of neuroendocrine cells and neuron factors in the ovary by zinc oxide nanoparticles. *Toxicol. Lett.* **2016**, *256*, 19–32. [CrossRef]
60. Akbulut, C.; Kotil, T.; Yön, N. Ultrastructural evaluation of oocyte envelopes of zebrafish (Danio Rerio) (Hamilton, 1822) after TiO_2 nanoparticle exposure. *Arch. Biol. Sci.* **2017**, *70*, 35. [CrossRef]
61. Ramsden, C.S.; Henry, T.B.; Handy, R.D. Sub-lethal effects of titanium dioxide nanoparticles on the physiology and reproduction of zebrafish. *Aquat. Toxicol.* **2013**, *126*, 404–413. [CrossRef]
62. Han, Z.; Yan, Q.; Ge, W.; Liu, Z.G.; Gurunathan, S.; De Felici, M.; Shen, W.; Zhang, X.F. Cytotoxic effects of ZnO nanoparticles on mouse testicular cells. *Int. J. Nanomed.* **2016**, *11*, 5187–5203. [CrossRef]
63. Chen, G.-H.; Song, C.-C.; Zhao, T.; Hogstrand, C.; Wei, X.-L.; Lv, W.-H.; Song, Y.-F.; Luo, Z. Mitochondria-Dependent Oxidative Stress Mediates ZnO Nanoparticle (ZnO NP)-Induced Mitophagy and Lipotoxicity in Freshwater Teleost Fish. *Environ. Sci. Technol.* **2022**, *56*, 2407–2420. [CrossRef]
64. Rajkumar, K.S.; Sivagaami, P.; Ramkumar, A.; Murugadas, A.; Srinivasan, V.; Arun, S.; Senthil Kumar, P.; Thirumurugan, R. Bio-functionalized zinc oxide nanoparticles: Potential toxicity impact on freshwater fish Cyprinus carpio. *Chemosphere* **2022**, *290*, 133220. [CrossRef] [PubMed]
65. Pei, X.; Jiang, H.; Xu, G.; Li, C.; Li, D.; Tang, S. Lethality of Zinc Oxide Nanoparticles Surpasses Conventional Zinc Oxide via Oxidative Stress, Mitochondrial Damage and Calcium Overload: A Comparative Hepatotoxicity Study. *Int. J. Mol. Sci.* **2022**, *23*, 6724. [CrossRef] [PubMed]
66. Chen, B.; Hong, W.; Tang, Y.; Zhao, Y.; Aguilar, Z.P.; Xu, H. Protective effect of the NAC and Sal on zinc oxide nanoparticles-induced reproductive and development toxicity in pregnant mice. *Food Chem. Toxicol.* **2020**, *143*, 111552. [CrossRef]
67. Yu, K.N.; Yoon, T.J.; Minai-Tehrani, A.; Kim, J.E.; Park, S.J.; Jeong, M.S.; Ha, S.W.; Lee, J.K.; Kim, J.S.; Cho, M.H. Zinc oxide nanoparticle induced autophagic cell death and mitochondrial damage via reactive oxygen species generation. *Toxicol. Vitr.* **2013**, *27*, 1187–1195. [CrossRef] [PubMed]
68. Roy, R.; Singh, S.K.; Chauhan, L.K.; Das, M.; Tripathi, A.; Dwivedi, P.D. Zinc oxide nanoparticles induce apoptosis by enhancement of autophagy via PI3K/Akt/mTOR inhibition. *Toxicol. Lett.* **2014**, *227*, 29–40. [CrossRef] [PubMed]
69. Mizushima, N.; Klionsky, D.J. Protein turnover via autophagy: Implications for metabolism. *Annu. Rev. Nutr.* **2007**, *27*, 19–40. [CrossRef] [PubMed]
70. Zhang, H.; Chen, F.; Li, Y.; Shan, X.; Yin, L.; Hao, X.; Zhong, Y. More serious autophagy can be induced by ZnO nanoparticles than single-walled carbon nanotubes in rat tracheal epithelial cells. *Environ. Toxicol.* **2021**, *36*, 238–248. [CrossRef]
71. Shen, J.; Yang, D.; Zhou, X.; Wang, Y.; Tang, S.; Yin, H.; Wang, J.; Chen, R.; Chen, J. Role of Autophagy in Zinc Oxide Nanoparticles-Induced Apoptosis of Mouse Leydig Cells. *Int. J. Mol. Sci.* **2019**, *20*, 4042. [CrossRef]
72. Wang, J.; Deng, X.; Zhang, F.; Chen, D.; Ding, W. ZnO nanoparticle-induced oxidative stress triggers apoptosis by activating JNK signaling pathway in cultured primary astrocytes. *Nanoscale Res. Lett.* **2014**, *9*, 117. [CrossRef]
73. Ahamed, M.; Akhtar, M.J.; Raja, M.; Ahmad, I.; Siddiqui, M.K.; AlSalhi, M.S.; Alrokayan, S.A. ZnO nanorod-induced apoptosis in human alveolar adenocarcinoma cells via p53, survivin and bax/bcl-2 pathways: Role of oxidative stress. *Nanomed.* **2011**, *7*, 904–913. [CrossRef]
74. Chen, S.X.; Yang, X.Z.; Deng, Y.; Huang, J.; Li, Y.; Sun, Q.; Yu, C.-P.; Zhu, Y.; Hong, W.S. Silver nanoparticles induce oocyte maturation in zebrafish (Danio rerio). *Chemosphere* **2017**, *170*, 51–60. [CrossRef] [PubMed]
75. Applerot, G.; Lipovsky, A.; Dror, R.; Perkas, N.; Nitzan, Y.; Lubart, R.; Gedanken, A. Enhanced Antibacterial Activity of Nanocrystalline ZnO Due to Increased ROS-Mediated Cell Injury. *Adv. Funct. Mater.* **2009**, *19*, 842–852. [CrossRef]
76. Mishra, P.K.; Mishra, H.; Ekielski, A.; Talegaonkar, S.; Vaidya, B. Zinc oxide nanoparticles: A promising nanomaterial for biomedical applications. *Drug Discov. Today* **2017**, *22*, 1825–1834. [CrossRef] [PubMed]
77. Zhou, J.; Peng, X.; Mei, S. Autophagy in Ovarian Follicular Development and Atresia. *Int. J. Biol. Sci.* **2019**, *15*, 726–737. [CrossRef] [PubMed]

78. Yadav, P.K.; Gupta, A.; Sharma, A.; Yadav, A.K.; Tiwari, M.; Pandey, A.N.; Prasad, S.; Shrivastav, T.G.; Chaube, S.K. Fate of the germ cells in mammalian ovary: A review. *J. Reprod. Health. Med.* **2020**, 1. [CrossRef]
79. Di Cerbo, A.; Palmieri, B. Review: The market of probiotics. *Pak. J. Pharm. Sci.* **2015**, *28*, 2199–2206.
80. Peluso, J.J. Progesterone signaling mediated through progesterone receptor membrane component-1 in ovarian cells with special emphasis on ovarian cancer. *Steroids* **2011**, *76*, 903–909. [CrossRef]
81. Peluso, J.J.; Gawkowska, A.; Liu, X.; Shioda, T.; Pru, J.K. Progesterone receptor membrane component-1 regulates the development and Cisplatin sensitivity of human ovarian tumors in athymic nude mice. *Endocrinology* **2009**, *150*, 4846–4854. [CrossRef]
82. Ahmed, I.S.; Rohe, H.J.; Twist, K.E.; Mattingly, M.N.; Craven, R.J. Progesterone receptor membrane component 1 (Pgrmc1): A heme-1 domain protein that promotes tumorigenesis and is inhibited by a small molecule. *J. Pharmacol. Exp. Ther.* **2010**, *333*, 564–573. [CrossRef]
83. Lin, S.-T.; Chou, H.-C.; Chang, S.-J.; Chen, Y.-W.; Lyu, P.-C.; Wang, W.-C.; Chang, M.D.-T.; Chan, H.-L. Proteomic analysis of proteins responsible for the development of doxorubicin resistance in human uterine cancer cells. *J. Proteom.* **2012**, *75*, 5822–5847. [CrossRef]
84. Patiño, R.; Thomas, P.; Yoshizaki, G. Ovarian follicle maturation and ovulation: An integrated perspective. *Fish Physiol. Biochem.* **2003**, *28*, 305–308. [CrossRef]
85. Zhu, Y.; Liu, D.; Shaner, Z.C.; Chen, S.; Hong, W.; Stellwag, E.J. Nuclear progestin receptor (pgr) knockouts in zebrafish demonstrate role for pgr in ovulation but not in rapid non-genomic steroid mediated meiosis resumption. *Front. Endocrinol. (Lausanne)* **2015**, *6*, 37. [CrossRef]
86. Morselli, E.; Tasdemir, E.; Maiuri, M.C.; Galluzzi, L.; Kepp, O.; Criollo, A.; Vicencio, J.M.; Soussi, T.; Kroemer, G. Mutant p53 protein localized in the cytoplasm inhibits autophagy. *Cell Cycle* **2008**, *7*, 3056–3061. [CrossRef] [PubMed]
87. Petitjean, A.; Achatz, M.I.; Borresen-Dale, A.L.; Hainaut, P.; Olivier, M. TP53 mutations in human cancers: Functional selection and impact on cancer prognosis and outcomes. *Oncogene* **2007**, *26*, 2157–2165. [CrossRef] [PubMed]
88. Raz, E. The function and regulation of vasa-like genes in germ-cell development. *Genome Biol.* **2000**, *1*, reviews1017. [CrossRef] [PubMed]
89. Gustafson, E.A.; Wessel, G.M. Vasa genes: Emerging roles in the germ line and in multipotent cells. *Bioessays* **2010**, *32*, 626–637. [CrossRef] [PubMed]
90. Hashimoto, H.; Sudo, T.; Mikami, Y.; Otani, M.; Takano, M.; Tsuda, H.; Itamochi, H.; Katabuchi, H.; Ito, M.; Nishimura, R. Germ cell specific protein VASA is over-expressed in epithelial ovarian cancer and disrupts DNA damage-induced G2 checkpoint. *Gynecol. Oncol.* **2008**, *111*, 312–319. [CrossRef] [PubMed]
91. Poon, J.; Wessel, G.M.; Yajima, M. An unregulated regulator: Vasa expression in the development of somatic cells and in tumorigenesis. *Dev. Biol.* **2016**, *415*, 24–32. [CrossRef]

antioxidants

MDPI

Article

Food-Grade Quercetin-Loaded Nanoemulsion Ameliorates Effects Associated with Parkinson's Disease and Cancer: Studies Employing a Transgenic *C. elegans* Model and Human Cancer Cell Lines

Sabya Sachi Das [1,†], Arunabh Sarkar [2,†], Siva Chander Chabattula [3], Priya Ranjan Prasad Verma [1], Aamir Nazir [2], Piyush Kumar Gupta [4,5], Janne Ruokolainen [6], Kavindra Kumar Kesari [5,6,7,*] and Sandeep Kumar Singh [1,*]

1 Department of Pharmaceutical Sciences and Technology, Birla Institute of Technology, Mesra, Ranchi 835215, Jharkhand, India; sabya2049@gmail.com (S.S.D.); prpverma@bitmesra.ac.in (P.R.P.V.)
2 Division of Neuroscience and Ageing Biology, CSIR-Central Drug Research Institute, Lucknow 226031, Uttar Pradesh, India; arunabh.sarkar.bt@gmail.com (A.S.); anazir@cdri.res.in (A.N.)
3 Stem Cell and Molecular Biology Laboratory, Department of Biotechnology, Indian Institute of Technology Madras, Chennai 600036, Tamil Nadu, India; siva.chabathula@gmail.com
4 Department of Life Sciences, School of Basic Sciences and Research, Sharda University, Plot No. 32-34, Knowledge Park III, Greater Noida 201310, Uttar Pradesh, India; piyush.kumar1@sharda.ac.in
5 Department of Biotechnology, Graphic Era Deemed to Be University, Dehradun 248002, Uttarakhand, India
6 Department of Applied Physics, School of Science, Aalto University, 00076 Espoo, Finland; janne.ruokolainen@aalto.fi
7 Department of Bioproducts and Biosystems, School of Chemical Engineering, Aalto University, 00076 Espoo, Finland
* Correspondence: kavindra.kesari@aalto.fi or kavindra_biotech@yahoo.co.in (K.K.K.); sandeep.singh@bitmesra.ac.in (S.K.S.)
† These authors contributed equally to this work.

Abstract: A nanosized food-grade quercetin-loaded nanoemulsion (QNE) system comprising capmul MCM NF (oil) and cremophor RH 40 (surfactant) was developed using a high-speed homogenization technique. The developed QNE was studied for its significant neuroprotective (anti-Parkinsonism) and cytotoxicity (anticancer) effects against *Caenorhabditis elegans* (*C. elegans*) strains and human cancer cells, respectively. HR-TEM studies revealed that the QNE was spherical with a mean globule size of ~50 nm. Selected area electron diffraction (SAED) studies results demonstrated that QNE was amorphous. In vivo results show that QNE potentially reduced the α-Syn aggregation, increased mitochondrial and fat content, and improved the lifespan in transgenic *C. elegans* strain NL5901. QNE significantly downregulated the reactive oxygen species (ROS) levels in wild-type *C. elegans* strain N2. In vitro results of the MTT assay show that QNE significantly exhibited chemotherapeutic effects in all treated human cancer cells in an order of cytotoxicity: HeLa cells > A549 cells > MIA PaCa-2 cells, based on the IC_{50} values at 24 h. Conclusively, the QNE showed improved solubility, targetability, and neuroprotective effects against the PD-induced *C. elegans* model, and also cytotoxicity against human cancer cells and could be potentially used as an anti-Parkinson's or anticancer agent.

Keywords: food-grade quercetin nanoemulsion; *Caenorhabditis elegans*; Parkinson's disease; neuroprotective effect; chemotherapeutic effect

1. Introduction

Dietary flavonoids are the major polyphenolic phytoconstituents that have exhibited numerous promising therapeutic effects in treating neurodegenerative diseases (NDDs), cancer, cardiovascular diseases, microbial infections and many others, mainly due to their free-radical scavenging and anti-oxidative properties [1]. Quercetin (QT) is one of the most essential dietary flavonoids and is primarily found in various herbal sources, including vegetables (onion, broccoli), fruits (apple, blueberry), and grains. Numerous studies have shown that QT exhibits multifaceted therapeutic applications in various NDDs and demonstrates potential pharmacological effects, including anticancer, antimicrobial, antiviral, cardiovascular diseases, and many others [2,3]. QT is one of the most potent natural antioxidants, which exhibits neuroprotective [4] and anticancer effects [5] due to its superior anti-oxidative properties, inhibitory actions against protein kinases, and regulatory action on several gene expressions. The anti oxidative properties of QT assists in counteracting the excessive formation of ROS, leading to cellular oxidative stress, a pathological condition associated with cancer, and several ageing-mediated neurological diseases [6,7]. Additionally, QT impacts the expression of glutathione S-transferase (a phase II metabolism enzyme), which is recognized as a potent marker for intracellular oxidative stress and influences cell signaling [8].

Parkinson's disease (PD) is the second most common NDD, which progresses slowly and is recognized by the accretion of Lewy neurites/bodies. Both Lewy neurites and Lewy bodies are primarily comprised of accumulated α-synuclein (α-Syn) proteins and post-translationally altered protein by-products. Atypical aggregation of Lewy bodies within the brain is associated with synaptic dysfunctions and the deprivation of dopaminergic neurons of the nigrostriatal dopamine pathway [9]. In addition, the phosphorylation of Serine 129 (S129), a principal constituent of α-Syn, contributes to the accumulation of α-Syn, causing homeostasis and the amalgamation of synaptic vesicle neuronal transmission imperfections [10]. Furthermore, the imbalance between ROS production and the antioxidant defensive system leads to oxidative stress, one of the significant factors in the pathogenesis of numerous diseases and cell ageing processes [11]. Oxidative stress is also presumed to be responsible for protein and gene alterations that are responsible for the hallmarks of various NDDs, including PD [12].

Most of the experimental information associated with QT originated either from in vitro or in vivo studies that include complex processes including uptake, metabolism, and interconnections between cells/tissue and organs within an entire animal model, which are sometimes limited [13]. Thus, to overcome these limitations and attain additional information about the biological effects, particularly associated with aging and stress resistance, researchers use *Caenorhabditis elegans* (*C. elegans*), a nematode, as an in vivo model [14]. *C. elegans* has a transparent body, exhibits orthologous genes and numerous basic conserved pathways from higher-order animals, and can be effortlessly cultured in an agar medium at room temperature. Moreover, *C. elegans* has a shorter lifespan that assists in conducting several biological assays within a limited time frame [15,16]. In addition, the genomic sequence of *C. elegans* and humans highly resembles each other [17].

In laboratory experiments, dietary *Escherichia coli* OP50 (*E. coli* OP50) is used as nutrition for *C. elegans*, which is ingested by pumping it within the mouth and directing it within the pharynx before passing into the intestine [18]. The hydrophilic behavior of the growth media and the food behavior (specificity for *E. coli* OP50) of *C. elegans* have restricted their usage as an in vivo model for studying assimilation, absorption, and therapeutic activities, particularly of hydrophobic moieties. However, these limitations could be overcome by establishing emulsion-based delivery systems and a perpetual pumping-in reflex within the pharynx of *C. elegans* [18]. Moreover, QT exhibits poor solubility and low mucosal permeability, leading to lower bioavailability; thus, it becomes necessary to encapsulate QT within a steady nanosystem to increase its bioavailability. To date, numerous nano-carrier-based approaches such as nanoemulsions, polymeric nanoparticles, liposomes, and others have been reported for the encapsulation of QT to achieve improved solubility, permeability, bioavailability, and diseased-site targetability [19].

Despite comprehensive research, the therapeutic possibilities for the management of PD are restricted, offering symptomatic relief only and cannot avoid disease progression completely. Therefore, the present study aimed to establish a food-grade nanoemulsion system for delivering QT into the transgenic *C. elegans* expressing human α-Syn (NL5901 strain) and to evaluate its neuroprotective and pharmacological actions. Also, the potential toxicity of the pure QT and QNE were observed in various carcinogenic cells, including A549 (lung carcinoma epithelial) cells, MIA PaCa-2 (human pancreatic cancer) cells, and HeLa (cervical cancer) cells using the MTT assay method. Moreover, the therapeutic effects of quercetin-loaded nanoemulsion in a transgenic *C. elegans* model have not been reported yet, thus, we believe that these findings would allow the development of novel emulsion-based systems as potential anti-parkinsonism and anticancer agents with improved bioavailability and biocompatibility.

2. Materials and Methods

2.1. Materials

Quercetin (QT), sodium azide, phosphotungstic acid (PTA, $H_3PW_{12}O_{40}$), 3-(4,5-dimethylthiazol-2-yl)-2,5-diphenyl tetrazolium bromide (MTT), sodium chloride (NaCl), and peptone were purchased from Sigma-Aldrich Chemicals, St. Louis, MO, USA. 2,7-Dichlorodihydrofluorescein diacetate (H2DCFDA) was obtained from Invitrogen, Waltham, MA, USA. Capmul MCM NF (CAP MCM NF) and cremophor RH40 (CR RH 40) were ex gratis from Gattefosse (Saint-Priest, Cedex, France) and BASF (Ludwigshafen, Germany), respectively. Sodium hydroxide (NaOH), doxorubicin hydrochloride (DOX), and organic solvents were procured by Merck, India. Agar was purchased from HIMEDIA, Mumbai, India. Glassware was acquired from Borosil, India. A549 (lung carcinoma epithelial) cells, MIA PaCa-2 (human pancreatic cancer) cells, and HeLa (cervical cancer) cells were purchased from the National Centre for Cell Science, India. These cells were maintained in 10% fetal bovine serum (FBS) comprising Roswell Park Memorial Institute (RPMI) media (Gibco, Waltham, MA, USA) and Dulbecco's Modified Eagle Medium (DMEM) in a humidified CO_2 incubator (Thermo Scientific, Waltham, MA, USA) at 37 °C. The cell culture plastics were procured from Corning, Corning, NY, USA. All other chemicals and reagents were of analytical grade and were used as such.

2.2. Formulation of Optimized QNE

The optimized quercetin-loaded nanoemulsion (QNE) was formulated as per our previously reported method [19]. In brief, the nanoemulsion comprised CAP MCM NF (oil) and CR RH 40 (surfactant) was prepared using simple mixing followed by a high-shear homogenization technique. Initially, the drug was solubilized in the oil phase, and then the oil phase was added dropwise to the aqueous phase containing surfactant, followed by constant stirring at 500 rpm using a magnetic stirrer (IKA C-MAG HS 7, Staufen, Germany). QNE was observed for stability and was homogenized at 8000 rpm for 10 min using a high-shear homogenizer (IKA T25, ULTRA TURRAX, Staufen, Germany). Further, the formulation was stored in a sterile environment till further analysis.

2.3. Morphological Findings Using HR-TEM Studies

For HR-TEM analysis, the concentrated QNE was diluted using Milli-Q water (1:10). The diluted sample was drop-cast over the carbon-coated copper grid (200 mesh) followed by negative staining using 2% *w/v* phosphotungstic acid (PTA) and was kept for drying at room temperature. Morphological and structural analysis of the optimized QNE was studied using high-resolution transmission electron microscopy (HR-TEM; JEM 2100F, JEOL-200, Peabody, MA, USA) with an accelerating potential of 200 kV. Further, SAED studies were performed to evaluate the physical properties of QNE, either crystalline or amorphous.

2.4. Preservation and Culturing of *C. elegans* Culture

In this study, an *E. coli* strain (OP50) was used by us as a food source for *C. elegans*. The OP50 was seeded appropriately to develop a bacterial lawn over the NGM plates. The growth media for the *C. elegans* culture was developed by adding NaCl (3 g), peptone (2.5 g), and agar (2.5 g) into deionized water (DI) water, and then the solution mixture was autoclaved at 50 °C. After autoclaving, 1 M $MgSO_4$ (1 mL), cholesterol (1 mL of

5 mg/mL stock), 1 M KH_2PO_4 (25 mL; 6.0), and 1 M $CaCl_2$ (1 mL) was added into the solution mixture. Further, the media was gently decanted into Petri plates (90 mm) in a sterile environment and was kept undisturbed till congealed. Once the media was properly congealed, the plates were sterilized under ultraviolet light and were stored at 4 °C till further use. Further, *E. coli*-OP50 (500 µL) was dispensed over the NGM plates using a spreader in a sterile environment. To attain an appropriate bacterial lawn, seeded plates were kept in the incubator at 22 °C overnight. The sub culturing of *C. elegans* strains was carried out using the pre-seeded NGM plates containing OP50, maintained at 22 °C.

2.5. Isolation of C. elegans *Embryo*

Gravid worms growing over the OP50 seeded NGM plates were harvested using M9 buffer. The worms or nematodes were transferred into a sterilized 15 mL conical tube, centrifuged (1500 rpm; 5 min), and the precipitates collected. The precipitated nematodes (pellets) were resuspended into M9B followed by washing (thrice) to remove any adhered bacteria over the worm surface. Finally, the pellets were treated with an axenizing solution composed of NaOCl (2 mL) and NaOH solution (1 M). The body of nematodes was dissolved by gently mixing the whole solution, causing the discharge of the embryos. The acquired embryos were centrifuged (1500 rpm; 5 min) to achieve pelleted embryos, followed by washing (thrice) using M9 buffer, and then dispersed uniformly over the experimental plates under aseptic conditions.

2.6. C. elegans *Strains, Staining, and Image Acquisition*

In the present study we have used significant strains including, N2: Bristol wild-type strain, NL5901: pkls2386 [unc-54p::alpha-synuclein::YFP + unc-119(+)].

The various biological changes in the untreated (control), QT-treated (1 mM), and QNE-treated (1 mM) nematodes were monitored using fluorescent microscopy techniques. Initially, the synchronized worms were washed (thrice) using M9 buffer for the removal of any adhered bacteria from the treatment plates. Then the collected worms were treated with sodium azide (100 mM) for their immobilization. The immobilized nematodes were mounted over clean and sterilized glass slides with the help of coverslips. Lastly, the fluorescence microscope (Carl Zeiss Axio Imager M3 was used for capturing the images of immobilized nematodes.

Moreover, for α-Syn protein aggregation experimentations, *C. elegans* strains NL5901 were used. Further, MitoTracker™ Red CMXRos and Nile Red staining dye were used to enumerate the treated worms' mitochondrial and fat content respectively. Image acquisition and quantification of images were performed using ZEN2010 image acquiring software and Image J software (Image J, National Institutes of Health, Bethesda, MD, USA).

2.7. C. elegans *Lifespan Assay*

Age-synchronized worms were obtained by applying the isolated embryos of gravid *C. elegans* onto treated and control plates. After 48 h, ~100 adult worms (L4 stage), observed under a stereo zoom microscope, were selected and relocated onto the freshly arranged feeding plates of both control and treated groups. Thenceforth, daily monitoring and counting of living, dead, and expurgated worms was executed, and during this process, counting was performed by taking two replicate plates for each group. An expurgated set of statistics were documented based on an overall count of mislaid nematodes or the nematodes near the edge of the plates. Further, based on the responses to moderate nudging over the nematodes' heads, the number of living and dead nematodes was recognized and documented each day. Furthermore, if no response was monitored, the nematode was considered to be dead. Regularly, *C. elegans* were relocated onto freshly arranged treated plates for 20 days and incubated in BOD incubators (22 °C). The grading of worms was executed from the egg phase till its death phase, and Kaplan–Meier survival curves were used for the analysis of the results.

2.8. ROS Estimation in *C. elegans* N2 Strain

The ROS estimation studies were performed in *C. elegans* N2 strain using H_2DCFDA. The untreated nematodes (control) and treated nematodes were washed using M9 buffer (thrice) and then with phosphate buffer saline (twice). The groups (~100 worms/100 mL media) were individually examined (n = 3) and they were added to the experimental wells (OptiPlate-96 F; PerkinElmer), with further addition of 100 mM of H_2DCFDA (100 µL) into each well. Estimation of the fluorescence intensity ($F_{int.}$) from individual wells was noted at three distinct durations, (i): before adding dye (D1), (ii): instantaneously after adding dye (D2), and (iii): one-hour post-incubation after adding dye (D3). The $F_{int.}$ was quantified using a multimode plate reader (Perkin Elmer, VICTOR X3) having excitation and emission wavelengths of 485 nm and 520 nm, respectively. The difference in the $F_{int.}$ was attained by deducting the values of D1 from D2 and subtracting the obtained value (D2-D1) from the value of D3. The $F_{int.}$ of untreated (control), QT-treated (1 mM), and QNE-treated (1 mM) worms were plotted as their mean value. Moreover, statistical significance was attained by Student's t-test (GraphPad Prism software, San Diego, CA, USA).

2.9. Cytotoxicity Study Using MTT Assay

The anticancer activity of pure QT and QNE against selective cancer cell lines (A549, MIA PaCa-2, and HeLa) were analyzed using an MTT assay. In brief, 5×10^3 cells (in each well) were seeded in a 96-wells plate and then were treated with varying concentrations (15 and 500 µg/mL) of different test samples (QT and QNE) under serial dilutions. The study was performed by considering the equivalent weight of the drug (500 µg) in both the test samples (pure QT and QNE), followed by serial dilutions. In addition, cells were also treated with DOX (positive control) with a varying concentration range (1.5 to 100 µg/mL). The treated wells were incubated in a CO_2 incubator maintained at 37 °C and were observed for 24, 48, and 72 h post-treatment. Later, the percentages of cell viability (% cell viability) for each sample were calculated by calculating the absorbance (Abs.) of samples using the following formula:

$$\mathbf{CV}\ (\%) = \frac{\mathbf{A_S} - \mathbf{A_B}}{\mathbf{A_N} - \mathbf{A_B}} \times \mathbf{100}$$

where, A_S is the Abs. of the sample, A_B is Abs. of the blank well and A_N is Abs. of the negative control. Further, the IC_{50} values were determined for all the tested samples and the positive and negative controls. The results were signified as mean ± SD and experiments were carried out in triplicate (n = 3).

2.10. Statistical Analysis

We performed at least two independent experiments for microscopy-mediated quantification assays to treat and study the 100 nematodes for individual groups, as reported in our published literature [20]. However, the $F_{int.}$ of nematodes was noted for all sets of slides. The characteristic images within each distinct experiment were randomly captured (n = 10). Finally, the quantification of the intensity of each image was performed by Image J analysis software. Further, a one-way ANOVA followed by Tukey's test was performed to examine the $F_{int.}$ for images of each set and ROS values, using GraphPad Prism 5 software; the results are represented as mean ± SD. Furthermore, the p-values are signified as * $p < 0.05$, ** $p < 0.01$, *** $p < 0.001$. For all the experiments, adult nematodes at the L4 stage were used.

Specifically, all the findings for anticancer studies (MTT assay) were analyzed using GraphPad Prism 9.0 and represented as mean ± SD (n = 3). The obtained results for pure QT and QNE were examined using multiple t-tests and two-way ANOVA for DOX analysis, respectively. Furthermore, the p-values are signified as * $p < 0.05$, ** $p < 0.01$, *** $p < 0.001$, **** $p < 0.0001$.

3. Results

3.1. Formulation and Morphological Assessment

The optimized quercetin-loaded nanoemulsion (QNE) was developed as per the method reported in our previously published literature [19]. The optimized QNE comprised of QT (10 mg), CAP MCM NF (250 mg), CR RH 40 (250 mg), with a volume made up to 10 mL using Milli-Q water. Morphological assessments of QNE were performed using HR-TEM. Negative (-ve) staining was performed using PTA (-ve stain) to attain distinct morphological findings. PTA is a typical -ve stain that generally works at a pH range of 6.0 to 8.0 [21]. As per the HR-TEM analysis, QNE were homogeneously distributed, and exhibited stability with a particle size of 50 nm, spherical appearance, and smoother surface (Figure 1A,B). These results are similar to earlier published results [22,23]. Bouchemal et al. reported that parameters including the viscosity of oil, HLB values of surfactants, and miscibility of solvent systems with an aqueous phase play a crucial role in governing the size and morphology of nanoemulsion systems [22]. Moreover, the results of SAED suggested that the QNE exhibited an amorphous nature, showing proper incorporation of the drug within the excipient core system (Figure 1C). Similar findings regarding the effect of excipients on the crystallinity of drug moieties were reported in earlier works from the literature [23,24].

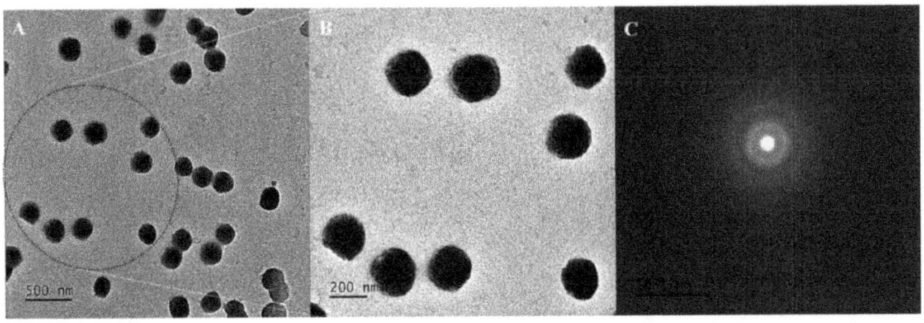

Figure 1. Morphological characterization of optimized QNE: HR-TEM image at 500 nm (**A**) and magnified area (showed with the red dotted area) at 200 nm scale bar (**B**); SAED pattern images (**C**).

3.2. QNE Decreases the α-Synuclein Aggregation in Transgenic C. elegans Strain NL5901

This study examined the neuroprotective effects of pure QT and QNE on α-Syn protein aggregation in transgenic *C. elegans* strain NL5901. NL5901 expresses human α-Syn in its muscle cell wall that is tagged with a yellow fluorescent protein. The microscopical findings (Figure 2) demonstrate that the mean $F_{int.}$ of untreated worms (only OP50) exhibited the highest level (5.495 ± 0.658) of α-Syn aggregation. However, the mean $F_{int.}$ of pure QT-treated worms (OP50 + QT) was less (3.47 ± 0.325) than the untreated worms and least (2.299 ± 0.012) in QNE-treated worms (OP50 + QNE). The results demonstrate that the optimized QNE downregulated the α-Syn expression levels more effectively than the pure QT in the transgenic *C. elegans* expressing human α-Syn (NL5901 strain). These findings suggest that the administration of QNE significantly enhanced the release of QT within the worms, leading to high targetability against α-Syn aggregations with improved bioavailability.

3.3. QNE Increases the Mitochondrial Content in Transgenic C. elegans Strain NL5901

Our study investigated the protective role of pure QT and QNE against mitochondrial content using transgenic *C. elegans* strain NL5901 as in vivo model. It was considered that the mean $F_{int.}$ was based on mitochondrial content, i.e., high mean $F_{int.}$ signifies higher mitochondrial content and vice-versa.

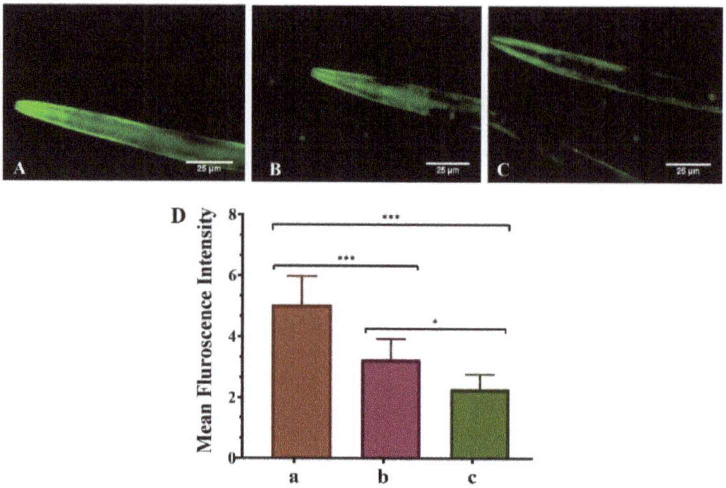

Figure 2. Effect of pure QT and QNE on α-Syn expression in transgenic *C. elegans* NL5901: (**A**) control (OP50 only), (**B**) worms treated with pure QT, (**C**) worms treated with QNE, and (**D**) mean $F_{int.}$ for (a) control (OP50 only), (b) worms treated with pure QT, (c) worms treated with QNE; (n = 10). One-way ANOVA followed by Tukey's test was performed for the quantification of graphically represented mean F_{int}. (mean ± SD; * $p < 0.05$, *** $p < 0.001$).

Results of the MitoTracker™ Red CMXRos and image acquisition (Figure 3) show that untreated worms (only OP50) exhibited the least mean $F_{int.}$ (1.375 ± 0.092), showing poor mitochondrial content. However, the mean $F_{int.}$ of pure QT-treated worms (OP50 + QT) was more (2.855 ± 0.544) than the untreated worms and was highest (3.080 ± 1.117) for QNE-treated worms (OP50 + QNE). Thus, the results signify that QNE elevated the overall mitochondrial content in the transgenic *C. elegans* expressing human α-Syn (NL5901 strain) compared with pure QT.

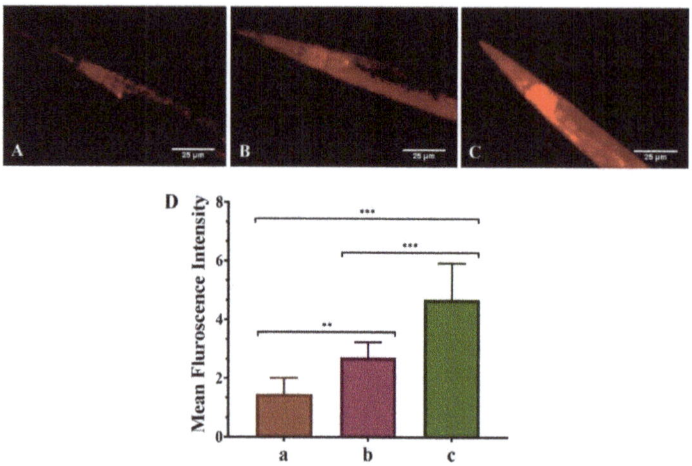

Figure 3. Effect of pure QT and QNE on the mitochondrial changes in transgenic *C. elegans* NL5901: (**A**) control (OP50 only), (**B**) worms treated with pure QT, (**C**) worms treated with QNE, and (**D**) mean $F_{int.}$ for (a) control (OP50 only), (b) worms treated with pure QT, (c) worms treated with QNE; (n = 10). One-way ANOVA followed by Tukey's test was performed for the quantification of graphically represented mean F_{int}. (mean ± SD; ** $p < 0.01$, *** $p < 0.001$).

3.4. QNE Increases the Fat Content in Transgenic *C. elegans* Strain NL5901

We explored the activity of both pure QT and QNE in regulating the fat content in the transgenic *C. elegans* strain NL5901 (Figure 4). Fat content was detected using Nile red as a staining dye. It was considered that mean $F_{int.}$ was based on fat content, i.e., high mean $F_{int.}$ signifies higher fat content and vice-versa. The results show that untreated worms (only OP50) exhibited the smallest mean $F_{int.}$ (1.44 ± 0.014), showing poor fat content. However, the mean $F_{int.}$ of pure QT-treated worms (OP50 + QT) was more (2.64 ± 0.113) than the untreated worms and was highest (4.595 ± 0.516) for QNE-treated worms (OP50 + QNE). Thus, the results signify that QNE elevated the overall fat content in transgenic *C. elegans* expressing human α-Syn (NL5901 strain).

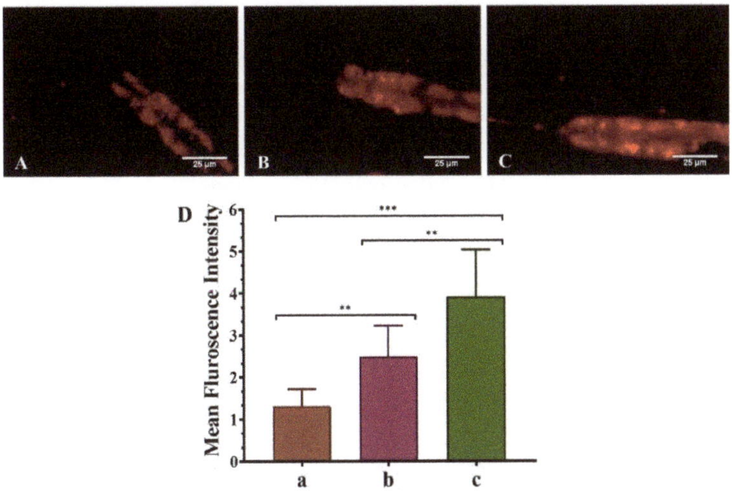

Figure 4. Effect of pure QT and QNE over the fat content in transgenic *C. elegans* NL5901: (**A**) control (OP50 only), (**B**) worms treated with pure QT, (**C**) worms treated with QNE, and (**D**) mean $F_{int.}$ for (a) control (OP50 only), (b) worms treated with pure QT, (c) worms treated with QNE; ($n = 10$). One-way ANOVA followed by Tukey's test was performed for the quantification of graphically represented mean F_{int}. (mean ± SD; ** $p < 0.01$, *** $p < 0.001$).

3.5. QNE Increases the Longevity in *C. elegans* NL5901 Strain and Downregulates the ROS Levels in Wild-Type *C. elegans* N2 Strain

It has been reported that treatment with QT efficiently prolonged the lifespan, inhibited age-associated motility delay, induced heat-stress tolerance, and reduced the production of intercellular and mitochondrial ROS in *C. elegans* strains [15]. Thus, we explored the effect of pure QT and QNE on the longevity of the treated *C. elegans* NL5901 strain. We observed that treatment with QNE significantly increased the longevity up to 24 days, whereas in QT-treated worms, the longevity was increased up to 22 days. In untreated *C. elegans* (control group) the lifespan was found to be up to 18 days (Figure 5A).

We further explored the effects of pure QT and QNE on the overall ROS content in wild-type *C. elegans* N2 strain. In our study, the estimation of ROS was performed using H_2DCFDA. It was expected that the treatment samples would exhibit ROS scavenging properties. The results of the ROS analysis show that the QNE (7.78 mean intensity) decreased the overall ROS content more efficiently than pure QT (13.06 mean intensity) in wild-type *C. elegans* (Figure 5B). Grunz and co-workers stated that QT (100 M; 48 h), a potent natural antioxidant, decreased levels of mitochondrial ROS in the *C. elegans* in vivo model by about 70% and also improved the lifespan (18.4%) [25].

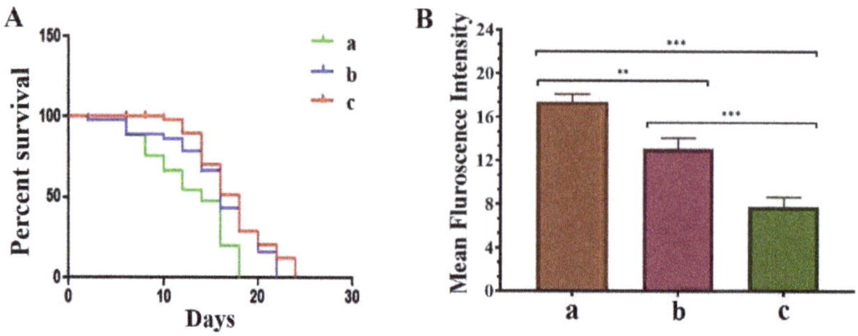

Figure 5. Effect of pure QT and QNE on: (**A**) percent survival of treated transgenic *C. elegans* NL5901 (a) control (NL5901 only), (b) worms treated with pure QT, and (c) worms treated with QNE; and (**B**) mean $F_{int.}$ of ROS level in *C. elegans* N2 for (a) control (OP50 only), (b) worms treated with pure QT, and (c) worms treated with QNE; (n = 10). One-way ANOVA followed by Tukey's test was performed for the quantification of graphically represented mean F_{int}. (mean ± SD; ** $p < 0.01$, *** $p < 0.001$).

3.6. QNE Potentially Reduced the Cell Viability of Treated Human Cancer Cells

The anticancer activity of free QT, QNE, and positive control (DOX) was analyzed using the MTT test on different cancer cell lines, A549, MIA PaCa-2, and HeLa. The IC_{50} values for all samples and the positive control (DOX) were calculated at 24 h (Figure 6).

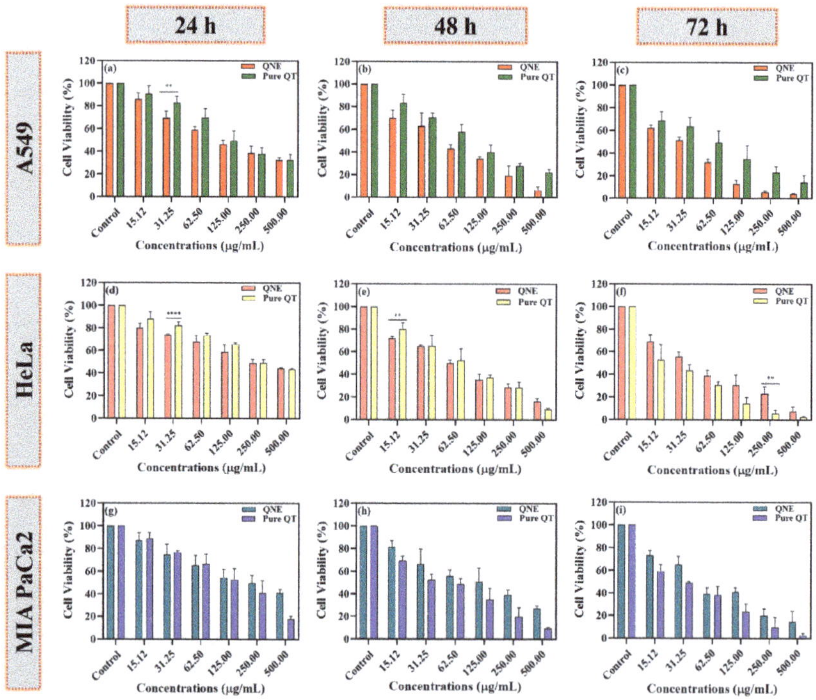

Figure 6. The percentages of cell viability of free QT- and QNE-treated cells were calculated in a dose- and time-dependent manner using the MTT test on different human cancer cells: A549 (**a–c**), HeLa (**d–f**), and MIA PaCa-2 cells (**g–i**). The data were analyzed using GraphPad Prism 9.0 software and represented as mean ± SD (n = 3). The obtained results for pure QT and QNE were further examined using multiple t-tests. The p-values are signified as ** $p < 0.01$, **** $p < 0.0001$.

However, the presence of surfactant and oil in QNE could have increased the cytotoxic potential of pure QT against the treated human cancer cells. The chemotherapeutic potential of QT is mainly due to its ability to promote cell viability loss, apoptosis, and autophagy through the modulation of various molecular pathways associated with cancer progression [26]. In our study, QNE showed potential cytotoxicity against treated HeLa cells (Figure 6a), A549 cells (Figure 6d), and MIA PaCa-2 cells (Figure 6g), with IC_{50} values of 34.25 ± 1.213 μg/mL, 40.33 ± 6.221 μg/mL, and 43.58 ± 9.160 μg/mL, respectively, at 24 hr. In addition, the pure QT-treated cells also exhibited potential chemotherapeutic activity against treated HeLa cells (Figure 6a), A549 cells (Figure 6d), and MIA PaCa-2 cells (Figure 6g), with IC_{50} values of 63.23± 1.884, 63.46 ± 8.485, and 84.14 ± 8.607, respectively, at 24 h. The IC_{50} values of pure QT-treated carcinogenic cells were found to be more than QNE-treated carcinogenic cells, signifying QNE exhibits superior activity at 24 h treatment. Moreover, similar findings were observed in earlier studies for HeLa cells [27,28], A549 cells [29,30], and MIA PaCa-2 cells [31,32]. Moreover, there were no significant differences between the pure QT and QNE against carcinogenic cells, except for few concentrations including: A549 (31.25 μg/mL; $p < 0.01$), HeLa cells (31.25 μg/mL; $p < 0.0001$) at 24 h; HeLa cells (15.12 μg/mL; $p < 0.01$) at 48 h; and HeLa cells (250 μg/mL; $p < 0.01$) at 72 h of treatment. This shows that QNE exhibited superior activity against HeLa cells and A549 cells at a lower concentration.

Overall, the results show that both QNE and pure QT exhibited cytotoxic effects against all the treated cancer cell lines in a dose- and time-dependent manner. QNE was found to be more toxic to cervical cancer (HeLa) cells, followed by lung (A549) and pancreatic (MIA PaCa-2) cancer cells (Figure 6). Moreover, DOX exhibited potent anticancer activity on all three tested human cancer cells in a dose- and time-dependent manner, indicating that cancer cells were not resistant (Figure S1).

4. Discussion

Quercetin (QT), a natural flavonoid and anti-oxidant, has exhibited potential neuroprotective (anti-parkinsonism) [4] and chemotherapeutic (anticancer) [5] effects. QT potentially inhibits intracellular and mitochondrial ROS, leading to reduced oxidative stress in neuronal cells [1]. Unfortunately, QT, whose neuroprotective and chemotherapeutic effects have been established in various studies, shows limitations due to its poor aqueous solubility and low oral bioavailability, which could be overcome through nanotechnological approaches [3]. Moreover, despite extensive research studies about PD, no potential medications have been reported with high therapeutic efficacy.

Here, we explored the neuroprotective and chemotherapeutic potential of the natural antioxidant (QT)-encapsulated nanoemulsion (QNE) system against *C. elegans* strains and human cancer cells, respectively. One of the essential facts about using food-grade excipients in QNE fabrication is that although QT is highly soluble in organic solvents like ethanol and DMSO, such solvents' usage produces adverse effects in *C. elegans* when administered directly [33]. Morphological findings demonstrated that the QNE exhibited a smoother and spherical appearance due to the proper blending of drugs within the excipient system [23]. This improved the solubility and stability of the drug, leading to improved bioavailability.

The progression of PD has been reported to be slow and is mainly recognized by the deposition of Lewy neurites/bodies, primarily comprised of accumulated α-Syn proteins. Here, we observed that QNE significantly downregulated α-Syn aggregations in the transgenic *C. elegans* expressing human α-Syn (NL5901 strain). This could be possibly due to the ability of QT to bind with α-Syn specifically through covalent bonds, resulting in the α-Syn–QT complex [34]. In an earlier study, the neuroprotective role of QT against synucleinopathies by efficiently hindering the aggregations of α-Syn has been reported [34]. In another study, researchers demonstrated that QT exhibits neuroprotective effects in SH-SY5Y (neuroblastoma-derived) cells against rotenone-induced neuronal injuries by modulating the process of autophagy [35].

Mitochondria exhibit a vital role in smooth neuronal functioning; however, loss of mitochondrial content and mitochondrial dysfunction has been reported as significant factor causing the neurodegeneration detected in PD. QT has been found to have a protective effect against impaired mitochondrial biosynthesis contributing to mitochondrial dysfunction in PD [36]. The results were identical to the previously published literature where the researchers explored the neuroprotective effects of QT in 6-hydroxydopamine(6-HD)-induced rats in vivo and 6-HD-treated PC12 (derived from rat pheochromocytoma) cells in vitro. These in vitro studies showed that QT (20 μM)-treated PC12 cells exhibited improved mitochondrial functions, decreased oxidative stress and α-Syn aggregations, and enhanced mitophagy marker levels. The in vivo findings revealed that QT inhibited neuronal death, mitochondrial damage, and α-Syn aggregation in PD rat models [37]. Moreover, higher intakes of cholesterol and polyunsaturated fatty acids (PUFA), particularly monounsaturated fatty acids (MUFA), might reduce the risk of PD in both men and women. Moreover, the FA are the primary constituents present in neuronal cell membranes and are vital for upholding their structural integrity and neurological functions [38,39]. Additionally, PUFAs play a critical role in maintaining the fluidity and permeability of the neuronal membrane, triggering phospholipases, reprocessing synaptic vesicles, and inhibiting ion channels [40]. Here, QNE significantly improved both mitochondrial and fat content in the treated transgenic *C. elegans* expressing human α-Syn (NL5901 strain).

Lifespan is a practical and supportive physiological factor that helps in assessing the biological effects of a compound in various animal models, either positive (increased longevity or non-toxic) or negative (reduced longevity or toxic) [41]. QNE potentially increased the longevity of the treated transgenic *C. elegans* expressing human α-Syn (NL5901 strain). Similar activities have been reported in earlier studies, where QT potentially prolonged the lifespan and increased stress tolerance in *C. elegans* [42–44].

Furthermore, mitochondria are susceptible to oxidative stress (majorly instigated due to ROS) and oxidative stress is responsible for the distraction of mitochondrial electron transport chains leading to reduced energy production by mitochondria. Thus, it becomes necessary to inactivate ROS using antioxidants and associated mechanisms [45]. In our study, QNE potentially downregulated the ROS level in the wild-type *C. elegans* N2 strain that could be responsible for neutralizing oxidative stress within the nematode. The mechanism behind the anti-oxidative effects of QT is due to the reaction of QT with free radicals, leading to the formation of a stable moiety with less reactivity, thus preserving the viability of cells [7].

In addition, the cytotoxic potential of QT has been well known, however, biological limitations of QT have restricted its direct usage [3]. Here, in our study, QT-encapsulated nanoemulsions exhibited potential cytotoxic effects against all the treated human cancer cells, including HeLa (cervical cancer) cells, A549 (lung carcinoma epithelial) cells, and MIA PaCa-2 (human pancreatic cancer) cells. El-Gogagry and co-workers reported that the cell viability of QT (10 μM)-treated cell lines after 48 h of treatment was found to be 81.70% $\pm$ 5.75 (C6 rat glioma cells), 56.09% $\pm$ 8.20 (B16F10 murine melanoma cells), 47.08% $\pm$ 8.73 (CT26 murine colon cancer cells), and 43.99% $\pm$ 3.95 (HeLa cells) [27]. In another study, QT-treated HeLa cells exhibited a significant reduction at 100 μM (24 h). In a study, QNE exhibited cytotoxicity against A549 cells (IC_{50}: 300 μg/mL; 48 h) in a dose- and time-dependent manner [29]. In another study, MTT assay findings stated that QT significantly decreased the cell viability of A549 cells (IC_{50}: 52.35 $\pm$ 2.44 μM) and MCF-7 breast cancer cells (IC_{50}: 41.78 $\pm$ 2.21 μM) in a dose-dependent manner [30]. Moreover, QT exhibited no toxicity against treated lymphocytes (similar dose), and thus, QT was found to be safe in non-cancer cells, explicitly targeting carcinogenic cells [28]. An earlier study demonstrated that QT (0–75 μM) reduced the cell numbers of both cells, including MIA PaCa-2 and BxPC-3 (temperately differentiated cells) after 48 h of treatment, with the smallest QT concentration of 10 μM [31]. In another study, QT intensely decreased cell counts, enhanced autophagy, and induced apoptosis in a dose-dependent manner in gemcitabine (GEM)-resistant MIA Paca-2 cells [32].

5. Conclusions

Taken together, we developed food-grade QT-loaded nanoemulsion (QNE) using a high-speed homogenization technique with improved solubility and oral bioavailability of quercetin. QNE were spherical with a globule size of ~50 nm (TEM studies) and were amorphous, signifying a complete blend of QT within the excipient system. Moreover, QNE decreased the α-synuclein expression, increased the mitochondrial and fat content, and improved the longevity in transgenic *C. elegans* strain NL5901. In addition, QNE downregulated the ROS levels in wild-type *C. elegans* strain N2. Furthermore, QNE exhibited superior cytotoxicity against all the treated cancer cell lines with an order of cytotoxicity: HeLa cells > A549 > MIA PaCa-2 cells. Also, DOX (positive control) exhibited potent anticancer activity on all three tested cells indicating that the cancer cells were not resistant. These findings could be used to set nanoplatforms encapsulating potential natural antioxidants with improved neuroprotective effects against neurological diseases like Parkinson's disease and also for targeting diverse cancer types. Moreover, findings at the pre-clinical and clinical levels could put forward a precise mechanism associated with quercetin nanocarriers in neurological diseases and cancer therapy.

Supplementary Materials: The following supporting information can be downloaded at: https://www.mdpi.com/article/10.3390/antiox11071378/s1, Figure S1: The percentage of cell viability with DOX was calculated in a dose- and time-dependent manner using the MTT test on different human cancer cells: A549 (a), HeLa (b), and MIA PaCa-2 cells (c). The data were analyzed using GraphPad Prism 9.0 software and represented as mean ± SD ($n = 3$). The obtained results for DOX were further examined using a two-way ANOVA analysis. The p-values were signified as * $p < 0.05$, ** $p < 0.01$, *** $p < 0.001$, **** $p < 0.0001$.

Author Contributions: Conceptualization, S.S.D., S.K.S.; methodology, S.S.D., A.S., S.C.C.; software, S.S.D., A.S., S.C.C.; formal analysis, S.K.S.; investigation, S.S.D., A.S., S.C.C.; resources, A.N., P.K.G.; data curation, A.N., J.R., S.K.S., P.K.G.; writing—original draft preparation, S.S.D.; writing—review and editing, S.S.D., A.S.; visualization, P.R.P.V., S.K.S.; supervision, P.R.P.V., A.N., P.K.G., J.R., S.K.S., K.K.K.; funding acquisition, K.K.K. All authors have read and agreed to the published version of the manuscript.

Funding: The APC was funded by Kavindra Kesari, Aalto University, Finland.

Institutional Review Board Statement: Not applicable.

Informed Consent Statement: Not applicable.

Data Availability Statement: Data is contained within the article and supplementary materials.

Acknowledgments: Authors sincerely acknowledge Devinder Yadav, Department of Metallurgical and Materials Engineering, Indian Institute of Technology, Patna for extending the facilities of HR-TEM.

Conflicts of Interest: The authors declare no conflict of interest.

References

1. Kumar, S.; Pandey, A.K. Chemistry and biological activities of flavonoids: An overview. *Sci. World J.* **2013**, *2013*, 162750. [CrossRef] [PubMed]
2. Batiha, G.E.; Beshbishy, A.M.; Ikram, M.; Mulla, Z.S.; El-Hack, M.E.A.; Taha, A.E.; Algammal, A.M.; Elewa, Y.H.A. The Pharmacological Activity, Biochemical Properties, and Pharmacokinetics of the Major Natural Polyphenolic Flavonoid: Quercetin. *Foods* **2020**, *9*, 374. [CrossRef] [PubMed]
3. Das, S.S.; Verma, P.R.P.; Singh, S.K. Quercetin-Loaded Nanomedicine as Nutritional Application. In *Nanomedicine for Bioactives*; Rahman, M., Beg, S., Kumar, V., Ahmad, F.J., Eds.; Springer: Singapore, 2020; pp. 259–301.
4. Costa, L.G.; Garrick, J.M.; Roque, P.J.; Pellacani, C. Mechanisms of Neuroprotection by Quercetin: Counteracting Oxidative Stress and More. *Oxid. Med. Cell Longev.* **2016**, *2016*, 2986796. [CrossRef] [PubMed]
5. Das, S.S.; Verma, P.R.P.; Kar, S.; Singh, S.K. Quercetin-Loaded Nanomedicine as Oncotherapy. In *Nanomedicine for Bioactives*; Rahman, M., Beg, S., Kumar, V., Ahmad, F.J., Eds.; Springer: Singapore, 2020; pp. 155–183.

6. Lei, X.; Chao, H.; Zhang, Z.; Lv, J.; Li, S.; Wei, H.; Xue, R.; Li, F.; Li, Z. Neuroprotective effects of quercetin in a mouse model of brain ischemic/reperfusion injury via anti-apoptotic mechanisms based on the Akt pathway. *Mol. Med. Rep.* **2015**, *12*, 3688–3696. [CrossRef]
7. Xu, D.; Hu, M.J.; Wang, Y.Q.; Cui, Y.L. Antioxidant Activities of Quercetin and Its Complexes for Medicinal Application. *Molecules* **2019**, *24*, 1123. [CrossRef] [PubMed]
8. Kampkotter, A.; Timpel, C.; Zurawski, R.F.; Ruhl, S.; Chovolou, Y.; Proksch, P.; Watjen, W. Increase of stress resistance and lifespan of *Caenorhabditis elegans* by quercetin. *Comp. Biochem. Physiol. B Biochem. Mol. Biol.* **2008**, *149*, 314–323. [CrossRef] [PubMed]
9. Henriquez, G.; Gomez, A.; Guerrero, E.; Narayan, M. Potential Role of Natural Polyphenols against Protein Aggregation Toxicity: *In Vitro, In Vivo*, and Clinical Studies. *ACS Chem. Neurosci.* **2020**, *11*, 2915–2934. [CrossRef]
10. Waxman, E.A.; Giasson, B.I. Characterization of kinases involved in the phosphorylation of aggregated alpha-synuclein. *J. Neurosci. Res.* **2011**, *89*, 231–247. [CrossRef] [PubMed]
11. Wallace, D.C.; Melov, S. Radicals r'aging. *Nat. Genet.* **1998**, *19*, 105–106. [CrossRef]
12. Forsberg, L.; de Faire, U.; Morgenstern, R. Oxidative stress, human genetic variation, and disease. *Arch. Biochem. Biophys.* **2001**, *389*, 84–93. [CrossRef]
13. Williamson, G.; Manach, C. Bioavailability and bioefficacy of polyphenols in humans. II. Review of 93 intervention studies. *Am. J. Clin. Nutr* **2005**, *81*, 243S–255S. [CrossRef] [PubMed]
14. Helmcke, K.J.; Avila, D.S.; Aschner, M. Utility of *Caenorhabditis elegans* in high throughput neurotoxicological research. *Neurotoxicol. Teratol.* **2010**, *32*, 62–67. [CrossRef] [PubMed]
15. Sugawara, T.; Sakamoto, K. Quercetin enhances motility in aged and heat-stressed *Caenorhabditis elegans* nematodes by modulating both HSF-1 activity, and insulin-like and p38-MAPK signalling. *PLoS ONE* **2020**, *15*, e0238528. [CrossRef]
16. Surco-Laos, F.; Cabello, J.; Gomez-Orte, E.; Gonzalez-Manzano, S.; Gonzalez-Paramas, A.M.; Santos-Buelga, C.; Duenas, M. Effects of O-methylated metabolites of quercetin on oxidative stress, thermotolerance, lifespan and bioavailability on *Caenorhabditis elegans*. *Food Funct.* **2011**, *2*, 445–456. [CrossRef]
17. Kim, Y.; Park, Y.; Hwang, J.; Kwack, K. Comparative genomic analysis of the human and nematode *Caenorhabditis elegans* uncovers potential reproductive genes and disease associations in humans. *Physiol. Genom.* **2018**, *50*, 1002–1014. [CrossRef] [PubMed]
18. Colmenares, D.; Sun, Q.; Shen, P.; Yue, Y.; McClements, D.J.; Park, Y. Delivery of dietary triglycerides to *Caenorhabditis elegans* using lipid nanoparticles: Nanoemulsion-based delivery systems. *Food Chem.* **2016**, *202*, 451–457. [CrossRef] [PubMed]
19. Das, S.S.; Verma, P.R.P.; Singh, S.K. Screening and preparation of quercetin doped nanoemulsion: Characterizations, antioxidant and anti-bacterial activities. *LWT* **2020**, *124*, 109141. [CrossRef]
20. Sarkar, A.; Hameed, R.; Mishra, A.; Bhatta, R.S.; Nazir, A. Genetic modulators associated with regulatory surveillance of mitochondrial quality control, play a key role in regulating stress pathways and longevity in *C. elegans*. *Life Sci.* **2022**, *290*, 120226. [CrossRef]
21. Cao, B.; Xu, H.; Mao, C. Transmission electron microscopy as a tool to image bioinorganic nanohybrids: The case of phage-gold nanocomposites. *Microsc. Res. Tech.* **2011**, *74*, 627–635. [CrossRef]
22. Bouchemal, K.; Briancon, S.; Perrier, E.; Fessi, H. Nano-emulsion formulation using spontaneous emulsification: Solvent, oil and surfactant optimisation. *Int. J. Pharm.* **2004**, *280*, 241–251. [CrossRef]
23. Kumari, S.; Kumaraswamy, R.V.; Choudhary, R.C.; Sharma, S.S.; Pal, A.; Raliya, R.; Biswas, P.; Saharan, V. Thymol nanoemulsion exhibits potential antibacterial activity against bacterial pustule disease and growth promotory effect on soybean. *Sci. Rep.* **2018**, *8*, 6650. [CrossRef] [PubMed]
24. Guinebretière, S.; Briançon, S.; Fessi, H.; Teodorescu, V.S.; Blanchin, M.G. Nanocapsules of biodegradable polymers: Preparation and characterization by direct high resolution electron microscopy. *Mater. Sci. Eng. C* **2002**, *21*, 137–142. [CrossRef]
25. Grunz, G.; Haas, K.; Soukup, S.; Klingenspor, M.; Kulling, S.E.; Daniel, H.; Spanier, B. Structural features and bioavailability of four flavonoids and their implications for lifespan-extending and antioxidant actions in *C. elegans*. *Mech. Ageing Dev.* **2012**, *133*, 1–10. [CrossRef] [PubMed]
26. Reyes-Farias, M.; Carrasco-Pozo, C. The Anti-Cancer Effect of Quercetin: Molecular Implications in Cancer Metabolism. *Int J. Mol. Sci.* **2019**, *20*, 3177. [CrossRef] [PubMed]
27. El-Gogary, R.I.; Rubio, N.; Wang, J.T.; Al-Jamal, W.T.; Bourgognon, M.; Kafa, H.; Naeem, M.; Klippstein, R.; Abbate, V.; Leroux, F.; et al. Polyethylene glycol conjugated polymeric nanocapsules for targeted delivery of quercetin to folate-expressing cancer cells in vitro and in vivo. *ACS Nano* **2014**, *8*, 1384–1401. [CrossRef]
28. Sundaram, M.K.; Raina, R.; Afroze, N.; Bajbouj, K.; Hamad, M.; Haque, S.; Hussain, A. Quercetin modulates signaling pathways and induces apoptosis in cervical cancer cells. *Biosci. Rep.* **2019**, *39*, BSR20190720. [CrossRef]
29. Arbain, N.H.; Salim, N.; Masoumi, H.R.F.; Wong, T.W.; Basri, M.; Abdul Rahman, M.B. *In vitro* evaluation of the inhalable quercetin loaded nanoemulsion for pulmonary delivery. *Drug Deliv. Transl. Res.* **2019**, *9*, 497–507. [CrossRef]
30. Yousuf, M.; Khan, P.; Shamsi, A.; Shahbaaz, M.; Hasan, G.M.; Haque, Q.M.R.; Christoffels, A.; Islam, A.; Hassan, M.I. Inhibiting CDK6 Activity by Quercetin Is an Attractive Strategy for Cancer Therapy. *ACS Omega* **2020**, *5*, 27480–27491. [CrossRef]
31. Angst, E.; Park, J.L.; Moro, A.; Lu, Q.Y.; Lu, X.; Li, G.; King, J.; Chen, M.; Reber, H.A.; Go, V.L.; et al. The flavonoid quercetin inhibits pancreatic cancer growth in vitro and in vivo. *Pancreas* **2013**, *42*, 223–229. [CrossRef]
32. Lan, C.Y.; Chen, S.Y.; Kuo, C.W.; Lu, C.C.; Yen, G.C. Quercetin facilitates cell death and chemosensitivity through RAGE/PI3K/AKT/mTOR axis in human pancreatic cancer cells. *J. Food Drug Anal.* **2019**, *27*, 887–896. [CrossRef]

33. Davies, A.G.; Pierce-Shimomura, J.T.; Kim, H.; VanHoven, M.K.; Thiele, T.R.; Bonci, A.; Bargmann, C.I.; McIntire, S.L. A central role of the BK potassium channel in behavioral responses to ethanol in *C. elegans*. *Cell* **2003**, *115*, 655–666. [CrossRef]
34. Zhu, M.; Han, S.; Fink, A.L. Oxidized quercetin inhibits alpha-synuclein fibrillization. *Biochim. Biophys. Acta* **2013**, *1830*, 2872–2881. [CrossRef] [PubMed]
35. Pakrashi, S.; Chakraborty, J.; Bandyopadhyay, J. Neuroprotective Role of Quercetin on Rotenone-Induced Toxicity in SH-SY5Y Cell Line Through Modulation of Apoptotic and Autophagic Pathways. *Neurochem. Res.* **2020**, *45*, 1962–1973. [CrossRef] [PubMed]
36. Ay, M.; Luo, J.; Langley, M.; Jin, H.; Anantharam, V.; Kanthasamy, A.; Kanthasamy, A.G. Molecular mechanisms underlying protective effects of quercetin against mitochondrial dysfunction and progressive dopaminergic neurodegeneration in cell culture and MitoPark transgenic mouse models of Parkinson's Disease. *J. Neurochem.* **2017**, *141*, 766–782. [CrossRef]
37. Wang, W.W.; Han, R.; He, H.J.; Li, J.; Chen, S.Y.; Gu, Y.; Xie, C. Administration of quercetin improves mitochondria quality control and protects the neurons in 6-OHDA-lesioned Parkinson's disease models. *Aging* **2021**, *13*, 11738–11751. [CrossRef]
38. Seidl, S.E.; Santiago, J.A.; Bilyk, H.; Potashkin, J.A. The emerging role of nutrition in Parkinson's disease. *Front. Aging Neurosci.* **2014**, *6*, 36. [CrossRef]
39. Tan, L.C.; Methawasin, K.; Tan, E.K.; Tan, J.H.; Au, W.L.; Yuan, J.M.; Koh, W.P. Dietary cholesterol, fats and risk of Parkinson's disease in the Singapore Chinese Health Study. *J. Neurol. Neurosurg. Psychiatry* **2016**, *87*, 86–92. [CrossRef]
40. Chianese, R.; Coccurello, R.; Viggiano, A.; Scafuro, M.; Fiore, M.; Coppola, G.; Operto, F.F.; Fasano, S.; Laye, S.; Pierantoni, R.; et al. Impact of Dietary Fats on Brain Functions. *Curr. Neuropharmacol.* **2018**, *16*, 1059–1085. [CrossRef]
41. Guerrero-Rubio, M.A.; Hernandez-Garcia, S.; Garcia-Carmona, F.; Gandia-Herrero, F. Flavonoids' Effects on *Caenorhabditis elegans'* Longevity, Fat Accumulation, Stress Resistance and Gene Modulation Involve mTOR, SKN-1 and DAF-16. *Antioxidants* **2021**, *10*, 438. [CrossRef]
42. Kampkotter, A.; Nkwonkam, C.G.; Zurawski, R.F.; Timpel, C.; Chovolou, Y.; Watjen, W.; Kahl, R. Investigations of protective effects of the flavonoids quercetin and rutin on stress resistance in the model organism *Caenorhabditis elegans*. *Toxicology* **2007**, *234*, 113–123. [CrossRef]
43. Pallauf, K.; Duckstein, N.; Rimbach, G. A literature review of flavonoids and lifespan in model organisms. *Proc. Nutr. Soc.* **2017**, *76*, 145–162. [CrossRef] [PubMed]
44. Pietsch, K.; Saul, N.; Menzel, R.; Sturzenbaum, S.R.; Steinberg, C.E. Quercetin mediated lifespan extension in *Caenorhabditis elegans* is modulated by age-1, daf-2, sek-1 and unc-43. *Biogerontology* **2009**, *10*, 565–578. [CrossRef] [PubMed]
45. Guo, C.; Sun, L.; Chen, X.; Zhang, D. Oxidative stress, mitochondrial damage and neurodegenerative diseases. *Neural Regen. Res.* **2013**, *8*, 2003–2014. [CrossRef] [PubMed]

antioxidants

MDPI

Article

Novel Copper-Zinc-Manganese Ternary Metal Oxide Nanocomposite as Heterogeneous Catalyst for Glucose Sensor and Antibacterial Activity

Mir Waqas Alam [1,2,*], Hassan S. Al Qahtani [3], Basma Souayeh [1,2], Waqar Ahmed [4], Hind Albalawi [5,*], Mohd Farhan [1,6], Alaaedeen Abuzir [1,2] and Sumaira Naeem [7]

1. Al Bilad Bank Scholarly Chair for Food Security in Saudi Arabia, The Deanship of Scientific Research, The Vice Presidency for Graduate Studies and Scientific Research, King Faisal University, Al-Ahsa 31982, Saudi Arabia; bsouayeh@kfu.edu.sa (B.S.); mfarhan@kfu.edu.sa (M.F.); aabuzir@kfu.edu.sa (A.A.)
2. Department of Physics, College of Science, King Faisal University, Al-Ahsa 31982, Saudi Arabia
3. EXPEC Advanced Research Centre, Saudi Aramco, Dhahran 31311, Saudi Arabia; hassan.alqahtani.2@aramco.com
4. Takasago i-Kohza, Malaysia-Japan International Institute of Technology, Universiti Teknologi Malaysia, Kuala Lumpur 54100, Malaysia; waqarum.ah@gmail.com
5. Department of Physics, College of Sciences, Princess Nourah bint Abdulrahman University (PNU), P.O. Box 84428, Riyadh 11671, Saudi Arabia
6. Department of Basic Sciences, Preparatory Year Deanship, King Faisal University, Al-Ahsa 31982, Saudi Arabia
7. Department of Chemistry, University of Gujrat, Gujrat 50700, Pakistan; sumaira.usman@uog.edu.pk

* Correspondence: wmir@kfu.edu.sa (M.W.A.); hmalbalawi@pnu.edu.sa (H.A.)

Abstract: A novel copper-zinc-manganese trimetal oxide nanocomposite was synthesized by the simple co-precipitation method for sensing glucose and methylene blue degradation. The absorption maximum was found by ultraviolet–visible spectroscopy (UV-Vis) analysis, and the bandgap was 4.32 eV. The formation of a bond between metal and oxygen was confirmed by Fourier Transform Infrared Spectroscopy (FT-IR) analysis. The average crystallite size was calculated as 17.31 nm by X-ray powder diffraction (XRD) analysis. The morphology was observed as spherical by scanning electron microscope (SEM) and high-resolution transmission electron microscopy (HR-TEM) analysis. The elemental composition was determined by Energy Dispersive X-ray Analysis (EDAX) analysis. The oxidation state of the metals present in the nanocomposites was confirmed by the X-ray photoelectron spectroscopy (XPS) analysis. The hydrodynamic diameter and zeta potential of the nanocomposite were 218 nm and −46.8 eV, respectively. The thermal stability of the nanocomposite was analyzed by thermogravimetry-differential scanning calorimetry (TG-DSC) analysis. The synthesized nanocomposite was evaluated for the electrochemical glucose sensor. The nanocomposite shows 87.47% of degradation ability against methylene blue dye at a 50 μM concentration. The trimetal oxide nanocomposite shows potent activity against *Escherichia coli*. In addition to that, the prepared nanocomposite shows strong antioxidant application where scavenging activity was observed to be 76.58 ± 0.30, 76.89 ± 0.44, 81.41 ± 30, 82.58 ± 0.32, and 84.36 ± 0.09 % at 31, 62, 125, 250, and 500 μg/mL, respectively. The results confirm the antioxidant potency of nanoparticles (NPs) was concentration dependent.

Keywords: absorption; glucose; methylene blue; sensor; trimetal oxide

1. Introduction

Presently, diabetes is considered one of the most common chronic diseases and is already declared a serious threat to a healthy lifestyle [1]. Several medical conditions are associated with diabetes, including heart diseases, tuberculosis, coeliac disease, and cystic fibrosis. These diseases can result in blindness and nephropathy that can even cause renal failure, nerve damage, foot ulcers, and cancer [2,3]. An abnormal level of glucose in the human body is a major source of diabetes, which comes from daily food products such as potatoes, fruit, and preservative food. Consuming food rich in glucose levels can increase blood sugar and, in turn, cause diabetes [4,5]. Therefore, due to daily increasing risks to health, it is important to develop a highly sensitive and simple technique to detect and monitor glucose levels for clinical diagnosis, medicine, and the food industry. In addition to that, the detection of glucose levels is also specifically important in several food products because glucose can cause browning due to dehydration and longer storage time. Moreover, monitoring glucose is also highly important in pharmaceutical products where several food products are being used [6]. Until now, metal oxides (MOs) and metal sulfides (MSs) have been used as advanced electrocatalysts for developing highly sensitive electrochemical sensors [7–9]. However, these sensors have drawbacks such as low detection limits [10–12]. Due to excellent electrical and chemical properties, several nanomaterials including metal oxides, nanoparticles, graphene, and carbon nanotubes are frequently used as electrochemical biosensors [13]. It has also been reported that a combination of two or several nanomaterials as nanocomposites further enhance these properties and are frequently used in biosensing applications [14]. High-performance ternary metal oxide nanocomposites such as $ZnO/MnO_2/Cu_2O$ [15], $ZnO/Fe_2O_3/MnO_2$ [16], and $ZnO/MnO_2/Gd_2O_3$ [17] have been reported for enhanced photocatalytic application. For the effective removal of organic contaminants, heterogenous photocatalysis is considered an important class of advanced oxidation processes [18]. To enhance the photocatalytic properties and glucose sensing, the ternary nano heterojunction combination with a compatible valence band can highly useful. Similarly, a Fe/La/Zn nanocomposite with graphene oxides was prepared by another group of researchers to analyze the photodegradation of phenylhydrazine, environmental remediation, and antimicrobial studies [19]. The undiscriminating usage of antimicrobial/antibacterial drugs for treating various infectious diseases has also attracted the attention of researchers to develop organic and inorganic nanomaterial agents. Extreme oxidative sensitivity and instability issues related to organic antibacterial nanoparticles pose a limitation to their usage and simultaneously suggest crossing this barrier by using inorganic materials for this purpose based on their capability to tolerate severe procedural conditions. Metal oxides are considered among the best choices to prepare antimicrobial medicines owing to their stability as well as their safety for humans, animals, and plants [20]. For example, the synthesis of one-dimensional (1D) MgO nanowires via the microwave hydrothermal method has gained remarkable attention in preparing antimicrobial medicines due to their enriched surface chemistry with special emphasis on the high surface area [21]. Silicon nanowires decorated with silver nanoparticles are also reported as synthetic one-dimensional semiconducting long-term antibacterial nanomaterials, which have been gaining interest in recent years [22]. Similarly, a green approach to biosynthesizing silver nanowires from commercial *Camellia sinesis* has been considered for their antibacterial properties against *Escherichia coli* and *Staphylococcus aureus*, which proved fatal for infectious microorganisms [23]. Nanocomposites, especially heterocyclic ones, are considered advantageous over metallic nanoparticles as they play the role of a junction between two or more nanoparticles due to their high versatility. They have a promising position in medicinal chemistry owing to their wide spectrum of activities [24], including photosensitizer (e.g., Ag/Ti/Zn Trimetallic Nanoparticles and Carbon Quantum Dots Nanocomposites) [25], antimicrobial [26], and antioxidant activity (e.g., bio-Ag/CdO/ZnO@MWCNTs nanocomposites) [27], by using several different methods. For antibacterial activities, zinc- and copper-doped TiO_2 nanoparticles have been reported. The results show that the doping of both the materials is considered an essential antibacterial agent, and strongly influenced photocatalytic degradation and antibacterial properties [28,29]. In addition, Polyvinylchloride coated with a combination of silver nanoparticles and zinc oxide nanowires also showed potential for antimicrobial applications [30].

Because of their high surface area, biocompatibility, and excellent electrical and catalytic properties, Cu-Zn-Mn nanocomposites are proven to be highly efficient sensors [31–33]. Due to the compatible band structure and narrow bandgap of Cu, Zn, and Mn, they are highly useful for photocatalytic applications [34]. Several methods, such as biosynthesis, the hydrothermal route, and screen-printing, have been used to prepare the ternary nanocomposite [35]. However, the co-precipitation method is a frequently used technique for developing a nanocomposite of mixed oxides. The application of the co-precipitation method in the current research area has shown a significant difference in the phase of calcined oxides with mixed nanocomposites [36].

Therefore, in the current study, the author aims to produce a copper-zinc-manganese ternary metal oxide nanocomposite as a heterogeneous catalyst via the co-precipitation method. The synthesized nanocomposite was evaluated for an electrochemical glucose sensor, photocatalytic degradation of methylene blue, and antioxidant and antibacterial applications.

2. Experimentation

2.1. Materials

The precursors, such as copper sulphate pentahydrate—$CuSO_4{\cdot}5H_2O$ (99%), zinc nitrate hexahydrate—$Zn(NO_3)_2{\cdot}6H_2O$ (99%), and manganese acetate tetrahydrate—$Mn(CH_3COO)_2{\cdot}4H_2O$ (99%) used for trimetal oxide nanomaterial synthesis, were purchased from Sigma Aldrich (St. Louis, MO, USA). An aqueous ammonia solution was used as the precipitating agent. D-glucose was used for glucose-sensing applications. Methylene blue was chosen as a pollutant for the degradation process. Double-distilled water was used as a solvent throughout the experiments.

2.2. Methods

Synthesis of Cu-Zn-Mn Mixed Trimetal Oxide

In a typical reaction process, 1 mM copper sulphate pentahydrate was dissolved in 30 mL of double-distilled water and stirred for 15 min. To that, 1 mM manganese acetate tetrahydrate in 30 mL of double-distilled water was added, and stirring was continued for 45 min. To the above solution, 1 mM zinc nitrate hexahydrate in 30 mL of double-distilled water was added and stirring was continued for one hour. To the above precursor solutions, 15 mL of an aqueous ammonia solution was added, and the pH was maintained at 12. The black-colored precipitates were obtained and washed via the centrifugation process several times with a 3:1 ratio of water and the ethanol mixture. Then the precipitates were dried at 80 °C and calcinated at 600 °C for 5 h. The black-colored precipitates were obtained as a final product and were stored for further characterization and application processes. Figure 1 depicts the synthesis of Cu-Zn-Mn mixed trimetal oxide nanoparticles.

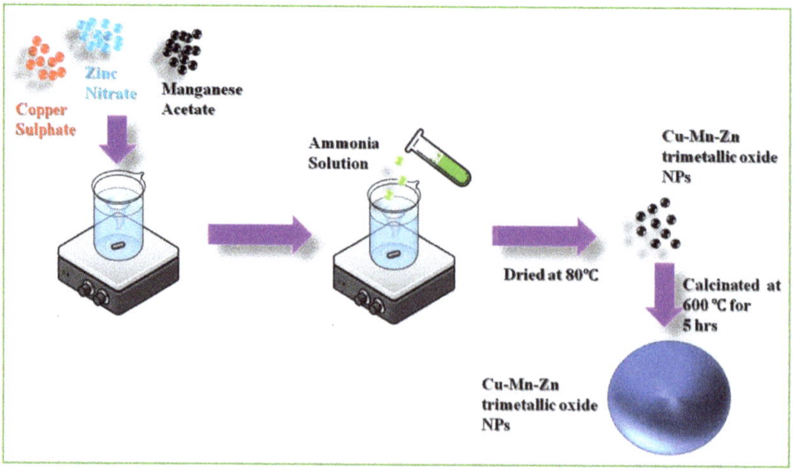

Figure 1. Synthesis of Cu-Zn-Mn mixed trimetal oxide nanoparticles (NPs).

2.3. Characterization

The crystalline phase, structure, and size of the synthesized trimetal oxide were found by X-ray powder diffraction (XRD) analysis performed with an Ultima IV Rigaku diffractometer (Rigaku, Tokyo, Japan) with Cu Kα as a radiation source (λ = 1.540 Å, 40 kV, 15 mA) and it was recorded in the range of 10–90°. The morphology and average particle size of the material were analyzed by SEM with EDX (Bruker, Billerica, MA, USA) at an operating voltage of 15 kV. The atomic and weight percentages were found using EDX analysis. XPS was performed using the PHI Versaprobe III (ULVAC-PHI, Inc., Chanhassen, MN, USA), which was recorded in the range of 0 to 1100 eV. HR-TEM analysis was performed using JEOL-2100 (JEOL Ltd., Tokyo, Japan). The FT-IR spectrometer (Jasco Inc., Tokyo, Japan) was used to determine the functional groups present in the nanocomposite and confirm the formation of a bond between metal and oxygen. The FT-IR analysis was recorded in the wavenumber range of 4000–400 cm^{-1} with KBr as a standard and a scanning speed of 2 cm^{-1}/s. The particle size and zeta potential were found using Dynamic Light Scattering (DLS) analysis. The synthesized nanomaterials were dispersed by the sonication process for 20 min in an ultrasonic bath and analyzed directly using a DLS instrument (Horiba, Tokyo, Japan) and the temperature was set to 25 °C during the analysis. The graphite electrode was used to perform and measure the zeta potential of the synthesized nanoparticles. The optical property was investigated by UV-Vis analysis using a JASCO spectrophotometer (Jasco Inc., Tokyo, Japan) and recorded in the range of 200–800 nm with a scanning speed of 1000 nm/min, and the bandgap was found using Tauc's plot. The thermal stability of the synthesized trimetal oxide nanocomposite was confirmed using the TG-6300 analyzer (Seiko Instruments Inc., Tokyo, Japan) under a nitrogen atmosphere.

2.4. Electrochemical Measurement

Electrochemical measurement was carried out for the glucose sensor application at room temperature. The standard three-electrode system (working electrode-prepared carbon paste electrode, reference electrode-Ag/AgCl electrode, and indicator electrode-platinum wire) was used for the electrochemical tests. 1 M KOH solution was used as an electrolyte and D-glucose was used as an analyte for glucose sensor measurement.

2.5. Photocatalytic Degradation of Dye Solution

The photocatalytic degradation of methylene blue (MB) dye as a pollutant was carried out under sunlight as an irradiation source in the presence of trimetal oxide as a photocatalyst. The degradation study was carried out in a batch reactor system. Briefly, 250 mL of the dye solution was taken in a borosilicate rectangular tray. The tray contained a known concentration (50 µM) of MB solution and 100 mg of the photocatalyst. After the addition of the photocatalyst, the pH of the solution was maintained at 7 $\pm$ 0.1 by adding the NaOH solution. Later, the solution was allowed to stir for 30 min using a magnetic stirrer in a dark room to attain the adsorption–desorption equilibrium of MB on the catalyst surface. The degradation of MB was carried out under direct sunlight and the intensity of the light was frequently measured. At particular time intervals, the degraded solution was continuously collected. The residual concentration of MB dye solution was measured at 662 nm using a UV-Vis spectrophotometer (Jasco Inc., Tokyo, Japan). The intensity of the sunlight was measured as 840–860 lux using a digital lux meter. The same protocol was followed for different concentrations, such as 75 and 100 µM dye solution.

2.6. Antioxidant Activity

DPPH Scavenging Activity

The antioxidant potency of the Cu-Zn-Mn mixed trimetal oxide nanocomposite was determined using a 1,1-diphenyl-2-picrylhydrazyl radical (DPPH) assay by following the protocols of [37]. To carry out the measurement, 100 µg of the Cu-Zn-Mn mixed trimetal oxide nanocomposite was mixed with 100 µL of ethanol and 50 µL of the DPPH solution and kept in a dark room for 30 min. The absorption value was observed at 518 nm for the prepared solution. Ascorbic acid was used as a standard antioxidant agent. Antioxidant activity was determined by calculating the percent (%) of inhibition by the following formula (Equation (1)):

$$\text{Scavenging effect (\%)} = [(A_c - A_s)/A_c] \times 100 \quad (1)$$

where A_c is the absorbance of the control and A_s is the absorbance of the sample.

2.7. Antibacterial Activity

The antibacterial efficacy of synthesized NPs was investigated against the pathogen *Escherichia coli*. The assessment of antibacterial activity was confirmed using the agar well diffusion method by adopting the protocols of (Burygin et al., 2009) with slight modifications [38].

3. Results and Discussion

3.1. XRD Analysis

The XRD pattern for the Cu-Zn-Mn mixed trimetal oxide nanocomposite is given in Figure 2. From the analysis, the 2θ value was observed at 30.19, 35.48, 53.42, 56.95, and 62.51°. Compared with JCPDS card No. (83-1665), the peak observed at 30.19, 35.48, 53.42, and 62.51° corresponded to the miller indices (200), (202), (314), and (020) for CuO and had a tetragonal phase. The peaks observed at 56.95 and 62.51° correspond to the miller indices (110) and (103), which confirmed the formation of ZnO, and it had a hexagonal phase. The formation of ZnO was confirmed by the JCPDS card No. 89-1397. According to JCPDS card No. 86-2337, the formation of MnO_2 was confirmed by the peaks at 30.19, 35.48, 56.95, and 62.51° with respect to the miller indices (011), (201), (341), and (112), and it had an orthorhombic phase. The average crystalline size of synthesized nanomaterial was found to be 17.31 nm. Juma et al. synthesized the CuO-NiO-ZnO mixed metal oxide, and XRD analysis was carried out. At a calcined temperature of 200 °C, the CuO and ZnO could be identified and NiO was not identified, which may be due to the Ni being in its hydroxide form. At a calcined temperature of 200 °C, CuO, ZnO, and NiO were well resolved, which confirmed that all the hydroxides were decomposed and converted to oxides [39].

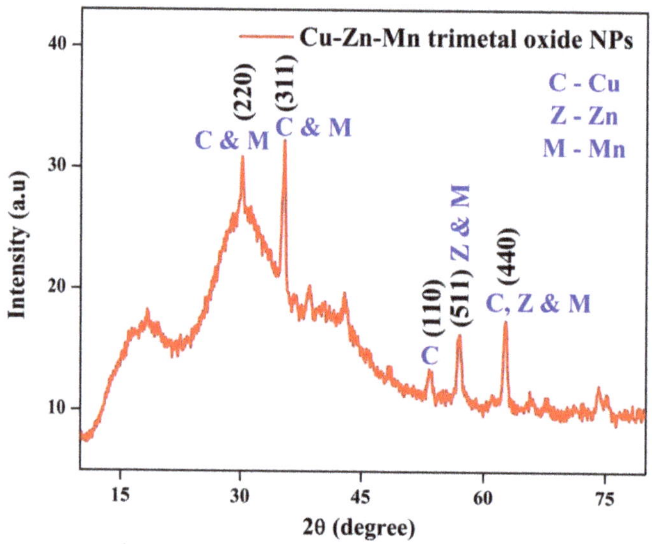

Figure 2. XRD pattern of Cu-Zn-Mn mixed trimetal oxide nanoparticles.

3.2. SEM-EDAX Analysis

Figure 3 shows the SEM analysis of the Cu-Zn-Mn mixed trimetal oxide nanocomposite (a) with 10 μm, (b) with 5 μm, (c) with 4 μm, and (d) the size distribution. The SEM analysis indicates the synthesized nanoparticle was non-uniformly spherical in morphology with some aggregation, which leads to enhancement of the particle size. The average particle size was found to be 92.33 nm with a total count of 965,632 particles with the aid of ImageJ software. The trimetal oxide has shown the agglomeration of particles, which is usual for all types of nanomaterials due to the involvement of strong interparticle contact-induced utilizing high surface energy. Enhessari et al. synthesized aggregated quasi-spherical $CuMn_2O_4$ nanoparticles with an average particle size of 39 nm [40]. According to Sanchez et al., the aggregation of the nanoparticles was reduced by increasing the reaction time [41].

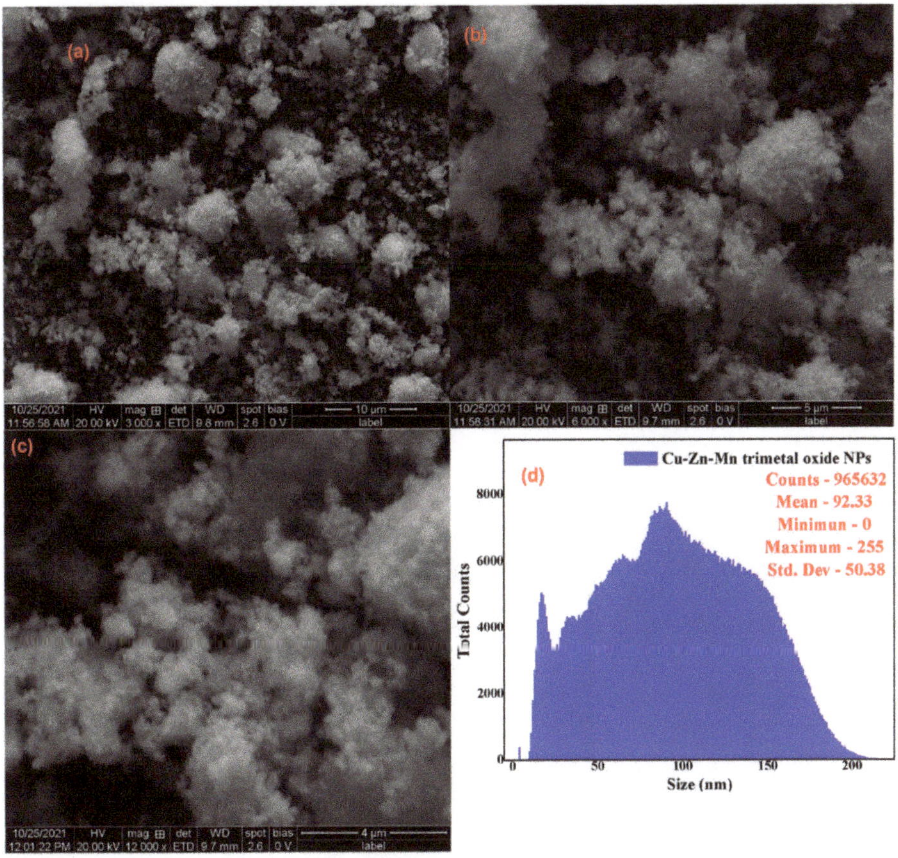

Figure 3. SEM of Cu-Zn-Mn mixed trimetal oxide nanoparticles. (**a**) 10 μm; (**b**) 5 μm; (**c**) 4 μm; (**d**) size distribution.

The atomic and weight percentage of the synthesized nanoparticle was found by using EDAX analysis. Figure 4 shows the EDAX of the Cu-Zn-Mn mixed trimetal oxide nanocomposite. The weight % age of Cu, Zn, Mn, and O was found to be 18.67, 23.44, 33.88, and 24.01, respectively. The atomic % age of Cu, Zn, Mn, and O was found to be 12.47, 13.42, 19.09, and 55.02, respectively. The error % of Cu, Zn, Mn, and O was found to be 0.43, 0.64, 0.87, and 2.96, respectively.

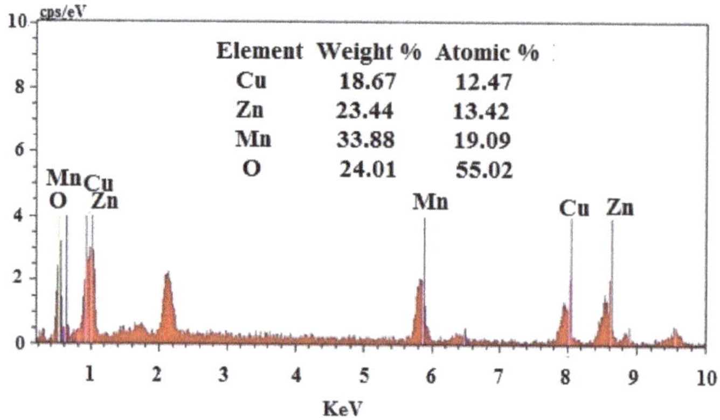

Figure 4. EDAX of Cu-Zn-Mn mixed trimetal oxide nanoparticles.

3.3. HR-TEM—SAED Analysis

The surface morphology of the synthesized Cu-Zn-Mn mixed trimetal oxide was analyzed by HR-TEM analysis (Figure 5). HR-TEM revealed that synthesized nanoparticles are spherical in morphology with agglomeration. Compared with XRD, the particle size was higher in HR-TEM (90 ± 3 nm), which may be due to the merging of particles to form larger particles. This shows that the formed particles are agglomerated, which is elucidated by the HR-TEM images of lattice fringes. The Selected area diffraction (SAED) model illustrates bright rings that prove the superior orientation of nanocrystals. The SAED pattern contains many rings with different radii, which shows that the Cu-Zn-Mn mixed trimetal oxide nanoparticles belong to a nanocrystalline structure. The diffraction rings matched with XRD results and the rings from inside to outside can be indexed to (220), (311), (110), (511), and (440) crystal planes.

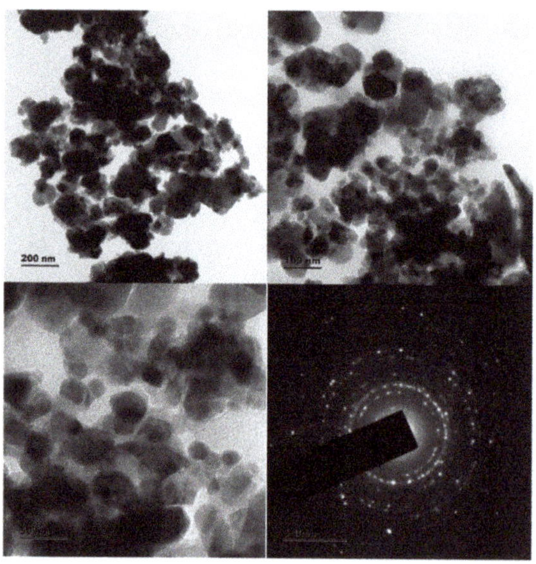

Figure 5. HR-TEM—SAED analysis of Cu-Zn-Mn mixed trimetal oxide nanoparticles.

3.4. XPS Analysis

The elemental composition and oxidation state of Cu-Zn-Mn mixed trimetal oxide nanocomposites were determined using XPS analysis in accordance with the binding energies of the various elements present on the material's surface, and the XPS spectrum was recorded between 0 and 1100 eV. Figure 6a shows the XPS survey scan of the Cu-Zn-Mn mixed trimetal oxide revealed the existence of Cu, Zn, Mn, O, and C. Figure 6b shows the Cu 2p core level consists of Cu $2p_{3/2}$ and Cu $2p_{1/2}$ at 933.6 eV and 953.5 eV, respectively, and it can be readily notified in the high-resolution spectrum of Cu 2p. At the same time, two characteristic satellite peaks at 941.90 eV and 961.26 eV can be clearly noticed, indicating the presence of Cu 3p [42]. Figure 6c shows the Mn 2p core level consists of Mn $2p_{3/2}$ and Mn $2p_{1/2}$ at 642.3 eV and 653.7 eV, respectively [43]. The characteristic peak appeared at 1021.3 eV and 1044.3 eV with respect to Zn $2p_{3/2}$ and Zn $2p_{1/2}$, respectively, for the Zn 2p core level region (Figure 6d) [44]. In the case of the O 1s core level (Figure 6e), the signal can be attributed to oxygen molecules attached to the different atoms. The peak at approximately 530.6 eV is ascribed to metal-oxygen bonds [45]. In the core level of C 1s (Figure 6f), the peak at approximately 284.8 eV is ascribed to the C-C bond based on the literature value [46].

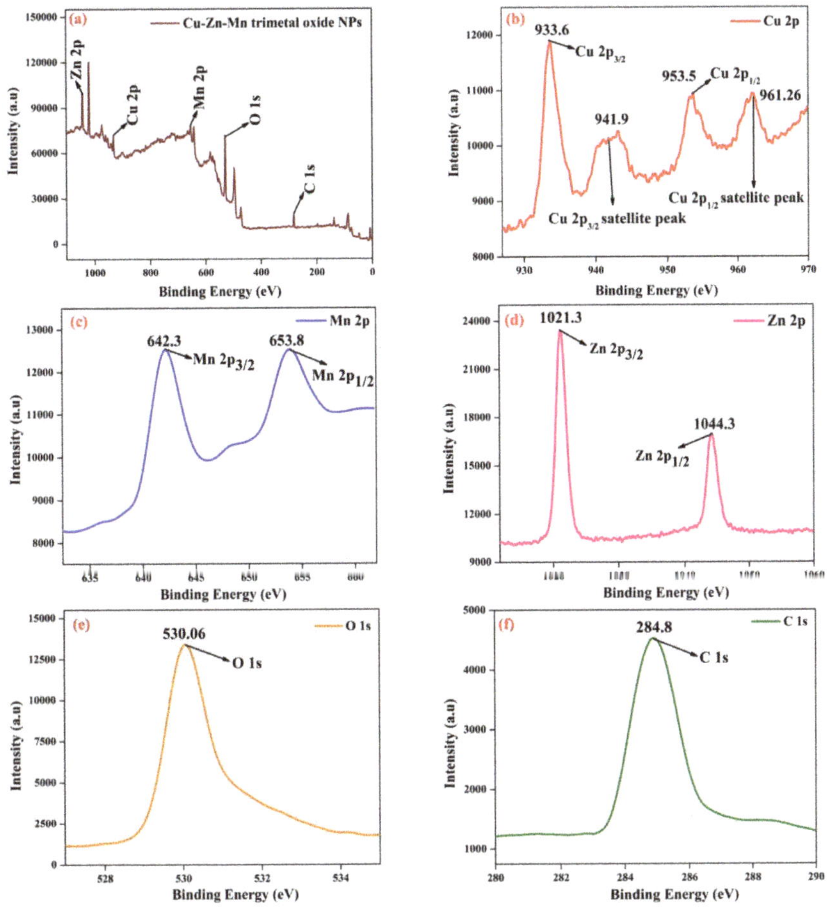

Figure 6. XPS of Cu-Zn-Mn mixed trimetal oxide nanoparticles. (**a**) survey scan of trimetal oxide; (**b**) Cu, (**c**) Mn, (**d**) Zn, (**e**) O, (**f**) C elements.

3.5. DLS Analysis

The hydrodynamic diameter of the Cu-Zn-Mn mixed trimetal oxide nanocomposite was found to be 218 nm. Figure 7a,b shows the DLS analysis and zeta potential of

Cu-Zn-Mn mixed trimetal oxide nanoparticles, respectively. The surface charge of the synthesized trimetal oxide was measured by zeta potential. The surface charge of the particle indicates the stability of trimetal oxide nanocomposite, which was found to be −46.8 mV. The zeta potential value in the range of >±30 mV shows the nanomaterial has sufficient repulsive force to attain better physical colloidal stability, and the zeta potential range of ±40 to 50 mV shows the nanomaterial has good stability [47].

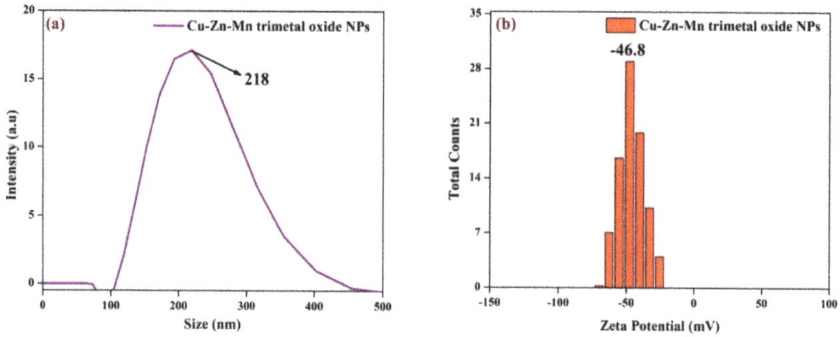

Figure 7. (**a**) Particle size and (**b**) Zeta potential of Cu-Zn-Mn mixed trimetal oxide nanoparticles.

3.6. UV-Vis Analysis

Figure 8 shows the UV-Vis spectrum of the Cu-Zn-Mn mixed trimetal oxide nanocomposite. The two peaks were observed in the UV region at wavelengths of 233 nm and 389 nm and these peaks correspond to the metal oxide. The two peaks observed in the spectrophotometer were owing to the interband fundamental edge transitions. The absorbance value moved towards the visible region, which was due to the presence of ZnO in the synthesized trimetal oxide nanocomposite. Similarly, copper-doped ZnO nanoparticles have an absorbance peak at 230 and 270 nm, which confirms the formation of a metal oxide. After doping the ZnO with Cu, the intensity of the absorbance peak increased, which was due to the zinc ions present in the crystal lattices leading to the alteration, especially in the extension of lattices [48]. Khalid et al. synthesized zinc-doped copper oxide nanoparticles, and the absorbance peak was observed at 390 nm with zinc doping, which was due to the d–d transition [49]. John Abel synthesized $CuMn_2O_4$ nanoparticles and the absorbance value was observed at 278 nm [50]. The optical bandgap of the Cu-Zn-Mn mixed oxide nanocomposite was found by Tauc's plot. From the Tauc relation, the bandgap of the synthesized nanocomposite was found to be 4.32 eV, which confirmed that the synthesized nanoparticle was a semiconductor in nature. The Tauc relation is shown in Equation (2):

$$(\alpha h\upsilon) \propto (h\upsilon - E_g)^n \quad (2)$$

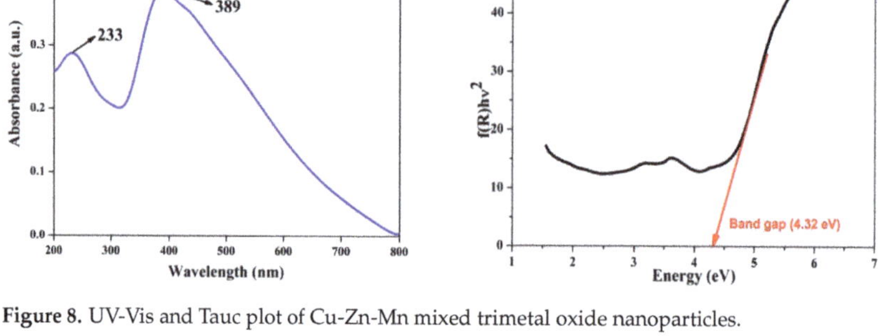

Figure 8. UV-Vis and Tauc plot of Cu-Zn-Mn mixed trimetal oxide nanoparticles.

3.7. FT-IR Analysis

The chemical bonding and functional group present in the synthesized Cu-Zn-Mn mixed-metal oxide nanoparticle was found using FT-IR analysis. Figure 9 shows the FT-IR analysis of the Cu-Zn-Mn mixed oxide nanocomposite. The band at 3429 cm^{-1} was assigned to the O-H stretching vibration, which was due to the moisture content present on the surface of the nanocomposite [51]. The C-H stretching vibration was confirmed by the peak at 2912 cm^{-1}. The peak appeared at 1634 cm^{-1} accredited to O-H bending vibration in the nanocomposite. The peak that appeared at 1403 cm^{-1} was attributed to the carboxy C-O stretching vibration [52]. The presence of C=C bending vibration present in the nanocomposite was confirmed by the peak that appeared at 908 cm^{-1}. The formation of the bond between metal and oxygen during nanoparticle formation was found by the peak appearing at 614 cm^{-1} [53].

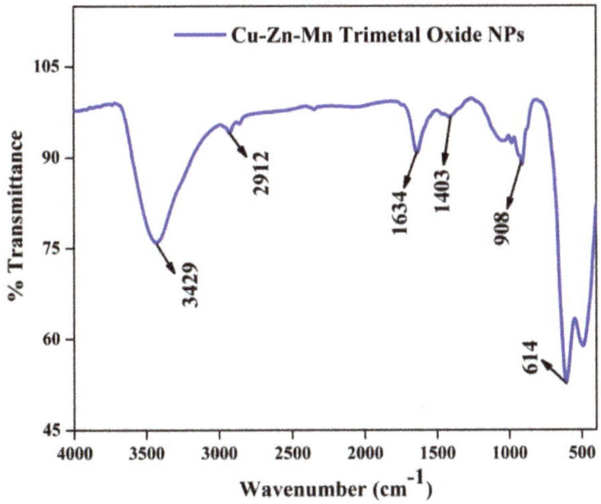

Figure 9. FT-IR of Cu-Zn-Mn mixed trimetal oxide nanoparticles.

3.8. TG-DSC Analysis

Figure 10 depicts the thermogravimetric analysis (TGA) and Differential scanning calorimetry (DSC) analysis of Cu-Zn-Mn trimetal oxide nanocomposite. The decomposition temperature of the synthesized material was found to be 67–148 and 436 °C, corresponding to a weight loss of 5.87 and 19.52%. The DSC curve illustrates the overlap of exothermic and endothermic peaks, approximately in the range of 200–270 °C. An endothermic peak was observed at 216 °C, and this might be due to the surface reaction initiated among metal nanoparticles. An exothermic peak was found at 258 °C, which may be due to the latent heat of crystallization, stabilization of crystal structure, and diffusion rearrangement of unstable atoms [54]. The removal of water molecules from the synthesized material was confirmed by the decomposition temperature in the range of 67–148 °C, which was observed from TGA analysis. Before 200 °C, the weight of synthesized nanoparticles steadily decreased while increasing the temperature without noticeable exothermic and endothermic peaks, which shows that there was no chemical reaction taking place. The peak at 436 °C was due to the decomposition of anions, which shows the conversion of hydroxide to the corresponding metal oxide nanoparticles, which was reliable considering the result of XRD. At the continuous temperature rise, there was no noticeable weight loss observed, which indicates that the nanoparticle was thermally stable after 450 °C, and 80% of the sample remained.

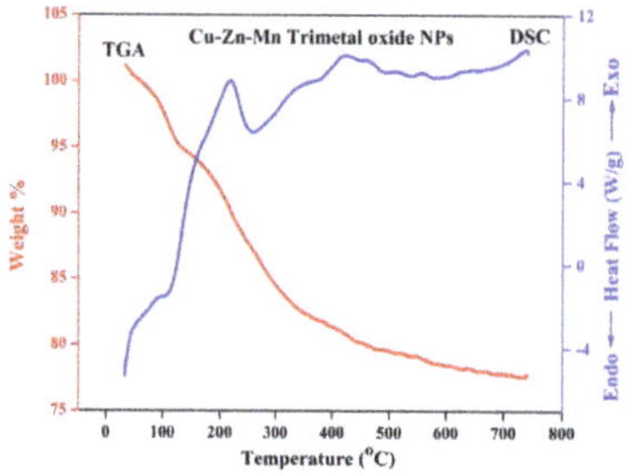

Figure 10. TG-DSC of Cu-Zn-Mn mixed trimetal oxide nanoparticles.

3.9. Glucose Sensor

Figure 11a shows the cyclic voltammetry (CV) of mixed trimetal oxide nanoparticles. The CV graph without glucose shows there is no proper appearance of peaks in oxidation, but during the reduction, the appearance of a small peak was observed at −0.7 V. During the sensing of glucose, oxidation and reduction peaks appeared. From Figure 11a, it is seen that, with an increased scan rate, the corresponding current peaks are increased; meanwhile, the oxidation peaks observed shifted slightly toward the positive side, and the reduction peaks shifted slightly towards the negative side of the potential. Figure 11b shows the CV results at different concentrations (1–5 mM) of the glucose analyte. A significant difference was observed between the cathodic and anodic peak intensities, which suggests the prepared materials have strong sensing applications [55]. By increasing the concentration of the analyte, a significant increase in the peak intensity was observed. As per these results, it is clearly seen that the prepared trimetal oxide nanoparticles are highly suitable for glucose sensing. As shown in Figure 11c, electrochemical impedance spectroscopy (EIS) studies were also investigated for the synthesized trimetal oxide nanoparticles to clearly recognize the resistance mechanism. The presence of a smaller area of the semi-circle for the electrode reveals that the ohmic resistance offered by the electrode in the basic medium is low due to its higher capacitance. For confirmation of the electrode process, Figure 11d shows the peak current vs. the square root of the scan rate where we can clearly observe a linear line, which indicates a diffusion-controlled reaction.

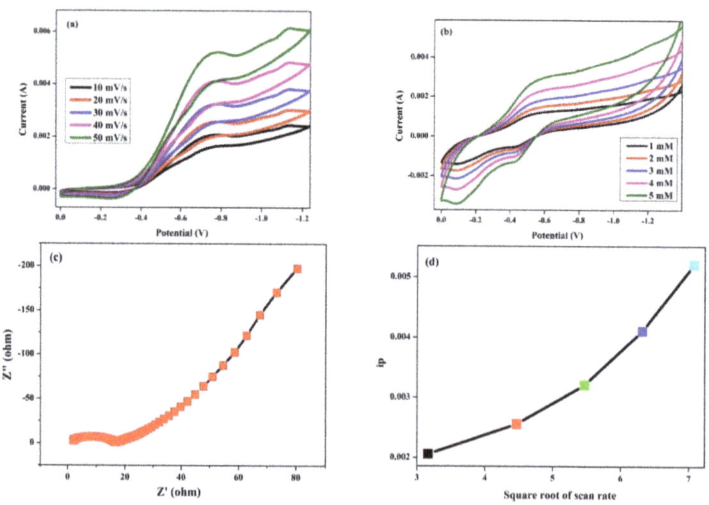

Figure 11. (**a**) CV graph of Cu-Zn-Mn mixed trimetal oxide nanoparticles with different scan rates, (**b**) CV graph with glucose at different concentrations, (**c**) Nyquist plots of the Cu-Zn-Mn mixed trimetal oxide, (**d**) plot of peak current vs. square root of scan rate.

3.10. Photocatalytic Degradation of MB Dye

The photocatalytic degradation efficiency of the synthesized Cu-Zn-Mn trimetal oxide nanocomposite was investigated against methylene blue dye as a pollutant and the reaction was carried out at neutral pH. The degraded solution was collected at different time intervals and tested using a UV-Vis spectrophotometer. Upon the degradation of the dye, three bands were observed at 661, 288, and 244 nm. Figure 12a–c shows the degradation of MB corresponding to concentrations of 50, 75, and 100 μM, respectively. The band observed at 661 nm in the visible region corresponds to a sulfur-nitrogen conjugated system. The intensity of the band gradually diminished as the degradation progressed, and this confirmed that the sulfur-nitrogen conjugated system was damaged during the degradation process. The color of the MB solution was slowly lightened during the constant irradiation of sunlight. The bands at 244 and 288 nm in the UV region indicate the phenothizine group present in the MB. This is owing to the oxidative decomposition and ring-opening reaction in phenothizine species. Photocatalysis generates a strong oxidation agent to break organic matter into CO_2 and H_2O in the presence of light and photocatalysts [56]. The degradation efficiency of nanoparticles was found to be 87.47, 83.6, and 81.02% with respect to 50, 75, and 100 μM. Figure 12d illustrates the degradation efficiency of synthesized nanoparticles. The % degradation was calculated using the following formula (Equation (3)).

$$\text{Degradation\%} = [(A0 - At)/A0] \times 100 \tag{3}$$

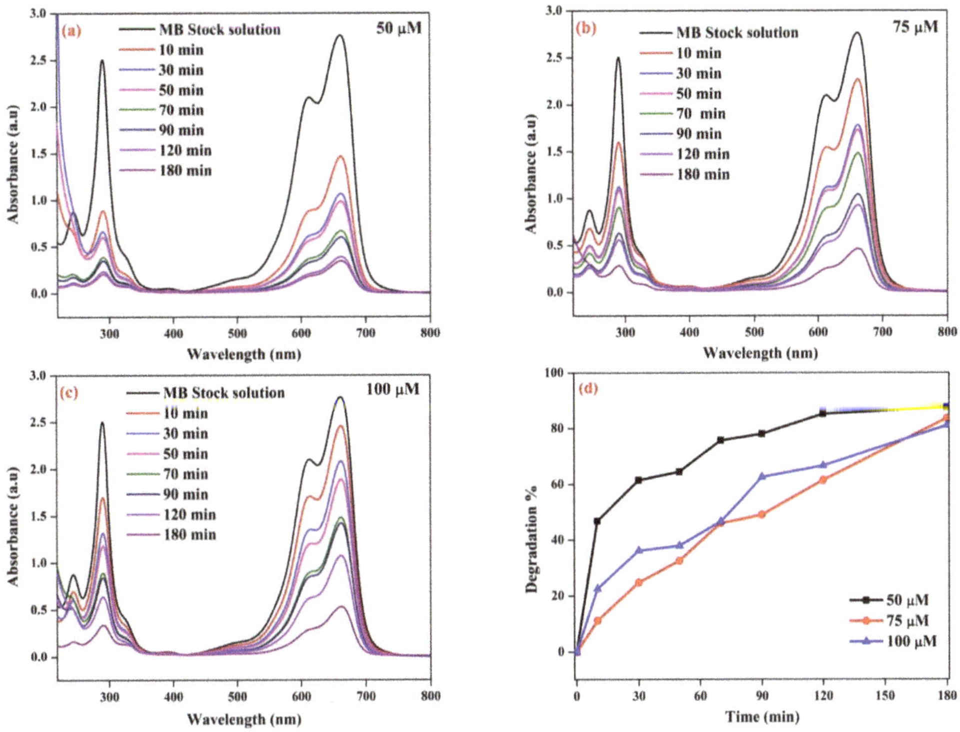

Figure 12. Photocatalytic degradation of methylene blue at (**a**) 50 μM, (**b**) 75 μM, and (**c**) 100 μM. (**d**) Degradation efficiency of Cu-Zn-Mn trimetal oxide NPs.

The absorbance value was decreased with the increased time of solar irradiation with the photocatalyst. The intensity of the blue color faded after the degradation of the dye solution. The degradation of dye was possible due to the generation of hole (h^+) and electron (e^-) pairs on the surface of the catalyst during the irradiation of sunlight. The e^- and h^+ pair interacts with a water molecule to produce a hydroxyl radical, which is responsible for breaking the hazardous dye constituents. Electrons present in the conduction band on the catalyst's surface convert molecular oxygen to superoxide ions and, finally, forms hydrogen peroxide. The hole produces a hydroxyl radical, which plays a key role in the breakage of dye molecules. The efficiency of the photocatalyst decreased with the increasing concentration of the dye. The efficiency was indirectly proportional to the concentration of the dye [57]. The rate constant (k) corresponding to 50, 75, and 100 μM was found to be 0.01089, 0.00953, and 0.009 and the linear regression coefficient (R^2) corresponding to 50, 75, and 100 μM was found to be 0.8554, 0.9661, and 0.9758 (Figure 13).

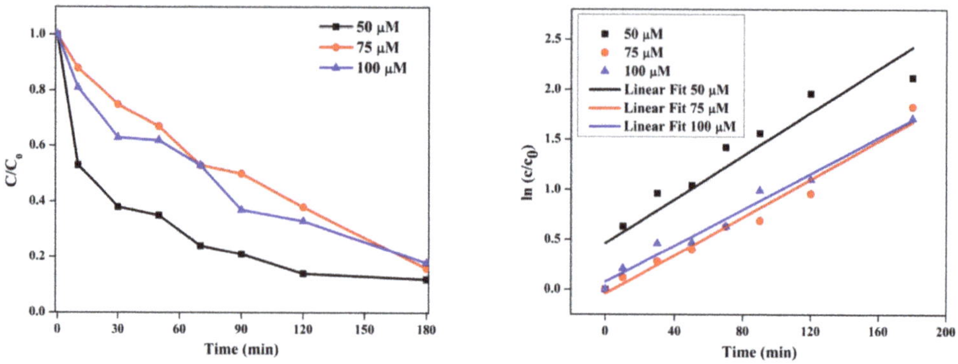

Figure 13. Plot of time vs. c/c_0 and time vs. ln c/c_0 for photocatalytic degradation of methylene blue dye.

Regeneration and Reusability

The regeneration and reusability of the photocatalyst are very important to evaluate the efficiency of the catalyst. After completion of the degradation process, the catalyst was collected from the reaction medium and further used for reusability study. To collect the catalyst, the degraded solution was centrifuged at 3000 rpm and the supernatant solution was discarded. Then the precipitate was thoroughly washed, thrice, with a 3:1 water:ethanol mixture to remove the pollutant. The obtained precipitate was washed and dried at 80 °C to remove the moisture content and impurities present in the catalyst. The collected catalyst underwent three reusability studies, and the efficiency of the catalyst was diminished during the studies. The efficiency % was reduced from 87 to 79 % after four cycles. This is due to the leaching of the catalyst during washing and drying. The weight of the catalyst was decreased, which leads to a decrease in the efficiency of the catalyst. Figure 14 illustrates the reusability of the catalyst for MB dye degradation.

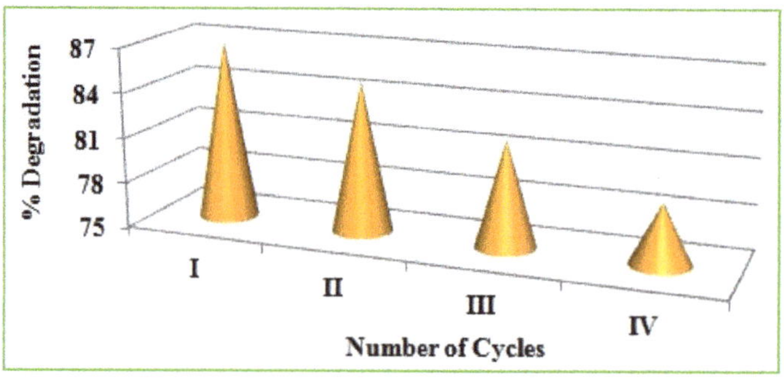

Figure 14. Reusability of catalyst for methylene blue degradation.

3.11. Antioxidant Activity

To determine the antioxidant potency of the Cu-Zn-Mn mixed trimetal oxide nanocomposite, ascorbic acid was used as a standard for DPPH assay. The scavenging activity of the NPs was increased with increasing concentrations of NPs. The scavenging activity was observed to be 76.58 ± 0.30, 76.89 ± 0.44, 81.41 ± 30, 82.58 ± 0.32, and 84.36 ± 0.09 % at 31, 62, 125, 250, and 500 μg/mL, respectively (Figure 15). The study confirmed that the antioxidant potency of NPs was concentration dependent.

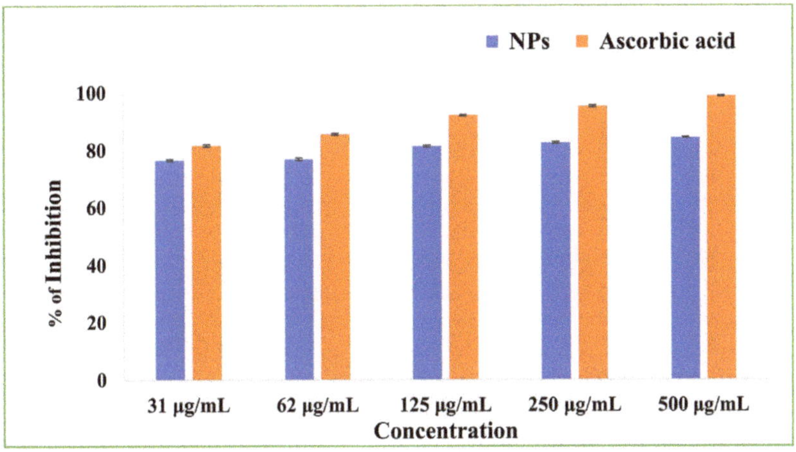

Figure 15. DPPH scavenging activity of Cu-Zn-Mn mixed trimetal oxide nanoparticles.

3.12. Antibacterial Activity

The results of the study suggested that the synthesized NPs showed potential antibacterial effects against *E. coli*. Figure 16 depicts the antibacterial activity of Cu-Zn-Mn mixed trimetal oxide nanoparticles against *E. coli*. The minimum and maximum zones of inhibition were noted as 12 mm and 16 mm at 25 and 100 μg/mL concentrations, respectively. At 50 and 75 μg/mL concentrations, the zone of inhibition was noted as 13.5 and 14.6 mm, respectively. Hence, it is clearly evidenced that the synthesized NPs for antibacterial activity were concentration-dependent and have the potency to inhibit the growth of pathogenic bacterial strains. The Gram-negative bacteria have an outer membrane made up of negatively charged lipopolysaccharide molecules. It seems that the synthesized nanomaterial passes through the cell wall of the bacteria, and it is damaged from the interior. The physical interaction took place between the bacterial cells and synthesized NPs, which creates the cell wall structure disruption, leading to the breakdown and, finally, bacterial death [58].

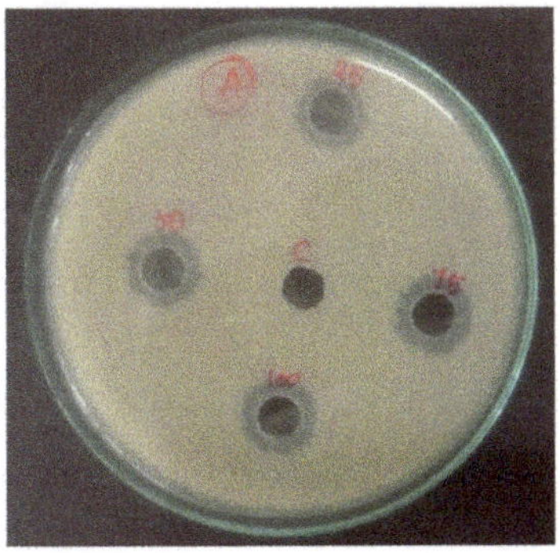

Figure 16. Antibacterial activity of Cu-Zn-Mn mixed trimetal oxide nanoparticles.

4. Conclusions

In summary, the Cu-Zn-Mn mixed trimetal oxide NPs were successfully synthesized, characterized, and investigated for a glucose sensor, photocatalytic degradation of methylene blue, and antioxidant and antibacterial activity. The synthesized nanoparticles were spherical with an average particle size of 92 nm. The semiconductor nature was confirmed by the bandgap value of 4.32 eV. The nanoparticles were thermally stable, confirmed by TG-DSC analysis. The hydrodynamic diameter and zeta potentials were 218 nm and −46.8 mV. The binding energy of the elements was found by XPS analysis. The degradation efficiency of the photocatalyst was found to be 87% against methylene blue. The antibacterial and antioxidant activity of the nanoparticles were concentration-dependent. The nanoparticles were active for glucose sensor application.

Author Contributions: Conceptualization, M.W.A. and B.S.; Data curation, M.F. and A.A.; Formal analysis, W.A. and S.N.; Funding acquisition, M.W.A. and H.A.; Investigation, H.S.A.Q., W.A. and S.N.; Methodology, H.S.A.Q. and W.A.; Project administration, M.W.A., H.A. and B.S.; Resources, M.W.A. and H.S.A.Q.; Software, M.F.; Supervision, M.W.A. and B.S.; Writing—original draft, M.W.A., H.S.A.Q. and B.S.; Writing—review & editing, M.W.A., W.A., S.N., A.A., M.F. and H.A. All authors have read and agreed to the published version of the manuscript.

Funding: This work was supported by Al Bilad Bank Scholarly Chair for Food Security in Saudi Arabia, the Deanship of Scientific Research, Vice Presidency for Graduate Studies and Scientific Research, King Faisal University, Saudi Arabia [Project No. CHAIR36] and Princess Nourah bint Abdulrahman University Project number (PNURSP2022R29).

Institutional Review Board Statement: Not applicable.

Informed Consent Statement: Not applicable.

Data Availability Statement: Data is contained within this article.

Acknowledgments: This work was supported by Al Bilad Bank Scholarly Chair for Food Security in Saudi Arabia, the Deanship of Scientific Research, Vice Presidency for Graduate Studies and Scientific Research, King Faisal University, Saudi Arabia [Project No. CHAIR36]. We thank the Princess Nourah bint Abdulrahman University Researchers for Supporting Project number (PNURSP2022R29), Princess Nourah bint Abdulrahman University, Riyadh, Saudi Arabia.

Conflicts of Interest: The authors declare no conflict of interest.

References

1. Hoo, X.F.; Abdul Razak, K.; Ridhuan, N.S.; Mohamad Nor, N.; Zakaria, N.D. Electrochemical glucose biosensor based on ZnO nanorods modified with gold nanoparticles. *J. Mater. Sci. Mater. Electron.* **2019**, *30*, 7460–7470. [CrossRef]
2. Steiner, M.; Duerkop, A.; Wolfbeis, O. Optical methods for sensing glucose. *Chem. Soc. Rev.* **2011**, *40*, 4805–4839. [CrossRef]
3. Coster, S.; Gulliford, M.C.; Seed, P.T.; Powrie, J.K.; Swaminathan, R. Monitoring blood glucose control in diabetes mellitus: A systematic review. *Health Technol. Assess.* **2000**, *4*, 1–93. [CrossRef]
4. Demiate, I.M.; Konkel, F.E.; Pedroso, R.A. Enzymatic determination of starch in doce de leite using dialysis. *Food Sci. Technol.* **2001**, *21*, 339–342. [CrossRef]
5. Xavier, J.; Lemaitre, R.N.; Rea, T.D.; Sotoodehnia, N.; Empana, J.; Siscovick, D.S. Diabetes, glucose level, and risk of sudden cardiac death. *Eur. Heart J.* **2005**, *26*, 2142–2147.
6. Mislovicova, D.; Michalkova, E.; Vikartovska, A. Immobilized glucose oxidase on different supports for biotransformation removal of glucose from oligosaccharide mixtures. *Process Biochem.* **2007**, *42*, 704–709. [CrossRef]
7. Beitollahi, H.; Tajik, S.; di Bartolomeo, A. Application of MnO2 nanorod-ionic liquid modified carbon paste electrode for the voltammetric determination of sulfanilamide. *Micromachines* **2022**, *13*, 598. [CrossRef]
8. Tajik, S.; Afshar, A.A.; Shamsaddini, S.; Askari, M.B.; Dourandish, Z.; Nejad, F.G.; Beitollahi, H.; di Bartolomeo, A. Fe_3O_4@MoS_2/rGO nanocomposite/ionic liquid modified carbon paste electrode for electrochemical sensing of Dasatinib in the presence of doxorubicin. *Ind. Eng. Chem. Res.* **2022**. [CrossRef]
9. Alam, M.W. Electrochemical sensing of dextrose and photocatalytic activities by nickel ferrite nanoparticles synthesized by probe sonication method. *Curr. Nanosci.* **2021**, *17*, 893–903. [CrossRef]
10. Li, M.; Zhao, Z.; Liu, X.; Xiong, Y.; Han, C.; Zhang, Y.; Bo, X.; Guo, L. Novel bamboo leaf shaped CuO nanorod@hollow carbon fibers derived from plant biomass for efficient and non-enzymatic glucose detection. *Analyst* **2015**, *140*, 6412–6420. [CrossRef]

11. Yin, H.; Zhu, J.; Chen, J.; Gong, J.; Nie, Q. Hierarchical $CuCo_2O_4$/C microspheres assembled with nanoparticle-stacked nanosheets for sensitive non-enzymatic glucose detection. *J. Mater. Sci.* **2018**, *53*, 11951–11961. [CrossRef]
12. Zhang, D.; Zhang, X.; Bu, Y.; Zhang, J.; Zhang, R. Copper cobalt sulfide structures derived from MOF precursors with enhanced electrochemical glucose sensing properties. *Nanomaterials* **2022**, *12*, 1394. [CrossRef]
13. Dourandish, Z.; Tajik, S.; Beitollahi, H.; Jahani, P.M.; Nejad, F.G.; Sheikhshoaie, I.; di Bartolomeo, A. A comprehensive review of metal organic framework: Synthesis, characterization, and investigation of their application in electrochemical biosensors for biomedical analysis. *Sensors* **2022**, *22*, 2238. [CrossRef]
14. Iqbal, T.; Irfan, F.; Afsheen, S.; Zafar, M.; Naeem, S.; Raza, A. Synthesis and characterization of Ag-TiO_2 nanocomposites to study their effect on seed germination. *Appl. Nanosci.* **2021**, *11*, 2043–2057. [CrossRef]
15. Hoseinpour, V.; Ghaemi, N. Novel ZnO-MnO_2-Cu_2O triple nanocomposite: Facial synthesis, characterization, antibacterial activity and visible light photocatalytic performance for dyes degradation-A comparative study. *Mater. Res. Express* **2018**, *5*, 085012. [CrossRef]
16. Tedla, H.; Diaz, I.; Kebede, T.; Taddesse, A.M. Synthesis, characterization and photocatalytic activity of zeolite supported ZnO/Fe_2O_3/MnO_2 nanocomposites. *J. Environ. Chem. Eng.* **2015**, *3*, 1586–1591. [CrossRef]
17. Pranesh, S.; Nagaraju, J. Nano sized ZnO/MnO_2/Gd_2O_3 ternary heterostructuctures for enhanced photocatalysis. *Curr. Nanomater.* **2020**, *5*, 36–46. [CrossRef]
18. Zou, X.; Dong, Y.; Ke, J.; Ge, H.; Chen, D.; Sun, H.; Cui, Y. Cobalt monoxide/tunsten trioxide p-n heterojunction boosting charge separation for efficient visible-light driven gaseous toluene degradation. *Chem. Eng. J.* **2020**, *400*, 125919. [CrossRef]
19. Sharma, G.; Garica-Penas, A.; Kumar, A.; Naushad, M.; Mola, G.T.; Alshehri, S.M.; Ahmed, J.; Alhokbany, N.; Stadler, F.J. Fe/La/Zn nanocomposite with graphene oxide for photodegradation of phenylhydrazine. *J. Mol. Liq.* **2019**, *285*, 362–374. [CrossRef]
20. Zhang, L.; Jiang, Y.; Ding, Y.; Povey, M.; York, D. Investigation into the antibacterial behaviour of suspensions of ZnO nanoparticles (ZnO nanofluids). *J. Nanopart. Res.* **2007**, *9*, 479–489. [CrossRef]
21. Al-Hazmi, F.; Alnowaiser, F.; Al-Ghamdi, A.A.; Al-Ghamdi, A.A.; Aly, M.M.; Al-Tuwirqi, R.M.; El-Tantawy, F. A new large-scale synthesis of magnesium oxide nanowires: Structural and antibacterial properties. *Superlattices Microstruct.* **2012**, *52*, 200–209. [CrossRef]
22. Lv, M.; Su, S.; He, Y.; Huang, Q.; Hu, W.; Li, D.; Fan, C.; Lee, S.T. Long-term antimicrobial effect of silicon nanowires decorated with silver nanoparticles. *Adv. Mater.* **2010**, *22*, 5463–5467. [CrossRef]
23. Flores-González, M.; Talavera-Rojas, M.; Soriano-Vargas, E.; Rodríguez-González, V. Practical mediated-assembly synthesis of silver nanowires using commercial Camellia sinensis extracts and their antibacterial properties. *New J. Chem.* **2018**, *42*, 2133–2139. [CrossRef]
24. Ringwal, S.; Bartwal, A.S.; Semwal, A.R.; Sati, S.C. Review on green synthesized nanocomposites and their biological activities. *J. Mt. Res.* **2021**, *16*, 181–186. [CrossRef]
25. Moradiya, M.A.; Khiriya, P.K.; Tripathi, G.K.; Bundela, P.; Khare, P.S. The investigation of Microwave assisted greener synthesis of Ag/Ti/Zn trimetallic nanoparticles and carbon quantum dots nanocomposites in the application of solar cell. *Lett. Appl. NanoBioSci.* **2022**, *11*, 3102–3110.
26. Vaseghi, Z.; Tavakoli, O.; Nematollahzadeh, A. Rapid biosynthesis of novel Cu/Cr/Ni trimetallic oxide nanoparticles with antimicrobial activity. *J. Environ. Chem. Eng.* **2018**, *6*, 1898–1911. [CrossRef]
27. Noushin, A.; Varasteh Moradi, A.; Sayyed Alangi, S.Z.; Hosseini, Z. Green synthesis and evaluation of antioxidant and antimicrobial activity of new dihydropyrroloazepines: Using bio-Ag/CdO/ZnO@MWCNTs nanocomposites as a reusable organometallic catalyst. *Appl. Organimetallic Chem.* **2021**, *35*, 6295. [CrossRef]
28. Moongraksathum, B.; Shang, J.-Y.; Chen, Y.-W. Photocatalytic Antibacterial Effectiveness of Cu-Doped TiO2 Thin Film Prepared via the Peroxo Sol-Gel Method. *Catalysts* **2018**, *8*, 352. [CrossRef]
29. Rajaramanan, T.; Shanmugaratnam, S.; Gurunanthanan, V.; Yohi, S.; Velauthapillai, D.; Ravirajan, P.; Senthilnanthanan, M. Cost Effective Solvothermal Method to Synthesize Zn-Doped TiO_2 Nanomaterials for Photovoltaic and Photocatalytic Degradation Applications. *Catalysts* **2021**, *11*, 690. [CrossRef]
30. Maharubin, S.; Nayak, C.; Phatak, O.; Kurhade, A.; Singh, M.; Zhou, Y.; Tan, G. Polyvinylchloride coated with silver nanoparticles and zinc oxide nanowires for antimicrobial applications. *Mater. Lett.* **2019**, *249*, 108–111. [CrossRef]
31. Marie, M.; Manoharan, A.; Kuchuk, A.; Ang, S.; Manasreh, M.O. Vertically grown zinc oxide nanorods functionalized with ferric oxide for *in vivo* and non-enzymatic glucose detection. *Nanotechnology* **2017**, *29*, 115501. [CrossRef] [PubMed]
32. Ahmad, R.; Tripathy, N.; Ahn, M.S.; Bhat, K.S.; Mahmoudi, T.; Wang, Y.; Yoo, J.; Kwon, D.; Yang, H.; Hahn, Y. Highly efficient non-enzymatic glucose sensor based on CuO modified vertically grown ZnO nanorods on electrode. *Sci. Rep.* **2017**, *7*, 5715. [CrossRef] [PubMed]
33. Chen, J.; de Zhang, W.; Ye, J. Non enzymatic electrochemical glucose sensor based on MnO2/MWNTs nanocomposite. *Electrochem. Commun.* **2008**, *10*, 1268–1271. [CrossRef]
34. Raha, S.; Mohanta, D.; Ahmaruzzaman, M. Novel CuO/Mn_3O_4/ZnO nanocomposite with superior photocatalytic activity for removal of rabeprazole from water. *Sci. Rep.* **2021**, *11*, 15187. [CrossRef] [PubMed]

35. Ogunyemi, S.O.; Zhang, M.; Abdallah, Y.; Ahmed, T.; Qiu, W.; Ali, M.; Yan, C.; Yang, Y.; Chen, J.; Li, B. The bio-synthesis of three metal oxide nanoparticles (ZnO, MnO_2, and MgO) and their antibacterial activity against the bacterial leaf blight pathogen. *Front. Microbiol.* **2020**, *11*, 588326. [CrossRef] [PubMed]
36. Yan, Q.; Cai, Z. Issues in preparation of metal-lignin nanocomposites by co-precipitation method. *J. Inorg. Organomet. Polym. Mater.* **2021**, *31*, 978–996. [CrossRef]
37. Alam, M.W.; Al Qahtani, H.S.; Aamir, M.; Abuzir, A.; Khan, M.S.; Albuhulayqah, M.; Mushtaq, S.; Zaidi, N.; Ramya, A. Phyto Synthesis of Manganese-Doped Zinc Nanoparticles Using Carica papaya Leaves: Structural Properties and Its Evaluation for Catalytic, Antibacterial and Antioxidant Activities. *Polymers* **2022**, *14*, 1827. [CrossRef]
38. Burygin, G.L.; Khlebtsov, B.N.; Shantrokha, A.N.; Dykman, L.A.; Bogatyrev, V.A.; Khlebtsov, N.G. On the enhanced antibacterial activity of antibiotics mixed with gold nanoparticles. *Nanoscale Res. Lett.* **2009**, *4*, 794–801. [CrossRef]
39. Juma, A.O.; Arbab, E.A.A.; Muiva, C.M.; Lepodise, L.M.; Mola, G.T. Synthesis and characterization of CuO-NiO-ZnO mixed metal oxide nanocomposite. *J. Alloys Compd.* **2017**, *723*, 866–872. [CrossRef]
40. Enhessari, M.; Salehabadi, A.; Maarofian, K.; Khanahmadzadeh, S. Synthesis and physicochemical properties of CuMn2O4 nanoparticles; a potential semiconductor for photoelectric devices. *Int. J. Bio-Inorg. Hybrid Nanomater.* **2016**, *5*, 115–120.
41. Sanchez, J.S.; Pendashteh, A.; Palma, J.; Anderson, M.; Marcilla, R. Porous NiCoMn trimetal oxide/graphene nanocomposites for high performance hybrid energy storage devices. *Electrochim. Acta* **2018**, *279*, 44–56. [CrossRef]
42. Guo, H.; Zhu, Q.; Wu, X.; Jiang, Y.; Xie, X.; Xu, A. Oxygen deficient ZnO1-x nanosheets with high visible light photocatalytic activity. *Nanoscale* **2015**, *7*, 7216–7223. [CrossRef] [PubMed]
43. Kosova, N.V.; Devyatkina, E.T.; Kaichev, V.V. Mixed layered Ni-Mn-Co hydroxides: Crystal structure, electronic state of ions, and thermal decomposition. *J. Power Source* **2007**, *174*, 735–740. [CrossRef]
44. Pal, S.; Maiti, S.; Maiti, U. Chattopadhyay, Low temperature solution processed ZnO/CuO heterojunction photocatalyst for visible light induced photo-degradation of organic pollutants. *Cryst. Eng. Comm.* **2015**, *17*, 1464–1476. [CrossRef]
45. Wu, Z.S.; Ren, W.; Wen, L.; Gao, L.; Zhao, J.; Chen, Z.; Zhou, G.; Li, F.; Cheng, H.M. Graphene anchored with Co_3O_4 nanoparticles as anode of lithium ion capacity and cyclic performance. *ACS Nano* **2010**, *4*, 3187–3194. [CrossRef]
46. Jerng, S.; Yu, D.S.; Lee, J.H.; Kim, C.; Yoon, S.; Chun, S. Graphitic carbon growth on crystalline and amorphous oxide substrates using molecular beam epitaxy. *Nanoscale Res. Lett.* **2011**, *6*, 565–571. [CrossRef]
47. Freitas, C.; Muller, R.H. Effect of light and temperature on zeta potential and physical stability in solid lipid nanoparticle (SLN (TM)) dispersions. *Int. J. Pharm.* **1998**, *168*, 221–229. [CrossRef]
48. Vanaja, A.; Suresh, M.; Jeevanandam, J.; Gousia, S.; Pavan, D.; Balaji, D.; Murthy, N.B. Copper-doped zinc oxide nanoparticles for the fabrication of white LEDs. *Prot. Met. Phys. Chem. Surf.* **2019**, *55*, 481–486. [CrossRef]
49. Khalid, A.; Ahmad, P.; Alharthi, A.I.; Muhammad, S.; Khandaker, M.U.; Rehman, M. Mohammad Rashed Iqbal Faruque, Israf Ud Din, Mshari A. Alotaibi, Khalid Alzimami, David A. Bradley, Structural, optical and antibacterial efficacy of pure and zinc doped copper oxide against pathogenic bacteria. *Nanomaterials* **2021**, *11*, 451. [CrossRef]
50. Abel, M.J.; Pramothkumar, A.; Senthilkumar, N.; Jothivenkatachalam, K.; Inbaraj, P.F.H.; Prince, J.J. Flake-like $CuMn_2O_4$ nanoparticles synthesized via co-precipitation method for photocatalytic activity. *Phys. B Condens. Matter* **2019**, *572*, 117–124.
51. Devi, S.M.; Nivetha, A.; Prabha, I. Role of citric acid/glycine-reinforced nanometal oxide for the enhancement of physio-chemical specifications in catalytic properties. *J. Supercond. Nov. Magn.* **2020**, *33*, 3893–3901. [CrossRef]
52. Shanmugam, V.; Jeyaperumal, K.S. Investigations of visible light driven Sn and Cu doped ZnO hybrid nanoparticles for photocatalytic performance and antibacterial activity. *Appl. Surf. Sci.* **2018**, *449*, 617–630. [CrossRef]
53. Ahmad, M.M.; Kotb, H.M.; Mushtaq, S.; Waheed-Ur-Rehman, M.; Maghanga, C.M.; Alam, M.W. Green synthesis of Mn+Cu bimetallic nanoparticles using vinca rosea extract and their antioxidant, antibacterial, and catalytic activities. *Crystals* **2022**, *12*, 72. [CrossRef]
54. Liu, X.; Wang, C.; Zheng, Z.; Liu, W. Synthesis and Characterization of ultra-fine bimetallic Ag-Cu nanoparticles as die attach materials. In Proceedings of the International Conference on Electronic Packaging Technology (ICEPT) 2016, Wuhan, China, 16–19 August 2016; pp. 206–208.
55. Alam, M.W.; Aamir, M.; Farhan, M.; Albuhulayqah, M.; Ahmad, M.M.; Ravikumar, C.R.; Kumar, V.G.D.; Murthy, H.C.A. Green synthesis of Ni-Cu-Zn based nanosized metal oxides for photocatalytic and sensor applications. *Crystals* **2021**, *11*, 1467. [CrossRef]
56. Lin, J.; Luo, Z.; Liu, J.; Li, P. Photocatalytic degradation of methylene blue in aqueous solution by using ZnO-SnO_2 nanocomposites. *Mater. Sci. Semicond. Process.* **2018**, *87*, 24–41. [CrossRef]
57. Koli, P.B.; Kapadnis, K.H.; Deshpande, U.G.; Patil, M.R. Fabrication and characterization of pure and modified Co_3O_4 nanocatalyst and their application for photocatalytic degradation of eosine blue dye: A comparative study. *J. Nanostruct. Chem.* **2018**, *8*, 453–463. [CrossRef]
58. Alzahrani, K.E.; Niazy, A.A.; Alswieleh, A.M.; Wahab, R.; El-Toni, A.M.; Alghamdi, H.S. Antibacterial activity of trimetal (CuZnFe) oxide nanoparticles. *Int. J. Nanomed.* **2018**, *13*, 77–87. [CrossRef]

antioxidants

MDPI

Article

β-Sitosterol Glucoside-Loaded Nanosystem Ameliorates Insulin Resistance and Oxidative Stress in Streptozotocin-Induced Diabetic Rats

Sherif M. Afifi [1,*], Naglaa M. Ammar [2], Rabab Kamel [3], Tuba Esatbeyoglu [4,*] and Heba A. Hassan [2]

1 Pharmacognosy Department, Faculty of Pharmacy, University of Sadat City, Sadat City 32897, Egypt
2 Therapeutic Chemistry Department, National Research Centre, 33 El Bohouth St., Dokki, Giza 12622, Egypt; nm.ammar@nrc.sci.eg (N.M.A.); ha.el-saud@nrc.sci.eg (H.A.H.)
3 Pharmaceutical Technology Department, National Research Centre, Cairo 12622, Egypt; rk.mahmoud@nrc.sci.eg
4 Department of Food Development and Food Quality, Institute of Food Science and Human Nutrition, Gottfried Wilhelm Leibniz University Hannover, Am Kleinen Felde 30, 30167 Hannover, Germany
* Correspondence: sherif.afifi@fop.usc.edu.eg (S.M.A.); esatbeyoglu@lw.uni-hannover.de (T.E.); Tel.: +49-511-762-5589 (T.E.)

Abstract: β-Sitosterol glucoside (SG), isolated from *Senecio petasitis* (Family Asteraceae), was loaded in self-nanoemulsifying drug delivery systems (SEDDS) in a trial to enhance its solubility and biological effect. Various co-surfactants were tested to prepare a successful SEDDS. The selected SG-loaded SEDDS had a droplet size of 134 ± 15.2 nm with a homogenous distribution (polydispersity index 0.296 ± 0.02). It also demonstrated a significant augmentation of SG in vitro release by 4-fold compared to the free drug suspension. The in vivo insulin sensitivity and antidiabetic effect of the prepared SG-loaded SEDDS were further assessed in streptozotocin-induced hyperglycemic rats. The hypoglycemic effect of SG-loaded nanosystem was evidenced by decreased serum glucose and insulin by 63.22% and 53.11%, respectively. Homeostasis model assessment-insulin resistance (HOMA-IR) index demonstrated a significant reduction by 5.4-fold in the diabetic group treated by SG-loaded nanosystem and exhibited reduced glucagon level by 40.85%. In addition, treatment with SG-loaded nanosystem significantly decreased serum MDA (malondialdehyde) and increased catalase levels by 38.31% and 64.45%, respectively. Histopathological investigations also supported the protective effect of SG-loaded nanosystem on the pancreas. The promising ability of SG-loaded nanosystem to ameliorate insulin resistance, protect against oxidative stress, and restore pancreatic β-cell secretory function warrants its inclusion in further studies during diabetes progression.

Keywords: antidiabetic; glucagon; insulin resistance; malondialdehyde; nanoemulsion; oxidative stress; release study; SEDDS; *Senecio petasitis*

1. Introduction

Diabetes mellitus (DM) is a metabolic disease marked by excessively high blood glucose levels because of insufficient endogenous insulin production or activity. As a result of increased intake of high-calorie meals and greater adoption of a sedentary lifestyle, its incidence has increased. It is a serious public health issue around the world. In 2017, more than 425 million people were diagnosed with diabetes [1]. Microvascular complications, such as nerve injury (neuropathy), renal system damage (nephropathy), eye damage (retinopathy), cardiovascular disease, stroke, and peripheral vascular disease, are all indications of diabetes complications [2]. Type 2 diabetes mellitus (T2DM) can cause long-term production of reactive oxygen species and damage to organs like the eyes, nerves, kidneys, and blood vessels if not treated properly [3]. Diet therapy, pharmacology, and insulin therapy are the basic treatment approaches for diabetes control, along with a large range of glucose-lowering medications that exert hypoglycemic effects through diverse mechanisms [4].

These therapy alternatives, however, have not gained much traction because they are frequently linked with limitations such as medication resistance, side effects, and toxicity. Due to the safe and non-toxic aspect of herbal-based medications, supplementation of hypoglycemia pharmaceutical drugs to treat DM is now a potential and unique therapeutic method, regardless of the presence of these hypoglycemic pharmacological drugs [5]. Insulin resistance is a condition in blunted response to insulin stimulation of target tissues [6], and it manifests as hyperglycemia and compensative hyper-insulinemia [7].

Senecio petasitis, also known as *Roldana petasitis* or velvet groundsel, is an evergreen shrub of the family Asteraceae/Compositae [8]. The daisy or Asteraceae family includes over 1900 genera, providing cooking oils and leaf vegetables, viz., sunflower seeds, artichokes, and lettuce [9]. The genus *Senecio*, meaning "old man" in Latin, is considered one of the largest genera of flowering plants, containing over 1500 species distributed almost worldwide [10]. The *Senecio* species has been used for the treatment of wounds and as vasodilator, anti-inflammatory, and antiemetic preparations in folk medicine [11]. The genus *Senecio* is a rich source of pyrrolizidine alkaloids, cacalolides, and eremophilanolides [12]. *S. petasitis* is native to Mexico and characterized by a yellow daisy-like flower [13]. Despite its therapeutic characteristics, viz., anti-parasitic, anti-inflammatory, anti-cancer, and immunomodulatory [14], β-sitosterol glucoside (SG) has received little attention as a natural product due to its low water solubility, which limits its bioavailability; however, this can be enhanced by incorporation into the proposed self-emulsifying delivery system. To the best of our knowledge, there were no studies reported the effect of SG on glucagon levels or insulin resistance in diabetic conditions [15].

Self-emulsifying drug delivery systems (SEDDS) is one of the nanotechnology-based platforms investigated to overcome the problem of poor bioavailability of aqueous insoluble active ingredients. This nanosystem is an isotropic mixture classified as a lipid-based one that is composed of the active agent, the oil, and the surfactant/co-surfactant. SEDDS forms a nanoemulsion upon dilution with the gastrointestinal tract fluids and hence can augment the drug absorption, bioavailability, and performance [16]. In addition, the surfactant used as an ingredient of the formula can interfere with the membranes lipid bilayer and enhance drug permeability through the biological membrane, along with decreasing the possible toxic effects encountered when using the surfactant in the free form [17]. Hence, besides offering a better drug bioavailability, a SEDDS provides different advantages comprising the ease of preparation and possibility of scaling-up without the need for complex procedures or high external energy [18].

The current study evaluated the impact of SG-loaded SEEDS on glucose homeostasis and insulin regulation in order to better understand the role of SG in diabetes management. For the first time, after treatment with SG-loaded nanosystem, we employed insulin tolerance tests (ITTs) to measure insulin sensitivity and the homeostatic model assessment (HOMA) to describe insulin resistance.

2. Materials and Methods

2.1. Plant Material

S. petasitis aerial parts were collected from El-Orman botanical garden in Cairo (Egypt). The plant was kindly identified by Prof. Dr. M. El-Gebally, a botanist specialist, and confirmed with published literature [10]. A voucher sample (SP-09-07-13-05) was kept in the Herbarium of El-Orman botanical garden, Cairo, Egypt.

2.2. Chemicals

Streptozotocin (STZ) (>98%), linoleic acid (LA), propylene glycol (PG), and Tween 80 (T80) were purchased from Sigma-Aldrich (St. Louis, MO, USA), and insulin (Actarapid) was purchased from a pharmacy. Acconon® MC8-2 EP/NF (polyoxyethylene-8 caprylic/capric glycerides) and Captex 200® (propylene glycol dicaprylocaprate) were kindly offered by ABITEC Corporations, Cleveland, OH, USA, while Labrafil® M1944LS (decyl polyglucoside) was a free sample from Gattefosse (Saint-Priest, France). All other chemicals used were of analytical grade.

2.3. Experimental Animals

Forty male Wistar albino rats, weighing 150–170 g, were obtained from the National Research Centre's animal house. Animal handling followed the Medical Ethical Committee of Egypt's National Research Centre's ethical guidelines. The animals were housed separately and given free access to food and water. The protocol of experimental conditions was accepted by the National Regulations on Animal Welfare and Institutional Animal Ethical Committee (IAEC) (Approval no: 6443042021).

2.4. Extraction and Isolation

The lyophilized pulverized aerial parts of *S. petasitis* (800 g) were extracted by ethanol (2 × 5 L), then the concentrated extract (90 g) was suspended in distilled water and fractionated using methylene chloride (3 × 400 mL). Column chromatography packed with silica gel (500 g, 70–230 mesh, 4 × 100 cm) was used to isolate the SG from methylene chloride fraction (30 g) through gradient elution of methylene chloride and increasing percentage of methanol. The eluted fractions were monitored using thin layer chromatography (TLC, 250 μm thickness, KGF Silica gel 60, Merck, Darmstadt, Germany) sprayed with 10% H_2SO_4. The fraction eluted with 80% methylene chloride yielded SG (95.6% purity) as white crystals precipitated by methanol.

2.5. Spectroscopic Characterization

Spectroscopic techniques such as infrared (IR), and proton nuclear magnetic resonance (^{1}H-NMR and ^{13}C-NMR) were employed to explore the structure of the SG. IR spectrum was acquired on a Shimadzu IR-400 spectrometer (Kyoto, Japan), and the ^{1}H-NMR and ^{13}C-NMR spectra were recorded in DMSO-d_6 on Bruker Ascend TM400/R (Rheinstetten, Germany) at 400 MHz and 100 MHz, respectively.

2.6. Preparation of SEDDS

The surfactant, co-surfactant, and oil combination (S/CoS/oil) with a ratio of 45:45:10 (*w*/*w*/*w*) was used to prepare the SEDDSs. Tween 80 (T80) and linoleic acid (LA) were used as the surfactant and oil, respectively, while propylene glycol (PG), Acconon® MC8-2 EP/NF (AC), Captex ®200 (C200), and Labrafil® M1944LS (LB) were used as the co-surfactants. The ternary mixtures were stirred by vortex mixing (Julabo Labortechnik, Seelbach, Germany) and left 21 h for equilibrium at room temperature to form homogenous isotropic mixtures [19].

2.7. Infinite Dilution Capacity

The infinite dilution capacity of the prepared systems was assessed based on the previously documented visual method [20]. Each tested system (1 g) was diluted gradually with 20 mL of distilled water at 37 ± 0.5 °C with continuous stirring using a magnetic stirrer. Only systems forming a clear nanoemulsion within 1 min were selected to continue the evaluation.

2.8. Percentage Transmittance

The percentage transmittance was measured at 560 nm using a Shimadzu UV spectrophotometer (2401/PC, Tokyo, Japan) and deionized water was used as a blank. The selected SEDDS formulation (1 mL) was diluted with distilled water (1:100).

2.9. Drug Loading

The drug-loaded SEDDS was prepared by adding SG to the selected system (10 mg/mL) with continuous stirring using a magnetic stirrer at 40 °C until the formation of a clear and transparent system.

2.10. Droplet Size Determination, Polydispersity Index, and Zeta Potential

The mean droplet size and the size distribution expressed as polydispersity index (PDI), in addition to the zeta potential (Z) of the selected system were measured using a Zetasizer (Nano-ZS, Malvern Instruments Ltd., Malvern, UK) after doing the suitable dilution with distilled water (1:10).

2.11. In Vitro Release Studies

Release studies were done by the dialysis bag diffusion method widely used to test drug release from nanosystems [21,22]. The cellulose membrane (12,000–14,000 MWT) was filled with 1 mL of the drug-loaded SEDDS or the drug suspension containing an equivalent amount of the drug, then both ends of the bags were tied, and the dialysis bags were placed in beakers containing 100 mL phosphate buffer (pH 6.8)/Tween 80 (2.5% *w*/*v*) [23] to assure sink conditions (rotation at 100 rpm for 24 h at 37.0 ± 0.1 °C). At different time intervals up to 24 h, samples (2 mL) were drawn and replaced with an equal volume of fresh medium. A similar set was run in parallel for the unmedicated SEDDS (blank) following the same experimental conditions to eliminate any possible interference. The cumulative amount of drug released was quantitatively determined at 266 nm using Shimadzu UV-2401PC and release profiles were plotted. The experiments were carried out in triplicate and data was expressed as mean value ± S.D.

2.12. Transmission Electron Microscopy (TEM)

The micro-morphological structure of the selected nanosystem was investigated by transmission electron microscopy (JEM-1 230; Jeol, Tokyo, Japan). A droplet of diluted preparation was placed on carbon film-coated copper grids and negatively stained with phosphotungstic acid solution 2% (*w*/*w*), and then allowed to dry before examination.

2.13. Induction of Diabetes

After acclimatization for a week, 40 rats were divided equally into five groups (8 rats for each) as follows: normal control (G1), streptozotocin (STZ)-induced diabetic control (G2), SG suspension-treated diabetic (20 mg/kg) (G3) [24], unmedicated nanosystem-treated diabetic group (G4), and medicated nanosystem-treated diabetic (G5).

The animals in the normal control group were fed normal chow pellets for the duration of the experiment. The remaining animals, on the other hand, were fed a high-fat diet (HFD) for two weeks to induce insulin resistance. The compositions of HFD were as follows: sucrose 20%, cholesterol 2.5%, lard fat 10%, and powdered normal chow pellets 67.5% [25], and 25% fructose in drinking water [26]. The diet was kept up until the end of the experiment. T2DM was next produced in the rats by giving them 45 mg/kg body weight (BW) of STZ (Sigma-Aldrich, St. Louis, MO, USA) [27]. STZ was freshly dissolved in 0.1 mol/L sodium citrate buffer for this experiment (pH 4.5). Rats with blood glucose levels above 250 mg/dL seven days after induction of diabetes were regarded to have T2DM. Once diabetes was proven, all treated groups (6 rats for each) were administered by gavage needle for 21 days.

2.14. Collection of Blood and Tissue Samples

At the end of the experimental period, blood samples were collected from the eyes of all rats. Blood was drawn through cardiac puncture and immediately stored on ice for 3 h before being centrifuged for 15 min at 3000 rpm. The serum was then isolated and kept at −80 °C until further examination. For histopathological analysis, a small sample of pancreatic tissue from each animal was cut and stored in a 10% neutral buffered formalin solution at room temperature. Throughout the preservation period, each pancreas tissue sample's neutral buffered formalin was replenished weekly.

2.15. Measurements of Biochemical Parameters

After 12-h fast, fresh blood samples were taken from the rats' tail veins. Plasma glucose levels were measured using a blood glucose meter. In serum rats, insulin levels were determined using an enzyme-linked immunosorbent assay (ELISA) with a rat insulin ELISA kit (ELR-Insulin, RayBio®, Norcross, GA, USA) and glucagon levels were determined using an enzyme-linked immunosorbent assay (ELISA) with a rat glucagon ELISA kit (E-EL-R0523, Elabscience®, Bethesda, MD, USA). The insulin sensitivity of diabetic rats was measured using the homeostasis model assessment-insulin resistance (HOMA-IR) equation [28]:

(Fasting plasma insulin (μIU/mL) × Fasting blood glucose (mg/dL))/405.

In the ITT experiment, after fasting for 8 h, the rats were intraperitoneally injected with insulin at 0.5 IU/kg body weight [29], and blood samples were obtained at 0, 15, 30, and 60 min to evaluate glucose levels.

2.16. Determination of Serum Malondialdehyde (MDA)

Lipid peroxidation levels were determined in serum colorimetrically by measuring the content of thiobarbituric acid reactive product, MDA at 534 nm according to the method of Ohkawa, et al. [30] by using MDA kit (Cat no MD 25 29, Biodiagnostic, Dokki, Giza, Egypt).

2.17. Determination of Serum Catalase

Serum Catalase levels were determined colorimetrically according to the method of Aebi [31] by using a catalase kit (Cat no CA 25 17, Biodiagnostic, Dokki, Giza, Egypt).

2.18. Histopathological Examination of Pancreatic Tissue

Autopsy samples were obtained from the pancreas of rats in various groups and preserved for 24 h in 10% formal saline. After washing with tap water, dehydration was accomplished using serial dilutions of alcohol (methyl, ethyl, and absolute ethyl). Specimens were rinsed in xylene and embedded in paraffin for 24 h at 56 °C in a hot air oven. By using a sledge microtome, paraffin bee wax tissue blocks were formed for sectioning at a thickness of 4 microns. The tissue sections were mounted on glass slides, deparaffinized, and stained with hematoxylin and eosin for examination under a light electric microscope [32].

2.19. Statistical Analysis

Using software program GraphPad Prism (version 8.0), the data was analyzed by one-way analysis of variance (ANOVA) followed by Tukey comparison test. The difference was considered significant when $p < 0.05$.

3. Results and Discussion

3.1. Structure Identification of β-Sitosterol Glucoside

The total extract of *S. petasitis* (F: Asteraceae) aerial parts was chromatography fractionated and then purified, resulting in white needle crystals. IR spectrum revealed bands at 3384 and 1719 cm^{-1} owing to hydroxyl and ester groups, respectively. ^{1}H-NMR (400 MHz, DMSO-d_6) spectrum (Figure S1) exhibited six methyl (CH_3) signals, viz., two singlets at δ 0.63 and 0.94, three doublets at δ 0.80 (J = 6.2 Hz), 0.84 (J = 6.1 Hz), and 0.87 (J = 3.1 Hz), in addition to one triplicate at δ 0.91 (J = 6.8 Hz). Moreover, singlet olefinic proton at δ 5.31 and doublet anomeric proton at δ 4.24 (J = 7.6 Hz) were detected. Regarding the ^{13}C-NMR (100 MHz, DMSO-d_6) spectrum, six methyl (CH_3) signals were noticed at δ 11.82, 19.02, 19.18, 12.03, 18.69, and 19.75. Olefinic and anomeric carbons exhibited signals at δ 121.25 and 100.81, respectively. The aforementioned spectroscopic data was in accordance with previously published findings [33,34], indicating the identity of the compound as β-sitosterol glucoside.

3.2. Assessment of Self-Emulsification

The selection of convenient components to prepare the SEDDS is necessary to obtain a safe and effective nanosystem for pharmaceutical use. The systems under investigation were prepared using the oil and the surfactant in combination with different co-surfactants. The comparison between them was done based on the self-emulsifying capacity of the systems. The successful SEDDS should form a monophasic clear liquid upon dilution with water to allow for the active ingredient to be in a solubilized form upon contact with the gastrointestinal fluid after oral intake. Previous studies proved the crucial role of the co-surfactant, as it can maintain a stable uni-phase oil/water emulsion and form a flexible dynamic layer by diminishing the interfacial tension of the surfactant, so the drug incorporated in this high-energy nanosystem can easily diffuse through the flexible film formed between the phases, which facilitates its partitioning [35]. In addition, it can reduce the required number of surfactants and hence decrease their possible harmful effect.

It was reported that in a conventional emulsion, the different phases tend to separate upon dilution to reduce the interfacial area and the system's free energy. Controversially, in case of the SEDDS, the emulsification process can occur spontaneously, as the free energy needed to form the nanoemulsion is low [36].

Based on the visual examination to test the self-emulsification process upon dilution, it was detected that among all the prepared systems, only the one prepared with PG as a co-surfactant formed a clear nanoemulsion. The higher hydrophilicity of PG (short chain) compared to the other tested co-surfactants can explain its greater success. It was proved that a surfactant/co-surfactant mixture with higher hydrophilicity or hydrophilic lipophilic balance (HLB value) will help the formation of O/W type nanoemulsions [37]. The use of PG as a co-surfactant has previously proved a success in the preparation of this type of nanocarrier [38,39]. In another study, it was indicated that PG was essential to promote microemulsion formation as it increased the interfacial fluidity of the surfactant. Because of its high hydrophilicity, PG molecules are expected to partition into the aqueous phase and can also be partially incorporated into the polar parts of the surfactant layer, which reduces the rigidity of the condensed interfacial film [40]. Hence, this SEDDS was selected to continue the study.

3.3. Percentage Transmittance

The percentage transmittance of the selected SEDDS after dilution with distilled water (1:100) was $99.28 \pm 0.20\%$. Such a value can prove the formation of a clear nanoemulsion and indicate the successful preparation of a self-emulsifying drug delivery system.

3.4. Droplet Size Determination

The mean droplet size of the selected SG-loaded SEDDS was found to be 134 ± 15.2 nm, as shown in Figure 1. The nanoemulsion droplet size is a crucial factor influencing the self-emulsification process, and a small size can enhance the stability and facilitate the emulsification of the nanosystem [19,41].

The PDI was found to be equal to 0.296 ± 0.02, such a small value (≤ 0.3) showing the monomodal size of the tested nanosystem which indicates a homogenous uniform distribution. The Zeta potential (Z) value was -18.8 ± 3.80 mV (Figure 2) which can indicate the physical stability of the tested drug-loaded SEDDS and a low tendency to aggregate.

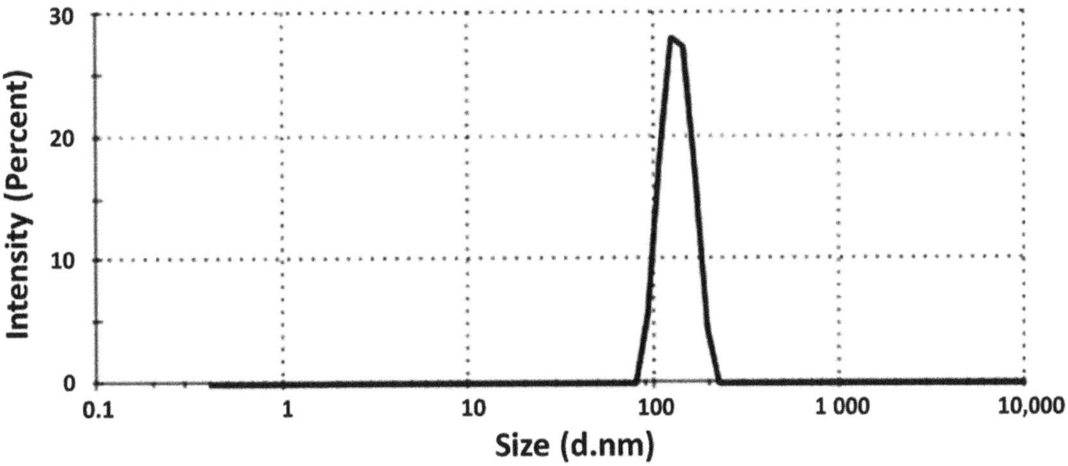

Figure 1. Particle size of the selected drug-loaded SEDDS.

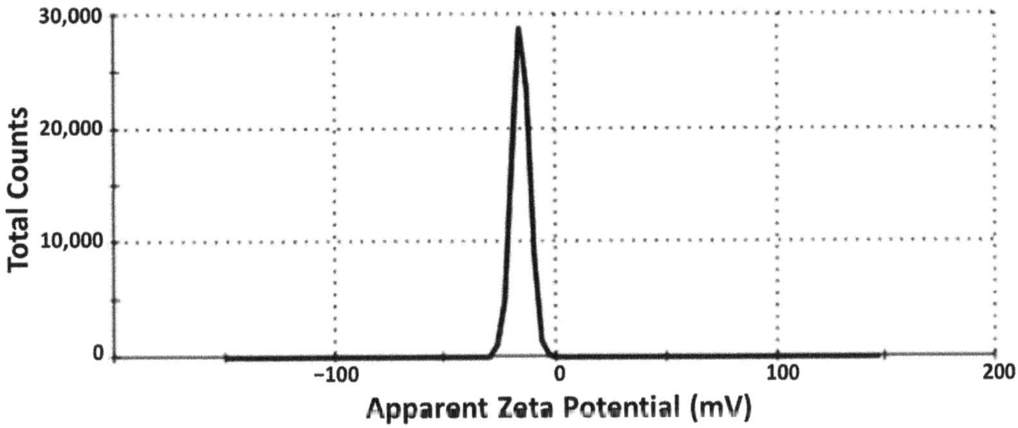

Figure 2. Zeta potential value of the selected drug-loaded SEDDS.

3.5. In Vitro Release Study

As seen in Figure 3, the prepared SG-loaded SEDDS significantly enhanced the drug release (~4-fold). After 24 h, the mean cumulative drug release was almost complete compared to only 25% in case of the free drug suspension, which can be explained by the capability of self-emulsifying drug delivery systems to solubilize aqueous insoluble drugs with the formation of fine-droplets nanoemulsions [19,42]. This can enhance drug absorption and bioavailability after oral administration and, in turn, ameliorate the biological efficacy.

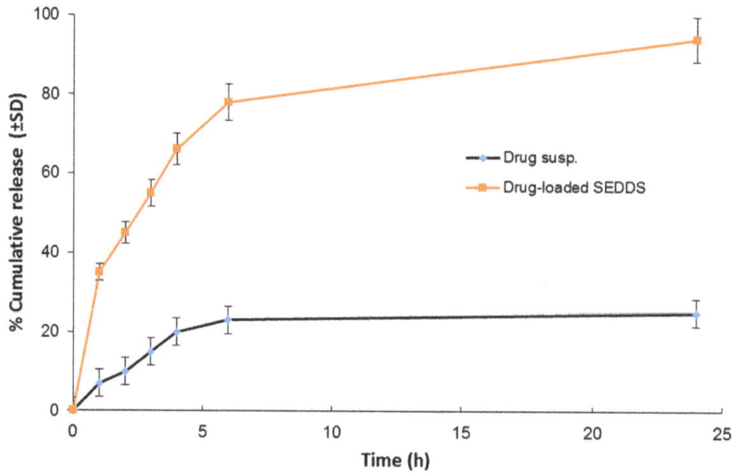

Figure 3. In vitro release study of the drug from the prepared SEDDS compared to the drug suspension.

3.6. Transmission Electron Microscopy

Figure 4 illustrates the microphotograph of the tested drug-loaded SEDDS. Almost spherical and separated dark spots, with a size approaching that was recorded by the Zetasizer, can be seen.

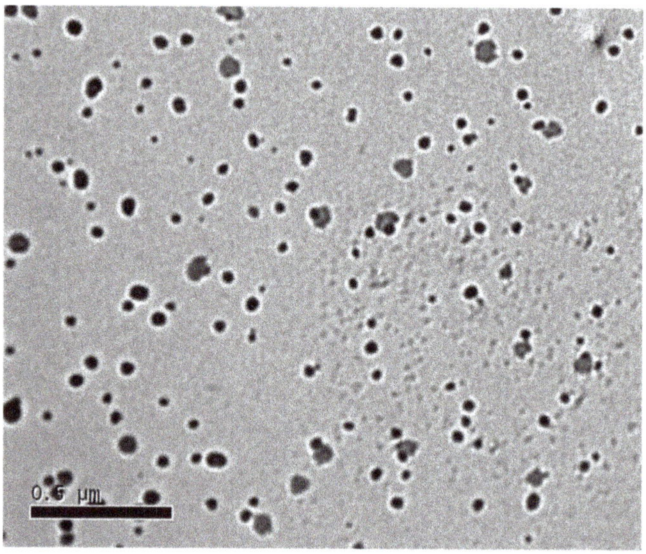

Figure 4. Transmission electron microscopy (TEM) photograph of the tested drug-loaded SEDDS.

All the displayed tests confirm the nanoencapsulation of the drug. In vivo studies comprising antidiabetic effect in streptozotocin-induced diabetic rats were performed to compare the efficacy of the drug-loaded SEDDS to the free drug suspension.

3.7. Effects of β-Sitosterol Glucoside on Body Weight and Serum Glucose

The effects of SG on body weight and serum glucose in STZ-induced diabetic rats were measured at the end of the experiment (Figure 5). There was a significant decrease ($p < 0.05$) in the body weight in the diabetic group with a reduction of 29.9% compared to the normal control group. On the other hand, the diabetic group treated with medicated nanosystem and drug suspension showed a significant increase ($p < 0.05$) in its weight (40.4% and 39.5%, respectively) compared to the diabetic control group (Figure 5A). Alternatively, there was a significant increase ($p < 0.05$) in the blood glucose level in the diabetic group compared to the control group and the diabetic group was ~4-fold higher than the normal control group. This level was significantly decreased ($p < 0.05$) in the diabetic group treated with medicated nanosystem and drug suspension when compared to the diabetic control group with a reduction of 63.2% and 47.1%, respectively (Figure 5B). The effect of medicated nanosystem on blood glucose was more comparable to drug suspension.

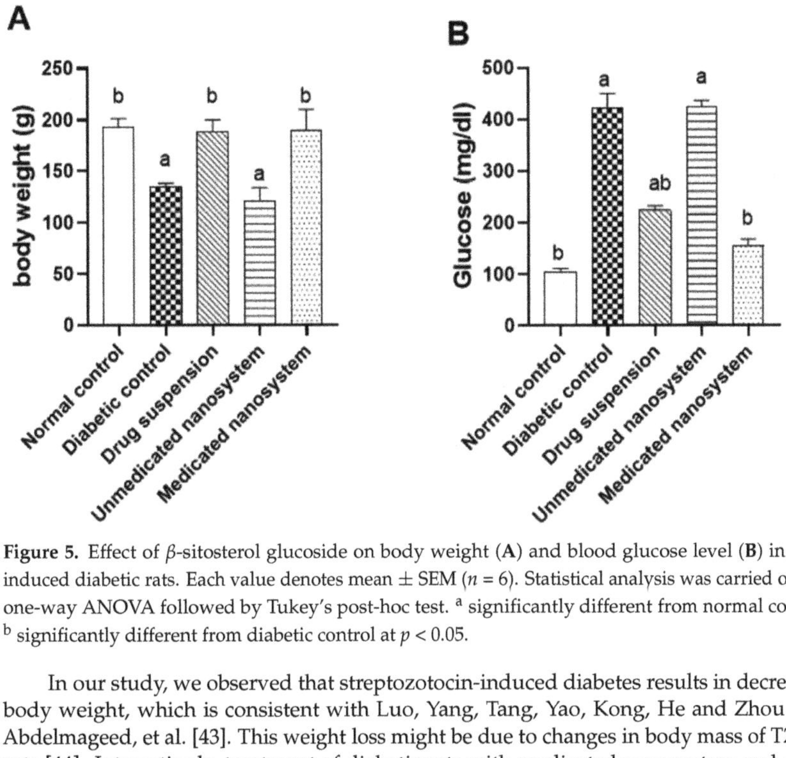

Figure 5. Effect of β-sitosterol glucoside on body weight (**A**) and blood glucose level (**B**) in STZ-induced diabetic rats. Each value denotes mean ± SEM ($n = 6$). Statistical analysis was carried out by one-way ANOVA followed by Tukey's post-hoc test. [a] significantly different from normal control. [b] significantly different from diabetic control at $p < 0.05$.

In our study, we observed that streptozotocin-induced diabetes results in decreased body weight, which is consistent with Luo, Yang, Tang, Yao, Kong, He and Zhou [25], Abdelmageed, et al. [43]. This weight loss might be due to changes in body mass of T2DM rats [44]. Interestingly, treatment of diabetic rats with medicated nanosystem and drug suspension improved body weight when compared with untreated diabetic rats.

T2DM is a complex metabolic disorder that is characterized by high blood glucose, mainly as a result of the dysfunctional secretion and action of insulin. To avoid complications, the major diabetes therapeutic interventions are to maintain blood glucose levels, improve β-cell function, and minimize insulin resistance. Meanwhile, drugs used to treat diabetic diseases must enhance glucose homeostasis and insulin sensitivity in addition to lowering blood glucose levels [45].

3.8. Effect of β-Sitosterol Glucoside on Serum Insulin, HOMA-IR, and Insulin Tolerance

The level of insulin was significantly increased ($p < 0.05$) in the diabetic group by about 2.16-fold (Figure 6A) compared to the normal control group. However, the medicated nanosystem group and drug suspension showed a lower level of insulin content than the diabetic control group with a reduction of 53.11% and 25.13%, respectively. Regarding HOMA-IR (Figure 6B), there was a significant elevation (8.3 fold higher) in the diabetic group compared to the normal control group ($p < 0.05$), indicating induction of insulin resistance. Upon treatment with medicated nanosystem and drug suspension, there was a significant reduction in HOMA-IR with a percentage decline of 81.60% and 58.75%, respectively, compared with the diabetic control group. However, the effect of medicated nanosystem on insulin resistance showed a more prominent effect.

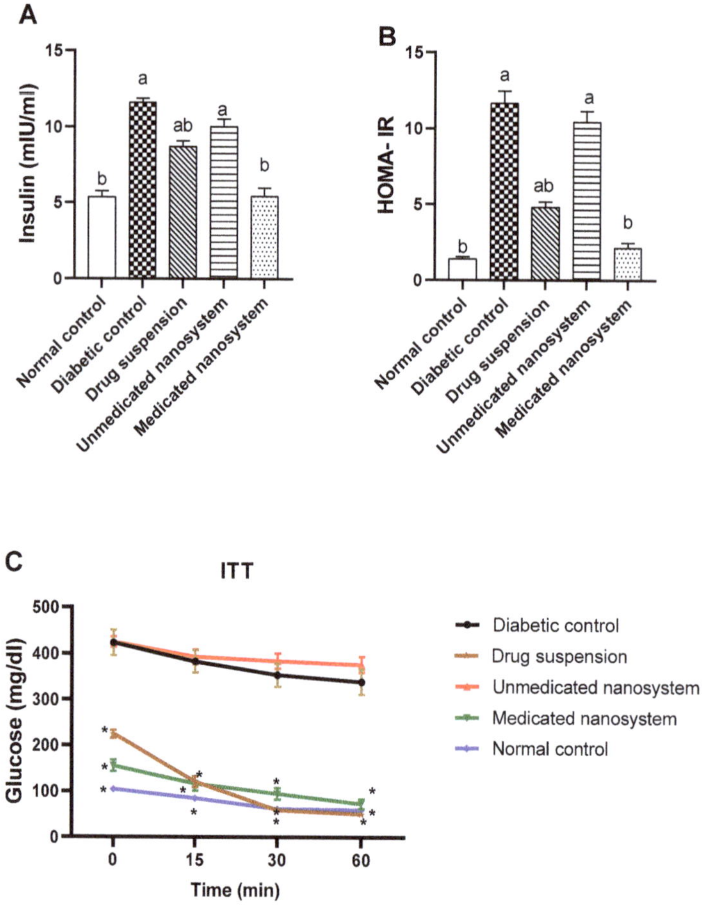

Figure 6. Effect of β-sitosterol glucoside on serum insulin (**A**), HOMA- IR (**B**), and ITT (**C**) in STZ-induced diabetic rats. Each value denotes mean ± SEM (n = 6). Statistical analysis was carried out by one-way ANOVA followed by Tukey's post-hoc test. [a] significantly different from normal control. [b] significantly different from diabetic control at $p < 0.05$. * significantly different from diabetic control at $p < 0.05$ for ITT.

In ITT, insulin administration (0.5 IU/kg, i.p.) to normal (G1), diabetic (G2), and treated animals (G3–G5) produced a decrease in blood glucose levels (Figure 6C), although the rate of decline in blood glucose was significantly higher in normal rats ($p < 0.05$, n = 6) compared to the diabetic untreated rats (Figure 6C). The blood glucose level in the medicated nanosystem group and drug suspension group were significantly lower ($p < 0.05$, n = 6) after insulin loading than the level in the diabetic rats at the 15-, 30-, and 60-min time points. These results indicate that medicated nanosystem and drug suspension enhanced insulin sensitivity and glucose utilization significantly ($p < 0.05$) over the complete period during the ITT compared to diabetic control rats.

In comparison to the control group (G1), the diabetic control group (G2) had significantly higher fasting glucose and insulin levels, as well as higher HOMA-IR values. T2DM is marked by a progressive loss of insulin action, referred to as insulin resistance, as well as compensatory hyperinsulinemia and fasting hyperglycemia [46]. The high HOMA-IR measurement reflects these two metabolic abnormalities. When compared to the diabetic control group, medicated nanosystem treatment group (G5) and drug suspension group (G3) lowered fasting hyperglycemia and basal insulin levels, as well as HOMA-IR values, implying its capacity to alleviate insulin resistance and restore β-cell secretory function. Medicated nanosystem group restored both insulin levels and HOMA-IR values to near normal and have the best effect. Moreover, medicated nanosystem treatment enhanced insulin sensitivity and promoted glucose utilization in T2DM rats, as shown by significant decreases in glucose levels in 15-, 30-, and 60-min time points in the ITT test. ITT evaluates insulin resistance and could be a useful tool for predicting the efficacy of insulin sensitizers [47].

3.9. Effects of β-Sitosterol Glucoside on Serum Malondialdehyde and Catalase Levels

Oxidative stress was assessed by measuring serum malondialdehyde and catalase levels. Compared with the normal control group, serum MDA content of the diabetic group was markedly elevated (1.7-fold) ($p < 0.05$) (Figure 7A), while serum catalase (Figure 7B) was significantly ($p < 0.05$) lower (0.57-fold) than those of normal control group. Medicated nanosystem and drug suspension treatment significantly suppressed lipid peroxidation levels (38.31% and 28.59%, respectively) in comparison with the diabetic untreated group. On the other hand, treatment with medicated nanosystem and drug suspension caused a significant increase in serum catalase levels (64.45% and 46.21%, respectively) compared to the diabetic control group. Oral administration of medicated nanosystem significantly ($p < 0.05$) restored these levels to near-normal values.

Insulin resistance, increasing β-cell dysfunction, poor glucose consumption, and T2DM have all been linked to oxidative stress [48]. Chronic hyperglycemia boosts tissue ROS and lipid peroxidation, impairing insulin action [49]. Moreover, antioxidant enzymes such as CAT play a crucial role in overcoming oxidative stress [50]. In the present study, as shown in Figure 7, in comparison to the normal control group, the serum of the diabetic control group exhibited a large increase in MDA, a lipid peroxidation product [51], and a significant decrease in catalase activity. These findings are supported by previous reports [52–54]. The medicated nanosystem-treated group mitigated oxidative stress in the serum of T2DM rats by decreasing the serum level of MDA and subsequently increasing the serum level of CAT.

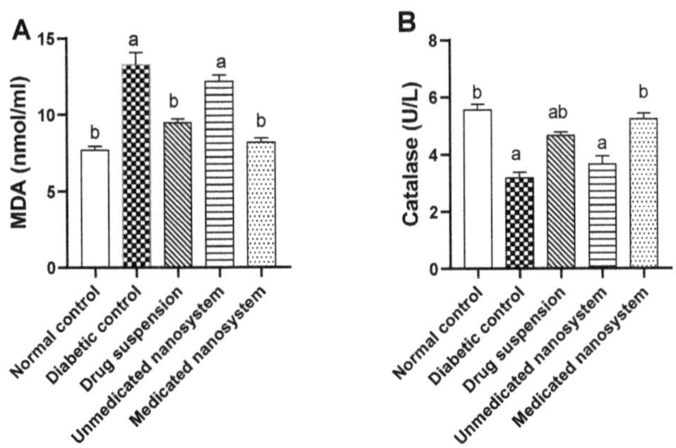

Figure 7. *Cont.*

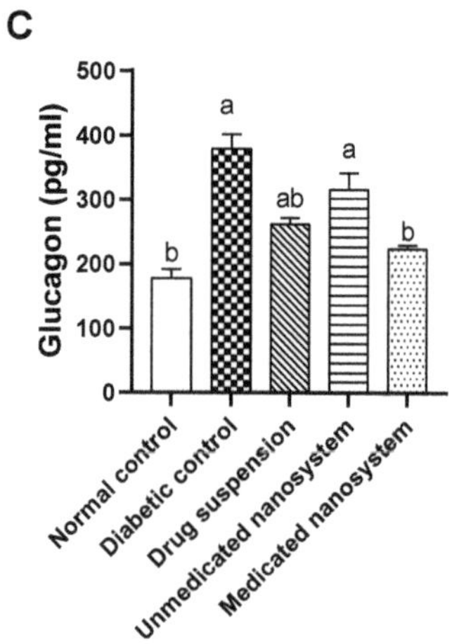

Figure 7. Effect of β-sitosterol glucoside on MDA (**A**), catalase (**B**), and glucagon levels (**C**) in STZ-induced diabetic rats. Each value denotes mean ± SEM ($n = 6$). Statistical analysis was carried out by one-way ANOVA followed by Tukey's post-hoc test. [a] significantly different from normal control. [b] significantly different from diabetic control at $p < 0.05$.

3.10. Effects of β-Sitosterol Glucoside on Serum Glucagon Levels

Further, the glucagon activity was investigated in the serum of tested groups (Figure 7C). Compared with normal control rats, glucagon level was significantly increased ($p < 0.05$, 2.13-fold) in diabetic untreated rats. On the other hand, glucagon levels were significantly decreased in diabetic rats treated with drug suspension (30.91%) and medicated nanosystem (40.85%) compared to the diabetic control group.

Further, to understand the mechanism of action of the SG, we measured the glucagon levels. The elevation of the activity of the glucagon in diabetic rats was reported in our study, and this finding is consistent with previous studies [55,56]. The upregulation of glucagon secretion may contribute to problems with glucose homeostasis [57].

Furthermore, increasing blood glucagon concentrations are linked to enhanced insulin resistance and raised glucose concentrations in both normal and T2DM participants [58], suggesting that glucagon may play a role in T2DM pathogenesis. In this study, medicated nanosystem administration reduced glucagon levels, implying that SG can alleviate insulin resistance, which is a complication of diabetes.

3.11. Effects of β-Sitosterol Glucoside on Pancreatic Histological Changes

Histological changes were screened to support results of the biochemical results. The photographs of histology sections are depicted in Figure 8. Histopathological examination revealed that the control group had a normal histological structure of the acini and duct system (Figure 8A). On the other hand, the diabetic group demonstrated atrophy and regression in the number of the islets of Langerhans cells with the surrounding intact acini (Figure 8B), in association with focal inflammatory cells infiltration and oedema surrounding the dilated blood vessels in the stroma between the lobules. SG suspension exhibited a remarkable recovery compared to diabetic untreated rats, with a mild degree of inflammation (Figure 8C). Treatment with blank (non-medicated nanosystem) resulted in atrophy and regression in the size contour of the islets of Langerhans cells (Figure 8D). Focal inflammatory cells infiltration was replaced by the regressed atrophied islet of Langerhans in the lobules. The interlobular stromal tissue showed focal oedema with inflammatory cells infiltration. Severe dilatation and congestion were detected in the stromal blood vessels associated with perivascular hemorrhages, oedema, and inflammatory cells infiltration. On the other hand, the medicated nanosystem (Figure 8E) has protected the tissue damage and there was no histopathological alteration in the islets of Langerhans cells and surrounding acini.

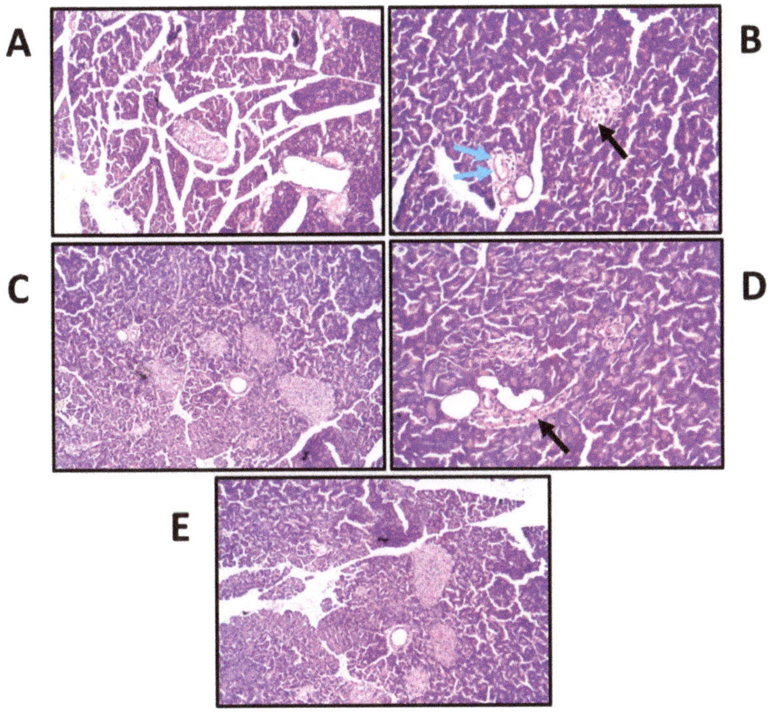

Figure 8. Histopathology of rat pancreatic tissue stained with hematoxylin and eosin determined by light electric microscopy (×40); (**A**): normal control revealing normal histological structure of cells; (**B**): diabetic control demonstrated atrophy (Black arrows), oedema (Blue arrows), and a drastic decrease in the number of the islets of Langerhans cells; (**C**): diabetic + drug suspension exhibited a remarkable recovery; (**D**): diabetic + unmedicated nanosystem resulted in atrophy (Black arrows) and regression in the size contour of the islets of Langerhans cells; and (**E**): diabetic + medicated nanosystem, revealing no histopathological alteration in the islets of Langerhans cells compared to normal control.

The protective effect of SG on cells of the islets of Langerhans is also confirmed by histopathology of pancreatic cells. The STZ-induced diabetic rats had atrophy and regression in the number of the islets of Langerhans cells, whereas rats given medicated nanosystem showed no alteration in islet growth and significantly reduced pancreatic β-cell damage.

In plants, phytosterols are essential metabolites reported as bioactive compounds against various pathogens and diseases [59]. Additionally, phytosterols are present in the human diet, and researchers have explored their absorption and metabolism [60,61]. It is recognized that SG is safe when taken orally, albeit with low bioavailability [62]; its incorporation into a self-nanoemulsifying delivery system enhanced the solubility and biological effect. Furthermore, our in vitro release findings indicate improved delivery of SG through increased dissolution and absorption. In vitro release study is a potent and valuable tool for monitoring clinical performance as a surrogate for in vivo pharmacokinetics [63]. Thus, a good linear relationship was observed upon investigating the in vitro/in vivo correlations [64,65].

Increasing oxidative stress aggravates diabetes and its complications. Therefore, antioxidants are commonly used as supplementary medicine especially in chronic diabetes [66]. SG was reported as an antioxidant inducing various therapeutic properties, viz., neuroprotective, analgesic, anti-inflammatory, and chemopreventive activities [14]. However, no studies reported any adverse effects of SG [67].

The current study focused on the efficacy of SG-loaded SEEDS on insulin resistance and glucagon levels for the first time in treating diabetes. Thus, experiments were designed to investigate these effects of SG in HFD-fed diabetic rats because HFD feeding causes insulin resistance and can be used to establish T2DM animal models [68]. A myriad of pathways and mechanisms can be considered as underlying reasons for enhanced insulin sensitivity and glucose homeostasis. For instance, insulin stimulates the translocation of GLUT4 (Glucose transporter type 4), which elevates glucose uptake in skeletal muscles. Thus, defective GLUT4 translocation exacerbates insulin resistance [69]. SG was reported to induce an estrogen like effect and increase GLUT4 translocation through PI-3K/AKT signaling in skeletal muscles [70]. In insulin resistance and obesity, c-Jun *N*-terminal kinase (JNK) is one of the most studied signal transducers [71]. SG was reported to possess an apoptotic effect in cancer cells through activating JNK signaling [72]. Nowadays, pharmacological management of diabetes is performed by inhibiting α-glucosidase and α-amylase, which aggressively delays the digestion of polysaccharides to absorbable simple sugars [73]. It was recently discovered that SG inhibited α-amylase and α-glucosidase [74], developing a potential hypoglycemic effect. By inducing inflammatory cytokines, NF-κB (Nuclear factor kappa B) may lower insulin sensitivity [75]. However, a recent study revealed that SG had no effect on the NF-κB signaling pathway [76]. Lastly, another study demonstrated the hypoglycemic effect of SG on improving some hematology parameters, viz., lipid profile, creatinine, and blood urea [77]. Therefore, the proposed mechanisms underlying the SG-induced effect on glucagon levels, insulin tolerance, and glucose homeostasis require further studies for clarification.

4. Conclusions

This study provides the first insight into β-sitosterol glucoside's effect on insulin resistance and glucagon levels in diabetes progression. β-Sitosterol glucoside extracted from *Senecio petasitis* was loaded in self-nanoemulsifying delivery systems to overcome its low aqueous solubility. The nanosystem showed an enhanced in vitro release of β-sitosterol glucoside compared to that of the drug suspension, providing a likely sensible model for pharmacokinetic aspect of β-sitosterol glucoside-loaded SEDDS in living organisms. The results from the HOMA-IR and ITTs revealed that β-sitosterol glucoside significantly improved insulin sensitivity and glucose utilization in diabetic rats. However, the hypoglycemic effect of β-sitosterol glucoside is regulated by a variety of enzymes and mechanisms. Future research work should investigate key markers in glycolysis, glycogen synthesis/degradation, gluconeogenesis, and glucose phosphorylation/dephosphorylation pathways. By being an antioxidant, β-sitosterol glucoside may partially attenuate hyperglycemia, though such a hypothesis should be confirmed by excessive further investigations. Additionally, whether β-sitosterol glucoside and its aglycone exhibit synergistic antidiabetic activities should be clarified later. The findings of the in vivo studies done using diabetic rats highlight the superior efficacy of the proposed β-sitosterol glucoside-loaded nanosystem compared to the free drug suspension in the suppression and control of T2DM by reducing oxidative stress and insulin resistance, indicating that it might be a promising biopharmaceutical candidate. In our histological study, we discovered that β-sitosterol glucoside not only reduces hyperglycemia but also attenuates pancreatic inflammation. Thus, it possesses huge potential for countering the deterioration of insulin resistance. Further clinical studies are recommended to unravel various pathways exerted by β-sitosterol glucoside, providing a new vision for the treatment of T2DM.

Supplementary Materials: The following supporting information can be downloaded at: https://www.mdpi.com/article/10.3390/antiox11051023/s1, Figure S1: ^{1}H-NMR spectrum of the isolated compound (β-Sitosterol glucoside) in DMSO-d_6.

Author Contributions: Conceptualization, S.M.A., N.M.A., R.K., T.E. and H.A.H.; methodology, S.M.A., N.M.A., R.K., T.E. and H.A.H.; formal analysis, S.M.A., N.M.A., R.K. and H.A.H.; investigation, S.M.A., N.M.A., R.K., T.E. and H.A.H.; writing—original draft preparation, S.M.A., N.M.A. and R.K.; writing—review and editing, S.M.A., N.M.A., R.K., T.E. and H.A.H.; funding acquisition, T.E. All authors have read and agreed to the published version of the manuscript.

Funding: The publication of this article was funded by the Open Access Fund of Leibniz Universität Hannover.

Institutional Review Board Statement: The study was carried out in accordance with the National Regulations on Animal Welfare and Institutional Animal Ethical Committee (IAEC) (approval no: 6443042021), guided by the Canadian Council on Animal Care.

Informed Consent Statement: Not applicable.

Data Availability Statement: All of the data is contained within the article and the Supplementary Materials.

Conflicts of Interest: The authors declare no conflict of interest.

References

1. Forouhi, N.G.; Wareham, N.J. Epidemiology of diabetes. *Medicine* **2019**, *47*, 22–27. [CrossRef]
2. Afroz, A.; Zhang, W.; Wei Loh, A.J.; Jie Lee, D.X.; Billah, B. Macro- and micro-vascular complications and their determinants among people with type 2 diabetes in Bangladesh. *Diabetes Metab. Syndr. Clin. Res. Rev.* **2019**, *13*, 2939–2946. [CrossRef] [PubMed]
3. Miaffo, D.; Ntchapda, F.; Mahamad, T.A.; Maidadi, B.; Kamanyi, A. Hypoglycemic, antidyslipidemic and antioxydant effects of *Vitellaria paradoxa* barks extract on high-fat diet and streptozotocin-induced type 2 diabetes rats. *Metab. Open* **2021**, *9*, 100071. [CrossRef] [PubMed]
4. Lorenzati, B.; Zucco, C.; Miglietta, S.; Lamberti, F.; Bruno, G. Oral hypoglycemic drugs: Pathophysiological basis of their mechanism of action oral hypoglycemic drugs: Pathophysiological basis of their mechanism of action. *Pharmaceuticals* **2010**, *3*, 3005–3020. [CrossRef]
5. Mandlik, R.V.; Naik, S.R.; Zine, S.; Ved, H.; Doshi, G. Antidiabetic activity of *Caulerpa racemosa*: Role of proinflammatory mediators, oxidative stress, and other biomarkers. *Planta Med. Int. Open* **2022**, *9*, e60–e71. [CrossRef]
6. Saltiel, A.R.; Kahn, C.R. Insulin signalling and the regulation of glucose and lipid metabolism. *Nature* **2001**, *414*, 799–806. [CrossRef]
7. Reaven, G.M. Insulin resistance/compensatory hyperinsulinemia, essential hypertension, and cardiovascular disease. *J. Clin. Endocrinol. Metab.* **2003**, *88*, 2399–2403. [CrossRef]
8. Iamonico, D. Alien taxa of the tribe Senecioneae (Asteraceae) in Italy: A nomenclatural synopsis. *Hacquetia* **2017**, *16*, 281–292. [CrossRef]
9. Gao, T.; Yao, H.; Song, J.; Zhu, Y.; Liu, C.; Chen, S. Evaluating the feasibility of using candidate DNA barcodes in discriminating species of the large Asteraceae family. *BMC Evol. Biol.* **2010**, *10*, 324. [CrossRef]
10. Funston, A.M. Taxonomic revision of Roldana (Asteraceae: Senecioneae), a genus of the southwestern USA, Mexico, and Central America. *Ann. Mo. Bot. Gard.* **2008**, *95*, 282–337. [CrossRef]
11. Yan, Y.; Lei, Z.; YuFang, W.; ManLi, C.; ChangHong, H.; YuCheng, G.; QingWen, S.; Kiyota, H. Chemical and pharmacological research on plants from the genus *Senecio*. *Chem. Biodivers.* **2011**, *8*, 13–72.
12. Portero, A.; González-Coloma, A.; Reina, M.; Díaz, C.E. Plant-defensive sesquiterpenoids from *Senecio* species with biopesticide potential. *Phytochem. Rev.* **2012**, *11*, 391–403. [CrossRef]
13. McDonald, J.A. Alpine flora of Cerro Quiexobra, Oaxaca, Mexico. *J. Bot. Res. Inst. Tex.* **2013**, *7*, 765–769.
14. López-Salazar, H.; Camacho-Díaz, B.H.; Ávila-Reyes, S.V.; Pérez-García, M.D.; González-Cortazar, M.; Arenas Ocampo, M.L.; Jiménez-Aparicio, A.R. Identification and quantification of β-sitosterol β-D-glucoside of an ethanolic extract obtained by microwave-assisted extraction from *Agave angustifolia* Haw. *Molecules* **2019**, *24*, 3926. [CrossRef]
15. Ambavade, S.D.; Misar, A.V.; Ambavade, P.D. Pharmacological, nutritional, and analytical aspects of β-sitosterol: A review. *Orient. Pharm. Exp. Med.* **2014**, *14*, 193–211. [CrossRef]
16. Neslihan Gursoy, R.; Benita, S. Self-emulsifying drug delivery systems (SEDDS) for improved oral delivery of lipophilic drugs. *Biomed. Pharmacother.* **2004**, *58*, 173–182. [CrossRef] [PubMed]
17. Scott Swenson, E.; Curatolo, W.J. Means to enhance penetration: (2) Intestinal permeability enhancement for proteins, peptides and other polar drugs: Mechanisms and potential toxicity. *Adv. Drug Deliv. Rev.* **1992**, *8*, 39–92. [CrossRef]

18. Tenjarla, S. Microemulsions: An overview and pharmaceutical applications. *Crit. Rev. Drug Carr. Syst.* **1999**, *16*, 461–521. [CrossRef]
19. Kamel, R.; Basha, M. Preparation and in vitro evaluation of rutin nanostructured liquisolid delivery system. *Bull. Fac. Pharm. Cairo Univ.* **2013**, *51*, 261–272. [CrossRef]
20. Khoo, S.-M.; Humberstone, A.J.; Porter, C.J.H.; Edwards, G.A.; Charman, W.N. Formulation design and bioavailability assessment of lipidic self-emulsifying formulations of halofantrine. *Int. J. Pharm.* **1998**, *167*, 155–164. [CrossRef]
21. Yang, S.C.; Lu, L.F.; Cai, Y.; Zhu, J.B.; Liang, B.W.; Yang, C.Z. Body distribution in mice of intravenously injected camptothecin solid lipid nanoparticles and targeting effect on brain. *J. Control. Release* **1999**, *59*, 299–307. [CrossRef]
22. D'Souza, S. A review of in vitro drug release test methods for nano-sized dosage forms. *Adv. Pharm.* **2014**, *2014*, 304757. [CrossRef] [PubMed]
23. Soleimanian, Y.; Goli, S.A.H.; Varshosaz, J.; di Cesare Mannelli, L.; Ghelardini, C.; Cirri, M.; Maestrelli, F. *β*-Sitosterol loaded nanostructured lipid carrier: Physical and oxidative stability, in vitro simulated digestion and hypocholesterolemic activity. *Pharmaceutics* **2020**, *12*, 386. [CrossRef] [PubMed]
24. Gupta, R.; Sharma, A.K.; Dobhal, M.P.; Sharma, M.C.; Gupta, R.S. Antidiabetic and antioxidant potential of *β*-sitosterol in streptozotocin-induced experimental hyperglycemia. *J. Diabetes* **2011**, *3*, 29–37. [CrossRef] [PubMed]
25. Luo, C.; Yang, H.; Tang, C.; Yao, G.; Kong, L.; He, H.; Zhou, Y. Kaempferol alleviates insulin resistance via hepatic IKK/NF-κB signal in type 2 diabetic rats. *Int. Immunopharmacol.* **2015**, *28*, 744–750. [CrossRef]
26. Kumar, S.A.; Magnusson, M.; Ward, L.C.; Paul, N.A.; Brown, L. Seaweed supplements normalise metabolic, cardiovascular and liver responses in high-carbohydrate, high-fat fed rats. *Mar. Drugs* **2015**, *13*, 788–805. [CrossRef]
27. El-Newary, S.A.; Afifi, S.M.; Aly, M.S.; Ahmed, R.F.; El Gendy, A.E.-N.G.; Abd-ElGawad, A.M.; Farag, M.A.; Elgamal, A.M.; Elshamy, A.I. Chemical profile of *Launaea nudicaulis* ethanolic extract and its antidiabetic effect in streptozotocin-induced rats. *Molecules* **2021**, *26*, 1000. [CrossRef]
28. Wallace, T.M.; Levy, J.C.; Matthews, D.R. Use and abuse of HOMA modeling. *Diabetes Care* **2004**, *27*, 1487–1495. [CrossRef]
29. Runtuwene, J.; Cheng, K.-C.; Asakawa, A.; Amitani, H.; Amitani, M.; Morinaga, A.; Takimoto, Y.; Kairupan, B.H.R.; Inui, A. Rosmarinic acid ameliorates hyperglycemia and insulin sensitivity in diabetic rats, potentially by modulating the expression of PEPCK and GLUT4. *Drug Des Devel* **2016**, *10*, 2193–2202. [CrossRef]
30. Ohkawa, H.; Ohishi, N.; Yagi, K. Assay for lipid peroxides in animal tissues by thiobarbituric acid reaction. *Anal. Biochem.* **1979**, *95*, 351–358. [CrossRef]
31. Aebi, H. Catalase in vitro. In *Methods in Enzymology*; Academic Press: Cambridge, MA, USA, 1984; Volume 105, pp. 121–126.
32. Bancroft, J.D.G.M. *Theory and Practice of Histological Techniques*; Churchill Livingstone: London, UK, 2008.
33. Vo, T.K.; Ta, Q.T.H.; Chu, Q.T.; Nguyen, T.T.; Vo, V.G. Anti-hepatocellular-cancer activity exerted by *β*-sitosterol and *β*-sitosterol-glucoside from *Indigofera zollingeriana* Miq. *Molecules* **2020**, *25*, 3021. [CrossRef] [PubMed]
34. Xu, H.; Li, Y.; Han, B.; Li, Z.; Wang, B.; Jiang, P.; Zhang, J.; Ma, W.; Zhou, D.; Li, X.; et al. Anti-breast-cancer activity exerted by *β*-sitosterol-D-glucoside from sweet potato via upregulation of microRNA-10a and via the PI3K–Akt signaling pathway. *J. Agric. Food Chem.* **2018**, *66*, 9704–9718. [CrossRef] [PubMed]
35. Lee, P.J.; Langer, R.; Shastri, V.P. Novel microemulsion enhancer formulation for simultaneous transdermal delivery of hydrophilic and hydrophobic drugs. *Pharm. Res.* **2003**, *20*, 264–269. [CrossRef] [PubMed]
36. Mercuri, A.; Passalacqua, A.; Wickham, M.S.J.; Faulks, R.M.; Craig, D.Q.M.; Barker, S.A. The effect of composition and gastric conditions on the self-emulsification process of ibuprofen-loaded self-emulsifying drug delivery systems: A microscopic and dynamic gastric model study. *Pharm. Res.* **2011**, *28*, 1540–1551. [CrossRef] [PubMed]
37. Kommuru, T.R.; Gurley, B.; Khan, M.A.; Reddy, I.K. Self-emulsifying drug delivery systems (SEDDS) of coenzyme Q10: Formulation development and bioavailability assessment. *Int. J. Pharm.* **2001**, *212*, 233–246. [CrossRef]
38. Kahlweit, M.; Busse, G.; Faulhaber, B.; Eibl, H. Preparing nontoxic microemulsions. *Langmuir* **1995**, *11*, 4185–4187. [CrossRef]
39. Kamel, R.; Mostafa, D.M. Rutin nanostructured lipid cosmeceutical preparation with sun protective potential. *J. Photochem. Photobiol. B Biol.* **2015**, *153*, 59–66. [CrossRef]
40. Kim, S.; Ng, W.K.; Shen, S.; Dong, Y.; Tan, R.B.H. Phase behavior, microstructure transition, and antiradical activity of sucrose laurate/propylene glycol/the essential oil of *Melaleuca alternifolia*/water microemulsions. *Colloids Surf. A Physicochem. Eng. Asp.* **2009**, *348*, 289–297. [CrossRef]
41. Kallakunta, V.R.; Bandari, S.; Jukanti, R.; Veerareddy, P.R. Oral self emulsifying powder of lercanidipine hydrochloride: Formulation and evaluation. *Powder Technol.* **2012**, *221*, 375–382. [CrossRef]
42. Pouton, C.W.; Porter, C.J.H. Formulation of lipid-based delivery systems for oral administration: Materials, methods and strategies. *Adv. Drug Deliv. Rev.* **2008**, *60*, 625–637. [CrossRef]
43. Abdelmageed, M.E.; Shehatou, G.S.G.; Suddek, G.M.; Salem, H.A. Protocatechuic acid improves hepatic insulin resistance and restores vascular oxidative status in type-2 diabetic rats. *Environ. Toxicol. Pharmacol.* **2021**, *83*, 103577. [CrossRef] [PubMed]
44. Swanston-Flatt, S.K.; Day, C.; Bailey, C.J.; Flatt, P.R. Traditional plant treatments for diabetes. Studies in normal and streptozotocin diabetic mice. *Diabetologia* **1990**, *33*, 462–464. [CrossRef] [PubMed]
45. Wilcox, G. Insulin and insulin resistance. *Clin. Biochem. Rev.* **2005**, *26*, 19–39. [PubMed]
46. Reaven, G.M. Compensatory hyperinsulinemia and the development of an atherogenic lipoprotein profile: The price paid to maintain glucose homeostasis in insulin-resistant individuals. *Endocrinol. Metab. Clin.* **2005**, *34*, 49–62. [CrossRef]

47. Kozawa, J.; Iwahashi, H.; Okita, K.; Okauchi, Y.; Imagawa, A.; Shimomura, I. Insulin tolerance test predicts the effectiveness of insulin sensitizers in japanese type 2 diabetic patients. *Diabetes Ther.* **2010**, *1*, 121–130. [CrossRef]
48. Ceriello, A.; Motz, E. Is oxidative stress the pathogenic mechanism underlying insulin resistance, diabetes, and cardiovascular disease? The common soil hypothesis revisited. *Arterioscler. Thromb. Vasc. Biol.* **2004**, *24*, 816–823. [CrossRef]
49. Nishikawa, T.; Araki, E. Impact of mitochondrial ROS production in the pathogenesis of diabetes mellitus and its complications. *Antioxid. Redox Signal.* **2007**, *9*, 343–353. [CrossRef]
50. Nimse, S.B.; Pal, D. Free radicals, natural antioxidants, and their reaction mechanisms. *RSC Adv.* **2015**, *5*, 27986–28006. [CrossRef]
51. Tsikas, D. Assessment of lipid peroxidation by measuring malondialdehyde (MDA) and relatives in biological samples: Analytical and biological challenges. *Anal. Biochem.* **2017**, *524*, 13–30. [CrossRef]
52. Veerapur, V.P.; Prabhakar, K.R.; Kandadi, M.R.; Srinivasan, K.K.; Unnikrishnan, M.K. Antidiabetic effect of *Dodonaea viscosa* aerial parts in high fat diet and low dose streptozotocin-induced type 2 diabetic rats: A mechanistic approach. *Pharm. Biol.* **2010**, *48*, 1137–1148. [CrossRef]
53. Strugała, P.; Dzydzan, O.; Brodyak, I.; Kucharska, A.Z.; Kuropka, P.; Liuta, M.; Kaleta-Kuratewicz, K.; Przewodowska, A.; Michałowska, D.; Gabrielska, J.; et al. Antidiabetic and antioxidative potential of the blue congo variety of purple potato extract in streptozotocin-induced diabetic rats. *Molecules* **2019**, *24*, 3126. [CrossRef] [PubMed]
54. Jamal Gilani, S.; Nasser Bin-Jumah, M.; Al-Abbasi, F.A.; Shahid Nadeem, M.; Afzal, M.; Sayyed, N.; Kazmi, I. Fustin ameliorates hyperglycemia in streptozotocin induced type-2 diabetes via modulating glutathione/superoxide dismutase/catalase expressions, suppress lipid peroxidation and regulates histopathological changes. *Saudi J. Biol. Sci.* **2021**, *28*, 6963–6971. [CrossRef] [PubMed]
55. Song, G.; Pacini, G.; Ahrén, B.; D'Argenio, D.Z. Glucagon increases insulin levels by stimulating insulin secretion without effect on insulin clearance in mice. *Peptides* **2017**, *88*, 74–79. [CrossRef] [PubMed]
56. Suanarunsawat, T.; Klongpanichapak, S.; Rungseesantivanon, S.; Chaiyabutr, N. Glycemic effect of stevioside and *Stevia rebaudiana* in streptozotocin-induced diabetic rats. *East. J. Med.* **2004**, *9*, 51–56.
57. Kulina, G.R.; Rayfield, E.J. The role of glucagon in the pathophysiology and management of diabetes. *Endocr Pract.* **2016**, *22*, 612–621. [CrossRef]
58. Færch, K.; Vistisen, D.; Pacini, G.; Torekov, S.S.; Johansen, N.B.; Witte, D.R.; Jonsson, A.; Pedersen, O.; Hansen, T.; Lauritzen, T.; et al. Insulin resistance is accompanied by increased fasting glucagon and delayed glucagon suppression in individuals with normal and impaired glucose regulation. *Diabetes* **2016**, *65*, 3473–3481. [CrossRef]
59. Nattagh-Eshtivani, E.; Barghchi, H.; Pahlavani, N.; Barati, M.; Amiri, Y.; Fadel, A.; Khosravi, M.; Talebi, S.; Arzhang, P.; Ziaei, R.; et al. Biological and pharmacological effects and nutritional impact of phytosterols: A comprehensive review. *Phytother. Res.* **2022**, *36*, 299–322. [CrossRef]
60. Richard, E.; Ostlund, J. Phytosterols in human nutrition. *Annu. Rev. Nutr.* **2002**, *22*, 533–549. [CrossRef]
61. Moreau, R.A.; Whitaker, B.D.; Hicks, K.B. Phytosterols, phytostanols, and their conjugates in foods: Structural diversity, quantitative analysis, and health-promoting uses. *Prog. Lipid Res.* **2002**, *41*, 457–500. [CrossRef]
62. Pegel, K.H.D. The importance of sitosterol and sitosterolin in human and animal nutrition. *S. Afr. J. Sci.* **1997**, *93*, 263–268.
63. Uppoor, V.R.S. Regulatory perspectives on in vitro (dissolution)/in vivo (bioavailability) correlations. *J. Control. Release* **2001**, *72*, 127–132. [CrossRef]
64. Cao, X.; Deng, W.; Fu, M.; Zhu, Y.; Liu, H.; Wang, L.; Zeng, J.; Wei, Y.; Xu, X.; Yu, J. Seventy-two-hour release formulation of the poorly soluble drug silybin based on porous silica nanoparticles: In vitro release kinetics and in vitro/in vivo correlations in beagle dogs. *Eur. J. Pharm. Sci.* **2013**, *48*, 64–71. [CrossRef] [PubMed]
65. Lu, Y.; Kim, S.; Park, K. In vitro–in vivo correlation: Perspectives on model development. *Int. J. Pharm.* **2011**, *418*, 142–148. [CrossRef] [PubMed]
66. Giacco, F.; Brownlee, M.; Schmidt, A.M. Oxidative stress and diabetic complications. *Circ. Res.* **2010**, *107*, 1058–1070. [CrossRef]
67. Villaseñor, I.M.; Angelada, J.; Canlas, A.P.; Echegoyen, D. Bioactivity studies on β-sitosterol and its glucoside. *Phytother. Res.* **2002**, *16*, 417–421. [CrossRef]
68. King, A.J. The use of animal models in diabetes research. *Br. J. Pharmacol.* **2012**, *166*, 877–894. [CrossRef]
69. Picatoste, B.; Yammine, L.; Leahey, R.A.; Soares, D.; Johnson, E.F.; Cohen, P.; McGraw, T.E. Defective insulin-stimulated GLUT4 translocation in brown adipocytes induces systemic glucose homeostasis dysregulation independent of thermogenesis in female mice. *Mol. Metab.* **2021**, *53*, 101305. [CrossRef]
70. Pandey, J.; Dev, K.; Chattopadhyay, S.; Kadan, S.; Sharma, T.; Maurya, R.; Sanyal, S.; Siddiqi, M.I.; Zaid, H.; Tamrakar, A.K. β-Sitosterol-D-glucopyranoside mimics estrogenic properties and stimulates glucose utilization in skeletal muscle cells. *Molecules* **2021**, *26*, 3129. [CrossRef]
71. Feng, J.; Lu, S.; Ou, B.; Liu, Q.; Dai, J.; Ji, C.; Zhou, H.; Huang, H.; Ma, Y. The role of JNk signaling pathway in obesity-driven insulin resistance. *Diabetes Metab. Syndr. Obes.* **2020**, *13*, 1399–1406. [CrossRef]
72. Gao, P.; Huang, X.; Liao, T.; Li, G.; Yu, X.; You, Y.; Huang, Y. Daucosterol induces autophagic-dependent apoptosis in prostate cancer via JNK activation. *Biosci. Trends* **2019**, *13*, 160–167. [CrossRef]
73. Teng, H.; Chen, L. α-Glucosidase and α-amylase inhibitors from seed oil: A review of liposoluble substance to treat diabetes. *Crit. Rev. Food Sci. Nutr.* **2017**, *57*, 3438–3448. [CrossRef] [PubMed]
74. Dehghan, H.; Salehi, P.; Amiri, M.S. Bioassay-guided purification of α-amylase, α-glucosidase inhibitors and DPPH radical scavengers from roots of *Rheum turkestanicum*. *Ind. Crops Prod.* **2018**, *117*, 303–309. [CrossRef]

75. Tang, T.; Zhang, J.; Yin, J.; Staszkiewicz, J.; Gawronska-Kozak, B.; Jung, D.Y.; Ko, H.J.; Ong, H.; Kim, J.K.; Mynatt, R.; et al. Uncoupling of inflammation and insulin resistance by NF-κB in transgenic mice through elevated energy expenditure 2. *J. Biol. Chem.* **2010**, *285*, 4637–4644. [CrossRef] [PubMed]
76. Youn, U.J.; Chang, L.C. Chemical constituents of fermented noni (Morinda citrifolia) juice exudates and their biological activity. *Nat. Prod. Sci.* **2017**, *23*, 16–20. [CrossRef]
77. Nualkaew, S.; Padee, P.; Talubmook, C. Hypoglycemic activity in diabetic rats of stigmasterol and sitosterol-3-O-β-D glucopyranoside isolated from *Pseuderanthemum palatiferum* (Nees) Radlk. leaf extract. *J. Med. Plants Res.* **2015**, *9*, 629–635.

antioxidants

MDPI

Article

Nanoparticles Based on Cross-Linked Poly(Lipoic Acid) Protect Macrophages and Cardiomyocytes from Oxidative Stress and Ischemia Reperfusion Injury

Chiara Bellini [1,2,†,‡], Salvatore Antonucci [1,†], Lucía Morillas-Becerril [3,†,§], Sara Scarpa [1,2], Regina Tavano [1,2], Fabrizio Mancin [3], Fabio Di Lisa [1,*] and Emanuele Papini [1,2,*]

1 Department of Biomedical Sciences, University of Padova, Via U. Bassi 58/b, 35121 Padova, Italy; chiara.bellini@ttk.elte.hu (C.B.); salvatore.antonucci@unipd.it (S.A.); sara.scarpa@studenti.unipd.it (S.S.); regina.tavano@unipd.it (R.T.)

2 CRIBI—Centre for Innovative Biotechnology Research, University of Padova, Via U. Bassi 58/b, 35121 Padova, Italy

3 Department of Chemical Sciences, University of Padova, Via F. Marzolo 1, 35121 Padova, Italy; lucia.morillasbecerril@unipd.it (L.M.-B.); fabrizio.mancin@unipd.it (F.M.)

* Correspondence: fabio.dilisa@unipd.it (F.D.L.); papinie@bio.unipd.it (E.P.)

† These authors contributed equally to this work.

‡ Current address: Hevesy György PhD School of Chemistry, Eötvös Loránd University, Pázmány Péter Sétány 1/A, 1117 Budapest, Hungary.

§ Current address: Department of Pharmaceutical Sciences, University of Milano, Via Golgi 19, 20133 Milano, Italy.

Abstract: The control of radical damage and oxidative stress, phenomena involved in a large number of human pathologies, is a major pharmaceutical and medical goal. We here show that two biocompatible formulations of Pluronic-stabilized, poly (lipoic acid)-based nanoparticles (NP) effectively antagonized the formation of radicals and reactive oxygen species (ROS). These NPs, not only intrinsically scavenged radicals in a-cellular DPPH/ABTS assays, but also inhibited the overproduction of ROS induced by tert-Butyl hydroperoxide (t-BHP) in tumor cells (HeLa), human macrophages and neonatal rat ventricular myocytes (NRVMs). NPs were captured by macrophages and cardiomyocytes much more effectively as compared to HeLa cells and non-phagocytic leukocytes, eventually undergoing intracellular disassembly. Notably, NPs decreased the mitochondrial ROS generation induced by simulated Ischemia/Reperfusion Injury (IRI) in isolated cardiomyocytes. NPs also prevented IRI-triggered cardiomyocyte necrosis, mitochondrial dysfunction, and alterations of contraction-related intracellular Ca^{2+} waves. Hence, NPs appear to be an effective and cardiomyocyte-selective drug to protect against damages induced by post-ischemic reperfusion.

Keywords: poly(lipoic acid); nanoparticles; ischemia and reperfusion injury

1. Introduction

Tissue and cell damage induced by high levels of radicals and reactive oxygen species (ROS) is linked to several pathological conditions and intoxications [1–5]. In this context, so-called Ischemia/Reperfusion Injury (IRI) has great clinical relevance. This is severe damage which can affect major organs, like the liver, heart, lungs, intestine, brain or kidneys. In particular, the damage is exacerbated by the restoration of blood flow (i.e., reperfusion) after a prolonged absence of tissue perfusion (i.e., ischemia), as reported in myocardial infarction, ischemic stroke, or in liver transplantations) [6]. Among the many mechanisms involved in IRI, a large increase in mitochondrial ROS formation is considered a hallmark and a major event responsible for causing tissue damage and death [7,8]. Indeed, although there are multiple potential sources of ROS in IRI, mitochondria represent a major one. They are abundant in the heart, and they contain several sites involved in ROS production (e.g., respiratory chain Complex I via Reverse Electron Transport or RET; monoamine oxidases, the translocation of p66Shc protein and the Permeability Transition Pore) [9].

Several agonists have been proposed to protect from oxidative stress and IRI [10,11]. Some of them have direct ROS scavenging actions, while others act by inducing an Nrf2-dependent increase in antioxidant defenses, resulting in anti-inflammatory and cytoprotective effects. However, despite positive results in experimental studies, such as in the case of cyclosporine A (CyA), no relevant candidates have emerged from clinical trials. This failure is likely due to several reasons. Some candidates target inflammation or the permeability transition pore (PTP), a protein complex of still uncertain molecular identity, involved in several diseases, including cardiac ischemia, and targeted by cyclophilin D and other inhibitors [12,13]. However, these agents tackle events downstream of reperfusion-induced oxidative stress leaving ROS formation unaltered [14–17]. This limitation is likely to be overridden by administration of small molecules with ROS scavenging ability. However, small drugs in general suffer from rapid clearance and low target specificity.

The nanoparticle (NP) approach may present special advantages compared to small drugs, for example, due to the possibility of reducing renal clearance, prolonging drug circulation, selectively targeting specific cells, and delivering the therapeutic principle only to the desired tissue and cells [18–23]. Most NP-based agents proposed for protecting against IRI are drug-delivery systems, where NPs act as biocompatible carriers of pharmacologically active compounds. For example, PLGA-NPs, albumin-based, or chitosan NPs were loaded with PTP inhibitors [24,25] or with antioxidant agents, such as quercetin, resveratrol or gallic acid [26–31]. However, in the case of PLGA-nanoparticles, it was demonstrated that the uptake by cardiomyocytes occurs after the insurgence of the oxidative stress deriving from the ischemic injury, and it was likely due to the cell damage induced by the oxidative stress. In several other cases, the intrinsic radical-scavenging action of the material forming the NPs, such as cerium dioxide, selenium, gold and carbon nanotubes, was exploited to counteract IRI oxidative stress [32,33]. However, the toxicological effects and the biocompatibility of these materials are likely to undermine the achievement of positive results [34,35]. These examples demonstrate the need for more efficient, selective, and biocompatible nanosystems for effective treatment of IRI.

Poly(lipoic acid) polymers and nanoparticles are an emerging class of biodegradable vectors capable to respond to local tissues environment [36,37]. The inclusion of disulfide units from lipoic acid in the nanoparticles' structure, translates in their redox-responsive behavior and eventual cargo release in presence of reducing agents, as observed for other particles [38–40]. We recently proposed a new concept of polylipoic acid-based NPs obtained by nanoprecipitation of di- or tri-lipoic acid derivatives in the presence of a pluronic surfactant followed by a Ring Opening Disulphide polymerization (RODEP) [41]. The resulting nanoparticles feature average diameters in the 100–200 nm range and a PEGylated surface, formed by the pluronic surfactant, which remains entangled in the polymeric matrix of the core. PEG coating is a well-recognized way to improve the colloidal stability of NPs and their biocompatibility and pharmacokinetics properties compared to equivalent uncoated NPs. Indeed, these NPs were found to be very stable in water and saline solutions. In addition, in vitro biological studies showed that these nanoparticles displayed both a reduced interaction with plasma proteins, including opsonins, and high biocompatibility. We also demonstrated that polylipoic nanoparticles underwent degradation, by thiol-induced depolymerization [42], in the presence of endogenous reducing agents such as glutathione, which is present in relatively high concentrations in the cells' cytosol, but not in the extracellular fluids. Results from in vivo experiments confirmed the low toxicity and revealed the ability of these nanoparticles to rapidly accumulate in the rat heart after injection. These observations suggested the possibility to use these poly-lipoic nanoparticles to contrast oxidative stress, and in particular IRI, in different cell lines due to their potential antioxidant activity. Indeed, not only are the lipoic acid molecules released upon nanoparticle degradation/reduction known antioxidants, but the disulphide bonds ubiquitous in the nanoparticle polymeric matrix before degradation can also have a ROS scavenging activity.

On these premises, we decided to investigate the potential of poly(lipoic acid) nanoparticles for scavenging free radicals in an abiotic measurement system to determine maximum antioxidant capacity while also testing in cellular types representative of the milieu encountered in organ-level ischemia. In particular, we used macrophages and NRVMs as a recognized and reliable model, keeping several crucial functional and structural features of adult cardiomyocytes from oxidative stress and IRI.

2. Materials and Methods

2.1. Cells

HeLa cells (obtained from DSB University of Padova, Padova, Italy) were maintained in Dulbecco's Modified Eagle Medium (DMEM, Gibco, Thermo Fisher Scientific, Waltham, MA, USA) supplemented with 10% FCS (*v*/*v*) (Euroclone®, Pero (MI), Italy) and antibiotics (penicillin and streptomycin, Invitrogen) at 37 °C in a humidified atmosphere containing 5% (*v*/*v*) CO_2; cells were split every 2–3 days.

Human macrophages were obtained from human monocytes, purified from buffy coats of healthy donors as previously described [43] by two sequential centrifugations on Ficoll and Percoll (GE Healthcare, Chicago, IL, USA) gradients, respectively, and differentiated for 7 days with 100 ng/mL macrophage colony-stimulating factor (M-CSF, BD Biosciences, Franklin Lakes, NJ, USA) in RPMI-1640 medium supplemented with 20% FCS (*v*/*v*) at 37 °C in a humidified atmosphere containing 5% (*v*/*v*) CO_2. The M2 phenotype was routinely assessed by *CD14, CD16, Cd80 and Cd163* expression. The peripheral blood mononuclear cells utilized in this study were derived from buffy coats obtained from healthy blood donors and anonymously provided by the Transfusion Centre of the Hospital of Padova. Written informed consent for the use of the buffy coats for research purposes was obtained from blood donors by the Transfusion Centre. Data related to human samples were all analyzed anonymously. Human leukocytes, provided by the Transfusion Centre of the Hospital of Padova, were obtained not as a consequence of experimentation on human beings, but as a consequence of voluntary and informed blood donation for transfusions; no approval of an ethics committee is needed in such cases at our institution.

Neonatal rat ventricular myocytes (NRVMs) were isolated from 1 to 3 days old Wistar rats as described previously [44]. Cardiomyocytes were plated in 0.1% porcine gelatin (Sigma-Aldrich, St Louis, MO, USA) coated plates at variable density (at least 2.5×10^5 cells/mL) in MEM supplemented with 10% FBS (*v*/*v*) (Thermo Fisher Scientific, Waltham, MA, USA), 1% penicillin/streptomycin (*v*/*v*) (Thermo Fisher Scientific), 1% non-essential amino acids (*v*/*v*) (Thermo Fisher Scientific, Waltham, MA, USA), 1 mM 5-Bromo-2-Deoxyuridine (Sigma-Aldrich, St Louis, MO, USA). Cells were maintained at 37 °C in the presence of 5% CO_2. The medium was changed to MEM supplemented with 1% FBS (*v*/*v*), 1% penicillin/streptomycin (*v*/*v*), and 1% non-essential amino acids (*v*/*v*) after 24 h of plating. The procedures relative to the isolation of primary cardiomyocytes from neonatal rats were approved by the local ethical committee of the University of Padova (Organism for Animal Welfare, OPBA) and by the Italian Ministry of Health (Ethical Approval Number: D2784.N.7RX).

2.2. DPPH Assay and ABTS Assay

To assess the intrinsic scavenging capacity of NPs DPPH and ABTS assays were performed. First, 100 μL of NPs at different concentrations (up to 400 μg/mL) were added to methanol buffer solution (60% methanol, 40% 0.1 M acetate buffer *v*/*v*, pH 5.5) were added to 50 μM DPPH radical (1,1-diphenyl-2-picrylhydrazyl) solution, and changes in optical density at 517 nm were measured every 120 s for 60 times. Results are indicated as percentage of antioxidant capacity inhibition (% DPPH scavenging). 7 mM ABTS (2,2′-azino-bis(3-ethylbenzothiazoline-6-sulfonic acid) solution and 2.46 mM potassium persulfate were mixed together and maintained for 18 h in the dark to obtain the radical molecule ABTS•+. Then, 100 μL of NPs at different concentrations (up to 400 μg/mL) in PBS solution were added to 0.28 mM ABTS•+ solution, and changes in optical density at 734 nm were measured every 60 s for 40 times at 30 °C. Results are indicated as percentage of antioxidant capacity inhibition (% ABTS scavenging). Butylated hydroxytoluene and water were used as positive and negative controls, respectively, in both assays.

2.3. Cellular Uptake Analysis

Cells were seeded into 24-well plates (5×10^4 cells/well HeLa, 2×10^6 cells/well human macrophages, 1.5×10^5 cells/well NRVM). On the day of the experiment, cells were treated with different concentrations of fluorescent-doped NPs (up to 400 μg/mL) in medium supplemented with 10% of FCS or HS; cells incubated with no nanoparticles were used as a negative control. Then, cells were washed in PBS, detached, centrifuged (1500 rpm, 5 min) and resuspended in FACS buffer (PBS containing 1% FCS and 0.1% NaN_3). Samples were analyzed by flow cytometry (BD FACSCantoII) and data processed through BD FACSDiva™ Software (BD).

2.4. Pulse–Chase Assay

For the pulse experiment, 2×10^6 macrophages were incubated with 400 μg/mL of F127@**1**-NP and F127@**2**-NP for different incubation times (5′, 10′, 20′, 40′, 60′, 120′ and 180′); cells were then washed with PBS, harvested, resuspended in FACS buffer (PBS supplemented with 1% FBS) and analyzed by flow cytometry. For the chase experiment, macrophages were incubated with 400 μg/mL of F127@**1**-NP and F127@**2**-NP for 10′; cells were then washed twice with PBS and incubated for different times with 10% FCS RPMI without nanoparticles; cells were then recovered, washed again with PBS, resuspended in FACS buffer and analyzed by flow cytometry.

NRVMs were seeded in either 24-well (pulse) or 96-well (chase) plates at density of 3×10^5 cells/mL. A pulse of 100 μM fluorescent-doped NPs was applied to cells at different timings, ranging from 5 min to 180 min. At the end of the pulse protocol, cells were harvested and resuspended in FACS buffer. Samples were analyzed by flow cytometry and data processed through BD FACSDiva™ Software (BD). Untreated cell fluorescence was subtracted from each sample and values are expressed as Mean Fluorescence Intensity (MFI).

For two given pulse periods (i.e., 5 min and 20 min), the chase phase was evaluated in NRVMs at different time points, ranging from 10 min to 180 min. Fluorescence was monitored using a plate reader (Tecan Infinite® M200 PRO). Data have been expressed as MFI normalized to basal value.

2.5. Estimation of ROS Production

ROS generation in cell systems was estimated using the fluorogenic probe CM-H_2DCFDA (Molecular Probes, Thermo Fisher Scientific, Waltham, MA, USA). Cells (1×10^4 cells/well HeLa, 1×10^5 cells/well human macrophages, 3×10^4 cells/well NRVM) were seeded in a 96-well plate and treated with NPs at different concentrations (up to 200 μg/mL) at different time points. Then, cells were washed in PBS and loaded with a 25 μM dye for 1 h in the dark at 37 °C. Afterwards, the cells were washed and incubated with tert-Butyl hydroperoxide (t-BHP, Sigma-Aldrich, St Louis, MO, USA) at different concentrations (up to 200 μM). The fluorescence increase was estimated on a plate reader (Tecan Infinite® M200 PRO) at 485 nm (λ excitation) and 527 nm (λ emission) for 1.5 h (2.5 h in NRVM experiments) [45].

2.6. Live Imaging

Experiments were carried out in HBSS at pH 7.4 (adjusted with NaOH) and at 37 °C. Images were acquired using an inverted fluorescence microscope (Leica DMI6000B equipped with DFC365FX camera) with PL APO 40x/1.25 oil objective. Fluorescence intensity was quantified using the Fiji distribution of the Java-based image processing program

ImageJ [46], and background signal was subtracted from all analyzed regions of interest. For Ca^{2+} imaging, traces were analyzed using the "Peak Analyzer" tool of Origin Pro 9.1. The experiments were performed in the presence or absence of 100 μg/mL NPs.

Ischemic injury was simulated in vitro as previously described [44]. Briefly, a 15 mm circular glass coverslip was placed on the center of cardiomyocyte monolayer to reduce availability of nutrients and O_2, thus inducing ischemic conditions. Reperfusion was simulated by removing the coverslip after 1 h of simulated ischemia.

To monitor mitochondrial ROS formation in NRVMs, cells were transfected with the genetically encoded H_2O_2 sensor Mito-HyPer (Evrogen, Moscow, Russia) [47]. NRVMs were plated on l-Plate 2-well black plates (Ibidi, Gräfelfing, Bayer, Germany) at a density of 1×10^5 cells/mL and transfected with Lipofectamine 3000 reagent (Sigma-Aldrich, St Louis, MO, USA). For each transfection, 2 μg of plasmid was diluted in 125 μL of Opti-MEM medium (Thermo Fisher Scientific) in the presence of 4 μL of P3000 reagent (Thermo Fisher Scientific, Waltham, MA, USA), and later combined with 5 μL of Lipofectamine 3000 (Thermo Fisher Scientific, Waltham, MA, USA). The DNA–lipid complexes were added to the cells and incubated at 37 °C in the presence of 5% CO_2. Transfected cells were used for experiments after 48 h. Images were collected before the ischemic injury and in the first 5′ after the reperfusion injury. Fluorescence values were expressed as HyPer ratio (488/410 nm).

To monitor mitochondrial membrane potential ($\Delta\Psi m$), cells were incubated with 25 nM tetramethyl rhodamine (TMRM, Thermo Fisher Scientific, Waltham, MA, USA) and 1.6 μM cyclosporin H for 30 min at 37 °C, in the presence of 5% CO_2. Cyclosporin H is necessary to block multidrug resistance glycoprotein (MDR) that otherwise would cause the release of TMRM into the extracellular space [48]. TMRM fluorescence intensity was monitored, and images were acquired during the whole experiment. Fluorescence values were normalized to basal value.

To monitor intracellular [Ca^{2+}] homeostasis, cells were incubated with 5 μM Fluo-4 AM ester (Thermo Fisher Scientific, Waltham, MA, USA), 0.01% *w*/*v* pluronic F-127 (Sigma-Aldrich, St Louis, MO, USA), and 250 μM sulfinpyrazone (Sigma-Aldrich, St Louis, MO, USA), for 20 min at 37 °C in a humidified incubator, followed by 20 min of de-esterification. Images have been collected before the ischemic injury and in the first minute after the reperfusion injury. Since the accumulation of Fluo-4 in NRVMs can vary from different preparations, data were normalized to the DMSO control.

2.7. Assessment of Cell Death

For anoxia/reoxygenation experiments, NRVMs were seeded in 24-well plates at density of 3×10^5 cells/mL and incubated in 118 mM NaCl, 5 mM KCl, 1.2 mM KH_2PO_4, 1.2 mM $MgSO_4$, 2 mM $CaCl_2$, 25 mM MOPS at pH 6.4 during anoxia or pH 7.4 during reoxygenation [44]. Cells were pre-treated with different concentrations of NPs (ranging from 10 to 200 μg/mL) and 2 μM CsA or 10 μM MitoTempo were used as positive controls. Anoxia was induced by adding 10 mM 2-deoxy-D-glucose (2-DG) and incubating cells in a BD GasPak™ EZ Anaerobe Gas-generating Pouch System with an indicator (BD Biosciences, Franklin Lakes, NJ, USA) at 37 °C for 12 h [44]. To induce reoxygenation, plates were removed from the GasPak™ pouch, 2-DG was replaced with 10 mM D-glucose, the pH was restored at 7.4. The plates were then incubated for 4 h in a humidified incubator at 37 °C. The release of LDH from NRVMs was measured to evaluate cell death in anoxia, reoxygenation and during the pre-treatment phase [49]. Supernatant aliquots were collected at every time point (3 h of pre-treatment, 12 h of anoxia, and 4 h of reoxygenation), and at the end of each experiment, intact cells were lysed by incubating them with 1% Triton X-100 (Sigma-Aldrich, St Louis, MO, USA) for 30 min. Between the collection of the reoxygenation supernatant and the lysis, cells were washed with PBS 1X to remove reoxygenation-derived LDH that could interfere with the analysis of the lysate.

2.8. Data Analysis

All values are expressed as mean ± SE. All data were normally distributed and comparison between groups was performed by either one-way or two-way ANOVA, followed by Tukey's post hoc multiple comparison. A value of $p < 0.05$ was considered significant.

3. Results

3.1. Synthesis and Characterization of 1- and 2-Poly(Lipoic Acid) NPs

Based on our previous screening [41], we selected derivatives **1** and **2** (Figure 1) as precursors to prepare the poly(lipoic acid) nanoparticles used in this study. They featured 1,8-octanediol and glycerol as spacers connecting respectively two and three lipoic acid molecules via ester linkages. Using these precursors, it was possible to explore the biological properties of nanoparticles characterized by different degrees of crosslinking. In particular, previous investigations revealed that less crosslinked F127@**1**-NP are more susceptible to degradation by endogenous thiols than F127@**2**-NP. The Rhodamine B/lipoic acid conjugate **3** was used, when necessary, as co-precursor for the fluorescent labeling of the nanoparticles [41]. Compounds **1**, **2** and **3** were prepared in good yields from commercially available precursors by standard synthetic protocols, as described in detail in [41].

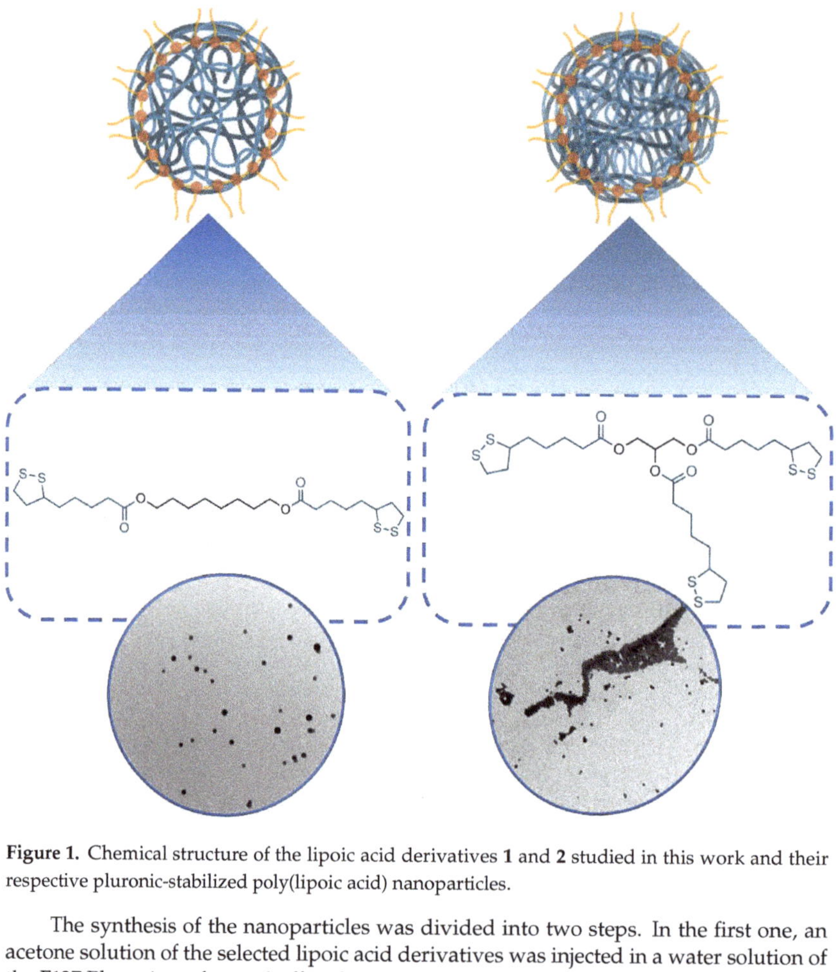

Figure 1. Chemical structure of the lipoic acid derivatives **1** and **2** studied in this work and their respective pluronic-stabilized poly(lipoic acid) nanoparticles.

The synthesis of the nanoparticles was divided into two steps. In the first one, an acetone solution of the selected lipoic acid derivatives was injected in a water solution of the F127 Pluronic surfactant buffered at pH 7 with PBS. The diffusion of acetone in water caused the formation of nanoparticles made by the aggregated precursors, stabilized by the F127 surfactant. In the second step, the polymerization and cross-linking of precursors in the nanoparticle core were induced by addition of 1-octanethiol and quenched after 30 min by addition of iodoacetamide. The nanoparticles were eventually purified by centrifugation and resuspension in water and PBS. Dynamic light scattering (DLS) analysis revealed that the batches of F127@**1**-NP and F127@**2**-NP obtained had average hydrodynamic diameters of 170–190 nm and 140–160 nm, respectively, with size dispersions in the 10–30% range (PDI values between 0.011 and 0.13, see Table S1). Larger size of F127@**2**-NP with respect to F127@**1**-NP agrees with previous reports and was attributed to the greater hydrophobicity of **2** with respect to **1**. Accordingly, co-polymerization with fluorescent derivative **3** resulted in a marginal decrease of the average particles size. TEM analysis confirmed the formation of spherical nanoparticles. Characterization data of a representative sample are reported in Figure S1A,B.

The stability of these nanoparticles upon prolonged storage (22 days) in water was studied using DLS, TEM and fluorescence spectroscopy. Hydrodynamic size, polydispersity index (PDI) and structure of both F127@**1**-NP and F127@**2**-NP, measured by DLS and TEM, did not significantly change over the same period of time (Figure S1E,F). The possible release of the co-polymerized **3** dye was investigated by measuring the fluorescence emission of the sample after centrifugation and resuspension in fresh solvent. No relevant emission decrease was observed for rhodamine-labeled F127@**2**-NPs, also, in this case, while only a small decrease was observed in the case of rhodamine-labeled F127@**1**-NPs after 3 weeks (Figure S1C,D, respectively).

3.2. Biocompatibility of Poly(Lipoic Acid) NPs

Consistent with previous data [17], F127@**1**-NP and F127@**2**-NP showed no cytotoxic or membrane destabilizing effects (Figure S2A–C). To ensure the biocompatibility of the NPs, the activation of the contact-triggered coagulation in human plasma (HP) and of the complement cascade in human serum (HS) was also considered (Figure S3A,B). Noticeably, NPs did not stimulate coagulation events, while only a weak induction of the complement cascade was observed in the presence of high concentrations (i.e., 400 μg/mL) of F127@**2**-NP. Consistently, both NPs formulations were virtually devoid of a protein hard corona in fetal calf serum (FCS), HP and HS (Figure S3C).

3.3. Radical Scavenging Activity of Poly(Lipoic Acid) NPs Compared with Free Lipoic Acid and Pluronic Acid in A-Cellular Assays

The radical scavenging efficacy of NPs was then tested using both the DPPH and ABTS radicals. Maximal antioxidant activities of F127@**1**-NP and F127@**2**-NP at 400 μg/mL concentration against the DPPH radical in methanol rich medium were 12% and 30%, respectively (Figure 2A). This activity was lower than that of the commonly used antioxidant BHT (20 μM; 48% scavenge), but significant. Dose-response and kinetics showed that the F127@**2**-NP was about 2–3 times more effective than F127@**1**-NP as DPPH scavenger. ABTS radical scavenging experiments made it possible to assess the nanoparticles' radical scavenging ability in a more physiological medium (PBS, pH 7.4), where the maximal activities were 12% and 19% for F127@**1**-NP and F127@**2**-NP, respectively, at 400 μg/mL concentration (Figure 2B). Again, ABTS radical neutralization by both NPs was inferior to that of the BHT positive control (38%). Dose-response and kinetics experiments showed that F127@**2**-NP was 1.4–1.7 times more effective as ABTS scavenger than F127@**1**-NP. It is interesting to note that the scavenging activity of NPs measured with the DPPH assay was better than that of their free constituents (lipoic acid and Pluronic surfactant). Conversely, in the ABTS assay, in more physiological conditions, the antiradical action of the sum of free lipoic acid and Pluronic was more effective than that of the equivalent amount of NPs (about 2 folds) (Figure S4). Conveniently, the release of Pluronic and lipoic acid is one of the results of the eventual degradation of NPs within cells after capture, suggesting that this could produce an improvement of intracellular protection from radical damage.

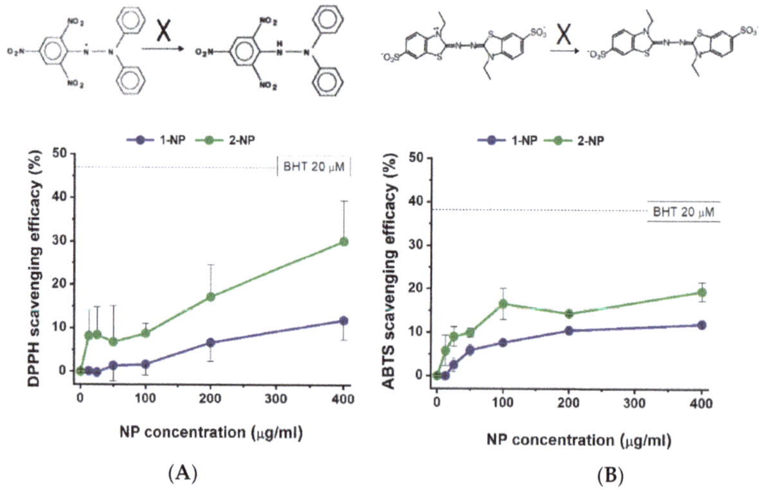

Figure 2. Organic radical scavenging efficacies of F127@**1**-NP and F127@**2**-NP. The indicated concentrations of NPs were incubated with DPPH (**A**) and ABTS (**B**) and the % neutralization (see top schemes) was estimated spectroscopically after 30 min incubation at 37 °C. Data are means ± SE (N = 4). The scavenging effect of BHT is indicated in the graphs for comparison.

3.4. Capture of Poly(Lipoic Acid) NPs by Different Cell Lines

Having established the radical scavenging ability of poly(lipoic acid) NPs, we investigated their internalization in different cell lines. Fluorescent labeled F127@**1**-NPs, incubated at different concentrations for 24 h, were captured by human primary macrophages and blood monocytes, and, although with reduced efficacy, by polymorphonuclear granulocytes (PMNGs). Conversely, lymphocytes captured NPs at very low levels (Figure S6A). This trend was confirmed by a time-course analysis at early times, which showed a rapid temperature-dependent initial phase of NP cell uptake, especially in macrophages (Figure S6B).

It is worth mentioning that these results showed that the mouse macrophagic cell line RAW 264.7, being extremely ineffective at NP capture, was an unreliable model for human macrophages.

NP association to macrophages, monocytes and lymphocytes was marginally modified when cells were incubated with FCS, HS or citrated HS (Figure S7), suggesting that these media have poor opsonic effect, in agreement with the lack of corona formation and complement activation by NPs (Figure S3B,C).

3.5. Capture and Antioxidative Effect of Poly(Lipoic Acid) NPs in Human Macrophage and HeLa Cells

Having established that human macrophages are a good target of our NPs, the interaction of these cells with fluorescent F127@**1**-NP and F127@**2**-NP was characterized in detail. Dose-response incubation with F127@**1**-NP for 3 h (Figure 3A) resulted in a cell-associated fluorescence signal about 3–4 times more intense than that observed after incubation with F127@**2**-NP, especially at higher doses (>100 μg/mL). This behavior was only slightly modified by the presence of HS, compared to FCS, in line with weak HS interaction on these NPs (Figure S8). The results of time-course experiments indicated that the F127@**1**-NP and F127@**2**-NP capture by macrophages was quite similar at early times (<20 min). However, a divergent increase of the F127@**1**-NP signal compared to the F127@**2**-NP was detected at longer times, accounting for the observed differences after 3 h incubation (Figure 3B). In addition, time-dependent uptake profiles were clearly biphasic. To discriminate whether this late fluorescence increase both in time- and concentration-dependent experiments was due to a true differential NP capture, macrophages fluorescence was measured after a 10 min pulse with the two NPs types, followed by different chase times. Interestingly, data indicated an increase of the cell fluorescence occurring after NP endocytosis (Figure 3C) for both the nanoparticles. This behavior can only be attributed to the decrease of the self-quenching of the Rhodamine dyes, due to their release in the cell environment following NP degradation. This effect seems more evident for the F127@**1**-NP compared with F127@**2**-NP, which is in agreement with previous data showing that thiol-induced NP degradation is faster in F127@**1**-NP than in F127@**2**-NP (Figure S1E,F; see also [41]).

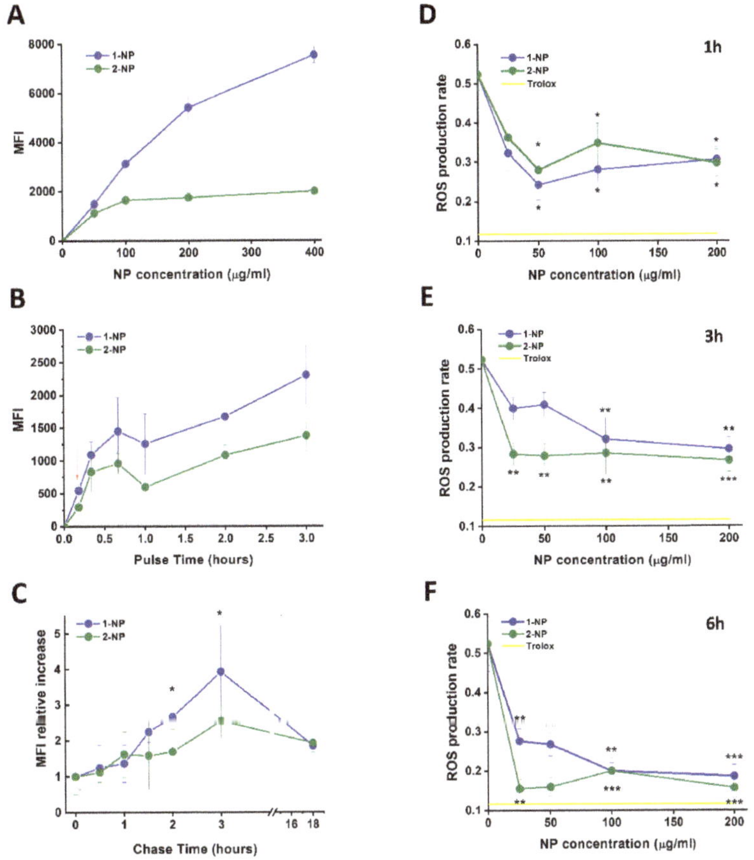

Figure 3. Capture, intracellular disassembly and antioxidative efficacies of F127@**1**-NP and F127@**2**-NP in t-BHP-treated human macrophages. (**A**) Cells were incubated with the indicated doses of fluorescently labeled F127@**1**-NP and F127@**2**-NP, for 3 h in DMEM plus 10% FCS and analyzed, after washing in NP-free medium, by flow cytofluorimetry. Data (Mean Fluorescence Intensity) are the mean of 4 independent experiments ± SE. (**B**) Cells were incubated with F127@**1**-NP and F127@**2**-NP (100 μg/mL) for the indicated time lapses and analyzed for their MFI by flow cytofluorimetry as above (data are mean ± SE, N = 4). The red arrow indicates the pulse–chase experiments described in panel (**C**). Cells were pulsed for 10 min as in panel (**B**), washed 3 times with PBS and further cashed in cell medium with no NPs for the indicated times. MFI acquired by flow cytometry after cell recovery are expressed as relative values compared to the MFI one after the pulse time (taken as 1). Data are

mean ± SE (N = 3). * Significance t < 0.05 of the difference between F127@**2**-NP and F127@**1**-NP at a given time. (**D–F**) Cells were treated with the shown concentrations of F127@**1**-NP and F127@**2**-NP for 1 h (**D**), 3 h (**E**), and 6 h (**F**). After washing, cells were incubated with the ROS-sensitive probe. The ROS production was induced using the oxidative agent t-BHP (100 μM). ROS production rate (ROS production/time) is reported as a function of NP dose. Data are mean ± SE (N = 4). Statistical significance of the difference compared with no NP samples: * t < 0.05; ** t < 001; *** t < 0.001. The inhibitory effect of the positive control Trolox (500 μM) is indicated as a yellow line.

Having shown that F127@**1**-NP and F127@**2**-NP are taken up by macrophages with similar efficiency, but differently degraded, we tested their antioxidant efficacy in these cells against an oxidative stress induced by the peroxide molecule t-BHP (Figure 3D–F). Pre-incubation of macrophages with NPs for 1 and 3 h reduced ROS formation upon subsequent t-BHP treatment, with an efficacy which was about half of that induced by the positive control Trolox. Interestingly, NP concentration doses as low as 25 μg/mL already gave quasi-maximal protective effects. Pre-preincubation of 6 h resulted in ROS prevention similar to that induced by Trolox (70% ROS inhibition). While the F127@**2**-NP and F127@**1**-NP anti-ROS activities in macrophages were comparable after 1-h preincubation, at longer preincubation times, F127@**2**-NP were significantly more effective.

Notably, at variance from cell-free assays, the antioxidant activity of F127@**1**-NP against t-BHP-derived reactive oxygen species (ROS) in macrophages was superior (~30% protection) than that elicited by free lipoic acid (~15%) (Figure S5).

Analogous experiments were also performed in HeLa neoplastic cell line, where ROS production induced by t-BHP was much reduced as compared to macrophages. Although cell-associated fluorescence values were reduced about 10-fold with respect to macrophages, their relative trend was quite similar to that seen in macrophages and was similarly not influenced by HS compared to FCS. Consequently, also in these cells, NPs inhibited t-BHP-induced ROS production, with a maximal efficacy of about 60% after a 6-h preincubation (Figure S11).

3.6. Uptake and Antioxidative Effects of Poly(Lipoic Acid) NPs in Neonatal Rat Ventricular Myocytes (NRVMs)

Having established the antioxidant efficacy of poly(lipoic acid) NPs in phagocytes and epithelial cells, we moved to test these particles in primary murine cardiomyocytes. Indeed, the oxidative injury of cardiac cells is involved in important pathological conditions, such as IRI.

Firstly, the uptake capacity of cardiomyocytes was evaluated. The fluorescence associated to neonatal rat ventricular myocytes (NRVMs) after incubation for 3 h with F127@**1**-NP was strikingly more intense than that due to F127@**2**-NP (Figure 4A). Time-dependent experiments revealed that, also with this cell line, the signal increase at early times showed a reduced capture rate, compared to macrophages at early times (<1 h), which was nevertheless similar for both F127@**1**-NP and F127@**2**-NP up to 60 min (Figure 4B). After this initial phase, fluorescence increased in both cases, but in a much more marked way in the presence of F127@**1**-NP compared to F127@**2**-NP. Pulse–chase experiments, again in line with what occurred in macrophages, demonstrated that the increase in fluorescence following internalization of F127@**1**-NP compared to F127@**2**-NP was due to cellular effects after internalization. However, in NRVMs the kinetics of fluorescence gain of internalized NPs, likely due to intracellular disassembly of the nanoparticles, was much more rapid (maximal effect after 0.5 h chase) (Figures 4C, S11A,B and S12A) as compared to human macrophages maximal effect (after 3 h chase). NRVMs pretreated with NPs were protected from t-BHP induced ROS production, similarly to macrophages. In these cells, almost maximal protection was achieved following only a 1 h pre-incubation with the lower concentration (i.e., 25 μg/mL) (Figure 4D). However, in NRVMs the F127@**2**-NP was slightly less effective than F127@**1**-NP, likely due to a more marked differential degradation rate in macrophages. Nevertheless, the maximal protective effect was about 80%, and no further protection was observed by increasing the pre-incubation time point (Figure 4E,F).

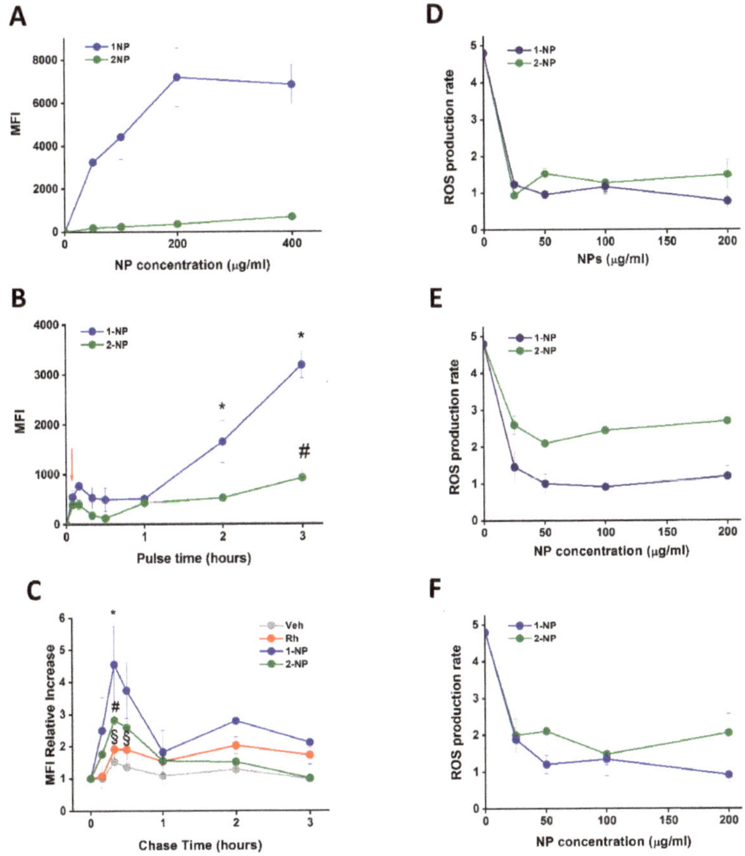

Figure 4. Capture, intracellular disassembly poly(lipoic acid) and antioxidative efficacies of F127@**1**-NP and F127@**2**-NP in t-BHP treated NRVMs. (**A**) Neonatal rat ventricular myocytes (NRVMs) were incubated with the indicated concentrations of fluorescently-labeled F127@**1**-NP and F127@**2**-NP for 3 h in DMEM plus 1% FCS and analyzed, after washings in NP-free medium, by flow cytofluorimetry. Data (Mean Fluorescence Intensity) are the mean of 3 independent experiments ± SE. (**B**) NRVMs were incubated with F127@**1**-NP and F127@**2**-NP (100 μg/mL) for the indicated time lapses and analyzed for their MFI by flow cytofluorimetry as above (data are mean ± SE, N = 3). * $p < 0.001$ vs. 5 min, # $p < 0.05$ vs. 5 min by two-way ANOVA with post hoc Tukey's multiple comparison test. The red arrow indicates the pulse time with NPs (5 min) used for pulse–chase experiments described in panel (**C**). Cells were pulsed for 5 min as in panel (**B**), washed 3 times with PBS and further chased in cell medium with no NPs for the indicated times. Equivalent amounts of the buffer (Veh) or the fluorophore rhodamine (Rh) were used as controls. MFI acquired by spectrofluorimetry after cell recovery are expressed as relative values compared to the MFI one after the pulse time (taken as 1). Data are mean ± SE (N = 3). * $p < 0.01$ vs. 5 min, # $p < 0.05$ vs. 5 min, § $p < 0.01$ vs. NPs by two-way ANOVA with post hoc Tukey's multiple comparison test. (**D–F**) NRVMs were preincubated with the shown concentrations of F127@**1**-NP and F127@**2**-NP for 1 h (**D**), 3 h (**E**) and 6 h (**F**), washed and further incubated with the CM-H_2DCFDA. The ROS production was initiated with t-BHP (100 μM). ROS production rate (ROS production/time) is reported as a function of NP dose. Data are mean ± SE (N = 3).

3.7. Poly(Lipoic Acid) NPs Protect NRVMs from Ischemia/Reperfusion Oxidative Injury

Having observed poly(lipoic acid) NP capture by primary NRVMs and their subsequent protection from chemically-induced oxidative stress, we investigated the possible prevention of the reperfusion damage in an in vitro model of IRI. NRVMs were pretreated with increasing concentrations of F127@**1**-NP or F127@**2**-NP, ranging from 10 to 200 μg/mL, and cells were subjected to anoxia/reoxygenation (A/R) protocol to simulate IRI. Both F127@**1**-NP and F127@**2**-NP at concentrations as low as 10 μg/mL protected cardiomyocytes against reoxygenation-induced loss of viability as shown by a decrease in lactate dehydrogenase (LDH) release (% LDH release: ~50% untreated vs. ~30% treated) (Figure 5A). The degree of protection was comparable with that afforded by MitoTempo (MT) and cyclosporine A (CsA). Of note, both NPs did not induce loss of viability in either pre-treatment or anoxic phase (Figure S12C,D).

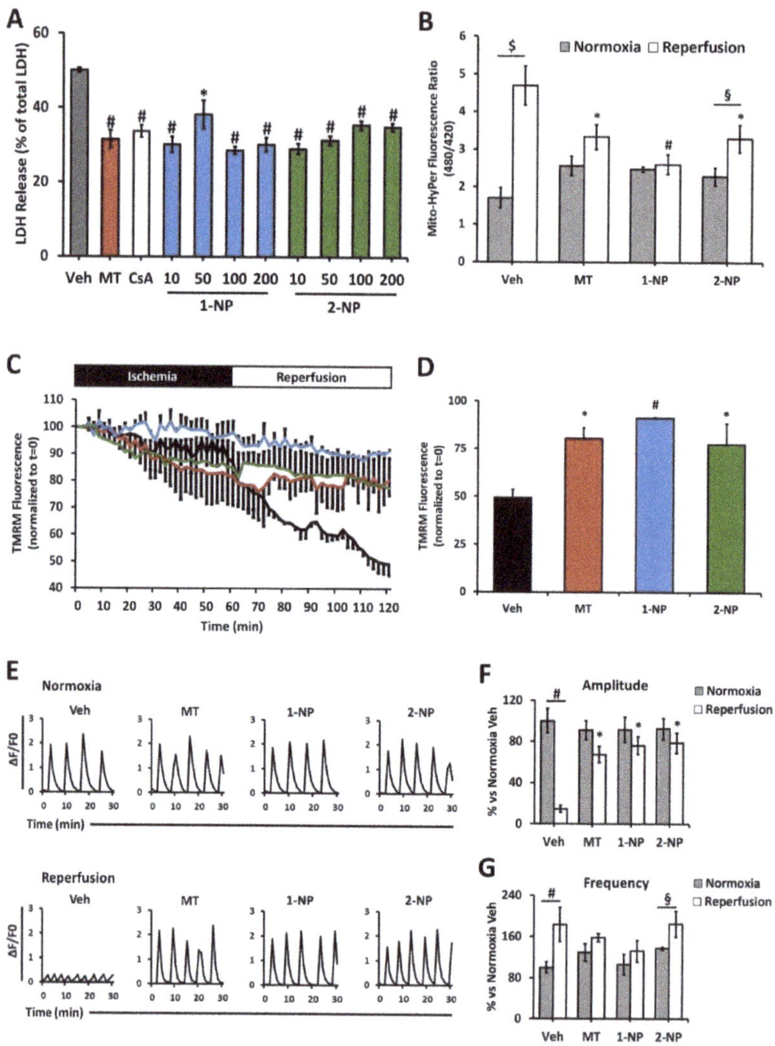

Figure 5. Poly(lipoic acid) NPs protect cardiomyocytes (RNVMs) from ischemia-reperfusion injury. (**A**) Cell death measured by LDH release in reoxygenation from isolated NRVMs. Cells were treated

with different concentrations of either F127@**1**-NP or F127@**2**-NP. MitoTempo (MT, 10 μM) or cyclosporin A (CsA, 2 μM) were used as positive control. * $p < 0.01$ vs. Veh, # $p < 0.001$ vs. Veh by one-way ANOVA with post hoc Tukey's multiple comparison test. (**B**) Mitochondrial H_2O_2 formation measured by Mito-HyPer in isolated NRVMs subjected to coverslip ischemia. Cells were treated with either F127@**1**-NP (100 μg/mL) or F127@**2**-NP (100 μg/mL). MitoTempo (MT 10 μM) was used as positive control. * $p < 0.01$ vs. Reoxygenation Veh, # $p < 0.001$ vs. Reoxygenation Veh, § $p < 0.05$, $ $p < 0.001$ by two-way ANOVA with post hoc Tukey's multiple comparison test. (**C**) Mitochondrial membrane potential ($\Delta\Psi$m) monitored by TMRM fluorescence in isolated NRVMs subjected to coverslip ischemia. Cells were treated with either F127@**1**-NP (100 μg/mL) or F127@**2**-NP (100 μg/mL). MitoTempo (MT 10 μM) was used as positive control. (**D**) $\Delta\Psi$m was quantified after 60 min of simulated reperfusion. * $p < 0.01$ vs. Veh, # $p < 0.001$ vs. Veh by one-way ANOVA with post hoc Tukey's multiple comparison test. (**E**) Representative intracellular [Ca^{2+}] transients during normoxia (upper panel) and reperfusion (lower panel) in isolated NRVMs subjected to coverslip ischemia. Cells were treated with either F127@**1**-NP (100 μg/mL) or F127@**2**-NP (100 μg/mL). MitoTempo (MT 10 μM) was used as positive control. (**F**) Transient amplitude average in spontaneous beating NRVMs. * $p < 0.001$ vs. Veh Reperfusion, # $p < 0.001$ by two-way ANOVA with post hoc Tukey's multiple comparison test. (**G**) Transient frequency average in spontaneous beating NRVMs. # $p < 0.001$, § $p < 0.05$ by two-way ANOVA with post hoc Tukey's multiple comparison test. Approximately 30 cells were analyzed per condition in each experiment. For LDH release, approximately 3–4 wells were analyzed per condition in each experiment. All the experiments were performed at least three times using different animal preparations. Data are expressed as mean ± SEM.

The burst of H_2O_2 production by mitochondria upon reperfusion was also inhibited by both F127@**1**-NP and F127@**2**-NP with an efficacy that was almost 100% in the case of the F127@**1**-NP and about 60% in the case of F127@**2**-NP, values comparable to that obtained with MT as a positive control (Figures 5B and S12E). Consistently, the drop in the mitochondrial membrane potential subsequent to reperfusion was prevented by both F127@**1**-NP and F127@**2**-NP, with efficacies comparable to, if not better than, that displayed by MT (Figures 5C,D and S12F). Eventually, the amplitude and the correct frequency of intracellular Ca^{2+} transients, which reflect the spontaneous contraction waves of NRVMs, were also preserved by both F127@**1**-NP and F127@**2**-NP preincubation, in spite of I/R damage (Figure 5E–G). In agreement with data obtained with t-BHP stress, the F127@**2**-NP were slightly less protective than the F127@**1**-NP against IRI.

4. Discussion

The present results highlight the antioxidative action of NPs made by cross-linked lipoic acid derivatives. Firstly, our study confirms the remarkable biocompatibility of these nanoparticles. Not only are they mainly composed of approved (F127) and endogenous (lipoic acid) building blocks, but they are also devoid of cellular toxicity and procoagulant activity, and complement activation. These results closely match those previously reported on these nanoparticles. In particular, it is remarkable to note the very small interaction with the plasma proteins, compared to other densely PEGylated nanoparticles. This resistance to protein adsorption may hence be attributed not only to the polymeric coating (PEG), but also to the influence that the specific core material used (polylipoic acid) may have on the coating molecules disposition and topology. This ability to escape plasma proteins is likely one of the factors at the basis of the high biocompatibility observed.

The second remarkable property is the relevant uptake by cardiomyocytes. This is indeed not so far from that exerted by scavenging M2 macrophages (here used) for F127@**1**-NP (17–34%) and even equal for F127@**2**-NP (91–124%). Moreover, NPs cardiomyocytes uptake is sensibly greater than that of lymphocytes and epithelial cells (5% for F127@**1**-NP and 13% for F127@**2**-NP, compared to M2 macrophages). This finding corroborates and helps to explain the results of previous in vivo studies with rats, which demonstrated a fast (maximum at 1 h after injection) and selective accumulation of these nanoparticles in the heart. In particular, detailed microscopy investigations demonstrated that the nanoparticles were taken up by the cardiomyocytes present in heart tissues, as confirmed by the present findings. It is important to note that, different from PLGA nanoparticles, uptake occurs in healthy cells, and hence it is not dependent on the presence of an oxidative stress. This would in principle make it possible to also target the initial ROS burst at the onset of post-ischemic reperfusion.

After uptake, nanoparticles undergo degradation, as revealed by the pulse and chase experiments. This process can occur both in endosomes, by hydrolytic degradation of the ester groups, or in the cytoplasm, by concurrent hydrolysis of the ester groups and reduction of the disulfide bonds. The result of this degradation is the release of both the payload and lipoic acid. Interestingly, degradation occurs with different degrees of efficiency in the different cell lines. Indeed, degradation is clearly observed in macrophages and cardiomyocytes; it is also present, albeit less efficient, in monocytes and in HeLa cells, and it appears to be absent in PMGNs. Such differences likely reflect the differences in the respective cell microenvironments. In particular, degradation in cardiomyocytes is noticeably faster than in macrophages, with the consequent quick release of the protective species. The degradation rate is also strongly influenced by the structure of nanoparticles. Indeed, the more crosslinked nature of F127@**2**-NP makes them more resistant to degradation both upon exposition to thiols, and inside the cells. Other factors, in particular the extent of water penetration, can influence this process. Again, precursor **2** is more lipophilic than **1**, and should offer more resistance to water penetration. It is to be mentioned that our analysis, although revealing NP disassembly, cannot establish whether lipoic and hypothetical payloads are quantitatively released from NPs in cardiomyocytes and other cells.

Remarkably, the degradation rate is not clearly paralleled by ROS scavenging activity. In cardiomyocytes, and less clearly in Hela cells, faster degrading F127@**1**-NP shows a slightly better performance than F127@**2**-NP. On the other hand, in macrophages, the trend is reversed. This behavior suggests that degradation is not straightforwardly related to ROS scavenging perfomance, likely because the disulfide groups widespread in the nanoparticles' cores are endowed with an antioxidant activity similar to that of lipoic acid.

Most remarkably, simulated reperfusion experiments on primary cardiomyocytes demonstrated a protective effect similar to that of leading cardioprotective compounds, highlighting the great potential of these nanoparticles.

5. Conclusions

At the end, not only do these soft NPs appear to be a good effective alternative to ceramic- or metal-based NPs as agents with intrinsic anti-oxidative effects, but they potentially allow for the development of more sophisticated drug systems. Indeed, while the NP matrix itself is active against ROS, it can at the same be loaded with pharmacologically active principles that are released only within cells, as Rhodamine was in this study. In addition, short-term accumulation of these NPs within the heart is independent of the physio pathological status of cells. This will allow them to act both as antioxidant particles and as a storage system of pharmacologically active principles, targeting simultaneously different stages of the IRI.

Supplementary Materials: The following supporting information can be downloaded at: https://www.mdpi.com/article/10.3390/antiox11050907/s1, Table S1. Nanoparticle size determined by DLS of F127@**1**-NPs and F127@**2**-NPs; Figure S1. Characterization of nanoparticles; Figure S2. Lack of F127@**1**-NP and F127@**2**-NP cytotoxicity; Figure S3. Coagulation, complement activation and corona formation assays performed with F127@**1**-NP and F127@**2**-NP; Figure S4. Organic radical scavenging efficacy evaluation of F127@**1**-NP, individual components for NP synthesis and different known antioxidants; Figure S5. Antioxidant activity of NPs against t-BHP-derived ROS in human macrophages; Figure S6. F127@**1**-NP uptake by human purified monocytes and lymphocytes, monocyte-derived macrophages, PMNGs and RAW 264.7 and HeLa cells; Figure S7. Dose-response uptake of F127@**1**-NP by macrophages, monocytes and lymphocytes in the presence of different percentage of FCS, HS or HP; Figure S8. Capture of F127@**1**-NP and F127@**2**-NP by human macrophages in the presence of FCS or HS; Figure S9. F127@**1**-NP and F127@**2**-NP scavenging activity in human macrophages in response to increasing concentration of t-BHP; Figure S10. Capture and scavenging activity of F127@**1**-NP and F127@**2**-NP in HeLa cells; Figure S11. Comparison between chase phases of nanoparticles; Figure S12. Effects of nanoparticles on cardiomyocytes.

Author Contributions: C.B. and L.M.-B. prepared and characterized the precursors and nanoparticles. C.B. performed most of the in vitro experiments. S.A. performed experiments on NRVM isolated cells. S.S. performed some in vitro experiments. R.T. supervised the in vitro experiments and performed the pulse chase experiment. E.P. contributed to the project design, funding and revised the manuscript. F.M., E.P. and F.D.L. designed research and supervised the project. All authors have read and agreed to the published version of the manuscript.

Funding: This project was partially founded by the European Union's Horizon 2020 research and innovation program, under the Marie Skłodowska-Curie grant agreement MMBio (No. 721613), Leducq Transatlantic Network of Excellence 16CVD04, the COST Action EU-CARDIOPROTECTION CA16225 and Progetto Strategico di Ateneo NAMECA, PRAT 2015 CPDA149379.

Institutional Review Board Statement: The study was conducted in accordance with the Declaration of Helsinki and the procedures relative to the isolation of primary cardiomyocytes from neonatal rats were approved by the local ethical committee of the University of Padova (Organism for Animal Welfare, OPBA) and by the Italian Ministry of Health (Ethical Approval Number: D2784.N.7RX).

Informed Consent Statement: The peripheral blood mononuclear cells utilized in this study were derived from buffy coats obtained from healthy blood donors and anonymously provided by the Transfusion Centre of the Hospital of Padova. Written informed consent for the use of the buffy coats for research purposes was obtained from blood donors by the Transfusion Centre. Data related to human samples were all analyzed anonymously. Human leu-kocytes, provided by the Transfusion Centre of the Hospital of Padova, were obtained not as a consequence of experimentation on human beings, but as a consequence of voluntary and informed blood donation for transfusions; no approval of an ethics committee is needed in such cases at our institution.

Data Availability Statement: Data is contained within the article and Supplementary Materials.

Conflicts of Interest: The authors declare no conflict of interest.

References

1. Sajadimajd, S.; Khazaei, M. Oxidative Stress and Cancer: The Role of Nrf2. *Curr. Cancer Drug Targets* **2018**, *18*, 538–557. [CrossRef] [PubMed]
2. Puspita, L.; Chung, S.Y.; Shim, J.-W. Oxidative stress and cellular pathologies in Parkinson's disease. *Mol. Brain* **2017**, *10*, 53. [CrossRef] [PubMed]
3. Peoples, J.N.; Saraf, A.; Ghazal, N.; Pham, T.T.; Kwong, J.Q. Mitochondrial dysfunction and oxidative stress in heart disease. *Exp. Mol. Med.* **2019**, *51*, 1–13. [CrossRef] [PubMed]
4. Checa, J.; Aran, J.M. Reactive Oxygen Species: Drivers of Physiological and Pathological Processes. *J. Inflamm. Res.* **2020**, *13*, 1057–1073. [CrossRef] [PubMed]
5. Singh, A.; Kukreti, R.; Saso, L.; Kukreti, S. Oxidative Stress: A Key Modulator in Neurodegenerative Diseases. *Molecules* **2019**, *24*, 1583. [CrossRef] [PubMed]
6. Ucar, B.; Ucar, G.; Saha, S.; Buttari, B.; Profumo, E.; Saso, L. Pharmacological Protection against Ischemia-Reperfusion Injury by Regulating the Nrf2-Keap1-ARE Signaling Pathway. *Antioxidants* **2021**, *10*, 823. [CrossRef]
7. Wu, M.-Y.; Yiang, G.-T.; Liao, W.-T.; Tsai, A.P.Y.; Cheng, Y.-L.; Cheng, P.-W.; Li, C.-Y.; Li, C.J. Current Mechanistic Concepts in Ischemia and Reperfusion Injury. *Cell. Physiol. Biochem.* **2018**, *46*, 1650–1667. [CrossRef]
8. Kalogeris, T.; Bao, Y.; Korthuis, R.J. Mitochondrial reactive oxygen species: A double edged sword in ischemia/reperfusion vs preconditioning. *Redox Biol.* **2014**, *2*, 702–714. [CrossRef]
9. Antonucci, S.; Di Lisa, F.; Kaludercic, N. Mitochondrial reactive oxygen species in physiology and disease. *Cell Calcium* **2021**, *94*, 102344. [CrossRef]
10. Neha, K.; Haider, R.; Pathak, A.; Yar, M.S. Medicinal prospects of antioxidants: A review. *Eur. J. Med. Chem.* **2019**, *178*, 687–704. [CrossRef]
11. Soares, R.O.S.; Losada, D.M.; Jordani, M.C.; Évora, P.; Castro-E-Silva, O. Ischemia/Reperfusion Injury Revisited: An Overview of the Latest Pharmacological Strategies. *Int. J. Mol. Sci.* **2019**, *20*, 5034. [CrossRef] [PubMed]
12. Bround, M.J.; Bers, D.M.; Molkentin, J.D. A 20/20 view of ANT function in mitochondrial biology and necrotic cell death. *J. Mol. Cell. Cardiol.* **2020**, *144*, A3–A13. [CrossRef] [PubMed]
13. Bernardi, P.; Di Lisa, F.; Fogolari, F.; Lippe, G. From ATP to PTP and Back. *Circ. Res.* **2015**, *116*, 1850–1862. [CrossRef] [PubMed]

14. Weinbrenner, C.; Liu, G.S.; Downey, J.M.; Cohen, M.V. Cyclosporine A limits myocardial infarct size even when administered after onset of ischemia. *Cardiovasc. Res.* **1998**, *38*, 676–684. [CrossRef]
15. Cung, T.-T.; Morel, O.; Cayla, G.; Rioufol, G.; Garcia-Dorado, D.; Angoulvant, D.; Bonnefoy-Cudraz, E.; Guérin, P.; Elbaz, M.; Delarche, N.; et al. Cyclosporine before PCI in Patients with Acute Myocardial Infarction. *N. Engl. J. Med.* **2015**, *373*, 1021–1031. [CrossRef]
16. Santos-Gallego, C.G.; Badimon, J.J.; Pottecher, J.; Diemunsch, P.; Geny, B.; Zografos, T.A.; Katritsis, D.G.; Mewton, N.; Bergerot, C.; Ovize, M.; et al. Cyclosporine before PCI in Acute Myocardial Infarction. *N. Engl. J. Med.* **2016**, *374*, 88–90. [CrossRef]
17. Monassier, L.; Ayme-Dietrich, E.; Aubertin-Kirch, G.; Pathak, A. Targeting myocardial reperfusion injuries with cyclosporine in the CIRCUS Trial—Pharmacological reasons for failure. *Fundam. Clin. Pharmacol.* **2015**, *30*, 191–193. [CrossRef]
18. Zang, X.; Zhou, J.; Zhang, X.; Han, Y.; Chen, X. Ischemia Reperfusion Injury: Opportunities for Nanoparticles. *ACS Biomater. Sci. Eng.* **2020**, *6*, 6528–6539. [CrossRef]
19. Guan, Y.; Yao, W.; Yi, K.; Zheng, C.; Lv, S.; Tao, Y.; Hei, Z.; Li, M. Nanotheranostics for the Management of Hepatic Ischemia-Reperfusion Injury. *Small* **2021**, *17*, 2007727. [CrossRef]
20. Zhao, T.; Wu, W.; Sui, L.; Huang, Q.; Nan, Y.; Liu, J.; Ai, K. Reactive oxygen species-based nanomaterials for the treatment of myocardial ischemia reperfusion injuries. *Bioact. Mater.* **2021**, *7*, 47–72. [CrossRef]
21. Chen, W.; Li, D. Reactive Oxygen Species (ROS)-Responsive Nanomedicine for Solving Ischemia-Reperfusion Injury. *Front. Chem.* **2020**, *8*, 732. [CrossRef] [PubMed]
22. Yoshitomi, T.; Nagasaki, Y. Self-Assembling Antioxidants for Ischemia & Reperfusion Injuries. *Antioxid. Redox Signal.* **2021**, *36*, 70–80. [CrossRef] [PubMed]
23. Yang, W.; Ding, H.; Qi, G.; Guo, J.; Xu, F.; Li, C.; Puglia, D.; Kenny, J.; Ma, P. Enhancing the Radical Scavenging Activity and UV Resistance of Lignin Nanoparticles via Surface Mannich Amination toward a Biobased Antioxidant. *Biomacromolecules* **2021**, *22*, 2693–2701. [CrossRef] [PubMed]
24. Ikeda, G.; Matoba, T.; Nakano, Y.; Nagaoka, K.; Ishikita, A.; Nakano, K.; Funamoto, D.; Sunagawa, K.; Egashira, K. Nanoparticle-Mediated Targeting of Cyclosporine a Enhances Cardioprotection against Ischemia-Reperfusion Injury through Inhibition of Mitochondrial Permeability Transition Pore Opening. *Sci. Rep.* **2016**, *6*, 20467. [CrossRef] [PubMed]
25. Ikeda, G.; Matoba, T.; Ishikita, A.; Nagaoka, K.; Nakano, K.; Koga, J.; Tsutsui, H.; Egashira, K. Nanoparticle-Mediated Simultaneous Targeting of Mitochondrial Injury and Inflammation Attenuates Myocardial Ischemia-Reperfusion Injury. *J. Am. Heart Assoc.* **2021**, *10*, e019521. [CrossRef] [PubMed]
26. Abdel-Wahhab, M.A.; Aljawish, A.; El-Nekeety, A.A.; Abdel-Aziem, S.H.; Hassan, N.S. Chitosan nanoparticles plus quercetin suppress the oxidative stress, modulate DNA fragmentation and gene expression in the kidney of rats fed ochratoxin A-contaminated diet. *Food Chem. Toxicol.* **2017**, *99*, 209–221. [CrossRef]
27. Sabourian, P.; Ji, J.; Lotocki, V.; Moquin, A.; Hanna, R.; Frounchi, M.; Maysinger, D.; Kakkar, A. Facile design of autogenous stimuli-responsive chitosan/hyaluronic acid nanoparticles for efficient small molecules to protein delivery. *J. Mater. Chem. B* **2020**, *8*, 7275–7287. [CrossRef]
28. Natesan, S.; Pandian, S.; Ponnusamy, C.; Palanichamy, R.; Muthusamy, S.; Kandasamy, R. Co-encapsulated resveratrol and quercetin in chitosan and peg modified chitosan nanoparticles: For efficient intra ocular pressure reduction. *Int. J. Biol. Macromol.* **2017**, *104*, 1837–1845. [CrossRef]
29. De Cristo Soares Alves, A.; Mainardes, R.; Khalil, N.M. Nanoencapsulation of gallic acid and evaluation of its cytotoxicity and antioxidant activity. *Mater. Sci. Eng. C Mater. Biol. Appl.* **2016**, *60*, 126–134. [CrossRef]
30. Mu, X.; Yan, C.; Tian, Q.; Lin, J.; Yang, S. BSA-assisted synthesis of ultrasmall gallic acid & Fe(III) coordination polymer nanoparticles for cancer theranostics. *Int. J. Nanomed.* **2017**, *12*, 7207–7223. [CrossRef]
31. Ni, D.; Wei, H.; Chen, W.; Bao, Q.; Rosenkrans, Z.T.; Barnhart, T.E.; Ferreira, C.A.; Wang, Y.; Yao, H.; Sun, T.; et al. Ceria Nanoparticles Meet Hepatic Ischemia-Reperfusion Injury: The Perfect Imperfection. *Adv. Mater.* **2019**, *31*, e1902956. [CrossRef] [PubMed]
32. Rana, T. Prospects and future perspectives of selenium nanoparticles: An insight of growth promoter, antioxidant and anti-bacterial potentials in productivity of poultry. *J. Trace Elem. Med. Biol.* **2021**, *68*, 126862. [CrossRef] [PubMed]
33. Keshavan, S.; Gupta, G.; Martin, S.; Fadeel, B. Multi-walled carbon nanotubes trigger lysosome-dependent cell death (pyroptosis) in macrophages but not in neutrophils. *Nanotoxicology* **2021**, *15*, 1125–1150. [CrossRef] [PubMed]
34. Mal, J.; Veneman, W.J.; Nancharaiah, Y.V.; van Hullebusch, E.D.; Peijnenburg, W.J.G.M.; Vijver, M.G.; Lens, P.N.L. A comparison of fate and toxicity of selenite, biogenically, and chemically synthesized selenium nanoparticles to zebrafish (*Danio rerio*) embryogenesis. *Nanotoxicology* **2017**, *11*, 87–97. [CrossRef]
35. Ma, Y.; Li, P.; Zhao, L.; Liu, J.; Yu, J.; Huang, Y.; Zhu, Y.; Li, Z.; Zhao, R.; Hua, S.; et al. Size-Dependent Cytotoxicity and Reactive Oxygen Species of Cerium Oxide Nanoparticles in Human Retinal Pigment Epithelia Cells. *Int. J. Nanomed.* **2021**, *16*, 5333–5341. [CrossRef]
36. Yang, H.; Shen, W.; Liu, W.; Chen, L.; Zhang, P.; Xiao, C.; Chen, X. PEGylated Poly(α-lipoic acid) Loaded with Doxorubicin as a pH and Reduction Dual Responsive Nanomedicine for Breast Cancer Therapy. *Biomacromolecules* **2018**, *19*, 4492–4503. [CrossRef]
37. Gu, F.; Hu, C.; Tai, Z.; Yao, C.; Tian, J.; Zhang, L.; Xia, Q.; Gong, C.; Gao, Y.; Gao, S. Tumour microenvironment-responsive lipoic acid nanoparticles for targeted delivery of docetaxel to lung cancer. *Sci. Rep.* **2016**, *6*, 36281. [CrossRef]

38. Maggini, L.; Cabrera, I.; Ruiz-Carretero, A.; Prasetyanto, E.A.; Robinet, E.; De Cola, L. Breakable mesoporous silica nanoparticles for targeted drug delivery. *Nanoscale* **2016**, *8*, 7240–7247. [CrossRef]
39. Picchetti, P.; Moreno-Alcántar, G.; Talamini, L.; Mourgout, A.; Aliprandi, A.; De Cola, L. Smart Nanocages as a Tool for Controlling Supramolecular Aggregation. *J. Am. Chem. Soc.* **2021**, *143*, 7681–7687. [CrossRef]
40. Talamini, L.; Picchetti, P.; Ferreira, L.M.; Sitia, G.; Russo, L.; Violatto, M.B.; Travaglini, L.; Alarcon, J.F.; Righelli, L.; Bigini, P.; et al. Organosilica Cages Target Hepatic Sinusoidal Endothelial Cells Avoiding Macrophage Filtering. *ACS Nano* **2021**, *15*, 9701–9716. [CrossRef]
41. Trzciński, J.W.; Morillas-Becerril, L.; Scarpa, S.; Tannorella, M.; Muraca, F.; Rastrelli, F.; Castellani, C.; Fedrigo, M.; Angelini, A.; Tavano, R.; et al. Poly(lipoic acid)-Based Nanoparticles as Self-Organized, Biocompatible, and Corona-Free Nanovectors. *Biomacromolecules* **2021**, *22*, 467–480. [CrossRef] [PubMed]
42. Gasparini, G.; Bang, E.-K.; Molinard, G.; Tulumello, D.V.; Ward, S.; Kelley, S.O.; Roux, A.; Sakai, N.; Matile, S. Cellular Uptake of Substrate-Initiated Cell-Penetrating Poly(disulfide)s. *J. Am. Chem. Soc.* **2014**, *136*, 6069–6074. [CrossRef] [PubMed]
43. Tavano, R.; Gabrielli, L.; Lubian, E.; Fedeli, C.; Visentin, S.; De Laureto, P.P.; Arrigoni, G.; Geffner-Smith, A.; Chen, F.; Simberg, D.; et al. C1q-Mediated Complement Activation and C3 Opsonization Trigger Recognition of Stealth Poly(2-methyl-2-oxazoline)-Coated Silica Nanoparticles by Human Phagocytes. *ACS Nano* **2018**, *12*, 5834–5847. [CrossRef] [PubMed]
44. Antonucci, S.; Mulvey, J.F.; Burger, N.; Di Sante, M.; Hall, A.R.; Hinchy, E.C.; Caldwell, S.; Gruszczyk, A.V.; Deshwal, S.; Hartley, R.; et al. Selective mitochondrial superoxide generation in vivo is cardioprotective through hormesis. *Free Radic. Biol. Med.* **2019**, *134*, 678–687. [CrossRef]
45. Tonolo, F.; Sandre, M.; Ferro, S.; Folda, A.; Scalcon, V.; Scutari, G.; Feller, E.; Marin, O.; Bindoli, A.; Rigobello, M.P. Milk-derived bioactive peptides protect against oxidative stress in a Caco-2 cell model. *Food Funct.* **2018**, *9*, 1245–1253. [CrossRef]
46. Schindelin, J.; Arganda-Carreras, I.; Frise, E.; Kaynig, V.; Longair, M.; Pietzsch, T.; Preibisch, S.; Rueden, C.; Saalfeld, S.; Schmid, B.; et al. Fiji: An open-source platform for biological-image analysis. *Nat. Methods* **2012**, *9*, 676–682. [CrossRef]
47. Solhjoo, S.; O'Rourke, B. Mitochondrial instability during regional ischemia & reperfusion underlies arrhythmias in monolayers of cardiomyocytes. *J. Mol. Cell. Cardiol.* **2014**, *78*, 90–99. [CrossRef]
48. Bernardi, P.; Scorrano, L.; Colonna, R.; Petronilli, V.; Di Lisa, F. Mitochondria and cell death. Mechanistic aspects and methodological issues. *JBIC J. Biol. Inorg. Chem.* **1999**, *264*, 687–701. [CrossRef]
49. Di Lisa, F.; Menabò, R.; Canton, M.; Barile, M.; Bernardi, P. Opening of the Mitochondrial Permeability Transition Pore Causes Depletion of Mitochondrial and Cytosolic NAD^+ and Is a Causative Event in the Death of Myocytes in Postischemic Reperfusion of the Heart. *J. Biol. Chem.* **2001**, *276*, 2571–2575. [CrossRef]

antioxidants

MDPI

Review

Solid Lipid Nanoparticles: Review of the Current Research on Encapsulation and Delivery Systems for Active and Antioxidant Compounds

Edy Subroto *, Robi Andoyo and Rossi Indiarto

Department of Food Industrial Technology, Faculty of Agro-Industrial Technology, Universitas Padjadjaran, Bandung 45363, Indonesia
* Correspondence: edy.subroto@unpad.ac.id

Abstract: Various active compounds are easily damaged, so they need protection and must be easily absorbed and targeted. This problem can be overcome by encapsulating in the form of solid lipid nanoparticles (SLNs). Initially, SLNs were widely used to encapsulate hydrophobic (non-polar) active compounds because of their matched affinity and interactions. Currently, SLNs are being widely used for the encapsulation of hydrophilic (polar) and semipolar active compounds, but there are challenges, including increasing their entrapment efficiency. This review provides information on current research on SLNs for encapsulation and delivery systems for active and antioxidant compounds, which includes various synthesis methods and applications of SLNs in various fields of utilization. SLNs can be developed starting from the selection of solid lipid matrices, emulsifiers/surfactants, types of active compounds or antioxidants, synthesis methods, and their applications or utilization. The type of lipid used determines crystal formation, control of active compound release, and encapsulation efficiency. Various methods can be used in the SLN fabrication of active compounds and hydrophilic/hydrophobic antioxidants, which have advantages and disadvantages. Fabrication design, which includes the selection of lipid matrices, surfactants, and fabrication methods, determines the characteristics of SLNs. High-shear homogenization combined with ultrasonication is the recommended method and has been widely used because of the ease of preparation and good results. Appropriate fabrication design can produce SLNs with stable active compounds and antioxidants that become suitable encapsulation systems for various applications or uses.

Keywords: nanoencapsulation; solid lipid nanoparticle; active compound; antioxidant; delivery system

1. Introduction

Utilization of lipid-based nanotechnology for encapsulation and delivery systems for active compounds can be applied in several models, including nanoliposomes, nanosuspensions, nanoemulsions, solid lipid nanoparticles (SLNs), and nanostructured lipid carriers (NLCs) [1–5]. SLNs are the most popular models because they can provide solid and stable nanoparticles, have a good delivery system, and can be modified with various lipid matrices, emulsifiers, core materials, and fabrication methods. SLNs were introduced in 1991 and are a better carrier system than conventional colloid systems [6–8]. SLNs have become an effective and stable model for encapsulation and delivery systems for liposomes, emulsions, and polymer nanoparticles mainly because of their ease of forming dispersion systems and adequate entrapment efficiency [9]. SLNs are colloidal carrier systems consisting of a lipid core with a high melting point and are coated with a liquid surfactant, where a surfactant with a concentration of about 0.5–5% can increase the dispersion stability of SLNs [8,10,11].

SLNs consist of main ingredients, namely solid lipids, surfactants/emulsifiers, and water or other solvents. The lipid used as the dispersed phase is a solid lipid that serves as a matrix material for the introduction of encapsulated compounds [12]. The types of solid lipids can be in the form of triglycerides, partial glycerides, free fatty acids, steroids, and waxes [4,13]. The phase change of liquid lipids to solid lipids has new benefits for SLN colloidal carrier systems, because it can improve control of the release kinetics of coated compounds and increase the stability of the formed lipophilic sites. The use of solid lipids can improve the control of the release of micronutrients trapped in lipids in the gastrointestinal system, compared to liquid lipids, and can maintain the stability of micronutrients from environmental conditions such as water, light, and oxygen [14–16]. In addition, the dense lipid matrix can slow the digestion of lipids, thereby allowing the release of the encapsulated compounds in a more sustainable or long-lasting manner. While in the emulsifying phase, the surfactant used is a liquid-type surfactant in order to form an O/W emulsion or the double emulsion (W/O/W), and at the same time, it can function as a stabilizer for SLN dispersion [17,18].

The selection of lipids and surfactants in the SLN synthesis/fabrication process affects the characteristics of SLNs, such as entrapment efficiency, particle size, stability, crystallinity, and pharmacokinetic properties such as bioavailability, release time, and absorption stability of the coated drug or active ingredient [19,20]. The methods that can be used for the fabrication of SLNs include high-speed homogenization combined with ultrasonication, high-pressure homogenization at high or low temperatures, evaporation or diffusion, solvent emulsification, and supercritical fluid extraction of emulsions [10,21]. The method for the fabrication of the selected SLNs must be adapted to the characteristics of the active ingredient to be encapsulated, so that the application is suitable for the objectives to be achieved [22,23].

The active ingredients encapsulated by SLNs include drugs, vitamins, minerals, antibiotics, and various polar, semipolar, and non-polar antioxidant compounds. The development of SLNs in antioxidant compounds has attracted attention, because SLNs are very effective in increasing antioxidant activity, bioavailability, and controlled release for absorption in the gastrointestinal system [24–26]. Various antioxidant compounds have been successfully encapsulated in SLNs using various methods, lipid matrices, and emulsifiers or surfactants. Hydrophobic antioxidant compounds are relatively easy to make into SLNs because of their affinity and suitable interactions between the lipid matrix and the core material [10,27–29]. Meanwhile, hydrophilic antioxidants require certain treatments to be encapsulated well, especially through the formation of emulsions, both single emulsion and double emulsion [30–32].

Antioxidant-loaded SLNs are becoming more of an object of interest, along with the increasing need for well-protected antioxidant compounds to improve the stability of foodstuffs and increasing interest by the pharmaceutical industry, due to their quality as a delivery system for optimal absorption [11,33,34]. In addition, specific discussions regarding the application of SLNs for antioxidant compounds are still limited. Therefore, this review aims to provide information on current research on SLNs, starting with an overview of various fabrication methods and their applications, especially for the encapsulation and delivery systems for various active compounds, especially antioxidant compounds, both non-polar (hydrophobic) and polar (hydrophilic) antioxidants.

2. Development of Lipid Nanoparticles Technology in the Form of Solid Lipid Nanoparticles (SLNs) and Nanostructured Lipid Carriers (NLCs)

Lipid nanoparticle formulation (LNF) as a delivery system provides many benefits related to the encapsulation of drugs and active compounds, providing kinetic stability and rigid structural morphology compared to other lipid-based vehicles, such as liposomes and emulsions in colloidal nanocarrier systems. Various kinds of LNFs can be developed, especially in the form of SLNs and NLCs [10,35–39]. SLNs are delivery systems with a solid lipid fraction to increase the bioavailability of micronutrients or active compounds that have low solubility [40–42]. SLNs are very good carriers for colloidal particles, such as emulsions, liposomes, micro-polymers, and nanoparticles [8,43]. SLNs consist of three main ingredients, namely active components or drugs, solid lipids, and surfactants. Surfactants act as a barrier between the lipid matrix on the outside of the particles. Solid lipids that can be used are saturated fats in the form of free fatty acids, mono- and diglycerides, triglycerides, and other fatty acid esters that act as binders of active substances or drugs in the lipid matrix [43–45].

SLNs are composed of a dense lipid matrix at physiological temperatures, surfactants, and sometimes added cosurfactants (such as solvents) [10,19,46]. SLNs can be synthesized by various methods, such as solvent emulsification/evaporation, cold homogenization, hot homogenization, high-pressure homogenization, high-shear homogenization, and ultrasound methods [39]. The synthesis/fabrication of SLNs must optimize the mixture of lipids used with surfactants and other materials, so that the resulting mixture can form a thermodynamically stable and transparent microemulsion [23,47]. However, the temperature used and preparation conditions can affect the functionality of SLNs. The use of high temperatures can also reduce the stability of the active compounds encapsulated in SLNs. In addition, the use of high temperatures during the preparation of SLNs and rapid cooling during solidification can lead to the formation of unstable lipid crystals and affect the entrapment efficiency [35,48].

The selection of appropriate lipids and surfactants can also affect micronutrient loading, stability during storage, particle size, and release behavior. The lipids used are biocompatible (e.g., glyceryl monostearate, tripalmitin, stearic acid, cetyl alcohol, Compritol 888, tristearin, etc.), in solid form at room temperature and body temperature. Surfactants that function as emulsifiers must be able to reduce the surface tension between the two phases, so that the hydrophilic groups as the head and the lipophilic groups that form the tail of the surfactant must have a suitable value of hydrophilic-lipophilic balance (HLB) [21]. SLNs, as micronutrient delivery systems, coat bioactive components, vitamins, minerals, and other active compounds to prevent these micronutrients from being damaged on the way to the absorption process in the intestine. SLNs in food products are generally used as a form of fortification with micronutrient components needed by the body [16,49].

2.1. The Superiority and Weakness of SLNs

SLNs are an emulsion system in the form of lipid nanoparticles, which was developed as an alternative carrier system that replaces previous methods such as emulsions, liposomes, and polymer nanoparticles [6,8,50]. SLNs are encapsulation and delivery systems that have been widely developed, because they have various advantages in various respects compared to other encapsulation systems. The advantages of the SLN delivery system are that it can control the release of active compounds, increase the stability of active compounds, combine hydrophilic and lipophilic components, avoid toxic drug carriers, and also avoid the use of organic solvents [51,52].

SLNs can also be produced on a large scale in a technically or economically feasible manner [53]. SLNs are easy to prepare, require low cost, have chemical versatility, easy lipid biodegradability, are less expensive than polymer carriers, are easier to obtain approval for, and have reliability and lipid biodegradability [54,55]. This potentially beneficial effect is due to several physicochemical characteristics associated with the physicochemical properties of the lipid phase. First, the rate of degradation of the active compound can be inhibited, because its movement in the solid lipid matrix is lower than in the liquid matrix. Second, degradation reactions of active compounds are prevented by inhibiting the accumulation of active compounds on the surface of lipid particles, due to the separation and control of the active ingredients and carrier lipids in the nanoparticles. Third, there is increased absorption of some free active compounds that are difficult to absorb, after incorporation into SLNs [56,57].

The physical properties of solid lipids greatly affect the characteristics of SLNs. The use of lipids with high melting temperatures can form SLNs with large sizes due to the high viscosity of the diffuse phase. The use of solid lipids with high melting points can also increase the polydispersity index, which indicates that the particle size of SLNs is not uniform [45,58]. The length of the fatty acid chains in lipids also influences the characteristics of the SLNs. The use of solid lipids that have long chains can reduce the zeta potential, which then causes the stability of the dispersion system to decrease. A decrease in zeta potential can cause SLN particles to easily stick to one another (agglomeration occurs), which results in larger particle size [47,59].

However, SLNs also have several weaknesses that make it necessary to carry out additional research and development; these include the limited number of components that can be bound, the appearance of component damage or leakage during storage due to changes in the crystallinity of solid lipids, low loading capacity for some active compounds, and the need for water in sufficient quantities to dissolve SLNs [60]. SLNs can also experience lipid particle growth due to agglomeration or coalescence between dispersed SLNs, unpredictable polymer transition dynamics, the emergence of a tendency towards unpredictable gelation processes, and low binding ability resulting from the dense lipid crystal structure [7,10]. This deficiency is then exploited and developed in the next generation of nanoparticles by combining with other materials, such as liquid lipids, to improve the microstructure in the nanoparticles, which are often known as nanostructured lipid carriers (NLCs) [10,61].

2.2. The Differences between SLNs and NLCs

NLCs are the further development of SLNs which have drawbacks: the low diffusion rate requires a longer release time; the high water content in the system can cause crystallization, which results in a decrease in the solubility of bioactive compounds, so that they are released suddenly or burst upon release [62,63]. Formulation in the form of NLCs was carried out to increase the loading of the active components in the lipid matrix, prevent leakage in the lipid matrix, improve effectiveness in increasing the loading of active compounds, and modulate the release of active compounds. This development or modification is carried out by mixing solid lipids and liquid lipids or oils [64,65]. The incorporation of active compounds or drugs into SLNs and NLCs can be described by three models, as shown in Figure 1.

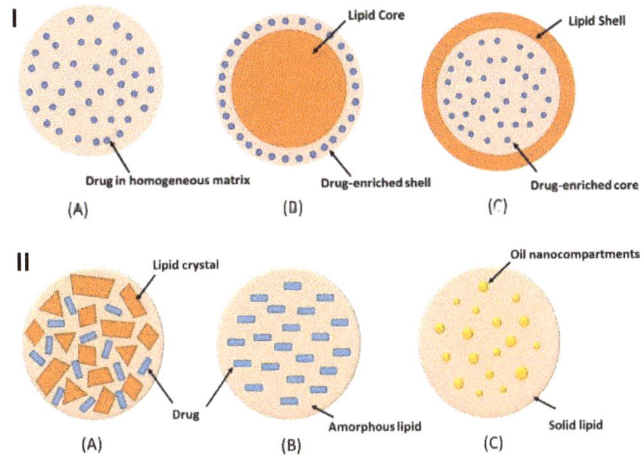

Figure 1. The active compounds or drug incorporation models of SLNs (**I**): homogeneous matrix (**A**), drug-enriched shell (**B**), and drug-enriched core (**C**); and NLCs (**II**): imperfect crystal type (**A**), amorphous type (**B**), and multiple-oil-in-fat-in-water type (**C**) [66].

Generally, the components in the formulation of NLCs consist of solid lipids, liquid lipids, surfactants, and cosurfactants. Commonly used solid lipids include glyceryl monostearate, glyceryl behenate, cetyl alcohol, and stearic acid [64,67]. Liquid lipids that can be used include isopropyl myristate and oleic acid. Commonly used surfactants are polysorbate 80 and poloxamer 188. Commonly used cosurfactants are ethanol, propylene glycol, glycerin, and sucrose stearate [68,69]. NLCs are formulated by forming a solid lipid matrix at room temperature and at body temperature, but inside the solid lipid matrix, there are portions filled with liquid lipids. The ratio of solid lipids and oils used in the formulation of stable NLCs can be 70:30 to 99.9:0.1 [38]. The different composition of NLCs that use liquid lipids causes additional gaps in the NLC structure, which makes the loading capacity of NLCs higher than that of SLNs. However, the shape of the nanoparticles in NLCs is less compact than that in SLNs. This is caused by the inhibition of crystallization by liquid lipids in NLCs. The morphological structure of the nanoparticles in SLNs and NLCs can be identified using a scanning electron microscope (SEM) and a transmission electron microscope (TEM), as shown in Figure 2.

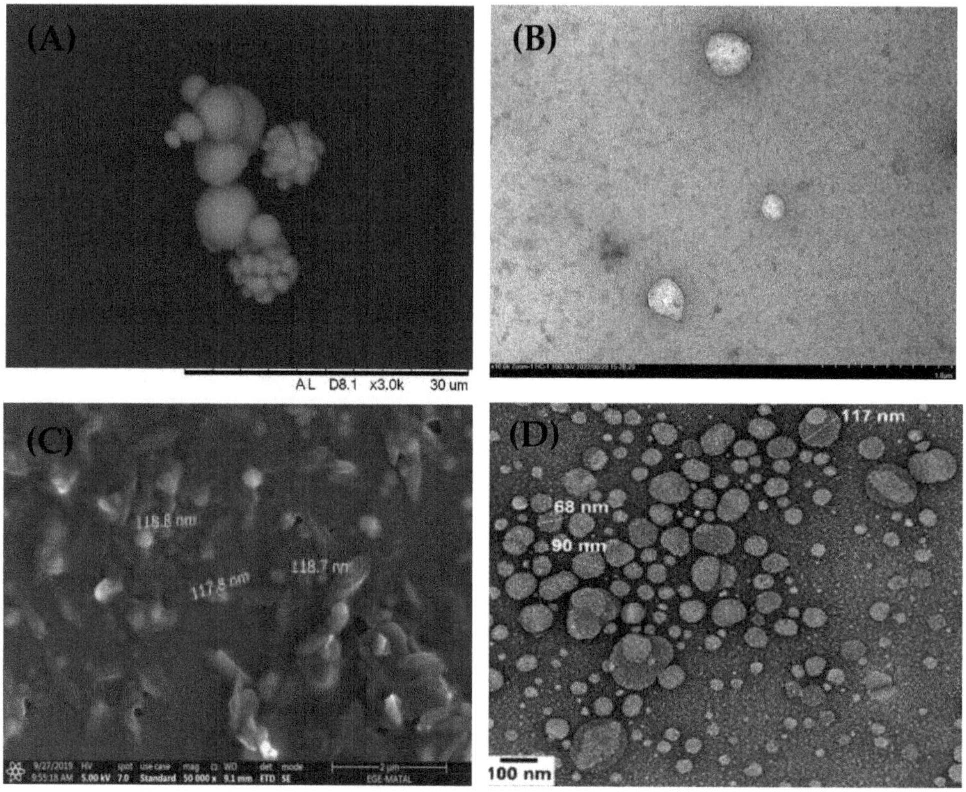

Figure 2. The morphological characterization of SLNs by SEM (**A**) and TEM (**B**) [45]. The morphological characterization of NLCs by SEM (**C**) [70], and TEM (**D**) [71].

NLCs of active compounds are widely used in the pharmaceutical field in drug delivery systems because of their ability to control the precise release of drugs or active compounds on the target, with their nanoparticle size also causing the bioactive components to be well-encapsulated [72,73]. The development of compatible NLCs in the food sector has not been widely carried out because it is related to the food safety standards of the ingredients used. The materials for making NLCs must be food-grade and included in the GRAS (Generally Recognized as Safe) category [62,74]. The differences between SLNs and NLCs can be seen in Table 1.

Table 1. The differences between SLNs and NLCs.

Characteristics	SLNs	NLCs
Ingredients	Solid lipids, surfactants, cosurfactants (optional), and active compounds	Solid lipids, liquid lipids, surfactants, cosurfactants (optional), and active compounds
Active compounds	Hydrophilic and hydrophobic compounds	Suitable for hydrophobic compounds
Crystal structure	Regular and perfect	Irregular, imperfection, lots of free space
Lipid matrix ability to bind to active compounds	Little/slight	More than SLNs
Application	Fortification	Supplementation
Cost	Inexpensive	Expensive
Fabrication difficulty	Easy	Difficult

NLCs have the advantage of being able to contain a greater number of drug molecules or active compounds than SLNs while minimizing damage to active compounds during storage, and can prevent particle coalescence [75]. However, the weakness of these NLCs is that there are some compounds that are not properly formulated in NLC preparations [76,77]. The high ability of NLCs to bind to active components makes NLCs suitable for use in drug delivery in high doses, so NLCs are effectively applied for supplementation compared to the fortification of food products. The release mechanism of NLCs incorporated in cream preparations can accelerate the diffusion process through the stratum corneum, which is facilitated by a matrix of NLCs that contain a lot of lipids due to their similar polarity properties [64,69]. In the preparation of the lipid matrix for NLCs, the crystal structure leads to many crystal imperfections, creating a lot of space for the placement of drug molecules and active compound molecules, whereas in SLNs, the crystal structure is more regular, so there tend to be fewer drug molecules in the lipid matrix [36,38].

3. Fabrication Methods for SLNs

There are various methods that can be used in the synthesis/fabrication of SLNs, including high-speed homogenization and ultrasonication, high-pressure homogenization at high or low temperatures, solvent evaporation, supercritical fluid extraction of emulsions (SFEE), multiple emulsions, and spray-drying [10,21].

3.1. High-Shear Homogenization/High-Speed Homogenization and Ultrasonication

High-shear homogenization/high-speed homogenization and ultrasonication is a very popular and relatively easy SLN fabrication method. The high-shear homogenization method was initially used to produce solid lipid nanodispersions, but the particle size formed after the dispersion was still micro-sized [78]. Higher stirring speed does not always significantly change the particle size but slightly increases the polydispersity index [79]. However, this method can be combined with ultrasonication by utilizing cavitation energy at high frequencies, which can help reduce dispersion particles to nano-sized. The high-shear homogenization method has several advantages; namely, it can be used for large-scale production, does not use organic solvents, and increases product stability and loading of drugs or active compounds [10,13]. The high-shear homogenization method is generally carried out at hot temperatures, so it is often also called the hot homogenization technique. The schematic representation of the ultrasonication method and high-speed homogenization can be seen in Figure 3.

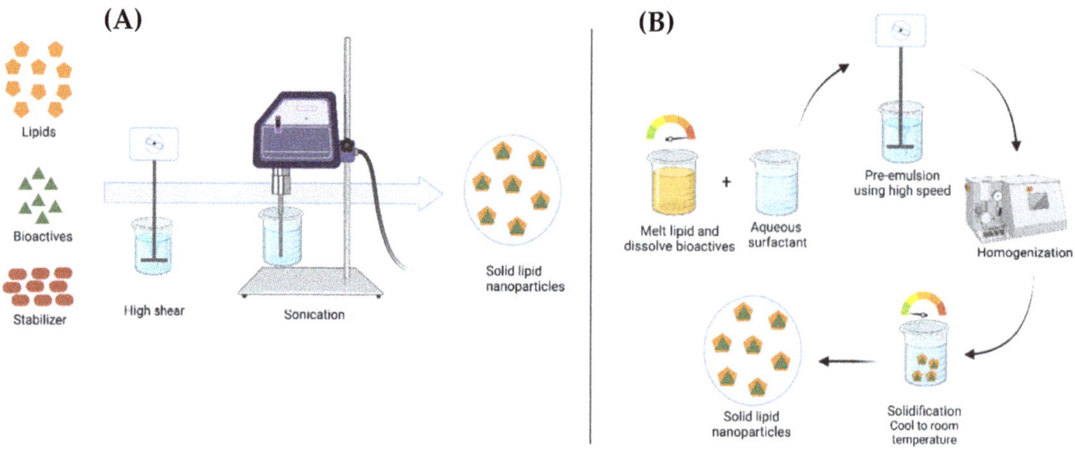

Figure 3. Schematic representation of ultrasonication method (**A**) and hot homogenization technique (**B**) [80].

The ultrasonication method and high-speed homogenization can be used in the fabrication of SLNs effectively [45,81,82]. The initial step is usually conducted by mixing the components of the active compounds that are put into the melted lipid, and then the liquid phase (which has been heated at the same temperature) is added to the previous mixture and emulsified with ultrasonication or by using a high-speed stirrer. Another way this can be conducted is by dripping the water phase on the lipid phase accompanied by high-speed stirring, and then an ultrasonicated pre-emulsion is obtained [83]. The production temperature is kept at least 5 °C above the melting point of the lipid to prevent recrystallization during the fabrication process. The nanoemulsion (o/w) obtained is filtered through a membrane to remove impurities carried during ultrasonication, and the resulting SLNs are then stored at 4 °C. Improvement of formulation stability can be conducted by the lyophilization process, which produces SLN powder by the freeze-drying process, and at a certain point, cryoprotectants such as trehalose or mannitol (5%) can be added to the SLNs as a form of protection [84].

Fabrication of SLNs with this method is relatively simple and does not require high concentrations of surfactants; the equipment used can be easily found in the laboratory [85]. This makes this method widely used for the application of SLNs as coatings and delivery systems for various drugs and active compounds. However, this method has a weakness; namely, the resulting particle size distribution is sometimes not uniform, thus affecting its stability during storage. In addition, this method also has the potential for metal contamination due to the ultrasonication process. The manufacture of SLNs with the ultrasonication method was then developed to form a stable formulation, where the combination of the ultrasonication method and high-speed homogenization at a high temperature can form smaller SLN particles by reducing the surface tension on the nanoparticles [81,86]. The ultrasonication method for SLN fabrication produces nanoparticles that are more optimal when combined with other methods, such as high-shear homogenization. Thus, the weakness of the ultrasonication method can be overcome [7,10].

The lipids used in the ultrasonication and high-speed homogenization methods include glyceryl behenate and tri-behenate (Compritol), glycerol monostearate (GMS), tristearin glyceride, and stearic acid [21]. At the same time, the surfactants that can be used are Poloxamer 188, Lecithin, and Tween [79,87]. The synthesis of SLNs using the ultrasonication method begins by dissolving the active compound to be encapsulated with melted lipid, and then the mixture is heated to 10 °C above the lipid melting point. The mixture of lipids and active compounds is then mixed into a liquid phase containing preheated surfactants and cosurfactants; the mixture is then heated to the same temperature as before and stirred slowly until a pre-emulsion is formed [52,87].

The pre-emulsion formed is then emulsified with an ultrasonicator at a stress efficiency of 35–40% for 3–5 min [87,88]. The combination of methods can be carried out before the ultrasonication process, as reported by Woo et al. [89] reported that the homogenization process can be carried out with a homogenizer on a mixture of lipids and surfactants before ultrasonication is carried out. The homogenization technique that can be conducted is high-shear homogenization or high-speed homogenization. Pre-emulsion with a high-shear homogenization treatment can be carried out at 13,000 rpm for 4 min [90], or stirred at 10,000 rpm using a high-speed homogenizer [79].

The emulsion formed after the ultrasonication process has a high temperature, so it needs to be poured into cold water (1–4 °C) and stirred using a magnetic stirrer for 3 min to crystallize the SLNs to obtain a nanoparticle suspension [79]. The crystallized SLNs are collected by centrifugation at 12,000 rpm for 60 min at 4 °C [88]. SLNs ware then lyophilized using a freeze-dryer and stored in a refrigerator [45,79]. High-shear homogenization combined with ultrasonication is the recommended method and has been widely used because of the ease of preparation and good results. Various uses of ultrasonication and high-shear homogenization methods in the fabrication of SLNs can be seen in Table 2.

Table 2. Various uses of ultrasonication and high-shear homogenization methods in the fabrication of SLNs of various active compounds.

Method/Treatment	Materials	Product Characteristics	References
Ultrasonication	Lipids: stearic acid; Surfactant: Tween 80; Cosurfactant: NaDC; Active substance: Ciprofloxacin	The particle size of SLNs is about 163–369 nm, EE of 51.25–90.08%, depending on lipid composition and surfactant.	[87]
Ultrasonication	Lipids: stearic acid;Active substance: Enrofloxacin	The SLN formed has an entrapment efficiency (EE) of 70.56% with diameter of 217.3 nm.	[88]
Hot homogenization and ultrasonication	Lipid: stearic acid; Surfactant: Tween 60; Active substance: salicylic acid	The particle size of SLNs is about 194–255 nm, EE values are in the range of 49–69%	[89]
Hot homogenization and ultrasonication	Lipid: stearic acid and fat rich in monolaurin; Surfactant: Tween 80; Active substance: Ferrous sulfate	The Z-average of SLNs ranges from 278.7 to 540.4 nm, polydispersity index of 0.88–1.24, and EE values are in the range of 99.7–99.9%	[45]
High-shear homogenization and ultrasonication	Lipids: stearic acid; Surfactant: Quillaja saponin; and Active substance: Imatinib mesylate,	The particle size of SLNs ranges from 143.5 to 641.9 nm, EE of 41–66.2%, polydispersity index (PI) of 0.127–0.237, and Zeta potential (ZP) of −2.43–0.95 mV.	[90]
High-shear homogenization and ultrasonication	Lipids: stearic acid; Surfactant: Tween80; Active substance: Voriconazole	The particle size of SLNs ranges from 286.6 to 313.1 nm, and ZP of −15 mV to −11 mV	[91]
High speed homogenization and ultrasonication	Lipid: stearic acid, Surfactant: Poloxamer 188, and Active substance: candesartan cilexetil (CDC)	The optimal SLN particle size is 197.9 nm, and ZP is about −21.3 mV	[79]
High speed homogenization and ultrasonication	Lipids: stearic acid, glycerol monostearate and Apifil®, Surfactants: Tego care and Planta care; active ingredients: Ceramide	Stable SLN ceramide has a loading capacity of 4% with Apifil® capacity of 4%, and Planta care 1% had a particle diameter of 113.5 nm and a polydispersity index (PI) of 0.263, and was stable for 2 months of storage with a ceramide content of 92.26%.	[52]

3.2. High-Pressure Homogenization

High-pressure homogenization (HPH) is one of the popular methods among the methods that have been developed. This method can be used by industry in the manufacture of SLNs on a large scale. The pressure used in this process ranges from 100 to 2000 bar, with fat content in the formula reaching 40% [92]. There are two approaches to SLN fabrication using the HPH method, namely, hot and cold processes [37]. In the hot homogenization process, the temperature conditions are set at 5–10 °C above the melting point of the fat used. The micronutrient components or active compounds are dissolved in the melted lipid and dispersed in the aqueous surfactant phase with an Ultra-Turrax mixer, which will form a pre-emulsion. The use of heat causes the viscosity to decrease due to an increase in temperature which results in smaller and more uniform particle sizes. In this process, the quality of the pre-emulsion affects the final product of nanoparticles. Therefore, temperature and pressure must be regulated to avoid degradation of the active ingredients contained [93,94].

In the cold homogenization method, the micronutrient components or active compounds are dissolved in melted lipids and then rapidly cooled with dry ice or liquid nitrogen [35,95]. The cooled fat is crushed by ball milling to produce microparticles (50–100 μm) which can be dispersed in the cold surfactant phase and form pre-suspensions. The pre-suspension is homogenized in a high-pressure reactor under cold conditions to make it a dispersion system. The HPH process is continued until nanoparticles are produced. The cold homogenization technique has been extended to solve the problem of the hot homogenization technique, especially to prevent damage to the active compounds due to the use of high temperatures [8,84].

3.3. Solvent Evaporation

SLN fabrication by this method is carried out by means of emulsification by adding fat that has been mixed in the o/w emulsion system. The lipophilic ingredients are then dissolved in a mixture of water and a non-polar organic solvent (cyclohexane). The organic solvent is evaporated under mechanical stirring or pressure-reducing treatment to obtain fat microparticles. The fat microparticles are precipitated again to produce nanoparticles [60]. Using this method, Sjostrom [96] produced cholesterol acetate nanoparticles with sizes between 25 and 100 nm with an emulsifier, namely lecithin/sodium glycocholate. These results have been proven by Westesen and Siekmann [97], who produced phospholipid-stabilized solid lipid nanoparticles with the formation of lipid o/w emulsions with good results.

The SLNs produced by this method are greatly affected by the combination of fat with surfactants or emulsifiers as well as the concentration of fat used in the formula. This method is suitable for use on active components that have thermosensitive properties due to the production process being carried out at low temperatures, and can be used to combine hydrophilic components with o/w/o emulsions [8,98]. However, the drawback of this method is that the use of organic solvents can be toxic, so it is necessary to look for non-toxic solvents [23,62,99].

3.4. Other Methods

Other fabrication methods that have been developed are the supercritical fluid technique, double-emulsion method, and spray-drying technique. The use of the supercritical fluid technique in SLN fabrication has the advantage of not using solvents, so that the fabrication process can be faster and safer than other methods that use solvents [100,101]. There are several innovations for nanoparticle fabrication, including SLNs, which can be produced quickly using supercritical carbon dioxide solutions (RESS) techniques. The use of carbon dioxide (99.99%) as a substitute for solvent in this method can produce SLNs with the best results [13,84]

The preparation of SLNs by the double-emulsion method is based on the evaporation of the emulsification of the solvent that has been used to incorporate the hydrophilic compound into the SLNs [102,103]. The double emulsion w/o/w can be made with a two-step process. First, a w/o microemulsion is prepared by adding a solution containing the active component to a mixture consisting of melted lipid and surfactant/cosurfactant, at a temperature slightly above the melting point of the lipid, to obtain a homogeneous microemulsion system. The surfactants used to form w/o emulsions can be lecithin or monoglycerides. Then, the w/o microemulsion formed is added to a mixture of water, surfactant, and cosurfactant to form a w/o/w double emulsion [43,45]. Generally, Tween 80 is used to form w/o/w emulsions. The preparation of SLNs by the double-emulsion method can be seen in Figure 4. Hydrophilic compounds that are added to SLNs need to be protected or stabilized with a stabilizer to prevent partitioning into the aqueous phase during the solvent evaporation process. SLNs are then centrifuged at 12,000× *g* for 30 min at a low temperature (±4 °C) [84].

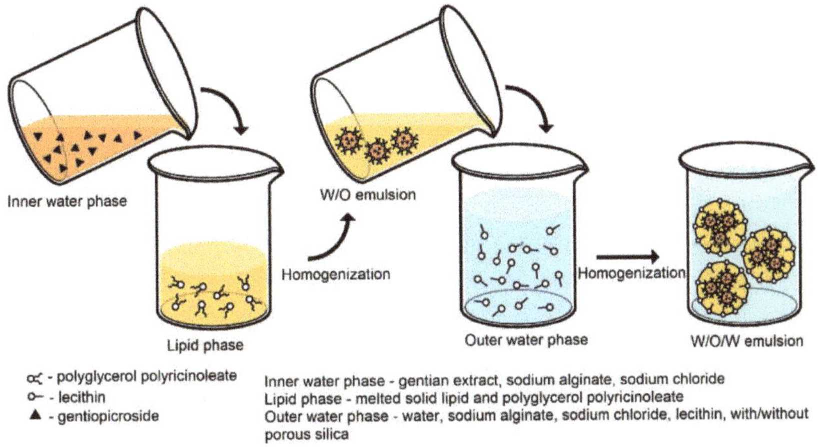

Figure 4. The preparation of SLNs by the double-emulsion method [104].

The use of the spray-dryer techniques is carried out as an alternative to the lyophilization process, in which the process changes SLNs from liquid to solid (powder) form [13,84]. Freitas and Müller [105] recommend using lipids with a melting point > 70 °C for spray-drying. The best results were obtained with a concentration of 1% SLNs in an aqueous trehalose solution or 20% trehalose in an ethanol–water mixture (10/90 *v*/*v*). The spray-drying technique is indeed cheaper when compared to lyophilization but causes particle aggregation due to high temperatures, shear strength, and partial melting of particles [106,107]. Therefore, it is necessary to use lipids with a high melting point or with the addition of trehalose [13,84].

Each method for fabricating SLNs has advantages and disadvantages, so adjustments are needed to the nature of the active ingredients used, the availability of tools and materials, and the costs involved. In general, a comparison of the advantages and disadvantages of several SLN fabrication methods can be seen in Table 3.

Table 3. Comparison of the advantages and disadvantages of several SLN fabrication methods.

Method	Advantages	Disadvantages	References
High-Pressure Homogenization	Low cost, can be produced on a small scale (laboratory) or large scale	It can cause damage to biomolecules, and on a large scale, it requires enormous energy and pressure.	[43,79]
Ultrasonication/High-Speed Homogenization	Effectively reduces surface tension, the process is easy and sustainable, can be commercialized	There is a potential for metal contamination due to the high rotational speed of the tool, and large-scale production requires a high investment.	[7,43]

Table 3. *Cont.*

Method	Advantages	Disadvantages	References
High-shear homogenization	Can be done without the use of solvents, and the process is easy	The particle size is relatively large and less uniform.	[10,79]
Solvent Evaporation Method	The resulting SLNs are stable and uniform, and commercialization can be carried out.	Requires a lot of energy, biomolecule damage can occur, and there is a potential for toxic solvents.	[46,60]
Supercritical Fluid Technique	Does not require a solvent; the particles formed are powdery.	Cost is high.	[43,84]
Double-Emulsion Method	Capable of incorporating hydrophilic components	Large-sized particles at the end of the fabrication	[43,46]
Spray-Drying Technique	Lower cost than lyophilization	Possibility of particle aggregation due to high temperatures	[46,84]

4. Applications of SLNs in Various Fields

Solid lipid nanoparticles (SLNs) have a very wide range of applications, including for topical, pulmonary, dermal, and parenteral drug delivery. These SLN application products have also been developed to minimize the toxic side effects of highly potent drugs and enhance treatment efficacy. Moreover, they have shown good potential in gene transfer, cosmetics, and food industries [10,84].

4.1. SLNs in Various Medical Fields and Cosmetics

The application of SLNs in the medical field is usually for oral drug administration in order to increase the bioavailability of drugs that initially have low bioavailability due to the poor water solubility of drugs [108]. In addition, the application of SLNs can also increase drug release in the body, increase residence time and lymphatic absorption, and potentially increase the bioavailability of drugs that are poorly soluble in water, especially lipophilic drugs [109,110].

SLNs can also be applied in the cosmetic and dermatological fields because of the similarity of the SLN formulation with the structure of the skin, and their application also does not show any interference and toxic effects when used topically [111–115]. The application of SLNs in this field is usually for sunscreen, anti-acne, and anti-aging skin care. SLNs can protect sensitive compounds against chemical degradation, increase skin moisture content, and can also penetrate active substances in the skin, inhibit UV, and hydrate the skin [10].

One of the mechanisms for releasing SLNs in the field of drug delivery occurs in the application of topical preparations, where SLNs can form an occlusive layer on the skin surface which is affected by the size of the SLNs, which are less than 400 nm [116]. When SLNs are applied to the skin surface, the water contained in the preparation will evaporate and leave an adhesive layer covering the skin, thereby reducing transepidermal water loss, which can cause the drug to penetrate into the deepest layers of the skin, reducing the corneocyte density and widening the inter-corneocyte gap [94,117].

4.2. SLNs in Various Food Products and as the Delivery System for Drugs or Active Compounds

Another application of SLNs is in the food sector, because they can be excellent potential carriers for sensitive compounds in the food industry to improve food quality and nutrition [118]. SLNs have also been applied for the fortification with nutrients that are easily damaged by environmental influences or nutrients that have an unfavorable taste and aftertaste that need to be protected or encapsulated in the form of SLNs [45]. In addition to carrying nutrients, SLNs have also been widely used as a drug delivery agent or as a carrier for other active compounds that are beneficial to health, such as medicinal compounds and antioxidants [119–121]. SLNs have been widely applied for delivery of drugs for neurological diseases and cancer, and for preventing antibiotic resistance, because this carrier can contain many antimicrobial drugs, increase drug absorption, and reduce bacterial efflux. SLNs are a good alternative in terms of functionality and biocompatibility, because they can directly reach the site of infection, increase drug bioavailability, and reduce toxicity or side effects [122].

SLNs are lipid-based drug delivery systems that have distinctive properties, such as large surface area, high drug loading, and protection of the drug or active compounds from the environment [84,98,123,124]. In addition, SLNs can increase the absorption efficiency or bioavailability of drug delivery systems. SLNs can have two advantages in drug delivery systems, namely in the effective protection of drugs and active compounds during the formulation process due to increased encapsulation efficiency; the effect of this system is preferred because of the increased release of drugs and active compounds due to the homogenization process in the production of SLNs [51,125,126].

The use of SLNs as an active compound delivery system is included in the solid fat material model, and the enriched nuclei are the desired active compounds. In drug delivery systems, molecular dispersion occurs in a solid lipid matrix when the particles are formed by surfactants or cosurfactants using cold homogenization techniques. Drug delivery with SLNs has a very strong interaction, especially in its lipid components [124,127]. In a drug delivery system with SLNs, the solid lipid core is formed after the lipid recrystallization temperature is reached, and the concentration of the SLN output will melt due to dispersion when the temperature decreases [84,128]. The essence of the drug delivery system with SLNs is the cooling of the nano- or microemulsion, which results in supersaturation of the drug delivery dissolved by the melting lipid approaching its saturation solubility, and precipitation will occur before lipid recrystallization. The extra cooling eventually leads to recrystallization of the lipid that surrounds the drug delivery system as a thin, membrane-like layer [8,129].

The development of the SLN system for various active compounds aims mainly to increase the loading capacity, solubility, and stability [8,130]. Several studies have been carried out on the utilization or application of SLNs related to the absorption and release of the active compound core ingredients in them. Pople and Singh [131] reported that SLNs that contains vitamin A have better release penetration than conventional preparations; namely, the concentration is doubled compared to conventional gels and also has good stability in its application to drug use. Another study, conducted by Kim et al. [132], showed that cyclosporin manufactured in the form of SLNs had good penetration and increased release two times higher than conventional preparations in vitro.

Lipid nanoparticles, including SLNs, have also been widely applied in mRNA delivery, especially used in mRNA vaccines, which have been proven safe and effective after going through clinical trials [133,134]. This development has also been applied to the provision of the vaccine against COVID-19, which was once a pandemic in various countries. Various lipid nanoparticle formulas for mRNA vaccines were developed, starting from the constituent lipid matrix, the surfactant used, and the encapsulated mRNA or active ingredient. Francis et al. [135] applied SLNs to non-viral DNA vaccine delivery to DNA vaccine candidates encoding the Urease alpha (UreA) using Monophosphoryl lipid A. It was found that SLNs have particle uptake by cells within 3 h in the endosome compartment. SLNs were able to stimulate the expression of the pro-inflammatory cytokine TNF-α in THP-1 cells. Lou et al. [136], encapsulating mRNA vaccine encoding the rabies virus glycoprotein (RVG) in the form of lipid nanoparticles using cationic lipids, found that lipid nanoparticles elicited strong humoral and cellular immune responses at a dose of 1.5 μg and have the potential to become and efficient form of mRNA vaccine delivery. The applications of solid lipid nanoparticles in various fields can be seen in Table 4.

Table 4. Applications of SLNs in various fields.

Field or Product Type	Fabrication Conditions	Product Characteristics	References
Skincare for hyperpigmentation	- Active ingredient: N-acetyl-d-glucosamine (NAG) - Method: high-shear homogenization - Lipid phase: hydrogenated castor oil, Peg-25, phosphatidylcholine, and cetyl palmitate - Water phase: purified water	- NAG can act as an emulsion stabilizer - Differences in concentration can affect the process of permeation and release of NAG into the skin, which can contribute to skin repair	[137]
Skincare	- Active ingredients: Epigallocatechin Gallate (EGCG), vitamin E, and Resveratrol. - Method: high-pressure homogenization - Solid lipids: compritol, phospholipon 80, and cetyl palmitate - Liquid lipids: sesame oil - Surfactant: Tween 80	Resveratrol and Vitamin E show results by providing protection against UV-induced parts to prevent degradation, but EGCG does not show the same results.	[138]
Photodynamic therapy	- Active ingredient: DH-I-180-3 - Method: solvent evaporation and hot homogenization - Lipids: Stearic acid and Capmull MCM C8 - Surfactant: poloxamer 188 - Cosurfactant: lecithin	The incorporation of DH-I-180-3 into SLNs enhances targeting efficacy and enhances photocytotoxicity.	[139]
Drug delivery	- Active ingredient: Oxyresveratrol (OXY) - Method: high-shear homogenization - Lipid phase: C888 - Water phase: Tween 80 and soy lecithin	Increases the bioavailability of OXY up to 125% compared to OXY that is not coated by SLN.	[140]
Drug delivery	- Active ingredient: hydrochlorothiazide (HCT) - Method: High-shear homogenization and ultrasonication - Surfactant: Precirol®ATO5, with two different surfactants, namely Tween 80 and Pluronic F68	- Use of Tween 80 elicits complete drug release at 150 min, without providing sustained release. - The use of pluronic F68 ensures a sustained release of more than 75% at the end of the test and a 1.8-fold increase over simple drug suspensions.	[119]
Drug delivery	- Active ingredient: Clarithromycin - Method: high-speed homogenization. - Lipid phase: stearic acid, tripalmitin, and glyceryl behenate - Surfactant: Tween 80	The best particle size was 318.0 nm with a polydispersity index of 0.228–0.472, and the Clarithromycin-SLNs showed extended release up to 48 h.	[141]
Drug delivery	- Active ingredient: Gliclazide - Method: high-shear homogenization. - Lipid phase: stearic acid - Surfactant: PEG 400 and Tween 80	Spherical-shaped particles with the best size of 745.8 nm, Polydispersity index of 0.776, and absorption efficiency of 75.29%.	[42]

Table 4. *Cont.*

Field or Product Type	Fabrication Conditions	Product Characteristics	References
Iron delivery	- Active ingredient: ferrous sulphate - Method: double emulsion and solvent evaporation. - Lipid phase: Stearic acid - Surfactant: Polyvinyl alcohol	The particle size of 300.3–495.1 nm, iron absorption indicates Caco-2 iron absorption up to 642.77 ng/mg cell protein or 24.9% greater than free ferrous sulphate, and ferrous sulphate-SLNs have the potential for iron delivery.	[142]
Encapsulation	- Active ingredients: Ferulic acid and tocopherol - Method: hot homogenization - Lipid phase: Glyceryl tristearate. - Surfactant: polysorbate 20.	- FA-SLN activity was stable during the entire storage period, and TOC-SLN activity increased with time - SLNs showed good stability and high antioxidant activity during 15 weeks of storage.	[121]
Encapsulation	- Active ingredients: ferrous sulfate - Method: ultrasonication and double emulsion - Lipid phase: glycerol monostearate and stearic acid - Surfactant: Tween 80 and span 80	The particles are spherical in shape with a size of 358 nm, a polydispersity index of 0.154, and an entrapment efficiency of 92.3%.	[143]
Fortification	- Active ingredients: gallic acid - Method: high-shear homogenization, ultrasonication, and double emulsion - Lipid phase: stearic acid and fat rich in monoacylglycerols and diacylglycerols - Surfactant: Tween 80	Gallic acid-SLNs, which was fortified with 5% in chocolate bars, increased the antioxidant activity and total phenolic content with an IC_{50} of 174.24 and had good organoleptic characteristics.	[45]
Skincare for cellulite	- Active ingredient: Caffeine - Method: hot homogenization - Lipid phase: Precirol	SLN containing caffeine showed good stability for 12 months of storage.	[144]
Skin allergy medication	- Active ingredient: Loratadine (LRT) - Method: High-pressure homogenization - Lipid phase: Precirol - Surfactants: TegoCare 450 and 1-hexadecanol	- Produces a particle size of 11–14 nm; the highest release rate was 0.021 mcg/mL/h - Stable on storage for 6 months	[145]
DNA Vaccine Delivery	- Active ingredient: DNA vaccine candidate encoding the Urease alpha (UreA) - Method: solvent-emulsification - Lipid phase: cholesteryl oleate, glyceryl trioleate, DOPE, DC-cholesterol, and monophosphoryl lipid A.	SLNs have particle uptake by cells within 3 h in the endosome compartment. SLNs were able to stimulate the expression of the pro-inflammatory cytokine TNF-α in THP-1 cells. Lipoplexes are compatible with being transfused efficiently in murine immune cells.	[135]
mRNA Vaccine Delivery	- Active ingredient: mRNA encoding prM-E from Zika, and mRNA encoding influenza HA genes - Method: solvent-emulsification - Lipid phase: ionizable lipid MC3, cholesterol, DSPC, and PEG lipid	Lipid nanoparticles elicit a strong immune response, and the tolerability of mRNA vaccines can be increased without affecting their potency.	[146]

Table 4. *Cont.*

Field or Product Type	Fabrication Conditions	Product Characteristics	References
mRNA Vaccine Delivery	- Active ingredient: mRNA vaccine encoding the rabies virus glycoprotein (RVG) - Method: solvent-emulsification - Lipid phase: 3ß-[N-(N′,N′-dimethylaminoethane)-carbamoyl]cholesterol (DC-Chol), DDA, DOTAP, DMTAP, DSTAP, and DOBAQ	Lipid nanoparticles elicited strong humoral and cellular immune responses at a dose of 1.5 µg. Lipid nanoparticles have the potential to become an efficient method for mRNA vaccine delivery.	[136]

5. Solid Lipid Nanoparticles for the Encapsulation of Antioxidant Compounds

SLNs have been widely applied to encapsulate various active compounds and antioxidants, both polar (hydrophilic), semipolar, and non-polar (hydrophobic) antioxidants [11,121,147]. Fabrication of SLNs of polar and semipolar antioxidant compounds requires surfactants or emulsifiers to bridge between lipid encapsulants and polar core materials. Meanwhile, non-polar antioxidant compounds tend to be more easily encapsulated in SLNs, along with the compatibility of the hydrophobicity properties between the lipid matrix and the core compound [128,148]. Various applications of SLNs for the encapsulation of non-polar antioxidant compounds can be seen in Table 5.

Table 5. Application of SLNs for the Encapsulation of Non-Polar Antioxidant Compounds.

Antioxidant Compound	Lipid Matrices	Fabrication Method	Characteristics of SLNs	References
β-Carotene	glyceryl monostearate, gelucire50/13, and phospholipid S-100	hot homogenization process with high-shear mixer	SLN increased the stability of antioxidant activity more than 3 times at 90 days. The bioavailability and efficacy also improved.	[120]
β-Carotene	fully hydrogenated sunflower oil	hot-melt high-pressure homogenization	β-Carotene formed 10 cis isomers, but did not affect the crystals of SLNs in the form of stable β-crystals.	[149]
Curcumin	Compritol 888, Tween 80, lecithin, Polysorbate 80	Micro-emulsification technique	Curcumin-SLN increased oral bioavailability and stability 32–155 times more than free curcumin, and sustained release.	[150]
Curcumin	Compritol® 888 ATO, soya lecithin	Hot-high-pressure homogenization	Curcumin-SLN had an entrapment efficiency of 75%, polydispersity index of 0.143, particle size of <200 nm, and a significant antimicrobial effect.	[151]
Curcumin	glycerol behenate (Compritol® 888 ATO)	Solvent evaporation method	Curcumin-pSLN has a high antioxidant activity of 3.73 ORAC Units compared to free curcumin of 1.6 ORAC Units, has a zeta potential of −30 mV, a particle size of less than 200 nm, and is stable during storage.	[152]
Alpha-tocopherol	Stearic acid	Hot homogenization by a high-shear homogenizer	SLN-alpha tocopherol had an in vitro release of 74.33% after 8 h. SLN was spherical in size <1000 nm and EE up to 98.67%.	[153]

Table 5. *Cont.*

Antioxidant Compound	Lipid Matrices	Fabrication Method	Characteristics of SLNs	References
Alpha-tocopherol	Glyceryl behenate (Compritol® 888)	Hot high homogenization with a high-pressure homogenizer	SLN-α-tocopherol has a particle size of 214.5 nm, zeta potential of −41.9 mV, α-tocopherol recovery rate of 75.4%, and was stable for 21 days at 6 °C, with polymorphic forms were α and β′.	[154]
Alpha-tocopherol and Ferulic acid	Glyceryl tristearate	ultrasound-assisted hot emulsification	SLN-Tocopherol and SLN-Ferulic acid with a lading of 2.5 mg/g were stable for 15 weeks, and significant radical scavenging activity was maintained.	[121]
Sesamol	Glyceryl monostearate, Sodium deoxycholate, and α-phosphatidylcholine	Microemulsion technique	Sesamol-SLN had an entrapment efficiency of 88.21% and a particle size of 127.9 nm. Application of the cream showed retention in the skin at minimum flux, and showed normalization of post-induced skin cancer.	[155]
Sesamol	Compritol 888, Soy Lecithin, and Tween 80	Microemulsion technique	Sesamol-SLN had a particle size of about 120.3 nm, and better hepatoprotection compared to free sesamol. Sesamol-SLN improved bioavailability, reduced toxicity and irritation, and controlled the effect of entrapped sesamol.	[156]
Umbelliferone (7-hydroxycoumarin)	Glyceryl Stearate and n-Hexadecyl Palmitate	high-shear homogenization	SLN had a particle size of about 173.4 nm, good entrapment efficiency (60.70%), and antioxidant properties of 75%.	[157]
Vitamin A	Cetyl alcohol, Tween 80, and Gelucire 44/14®	hot homogenization	Vitamin A-SLNs have an entrapment efficiency of >90%, a particle size of about 40 nm, an average size of 30–50 nm in the spherical form, and vitamin A-SLNs have stability >2 times compared to free vitamin A.	[158]
Astaxanthin	lipid phase: stearic acid, surfactant: Poloxamer	solvent-diffusion method	Astaxanthin-SLNs have a particle size of <200 nm, were able to maintain the stability of astaxanthin during 6 months of storage, and were able to improve antioxidant capacity more than free astaxanthin.	[159]
Ascorbyl Palmitate (AP)	Lipid phase: Glyceryl monostearate (GMS), Surfactant: Pluronic-F68	Ultrasonic method	SLN-AP had a cytotoxic effect at lower concentrations than in the form of AA or DHA. Formulation of SLN-AP with 3% Pluronic F-68 produced SLNs with good physicochemical characteristics and stable antioxidants but need further optimization because of their intrinsic cytotoxicity.	[160]

Various types of antioxidant compounds have been successfully encapsulated in the form of SLNs with various types of lipid matrices and fabrication methods. Jain et al. [120] have succeeded in making SLN β-Carotene with a lipid matrix in the form of glyceryl monostearate and phospholipid S-100 emulsifier, using the hot homogenization process by the high-shear mixer method. The SLNs obtained were able to increase the stability of the antioxidant β-Carotene 3 times higher than without encapsulation, and SLNs also increased the bioavailability and efficacy of β-Carotene. Schjoerring-Thyssen et al. [149] also succeeded in synthesizing SLNs of β-Carotene, using the hot-melt high-pressure homogenization method, with fully hydrogenated sunflower oil as a lipid matrix. The SLNs of β-Carotene obtained have stable crystals in the form of β-crystals.

SLNs are also effective for encapsulating the active compound curcumin, which is an antioxidant [152,161]. Curcumin can be encapsulated in the form of SLNs using the micro-emulsification technique method with Compritol 888 as a lipid matrix and assisted by emulsifiers in the form of Tween 80, lecithin, and polysorbate 80. Curcumin-SLNs increased oral bioavailability and stability up to 155 times more than free curcumin [150]. Shandu et al. [151] also succeeded in encapsulating curcumin in the form of SLNs using the hot-high-pressure homogenization method with a lipid matrix in the form of Compritol® 888 ATO and an emulsifier in the form of soya lecithin. Curcumin-SLNs have an entrapment efficiency of 75% and have a significant antimicrobial effect.

SLNs are also effective for encapsulating tocopherols as a source of antioxidants. Shylaja and Mathew [153] succeeded in synthesizing SLN-alpha tocopherol, using the method of hot homogenization with a high-shear homogenizer and stearic acid as the lipid matrix. SLN tocopherol has an in vitro release of 74.33%, entrapment efficiency of up to 98.67%, and is stable during storage. SLN-alpha tocopherol can also be synthesized using the hot high homogenization with the high-pressure homogenizer method with a lipid matrix in the form of glyceryl behenate, which produces SLNs with a high α-tocopherol recovery rate, stable during storage [154]. At the same time, Oehlke et al. [121] succeeded in encapsulating alpha-tocopherol and ferulic acid in the form of SLNs with a lipid matrix in the form of glyceryl tristearate, using the ultrasound-assisted hot emulsification method. The SLNs obtained were stable for 15 weeks, and the significant radical scavenging activity was maintained.

Other antioxidant compounds were also successfully encapsulated in the form of SLNs, including sesamol, which was encapsulated using the microemulsion technique with a lipid matrix in the form of glyceryl monostearate and an emulsifier in the form of α-phosphatidylcholine. Sesamol-SLNs applied to cream manufacture showed retention in the skin with minimal flux and showed normalization of post-induced skin cancer [155]. Meanwhile, Lacatusu et al. [157] encapsulated umbelliferone using n-Hexadecyl palmitate and glyceryl stearate with the high-shear homogenization method; it was found that the SLNs had a good entrapment efficiency and antioxidant properties up to 75%. SLN technology still has many opportunities to encapsulate various other non-polar active compounds, because the affinity and hydrophobicity properties are very suitable for the solid lipid matrix used. However, SLN fabrication for the encapsulation of non-polar antioxidant compounds needs to pay attention to several factors that can have an effect. The selected fabrication method should avoid using too high temperatures to keep the antioxidant compounds from being damaged. The lipid used should have high lipophilicity. The more lipophilic a solid lipid is, the more it can accommodate more lipophilic active ingredients [162]. If using a surfactant, one must be chosen that has a low HLB in order to homogenize the system, which is dominated by hydrophobic compounds [17].

SLNs have also been widely applied to encapsulate various polar (hydrophilic) and semipolar antioxidant compounds [163–166]. Antioxidant compounds that are polar tend to be more difficult to encapsulate in SLNs due to differences in polarity between the lipid matrix and the core compounds, thus requiring a suitable emulsifier and appropriate fabrication techniques or methods for high-efficiency entrapment, small particle size, and homogeneous or uniform [11,167]. Most of the active compounds that are antioxidants are polar or semipolar in nature, such as from a group of phenolic compounds, flavonoids, water-soluble vitamins, and several essential minerals. Therefore, researchers are trying to continue to develop various applications of SLNs for the encapsulation of polar and semipolar antioxidant compounds, which can be seen in Table 6.

Table 6. Application of SLNs for the Encapsulation of Polar and Semipolar Antioxidant Compounds.

Antioxidant Compound	Lipid Matrices	Fabrication Method	Characteristics of SLNs	References
Epigallocatechin-3-gallate (EGCG)	Cocoa butter	Hot homogenization method	EGCG-SLNs had an entrapment efficiency of about 68.5%, particle size between 108 and 122 nm, and increased shelf life.	[168]
Epigallocatechin-3-gallate (EGCG)	Glycerol monostearate, poloxamer 188, poly-oxyethylene stearate	Hot melt homogenization	SLN-EGCG had a particle size of about 300.2 nm, an entrapment efficiency of about 81%, and was able to improve the bioavailability and stability of EGCG.	[163]
Epigallocatechin-3-gallate (EGCG)	Stearic acid, Tripalmitin, and tristearin	Emulsion-solvent evaporation method	EGCG-SLNs had cytotoxicity of 3.8 folds higher against human prostate cancer cells of DU-145 and 8.1 folds higher against human breast cancer cells of MDA-MB 231 compared to free EGCG.	[169]
Myricitrin	Compritol®888 and oleic acid	Cold homogenization	SLN-myricitrin had antioxidant, antidiabetic, and antiapoptotic effects in vivo and in vitro.	[170]
Myricitrin	Compritol®888 and oleic acid	Cold homogenization	SLN-myricitrin reduced oxidative stress and increased antioxidant enzymes level	[171]
Resveratrol	Glyceryl behenate (Compritol®888)	High-shear homogenization	Resveratrol-SLNs had an antioxidant activity that can reduce ROS effectively. Resveratrol-SLNs had a particle size of about 287.2 nm, ZP was −15.3 mV, and the drug was trapped in the SLNs efficiently.	[172]
Resveratrol	Cetyl palmitate, polysorbate 60	High-shear homogenization and the ultrasound method	Resveratrol-SLNs increased oral bioavailability, stability, and sustained release.	[173]
Gallic acid	Stearic acid and fat rich in monolaurin	Double emulsion assisted by high-speed homogenization and ultrasonication	Gallic acid-SLNs had particle size of 224.4–3596.3 nm, entrapment efficiency of about 93.75%, polydispersity index of about 0.85, and were able to increase the antioxidant activity of chocolate bar.	[164]
Quercetin	Glyceryl monostearate, Tween-80, Soya Lecithin	Emulsification and low-temperature solidification	SLN-Quercetin had a spherical shape, with zeta potential of −32.2 mV, drug loading of 13,2%, entrapment efficiency of about 91.1%, a particle size of 155.3 nm, and relative bioavailability of 571.4%.	[174]
Phenolic and flavonoids of *Prunus persica* (L.) ethanolic extract (PPEE)	Glyceryl monostearate, Tween 80	Solvent evaporation method	PPEE-SLNs increased the antioxidant activity, anti-tyrosinase, anti-collagenase, and anti-elastase more than free PPEE.	[165]
Coenzyme Q-10	Cetyl palmitate or stearic acid	High-speed & high-pressure homogenization	Particle sizes were 100 nm and 50 nm, with polydispersity index between 0.20 and 0.11	[175]
Coenzyme Q-10	Glyceryl behenate (Compritol®888)	High-shear homogenization	SLN-Coenzyme Q10 was able to enhance cell proliferation more than free Coenzyme Q10, but no better than liposomes; less effective against ROS accumulation.	[176]
Ofloxacin	Palmitic acid	Hot homogenization and ultrasonication	SLNs had an encapsulation efficiency of 41.36%, loading capacity of 4.40%, diameter of 156.33 nm, zeta potential of about −22.70 mv, and polydispersity index of 0.26. SLNs increased the residence time up to 43.44 h and improved the bioavailability 2.27-fold.	[177]

Table 6. *Cont.*

Antioxidant Compound	Lipid Matrices	Fabrication Method	Characteristics of SLNs	References
Tetrandrine	Glyceryl behenate, Stearyl amine, and PEG stearate	Emulsion evaporation-solidification at low temperature	Tetrandrine-loaded SLNs retained the drug entity better than free tetrandrine, had an average diameter of 18.77 nm, a zeta potential of −8.71, an AUC value 2-fold higher than free tetrandrine, and had no significant toxicity.	[178]
Anthocyanins	Palmitic acid, Pluronic F127, Span 85, and egg lecithin	Microemulsion-dilution method	Anthocyanin-SLNs had an entrapment efficiency of about 89.2, a particle size of 455 nm, and revealed spherical morphology.	[179]
Ascorbic acid (AA)	Compritol® and Tween 80	hot homogenization method	AA-SLNs showed sustained release, high cytotoxic activity against H-Ras 5RP7 cells, high entrapment efficiency, more efficient cellular uptake, and induced apoptosis.	[166]
Grape seed extract (GSE) rich in Proanthocyanidins	Gelucire® 50/13 and Tween 85	melt-emulsification method	GSE-SLNs had good loading efficiency of about 0.058 mg/mg, a particle size of 243, stable antioxidant activity, and favorable properties for lung delivery.	[180]

Phenolic, polyphenolic, and flavonoid compounds are polar-semipolar active compounds that are abundant in various plants and have high antioxidant activity [181,182]. Many efforts have been made to protect and stabilize the antioxidant activity of phenolic and polyphenolic compounds, including through encapsulation in the form of SLNs. Epigallocatechin-3-gallate (EGCG) has been successfully encapsulated in the form of SLNs by various methods and lipid matrices. Shtay et al. [168] synthesized EGCG-SLNs, using the hot homogenization method and cocoa butter as a lipid matrix; they obtained EGCG-SLNs with an entrapment efficiency of 68.5% and increased the shelf life. Ramesh and Mandal [163] synthesized EGCG SLNs, using the same method but with a lipid matrix glycerol monostearate and an emulsifier in the form of poloxamer 188; SLNs were obtained with the entrapment efficiency of 81% and were able to increase the bioavailability and stability of EGCG. Meanwhile, Radhakrishnan et al. [169] synthesized EGCG-SLNs, using the emulsion-solvent evaporation method with lipid matrices in the form of stearic acid, tripalmitin, and tristearin; the obtained EGCG-SLNs had cytotoxicity of 8.1-fold higher against MDA-MB 231 human breast cancer cells compared to free EGCG. The myricitrin polyphenol compound has also been successfully fabricated in the form of SLNs, which were able to improve its bioactivity. Ahangarpour et al. [170] reported that myricitrin was encapsulated using lipid matrices in the form of Compritol® 888 and oleic acid with the cold homogenization method, showing that SLN-myricitrin had antioxidant, antidiabetic, and antiapoptotic effects in vivo and in vitro. SLN-myricitrin applied to type-2 diabetic male mice showed that SLN-myricitrin reduced oxidative stress and increased antioxidant enzyme levels [171].

Phenolic compounds that have high antioxidant activity include resveratrol, gallic acid, and quercetin. These compounds need to be protected for their bioactivity, including through encapsulation in the form of SLNs. Gokce et al. [172] succeeded in fabricating resveratrol-SLNs with glyceryl behenate as a lipid matrix, using high-shear homogenization. Resveratrol-SLNs were effective in reducing ROS accumulation and exerting antioxidant activity, and the drug in the shell model was relevant. Another study by Neves et al. [173] reported that resveratrol-SLNs could be fabricated with cetyl palmitate as a lipid matrix and polysorbate 60 as an emulsifier, using a combination of high-shear homogenization and the ultrasound method. Resveratrol-SLNs increased oral bioavailability, stability, and sustained release. Gallic acid phenolic compounds were also successfully fabricated in the form of SLNs by Subroto et al. [164]; they used stearic acid and fat rich in monolaurin, using the double-emulsion method assisted by high-speed homogenization and ultrasonication. In this fabrication, fat-rich monolaurin acts as a solid lipid that is healthy as well as an emulsifier due to the same properties as other monoacylglycerols, which act as surfactants [183–185]. Gallic acid-SLNs had an entrapment efficiency of 93.75% and were able to increase the antioxidant activity of a chocolate bar. Meanwhile, the phenolic quercetin compound was successfully fabricated in the form of SLNs by Li et al. [174] with glyceryl monostearate, using the method of emulsification and low-temperature solidification. SLN-Quercetin had a particle size of about 155.3 nm, with a spherical shape, entrapment efficiency of 91.1%, and relative bioavailability of 571.4%.

One of the antioxidant compounds that have high activity and can be produced by the human body is ubiquinone or coenzyme Q10. Coenzyme Q10 is semipolar, and the compound is also effective and stable when encapsulated in the form of SLNs. Farboud et al. [175] fabricated Coenzyme Q10-SLNs with cetyl palmitate and stearic acid, using the high-speed and high-pressure homogenization method to obtain SLNs with particle sizes 50–100 nm; and polydispersity index was 0.11–0.20. At the same time, Gokce et al. [176] reported that Coenzyme Q10-SLNs, which were fabricated with glyceryl behenate using high-shear homogenization, were able to enhance cell proliferation more than free Coenzyme Q10, but performed no better than liposomes.

Water-soluble high-activity antioxidant compounds that are easy to find are anthocyanins and vitamin C or ascorbic acid. These compounds can also be encapsulated in the form of SLNs. Ravanfar et al. [179] reported that anthocyanin-SLNs could be fabricated with palmitic acid, pluronic F127, egg lecithin, and span 85, using the microemulsion dilution method to obtain anthocyanin-SLNs that had entrapment efficiency of 89.2 and effectively increased stability. Meanwhile, ascorbic acid-SLNs were successfully fabricated by Güney et al. [166] with compritol® and Tween 80, using the hot homogenization method. Ascorbic acid-SLNs showed high entrapment efficiency, sustained release, high cytotoxic activity against H-Ras 5RP7 cells compared to free AA, more efficient cellular uptake, and induced apoptosis.

The success of SLN fabrication for polar antioxidant compounds is determined by the method chosen. The method used should not involve high temperatures to avoid thermal damage. The preferred method is primarily emulsion formation, such as double emulsion (W1/O/W2). Emulsion formation will help SLN homogeneity and increase entrapment efficiency [45,186]. The selection of the right type of surfactant also determines the success of SLN fabrication. The more polar the encapsulated antioxidant compound, the more surfactant or emulsifier with a higher HLB is needed, so that it can improve the homogeneity of the emulsion system, lead to a smaller particle size, and increase absorption efficiency [187].

6. Conclusions and Future Research

Solid lipid nanoparticles can be used as an encapsulation system and delivery system for various active compounds that tend to be lipophilic, but currently, it has been widely applied to hydrophilic active compounds by various methods, especially by forming a double emulsion w/o/w or by using an emulsifier. The success of SLN fabrication is largely determined by several factors, such as the choice of the fabrication method, the type of lipid matrices used, and the selection of surfactants or emulsifiers, as well as the preparation conditions and processes used. SLN fabrication has been effective in coating various active compounds. SLNs have been applied to various active compounds such as drugs, minerals, and various polar, semipolar, and non-polar antioxidant compounds, but several combinations of materials and processes need to be carried out to produce more stable SLNs and high entrapment efficiency.

Antioxidant compounds have attracted the attention of researchers, along with the need for antioxidants that are stable and have high bioavailability to prevent and treat various degenerative diseases. Various antioxidant compounds are numerous and have the potential to continue to be developed for fabrication in the form of SLNs using various types of lipid matrices, emulsifiers, and various methods or combinations thereof. These antioxidant-SLNs play a very large role in various fields of food, pharmaceuticals, and cosmetics to provide high-activity, stable antioxidant compounds, and to become the right delivery system for various treatments and fulfillment of appropriate nutrition. Aspects that are still a challenge in the future include efforts to make fabrication economically efficient, studies on increasing biocompatibility with other components, achieving active compounds on target, and clinical trials before they are used by the public.

Author Contributions: Conceptualization, E.S., R.A. and R.I.; methodology, E.S. and R.I.; software, R.I.; validation, R.A. and R.I.; formal analysis, E.S. and R.A.; investigation, E.S., R.A. and R.I.; resources, E.S.; data curation, E.S.; writing—original draft preparation, E.S.; writing—review and editing, R.A. and R.I.; visualization, E.S. and R.I.; supervision, R.A.; project administration, E.S.; funding acquisition, E.S. All authors have read and agreed to the published version of the manuscript.

Funding: This article was supported by Universitas Padjadjaran, Indonesia.

Institutional Review Board Statement: Not applicable.

Informed Consent Statement: Not applicable.

Data Availability Statement: Not applicable.

Acknowledgments: The authors would like to thank the Rector of Universitas Padjadjaran and The Ministry of Education, Culture, Research, and Technology of the Republic of Indonesia.

Conflicts of Interest: The authors declare no conflict of interest.

References

1. Hallan, S.S.; Sguizzato, M.; Esposito, E.; Cortesi, R. Challenges in the Physical Characterization of Lipid Nanoparticles. *Pharmaceutics* **2021**, *13*, 549. [CrossRef]
2. Fathi, M.; Mozafari, M.R.; Mohebbi, M. Nanoencapsulation of Food Ingredients Using Lipid Based Delivery Systems. *Trends Food Sci. Technol.* **2012**, *23*, 13–27. [CrossRef]
3. Indiarto, R.; Indriana, L.P.A.; Andoyo, R.; Subroto, E.; Nurhadi, B. Bottom–up Nanoparticle Synthesis: A Review of Techniques, Polyphenol-Based Core Materials, and Their Properties. *Eur. Food Res. Technol.* **2022**, *248*, 1–24. [CrossRef]
4. Maravajhala, V.; Papishetty, S.; Bandlapalli, S. Nanotechnology in Development of Drug Delivery System. *Int. J. Pharm. Sci.* **2012**, *3*, 84–96.
5. Matei, A.-M.; Caruntu, C.; Tampa, M.; Georgescu, S.R.; Matei, C.; Constantin, M.M.; Constantin, T.V.; Calina, D.; Ciubotaru, D.A.; Badarau, I.A.; et al. Applications of Nanosized-Lipid-Based Drug Delivery Systems in Wound Care. *Appl. Sci.* **2021**, *11*, 4915. [CrossRef]
6. Alsaad, A.A.A.; Hussien, A.A.; Gareeb, M.M. Solid Lipid Nanoparticles (SLN) as a Novel Drug Delivery System: A Theoretical Review. *Syst. Rev. Pharm.* **2020**, *11*, 259–273. [CrossRef]
7. Ekambaram, P.; Sathali, A.H.; Priyanka, K. Solid Lipid Nanoparticles–A Review. *Int. J. Appl. Pharm.* **2012**, *2*, 80–102.
8. Mishra, V.; Bansal, K.K.; Verma, A.; Yadav, N.; Thakur, S.; Sudhakar, K.; Rosenholm, J.M. Solid Lipid Nanoparticles: Emerging Colloidal Nano Drug Delivery Systems. *Pharmaceutics* **2018**, *10*, 191. [CrossRef]
9. Mirchandani, Y.; Patravale, V.B.S.B. Solid Lipid Nanoparticles for Hydrophilic Drugs. *J. Control. Release* **2021**, *335*, 457–464. [CrossRef]
10. Naseri, N.; Valizadeh, H.; Zakeri-Milani, P. Solid Lipid Nanoparticles and Nanostructured Lipid Carriers: Structure Preparation and Application. *Adv. Pharm. Bull.* **2015**, *5*, 305–313. [CrossRef]
11. Borges, A.; de Freitas, V.; Mateus, N.; Fernandes, I.; Oliveira, J. Solid Lipid Nanoparticles as Carriers of Natural Phenolic Compounds. *Antioxidants* **2020**, *9*, 998. [CrossRef] [PubMed]
12. Jaspreet, K.; Gurpreet, S.; Seema, S.; Rana, A. Innovative Growth in Developing New Methods for Formulating Solid Lipid Nanoparticles and Microparticles. *J. Drug Deliv. Ther.* **2012**, *2*, 146–150.
13. Mukherjee, S.; Ray, S.; Thakur, R.S. Solid Lipid Nanoparticles: A Modern Formulation Approach in Drug Delivery System. *Indian J. Pharm. Sci.* **2009**, *71*, 349–358. [CrossRef] [PubMed]
14. McClements, D.J. The Biophysics of Digestion: Lipids. *Curr. Opin. Food Sci.* **2018**, *21*, 1–6. [CrossRef]
15. McClements, D.J. Edible Lipid Nanoparticles: Digestion, Absorption, and Potential Toxicity. *Prog. Lipid Res.* **2013**, *52*, 409–423. [CrossRef]
16. Joye, I.J.; Davidov-Pardo, G.; McClements, D.J. Nanotechnology for Increased Micronutrient Bioavailability. *Trends Food Sci. Technol.* **2014**, *40*, 168–182. [CrossRef]
17. McClements, D.J.; Jafari, S.M. Improving Emulsion Formation, Stability and Performance Using Mixed Emulsifiers: A Review. *Adv. Colloid Interface Sci.* **2018**, *251*, 55–79. [CrossRef]

18. Sharipova, A.A.; Aidarova, S.B.; Mutaliyeva, B.Z.; Babayev, A.A.; Issakhov, M.; Issayeva, A.B.; Madybekova, G.M.; Grigoriev, D.O.; Miller, R. The Use of Polymer and Surfactants for the Microencapsulation and Emulsion Stabilization. *Colloids Interfaces* **2017**, *1*, 3. [CrossRef]
19. Geszke-Moritz, M.; Moritz, M. Solid Lipid Nanoparticles as Attractive Drug Vehicles: Composition, Properties and Therapeutic Strategies. *Mater. Sci. Eng. C* **2016**, *68*, 982–994. [CrossRef]
20. Lima, A.M.; Pizzol, C.D.; Monteiro, F.B.F.; Creczynski-Pasa, T.B.; Andrade, G.P.; Ribeiro, A.O.; Perussi, J.R. Hypericin Encapsulated in Solid Lipid Nanoparticles: Phototoxicity and Photodynamic Efficiency. *J. Photochem. Photobiol. B Biol.* **2013**, *125*, 146–154. [CrossRef]
21. Anjum, R.; Lakshmi, P.K. A Review on Solid Lipid Nanoparticles; Focus on Excipients and Formulation Techniques. *Int. J. Pharm. Sci. Res.* **2019**, *10*, 4090–4099. [CrossRef]
22. Assali, M.; Zaid, A.-N. Features, Applications, and Sustainability of Lipid Nanoparticles in Cosmeceuticals. *Saudi Pharm. J.* **2022**, *30*, 53–65. [CrossRef] [PubMed]
23. Duong, V.A.; Nguyen, T.T.L.; Maeng, H.J. Preparation of Solid Lipid Nanoparticles and Nanostructured Lipid Carriers for Drug Delivery and the Effects of Preparation Parameters of Solvent Injection Method. *Molecules* **2020**, *25*, 4781. [CrossRef] [PubMed]
24. Lin, C.-H.; Chen, C.-H.; Lin, Z.-C.; Fang, J.-Y. Recent Advances in Oral Delivery of Drugs and Bioactive Natural Products Using Solid Lipid Nanoparticles as the Carriers. *J. Food Drug Anal.* **2017**, *25*, 219–234. [CrossRef] [PubMed]
25. Wang, S.; Su, R.; Nie, S.; Sun, M.; Zhang, J.; Wu, D.; Moustaid-Moussa, N. Application of Nanotechnology in Improving Bioavailability and Bioactivity of Diet-Derived Phytochemicals. *J. Nutr. Biochem.* **2014**, *25*, 363–376. [CrossRef] [PubMed]
26. Ganesan, P.; Ramalingam, P.; Karthivashan, G.; Ko, Y.T.; Choi, D.K. Recent Developments in Solid Lipid Nanoparticle and Surface-Modified Solid Lipid Nanoparticle Delivery Systems for Oral Delivery of Phyto-Bioactive Compounds in Various Chronic Diseases. *Int. J. Nanomed.* **2018**, *13*, 1569–1583. [CrossRef]
27. Gonçalves, C.; Ramalho, M.J.; Silva, R.; Silva, V.; Marques-Oliveira, R.; Silva, A.C.; Pereira, M.C.; Loureiro, J.A. Lipid Nanoparticles Containing Mixtures of Antioxidants to Improve Skin Care and Cancer Prevention. *Pharmaceutics* **2021**, *13*, 2042. [CrossRef]
28. López-Martínez, A.; Rocha-Uribe, A. Antioxidant Hydrophobicity and Emulsifier Type Influences the Partitioning of Antioxidants in the Interface Improving Oxidative Stability in O/W Emulsions Rich in n-3 Fatty Acids. *Eur. J. Lipid Sci. Technol.* **2018**, *120*, 1700277. [CrossRef]
29. Aanisah, N.; Sulistiawati, S.; Djabir, Y.Y.; Asri, R.M.; Sumarheni, S.; Chabib, L.; Hamzah, H.; Permana, A.D. Development of Solid Lipid Nanoparticle-Loaded Polymeric Hydrogels Containing Antioxidant and Photoprotective Bioactive Compounds of Safflower (*Carthamus tinctorius* L.) for Improved Skin Delivery. *Langmuir* **2023**, *39*, 1838–1851. [CrossRef]
30. Jiménez-Colmenero, F. Potential Applications of Multiple Emulsions in the Development of Healthy and Functional Foods. *Food Res. Int.* **2013**, *52*, 64–74. [CrossRef]
31. Lu, W.; Kelly, A.L.; Miao, S. Emulsion-Based Encapsulation and Delivery Systems for Polyphenols. *Trends Food Sci. Technol.* **2016**, *47*, 1–9. [CrossRef]
32. Molet-Rodríguez, A.; Martín-Belloso, O.; Salvia-Trujillo, L. Formation and Stabilization of W1/O/W2 Emulsions with Gelled Lipid Phases. *Molecules* **2021**, *26*, 312. [CrossRef] [PubMed]
33. Campos, D.A.; Madureira, A.R.; Sarmento, B.; Pintado, M.M.; Gomes, A.M. Technological Stability of Solid Lipid Nanoparticles Loaded with Phenolic Compounds: Drying Process and Stability along Storage. *J. Food Eng.* **2017**, *196*, 1–10. [CrossRef]
34. Sridhar, K.; Inbaraj, B.S.; Chen, B.-H. Recent Advances on Nanoparticle Based Strategies for Improving Carotenoid Stability and Biological Activity. *Antioxidants* **2021**, *10*, 713. [CrossRef]
35. Tang, C.-H.; Chen, H.-L.; Dong, J.-R. Solid Lipid Nanoparticles (SLNs) and Nanostructured Lipid Carriers (NLCs) as Food-Grade Nanovehicles for Hydrophobic Nutraceuticals or Bioactives. *Appl. Sci.* **2023**, *13*, 1726. [CrossRef]
36. Ghasemiyeh, P.; Mohammadi-Samani, S. Solid Lipid Nanoparticles and Nanostructured Lipid Carriers as Novel Drug Delivery Systems: Applications, Advantages and Disadvantages. *Res. Pharm. Sci.* **2018**, *13*, 288–303. [CrossRef] [PubMed]
37. Shinde, P.B.; Gunvantrao, D.S.; Vivekanand, S.M. Lipid Based Nanoparticles: SLN/NLCs-Formulation Techniques, Its Evaluation and Applications. *Int. J. Creat. Innov. Res. All Stud.* **2019**, *1*, 20–31.
38. Weber, S.; Zimmer, A.; Pardeike, J. Solid Lipid Nanoparticles (SLN) and Nanostructured Lipid Carriers (NLC) for Pulmonary Application: A Review of the State of the Art. *Eur. J. Pharm. Biopharm.* **2014**, *86*, 7–22. [CrossRef]
39. Gordillo-Galeano, A.; Mora-Huertas, C.E. Solid Lipid Nanoparticles and Nanostructured Lipid Carriers: A Review Emphasizing on Particle Structure and Drug Release. *Eur. J. Pharm. Biopharm.* **2018**, *133*, 285–308. [CrossRef]
40. Hu, L.; Tang, X.; Cui, F. Solid Lipid Nanoparticles (SLNs) to Improve Oral Bioavailability of Poorly Soluble Drugs. *J. Pharm. Pharmacol.* **2004**, *56*, 1527–1535. [CrossRef]
41. Weiss, J.; Decker, E.A.; McClements, D.J.; Kristbergsson, K.; Helgason, T.; Awad, T. Solid Lipid Nanoparticles as Delivery Systems for Bioactive Food Components. *Food Biophys.* **2008**, *3*, 146–154. [CrossRef]
42. Amalia, A.; Jufri, M.; Anwar, E. Preparation and Characterization of Solid Lipid Nanoparticle (SLN) of Gliclazide. *J. Ilmu Kefarmasian Indones.* **2015**, *13*, 108–114.
43. Yadav, N.; Khatak, S.; Vir, U.; Sara, S. Solid Lipid Nanoparticles–A Review. *Int. J. Appl. Pharm.* **2013**, *5*, 8–18.
44. Basso, J.; Mendes, M.; Cova, T.; Sousa, J.; Pais, A.; Fortuna, A.; Vitorino, R.; Vitorino, C. A Stepwise Framework for the Systematic Development of Lipid Nanoparticles. *Biomolecules* **2022**, *12*, 223. [CrossRef] [PubMed]

45. Subroto, E.; Andoyo, R.; Indiarto, R.; Wulandari, E.; Wadhiah, E.F.N. Preparation of Solid Lipid Nanoparticle-Ferrous Sulfate by Double Emulsion Method Based on Fat Rich in Monolaurin and Stearic Acid. *Nanomaterials* **2022**, *12*, 3054. [CrossRef]
46. Basha, S.K.; Dhandayuthabani, R.; Muzammil, M.S.; Kumari, V.S. Solid Lipid Nanoparticles for Oral Drug Delivery. *Mater. Today Proc.* **2019**, *36*, 313–324. [CrossRef]
47. Musielak, E.; Feliczak-Guzik, A.; Nowak, I. Optimization of the Conditions of Solid Lipid Nanoparticles (SLN) Synthesis. *Molecules* **2022**, *27*, 2202. [CrossRef] [PubMed]
48. Bertoni, S.; Passerini, N.; Albertini, B. Liquid Lipids Act as Polymorphic Modifiers of Tristearin-Based Formulations Produced by Melting Technologies. *Pharmaceutics* **2021**, *13*, 1089. [CrossRef]
49. Blanco-Llamero, C.; Fonseca, J.; Durazzo, A.; Lucarini, M.; Santini, A.; Señoráns, F.J.; Souto, E.B. Nutraceuticals and Food-Grade Lipid Nanoparticles: From Natural Sources to a Circular Bioeconomy Approach. *Foods* **2022**, *11*, 2318. [CrossRef]
50. Müller, R.H.; Mäder, K.; Gohla, S. Solid Lipid Nanoparticles (SLN) for Controlled Drug Delivery–A Review of the State of the Art. *Eur. J. Pharm. Biopharm.* **2000**, *50*, 161–177. [CrossRef]
51. Dhiman, N.; Awasthi, R.; Sharma, B.; Kharkwal, H.; Kulkarni, G.T. Lipid Nanoparticles as Carriers for Bioactive Delivery. *Front. Chem.* **2021**, *9*, 580118. [CrossRef] [PubMed]
52. Jafar, G.; Darijanto, S.T.; Mauludin, R. Formulasi Solid Lipid Nanoparticle Ceramide. *J. Pharmascience* **2015**, *2*, 80–87.
53. Bayón-Cordero, L.; Alkorta, I.; Arana, L. Application of Solid Lipid Nanoparticles to Improve the Efficiency of Anticancer Drugs. *Nanomaterials* **2019**, *9*, 474. [CrossRef] [PubMed]
54. Feng, L.; Mumper, R.J. A Critical Review of Lipid-Based Nanoparticles for Taxane Delivery. *Cancer Lett.* **2013**, *334*, 157–175. [CrossRef] [PubMed]
55. Pardeshi, C.; Rajput, P.; Belgamwar, V.; Tekade, A.; Patil, G.; Chaudhary, K.; Sonje, A. Solid Lipid Based Nanocarriers: An Overview. *Acta Pharm.* **2012**, *62*, 433–472. [CrossRef] [PubMed]
56. Das, S.; Chaudhury, A. Recent Advances in Lipid Nanoparticle Formulations with Solid Matrix for Oral Drug Delivery. *AAPS PharmSciTech* **2011**, *12*, 62–76. [CrossRef]
57. Lingayat, V.J.; Zarekar, N.S.; Shendge, R.S. Solid Lipid Nanoparticles: A Review. *Nanosci. Nanotechnol. Res.* **2017**, *5*, 67–72. [CrossRef]
58. Bahari, L.A.S.; Hamishehkar, H. The Impact of Variables on Particle Size of Solid Lipid Nanoparticles and Nanostructured Lipid Carriers; A Comparative Literature Review. *Adv. Pharm. Bull.* **2016**, *6*, 143–151. [CrossRef]
59. Shi, L.; Li, Z.; Yu, L.; Jia, H.; Zheng, L. Effects of Surfactants and Lipids on the Preparation of Solid Lipid Nanoparticles Using Double Emulsion Method. *J. Dispers. Sci. Technol.* **2011**, *32*, 254–259. [CrossRef]
60. Deshpande, A.; Mohamed, M.; Daftardar, S.B.; Patel, M.; Boddu, S.H.S.; Nesamony, J. Solid Lipid Nanoparticles in Drug Delivery: Opportunities and Challenges. In *Emerging Nanotechnologies for Diagnostics, Drug Delivery and Medical Devices*; Elsevier: Amsterdam, The Netherlands, 2017; pp. 291–330, ISBN 9780323429979.
61. Iqbal, M.A.; Md, S.; Sahni, J.K.; Baboota, S.; Dang, S.; Ali, J. Nanostructured Lipid Carriers System: Recent Advances in Drug Delivery. *J. Drug Target.* **2012**, *20*, 813–830. [CrossRef]
62. Rohmah, M.; Raharjo, S.; Hidayat, C.; Martien, R. Application of Response Surface Methodology for the Optimization of β-Carotene-Loaded Nanostructured Lipid Carrier from Mixtures of Palm Stearin and Palm Olein. *JAOCS J. Am. Oil Chem. Soc.* **2019**, *97*, 213–223. [CrossRef]
63. Müller, R.H.; Radtke, M.; Wissing, S.A. Solid Lipid Nanoparticles (SLN) and Nanostructured Lipid Carriers (NLC) in Cosmetic and Dermatological Preparations. *Adv. Drug Deliv. Rev.* **2002**, *54*, 131–155. [CrossRef] [PubMed]
64. Elmowafy, M.; Al-Sanea, M.M. Nanostructured Lipid Carriers (NLCs) as Drug Delivery Platform: Advances in Formulation and Delivery Strategies. *Saudi Pharm. J.* **2021**, *29*, 999–1012. [CrossRef] [PubMed]
65. Severino, P.; Andreani, T.; Macedo, A.S.; Fangueiro, J.F.; Santana, M.H.A.; Silva, A.M.; Souto, E.B. Current State-of-Art and New Trends on Lipid Nanoparticles (SLN and NLC) for Oral Drug Delivery. *J. Drug Deliv.* **2012**, *2012*, 760891. [CrossRef] [PubMed]
66. Chutoprapat, R.; Kopongpanich, P.; Chan, L.W. A Mini-Review on Solid Lipid Nanoparticles and Nanostructured Lipid Carriers: Topical Delivery of Phytochemicals for the Treatment of Acne Vulgaris. *Molecules* **2022**, *27*, 3460. [CrossRef] [PubMed]
67. Sharma, A.; Baldi, A. Nanostructured Lipid Carriers: A Review Journal. *J. Dev. Drugs* **2018**, *7*, 1.
68. Fanun, M. Propylene Glycol and Ethoxylated Surfactant Effects on the Phase Behavior of Water/Sucrose Stearate/Oil System. *J. Dispers. Sci. Technol.* **2007**, *28*, 1244–1253. [CrossRef]
69. Sriarumtias, F.F.; Tarini, S.; Damayanti, S. Formulasi Dan Uji Potensi Antioksidan Nanostructured Lipid Carrier (NLC) Retinil Palmitat. *Acta Pharm. Indones.* **2017**, *42*, 25–31. [CrossRef]
70. Gundogdu, E.; Demir, E.-S.; Ekinci, M.; Ozgenc, E.; Ilem-Ozdemir, D.; Senyigit, Z.; Gonzalez-Alvarez, I.; Bermejo, M. An Innovative Formulation Based on Nanostructured Lipid Carriers for Imatinib Delivery: Pre-Formulation, Cellular Uptake and Cytotoxicity Studies. *Nanomaterials* **2022**, *12*, 250. [CrossRef]
71. Calderon-Jacinto, R.; Matricardi, P.; Gueguen, V.; Pavon-Djavid, G.; Pauthe, E.; Rodriguez-Ruiz, V. Dual Nanostructured Lipid Carriers/Hydrogel System for Delivery of Curcumin for Topical Skin Applications. *Biomolecules* **2022**, *12*, 780. [CrossRef]
72. Javed, S.; Mangla, B.; Almoshari, Y.; Sultan, M.H.; Ahsan, W. Nanostructured Lipid Carrier System: A Compendium of Their Formulation Development Approaches, Optimization Strategies by Quality by Design, and Recent Applications in Drug Delivery. *Nanotechnol. Rev.* **2022**, *11*, 1744–1777. [CrossRef]
73. Chauhan, I.; Yasir, M.; Verma, M.; Singh, A.P. Nanostructured Lipid Carriers: A Groundbreaking Approach for Transdermal Drug Delivery. *Adv. Pharm. Bull.* **2020**, *10*, 150–165. [CrossRef] [PubMed]

74. Babazadeh, A.; Ghanbarzadeh, B.; Hamishehkar, H. Formulation of Food Grade Nanostructured Lipid Carrier (NLC) for Potential Applications in Medicinal-Functional Foods. *J. Drug Deliv. Sci. Technol.* **2017**, *39*, 50–58. [CrossRef]
75. Nguyen, V.H.; Thuy, V.N.; Van, T.V.; Dao, A.H.; Lee, B.-J. Nanostructured Lipid Carriers and Their Potential Applications for Versatile Drug Delivery via Oral Administration. *OpenNano* **2022**, *8*, 100064. [CrossRef]
76. Gaba, B.; Fazil, M.; Ali, A.; Baboota, S.; Sahni, J.K.; Ali, J. Nanostructured Lipid (NLCs) Carriers as a Bioavailability Enhancement Tool for Oral Administration. *Drug Deliv.* **2015**, *22*, 691–700. [CrossRef]
77. Esposito, E.; Sguizzato, M.; Drechsler, M.; Mariani, P.; Carducci, F.; Nastruzzi, C.; Valacchi, G.; Cortesi, R. Lipid Nanostructures for Antioxidant Delivery: A Comparative Preformulation Study. *Beilstein J. Nanotechnol.* **2019**, *10*, 1789–1801. [CrossRef] [PubMed]
78. Souto, E.B.; Doktorovova, S.; Zielinska, A.; Silva, A.M. Key Production Parameters for the Development of Solid Lipid Nanoparticles by High Shear Homogenization. *Pharm. Dev. Technol.* **2019**, *24*, 1181–1185. [CrossRef]
79. Mahajan, A.; Kaur, S. Design, Formulation, and Characterization of Stearic Acid-Based Solid Lipid Nanoparticles of Candesartan Cilexetil to Augment Its Oral Bioavailability. *Asian J. Pharm. Clin. Res.* **2018**, *11*, 344–350. [CrossRef]
80. Subramanian, P. Lipid-Based Nanocarrier System for the Effective Delivery of Nutraceuticals. *Molecules* **2021**, *26*, 5510. [CrossRef]
81. Sastri, K.T.; Radha, G.V.; Pidikiti, S.; Vajjhala, P. Solid Lipid Nanoparticles: Preparation Techniques, Their Characterization, and an Update on Recent Studies. *J. Appl. Pharm. Sci.* **2020**, *10*, 126–141. [CrossRef]
82. Ganesan, P.; Narayanasamy, D. Lipid Nanoparticles: Different Preparation Techniques, Characterization, Hurdles, and Strategies for the Production of Solid Lipid Nanoparticles and Nanostructured Lipid Carriers for Oral Drug Delivery. *Sustain. Chem. Pharm.* **2017**, *6*, 37–56. [CrossRef]
83. Yukuyama, M.N.; Ghisleni, D.D.M.; Pinto, T.J.A.; Bou-Chacra, N.A. Nanoemulsion: Process Selection and Application in Cosmetics–A Review. *Int. J. Cosmet. Sci.* **2016**, *38*, 13–24. [CrossRef] [PubMed]
84. Dolatabadi, J.E.N.; Valizadeh, H.; Hamishehkar, H. Solid Lipid Nanoparticles as Efficient Drug and Gene Delivery Systems: Recent Breakthroughs. *Adv. Pharm. Bull.* **2015**, *5*, 151–159. [CrossRef] [PubMed]
85. Sinha, V.R.; Srivastava, S.; Goel, H.; Jindal, V. Solid Lipid Nanoparticles (SLN'S) -Trends and Implications in Drug Targeting. *Int. J. Adv. Pharm. Sci.* **2010**, *1*, 212–238. [CrossRef]
86. Khairnar, S.V.; Pagare, P.; Thakre, A.; Nambiar, A.R.; Junnuthula, V.; Abraham, M.C.; Kolimi, P.; Nyavanandi, D.; Dyawanapelly, S. Review on the Scale-Up Methods for the Preparation of Solid Lipid Nanoparticles. *Pharmaceutics* **2022**, *14*, 1886. [CrossRef] [PubMed]
87. Alarifi, S.; Massadeh, S.; Al-Agamy, M.; Al Aamery, M.; Al Bekairy, A.; Yassin, A.E. Enhancement of Ciprofloxacin Activity by Incorporating It in Solid Lipid Nanoparticles. *Trop. J. Pharm. Res.* **2020**, *19*, 909–918. [CrossRef]
88. Xie, S.; Zhu, L.; Dong, Z.; Wang, X.; Wang, Y.; Li, X.; Zhou, W.Z. Preparation, Characterization and Pharmacokinetics of Enrofloxacin-Loaded Solid Lipid Nanoparticles: Influences of Fatty Acids. *Colloids Surf. B Biointerfaces* **2011**, *83*, 382–387. [CrossRef]
89. Woo, J.O.; Misran, M.; Lee, P.F.; Tan, L.P. Development of a Controlled Release of Salicylic Acid Loaded Stearic Acid-Oleic Acid Nanoparticles in Cream for Topical Delivery. *Sci. World J.* **2014**, *2014*, 205703. [CrossRef]
90. Karthik, S.; Raghavan, C.V.; Marslin, G.; Rahman, H.; Selvaraj, D.; Balakumar, K.; Franklin, G. Quillaja Saponin: A Prospective Emulsifier for the Preparation of Solid Lipid Nanoparticles. *Colloids Surf. B Biointerfaces* **2016**, *147*, 274–280. [CrossRef]
91. Kelidari, H.R.; Babaei, R.; Nabili, M.; Shokohi, T.; Saeedi, M.; Gholami, S.; Moazeni, M.; Nokhodchi, A. Improved Delivery of Voriconazole to Aspergillus Fumigatus through Solid Lipid Nanoparticles as an Effective Carrier. *Colloids Surf. A Physicochem. Eng. Asp.* **2018**, *558*, 338–342. [CrossRef]
92. Mehnert, W.; Mäder, K. Solid Lipid Nanoparticles: Production, Characterization and Applications. *Adv. Drug Deliv. Rev.* **2001**, *47*, 165–196. [CrossRef] [PubMed]
93. Mesa, J.; Hinestroza-Córdoba, L.I.; Barrera, C.; Seguí, L.; Betoret, E.; Betoret, N. High Homogenization Pressures to Improve Food Quality, Functionality and Sustainability. *Molecules* **2020**, *25*, 3305. [CrossRef] [PubMed]
94. Rahmi, D. Lemak Padat Nanopartikel; Sintesis Dan Aplikasi. *J. Kim. dan Kemasan* **2010**, *32*, 27. [CrossRef]
95. Garg, U.; Jain, K. Dermal and Transdermal Drug Delivery through Vesicles and Particles: Preparation and Applications. *Adv. Pharm. Bull.* **2022**, *12*, 45–57. [CrossRef]
96. Sjöström, B.; Bergenståhl, B. Preparation of Submicron Drug Particles in Lecithin-Stabilized o/w Emulsions I. Model Studies of the Precipitation of Cholesteryl Acetate. *Int. J. Pharm.* **1992**, *88*, 53–62. [CrossRef]
97. Westesen, K.; Siekmann, B. Investigation of the Gel Formation of Phospholipid-Stabilized Solid Lipid Nanoparticles. *Int. J. Pharm.* **1997**, *151*, 35–45. [CrossRef]
98. Xu, L.; Wang, X.; Liu, Y.; Yang, G.; Falconer, R.J.; Zhao, C.-X. Lipid Nanoparticles for Drug Delivery. *Adv. NanoBiomed Res.* **2022**, *2*, 2100109. [CrossRef]
99. Pooja, D.; Tunki, L.; Kulhari, H.; Reddy, B.B.; Sistla, R. Optimization of Solid Lipid Nanoparticles Prepared by a Single Emulsification-Solvent Evaporation Method. *Data Br.* **2016**, *6*, 15–19. [CrossRef]
100. Chattopadhyay, P.; Shekunov, B.Y.; Yim, D.; Cipolla, D.; Boyd, B.; Farr, S. Production of Solid Lipid Nanoparticle Suspensions Using Supercritical Fluid Extraction of Emulsions (SFEE) for Pulmonary Delivery Using the AERx System. *Adv. Drug Deliv. Rev.* **2007**, *59*, 444–453. [CrossRef]
101. Campardelli, R.; Cherain, M.; Perfetti, C.; Iorio, C.; Scognamiglio, M.; Reverchon, E.; Porta, G.D. Lipid Nanoparticles Production by Supercritical Fluid Assisted Emulsion–Diffusion. *J. Supercrit. Fluids* **2013**, *82*, 34–40. [CrossRef]
102. Iqbal, M.; Zafar, N.; Fessi, H.; Elaissari, A. Double Emulsion Solvent Evaporation Techniques Used for Drug Encapsulation. *Int. J. Pharm.* **2015**, *496*, 173–190. [CrossRef]

103. Nabi-Meibodi, M.; Navidi, B.; Navidi, N.; Vatanara, A.; Reza Rouini, M.; Ramezani, V. Optimized Double Emulsion-Solvent Evaporation Process for Production of Solid Lipid Nanoparticles Containing Baclofene as a Lipid Insoluble Drug. *J. Drug Deliv. Sci. Technol.* **2013**, *23*, 225–230. [CrossRef]
104. Mudrić, J.; Šavikin, K.; Đekić, L.; Pavlović, S.; Kurćubić, I.; Ibrić, S.; Đuriš, J. Development of Lipid-Based Gastroretentive Delivery System for Gentian Extract by Double Emulsion–Melt Dispersion Technique. *Pharmaceutics* **2021**, *13*, 2095.
105. Freitas, C.; Müller, R.H. Spray-Drying of Solid Lipid Nanoparticles (SLNTM). *Eur. J. Pharm. Biopharm.* **1998**, *46*, 145–151. [CrossRef]
106. Ristroph, K.D.; Feng, J.; McManus, S.A.; Zhang, Y.; Gong, K.; Ramachandruni, H.; White, C.E.; Prud'homme, R.K. Spray Drying OZ439 Nanoparticles to Form Stable, Water-Dispersible Powders for Oral Malaria Therapy. *J. Transl. Med.* **2019**, *17*, 97. [CrossRef] [PubMed]
107. James, O.; Oloo, F.; Ng'etich, J.; Kivunzya, M.; Omwoyo, W.; Gathirwa, J. Comparison of Freeze and Spray Drying to Obtain Primaquine-Loaded Solid Lipid Nanoparticles. *J. Nanotoxicol. Nanomed.* **2017**, *2*, 31–50. [CrossRef]
108. Silva, A.C.; Kumar, A.; Wild, W.; Ferreira, D.; Santos, D.; Forbes, B. Long-Term Stability, Biocompatibility and Oral Delivery Potential of Risperidone-Loaded Solid Lipid Nanoparticles. *Int. J. Pharm.* **2012**, *436*, 798–805. [CrossRef] [PubMed]
109. Jacob, S.; Nair, A.B.; Shah, J.; Gupta, S.; Boddu, S.H.S.; Sreeharsha, N.; Joseph, A.; Shinu, P.; Morsy, M.A. Lipid Nanoparticles as a Promising Drug Delivery Carrier for Topical Ocular Therapy–An Overview on Recent Advances. *Pharmaceutics* **2022**, *14*, 533. [CrossRef]
110. Mu, H.; Holm, R.; Müllertz, A. Lipid-Based Formulations for Oral Administration of Poorly Water-Soluble Drugs. *Int. J. Pharm.* **2013**, *453*, 215–224. [CrossRef]
111. Sguizzato, M.; Esposito, E.; Cortesi, R. Lipid-Based Nanosystems as a Tool to Overcome Skin Barrier. *Int. J. Mol. Sci.* **2021**, *22*, 8319. [CrossRef]
112. Ahmad, J. Lipid Nanoparticles Based Cosmetics with Potential Application in Alleviating Skin Disorders. *Cosmetics* **2021**, *8*, 84. [CrossRef]
113. Rubiano, S.; Echeverri, J.D.; Salamanca, C.H. Solid Lipid Nanoparticles (SLNs) with Potential as Cosmetic Hair Formulations Made from Otoba Wax and Ultrahigh Pressure Homogenization. *Cosmetics* **2020**, *7*, 42. [CrossRef]
114. Souto, E.B.; Müller, R.H. Cosmetic Features and Applications of Lipid Nanoparticles (SLN®, NLC®). *Int. J. Cosmet. Sci.* **2008**, *30*, 157–165. [CrossRef]
115. Wissing, S.A.; Müller, R.H. Cosmetic Applications for Solid Lipid Nanoparticles (SLN). *Int. J. Pharm.* **2003**, *254*, 65–68. [CrossRef]
116. Souto, E.B.; Fangueiro, J.F.; Fernandes, A.R.; Cano, A.; Sanchez-Lopez, E.; Garcia, M.L.; Severino, P.; Paganelli, M.O.; Chaud, M.V.; Silva, A.M. Physicochemical and Biopharmaceutical Aspects Influencing Skin Permeation and Role of SLN and NLC for Skin Drug Delivery. *Heliyon* **2022**, *8*, e08938. [CrossRef] [PubMed]
117. Nugraha, M.W.; Iswandana, R.; Jufri, M. Preparation, Characterization, and Formulation of Solid Lipid Nanoparticles Lotion from Mulberry Roots (Morus Alba L.). *Int. J. Appl. Pharm.* **2020**, *12*, 182–186. [CrossRef]
118. Lai, F.; Wissing, S.A.; Müller, R.H.; Fadda, A.M. *Artemisia arborescens* L. Essential Oil-Loaded Solid Lipid Nanoparticles for Potential Agricultural Application: Preparation and Characterization. *AAPS PharmSciTech* **2006**, *7*, 2. [CrossRef]
119. Cirri, M.; Mennini, N.; Maestrelli, F.; Mura, P.; Ghelardini, C.; di Cesare Mannelli, L. Development and in Vivo Evaluation of an Innovative "Hydrochlorothiazide-in Cyclodextrins-in Solid Lipid Nanoparticles" Formulation with Sustained Release and Enhanced Oral Bioavailability for Potential Hypertension Treatment in Pediatrics. *Int. J. Pharm.* **2017**, *521*, 73–83. [CrossRef]
120. Jain, A.; Sharma, G.; Thakur, K.; Raza, K.; Shivhare, U.S.; Ghoshal, G.; Katare, O.P. Beta-Carotene-Encapsulated Solid Lipid Nanoparticles (BC-SLNs) as Promising Vehicle for Cancer: An Investigative Assessment. *AAPS PharmSciTech* **2019**, *20*, 100. [CrossRef]
121. Oehlke, K.; Behsnilian, D.; Mayer-Miebach, E.; Weidler, P.G.; Greiner, R. Edible Solid Lipid Nanoparticles (SLN) as Carrier System for Antioxidants of Different Lipophilicity. *PLoS ONE* **2017**, *12*, e0171662. [CrossRef]
122. Mendoza-Muñoz, N.; Urbán-Morlán, Z.; Leyva-Gómez, G.; De La Luz Zambrano-Zaragoza, M.; Piñón-Segundo, E.; Quintanar-Guerrero, D. Solid Lipid Nanoparticles: An Approach to Improve Oral Drug Delivery. *J. Pharm. Pharm. Sci.* **2021**, *24*, 509–532. [CrossRef] [PubMed]
123. Lu, H.; Zhang, S.; Wang, J.; Chen, Q. A Review on Polymer and Lipid-Based Nanocarriers and Its Application to Nano-Pharmaceutical and Food-Based Systems. *Front. Nutr.* **2021**, *8*, 783831. [CrossRef]
124. Satapathy, M.K.; Yen, T.-L.; Jan, J.-S.; Tang, R.-D.; Wang, J.-Y.; Taliyan, R.; Yang, C.-H. Solid Lipid Nanoparticles (SLNs): An Advanced Drug Delivery System Targeting Brain through BBB. *Pharmaceutics* **2021**, *13*, 1183. [CrossRef] [PubMed]
125. Adepu, S.; Ramakrishna, S. Controlled Drug Delivery Systems: Current Status and Future Directions. *Molecules* **2021**, *26*, 5905. [CrossRef] [PubMed]
126. Ana, R.D.; Fonseca, J.; Karczewski, J.; Silva, A.M.; Zielińska, A.; Souto, E.B. Lipid-Based Nanoparticulate Systems for the Ocular Delivery of Bioactives with Anti-Inflammatory Properties. *Int. J. Mol. Sci.* **2022**, *23*, 12102. [CrossRef]
127. Montoto, S.S.; Muraca, G.; Ruiz, M.E. Solid Lipid Nanoparticles for Drug Delivery: Pharmacological and Biopharmaceutical Aspects. *Front. Mol. Biosci.* **2020**, *7*, 587997. [CrossRef] [PubMed]
128. Sakellari, G.I.; Zafeiri, I.; Batchelor, H.; Spyropoulos, F. Formulation Design, Production and Characterisation of Solid Lipid Nanoparticles (SLN) and Nanostructured Lipid Carriers (NLC) for the Encapsulation of a Model Hydrophobic Active. *Food Hydrocoll. Health* **2021**, *1*, 100024. [CrossRef]

129. Sharma, A.; Arora, K.; Mohapatra, H.; Sindhu, R.K.; Bulzan, M.; Cavalu, S.; Paneshar, G.; Elansary, H.O.; El-Sabrout, A.M.; Mahmoud, E.A.; et al. Supersaturation-Based Drug Delivery Systems: Strategy for Bioavailability Enhancement of Poorly Water-Soluble Drugs. *Molecules* **2022**, *27*, 2969. [CrossRef]
130. Duan, Y.; Dhar, A.; Patel, C.; Khimani, M.; Neogi, S.; Sharma, P.; Kumar, N.S.; Vekariya, R.L. A Brief Review on Solid Lipid Nanoparticles: Part and Parcel of Contemporary Drug Delivery Systems. *RSC Adv.* **2020**, *10*, 26777–26791. [CrossRef]
131. Pople, P.V.; Singh, K.K. Development and Evaluation of Topical Formulation Containing Solid Lipid Nanoparticles of Vitamin A. *AAPS PharmSciTech* **2006**, *7*, E63–E69. [CrossRef]
132. Kim, S.T.; Jang, D.J.; Kim, J.H.; Park, J.Y.; Lim, J.S.; Lee, S.Y.; Lee, K.M.; Lim, S.J.; Kim, C.K. Topical Administration of Cyclosporin A in a Solid Lipid Nanoparticle Formulation. *Pharmazie* **2009**, *64*, 510–514. [CrossRef]
133. Hou, X.; Zaks, T.; Langer, R.; Dong, Y. Lipid Nanoparticles for MRNA Delivery. *Nat. Rev. Mater.* **2021**, *6*, 1078–1094. [CrossRef]
134. Akinc, A.; Maier, M.A.; Manoharan, M.; Fitzgerald, K.; Jayaraman, M.; Barros, S.; Ansell, S.; Du, X.; Hope, M.J.; Madden, T.D.; et al. The Onpattro Story and the Clinical Translation of Nanomedicines Containing Nucleic Acid-Based Drugs. *Nat. Nanotechnol.* **2019**, *14*, 1084–1087. [CrossRef] [PubMed]
135. Francis, J.E.; Skakic, I.; Dekiwadia, C.; Shukla, R.; Taki, A.C.; Walduck, A.; Smooker, P.M. Solid Lipid Nanoparticle Carrier Platform Containing Synthetic TLR4 Agonist Mediates Non-Viral DNA Vaccine Delivery. *Vaccines* **2020**, *8*, 551. [CrossRef] [PubMed]
136. Lou, G.; Anderluzzi, G.; Schmidt, S.T.; Woods, S.; Gallorini, S.; Brazzoli, M.; Giusti, F.; Ferlenghi, I.; Johnson, R.N.; Roberts, C.W.; et al. Delivery of Self-Amplifying MRNA Vaccines by Cationic Lipid Nanoparticles: The Impact of Cationic Lipid Selection. *J. Control. Release* **2020**, *325*, 370–379. [CrossRef] [PubMed]
137. Marto, J.; Sangalli, C.; Capra, P.; Perugini, P.; Ascenso, A.; Gonçalves, L.; Ribeiro, H. Development and Characterization of New and Scalable Topical Formulations Containing N-Acetyl-d-Glucosamine-Loaded Solid Lipid Nanoparticles. *Drug Dev. Ind. Pharm.* **2017**, *43*, 1792–1800. [CrossRef] [PubMed]
138. Chen, J.; Wei, N.; Lopez-Garcia, M.; Ambrose, D.; Lee, J.; Annelin, C.; Peterson, T. Development and Evaluation of Resveratrol, Vitamin E, and Epigallocatechin Gallate Loaded Lipid Nanoparticles for Skin Care Applications. *Eur. J. Pharm. Biopharm.* **2017**, *117*, 286–291. [CrossRef]
139. Park, J.H.; Ban, S.J.; Ahmed, T.; Choi, H.S.; Yoon, H.E.; Yoon, J.H.; Choi, H.K. Development of DH-I-180-3 Loaded Lipid Nanoparticle for Photodynamic Therapy. *Int. J. Pharm.* **2015**, *491*, 393–401. [CrossRef]
140. Sangsen, Y.; Wiwattanawongsa, K.; Likhitwitayawuid, K.; Sritularak, B.; Wiwattanapatapee, R. Modification of Oral Absorption of Oxyresveratrol Using Lipid Based Nanoparticles. *Colloids Surf. B Biointerfaces* **2015**, *131*, 182–190. [CrossRef]
141. Öztürk, A.A.; Aygül, A.; Şenel, B. Influence of Glyceryl Behenate, Tripalmitin and Stearic Acid on the Properties of Clarithromycin Incorporated Solid Lipid Nanoparticles (SLNs): Formulation, Characterization, Antibacterial Activity and Cytotoxicity. *J. Drug Deliv. Sci. Technol.* **2019**, *54*, 101240. [CrossRef]
142. Zariwala, M.G.; Elsaid, N.; Jackson, T.L.; Corral López, F.; Farnaud, S.; Somavarapu, S.; Renshaw, D. A Novel Approach to Oral Iron Delivery Using Ferrous Sulphate Loaded Solid Lipid Nanoparticles. *Int. J. Pharm.* **2013**, *456*, 400–407. [CrossRef] [PubMed]
143. Hatefi, L.; Farhadian, N. A Safe and Efficient Method for Encapsulation of Ferrous Sulfate in Solid Lipid Nanoparticle for Non-Oxidation and Sustained Iron Delivery. *Colloids Interface Sci. Commun.* **2020**, *34*, 100227. [CrossRef]
144. Hamishehkar, H.; Shokri, J.; Fallahi, S.; Jahangiri, A.; Ghanbarzadeh, S.; Kouhsoltani, M. Histopathological Evaluation of Caffeine-Loaded Solid Lipid Nanoparticles in Efficient Treatment of Cellulite. *Drug Dev. Ind. Pharm.* **2015**, *41*, 1640–1646. [CrossRef] [PubMed]
145. Uner, M.; Karaman, E.F.; Aydoğmuş, Z. Solid Lipid Nanoparticles and Nanostructured Lipid Carriers of Loratadine for Topical Application: Physicochemical Stability and Drug Penetration through Rat Skin. *Trop. J. Pharm. Res.* **2014**, *13*, 653–660. [CrossRef]
146. Hassett, K.J.; Benenato, K.E.; Jacquinet, E.; Lee, A.; Woods, A.; Yuzhakov, O.; Himansu, S.; Deterling, J.; Geilich, B.M.; Ketova, T.; et al. Optimization of Lipid Nanoparticles for Intramuscular Administration of MRNA Vaccines. *Mol. Ther. Nucleic Acids* **2019**, *15*, 1–11. [CrossRef] [PubMed]
147. Van Tran, V.; Loi Nguyen, T.; Moon, J.-Y.; Lee, Y.-C. Core-Shell Materials, Lipid Particles and Nanoemulsions, for Delivery of Active Anti-Oxidants in Cosmetics Applications: Challenges and Development Strategies. *Chem. Eng. J.* **2019**, *368*, 88–114. [CrossRef]
148. Rezaei, A.; Fathi, M.; Jafari, S.M. Nanoencapsulation of Hydrophobic and Low-Soluble Food Bioactive Compounds within Different Nanocarriers. *Food Hydrocoll.* **2019**, *88*, 146–162. [CrossRef]
149. Schjoerring-Thyssen, J.; Olsen, K.; Koehler, K.; Jouenne, E.; Rousseau, D.; Andersen, M.L. Morphology and Structure of Solid Lipid Nanoparticles Loaded with High Concentrations of β-Carotene. *J. Agric. Food Chem.* **2019**, *67*, 12273–12282. [CrossRef]
150. Kakkar, V.; Singh, S.; Singla, D.; Kaur, I.P. Exploring Solid Lipid Nanoparticles to Enhance the Oral Bioavailability of Curcumin. *Mol. Nutr. Food Res.* **2011**, *55*, 495–503. [CrossRef]
151. Sandhu, S.K.; Kumar, S.; Raut, J.; Singh, M.; Kaur, S.; Sharma, G.; Roldan, T.L.; Trehan, S.; Holloway, J.; Wahler, G.; et al. Systematic Development and Characterization of Novel, High Drug-Loaded, Photostable, Curcumin Solid Lipid Nanoparticle Hydrogel for Wound Healing. *Antioxidants* **2021**, *10*, 725. [CrossRef]
152. Santonocito, D.; Sarpietro, M.G.; Carbone, C.; Panico, A.; Campisi, A.; Siciliano, E.A.; Sposito, G.; Castelli, F.; Puglia, C. Curcumin Containing PEGylated Solid Lipid Nanoparticles for Systemic Administration: A Preliminary Study. *Molecules* **2020**, *25*, 2991. [CrossRef]
153. Shylaja, P.A.; Mathew, M.M. Preparation and Characterization of Alpha Tocopherol Loaded Solid Lipid Nanoparticles by Hot Homogenization Method. *Int. J. Pharm. Pharm. Res.* **2016**, *7*, 437–448.

154. de Carvalho, S.M.; Noronha, C.M.; Floriani, C.L.; Lino, R.C.; Rocha, G.; Bellettini, I.C.; Ogliari, P.J.; Barreto, P.L.M. Optimization of α-Tocopherol Loaded Solid Lipid Nanoparticles by Central Composite Design. *Ind. Crops Prod.* **2013**, *49*, 278–285. [CrossRef]
155. Geetha, T.; Kapila, M.; Prakash, O.; Deol, P.K.; Kakkar, V.; Kaur, I.P. Sesamol-Loaded Solid Lipid Nanoparticles for Treatment of Skin Cancer. *J. Drug Target.* **2015**, *23*, 159–169. [CrossRef] [PubMed]
156. Singh, N.; Khullar, N.; Kakkar, V.; Kaur, I.P. Sesamol Loaded Solid Lipid Nanoparticles: A Promising Intervention for Control of Carbon Tetrachloride Induced Hepatotoxicity. *BMC Complement. Altern. Med.* **2015**, *15*, 142. [CrossRef]
157. Lacatusu, I.; Badea, N.; Murariu, A.; Oprea, O.; Bojin, D.; Meghea, A. Antioxidant Activity of Solid Lipid Nanoparticles Loaded with Umbelliferone. *Soft Mater.* **2013**, *11*, 75–84. [CrossRef]
158. Argimón, M.; Romero, M.; Miranda, P.; Mombrú, Á.W.; Miraballes, I.; Zimet, P.; Pardo, H. Development and Characterization of Vitamin A-Loaded Solid Lipid Nanoparticles for Topical Application. *J. Braz. Chem. Soc.* **2017**, *28*, 1177–1184. [CrossRef]
159. Santonocito, D.; Raciti, G.; Campisi, A.; Sposito, G.; Panico, A.; Siciliano, E.A.; Sarpietro, M.G.; Damiani, E.; Puglia, C. Astaxanthin-Loaded Stealth Lipid Nanoparticles (AST-SSLN) as Potential Carriers for the Treatment of Alzheimer's Disease: Formulation Development and Optimization. *Nanomaterials* **2021**, *11*, 391. [CrossRef]
160. Ledinski, M.; Marić, I.; Peharec Štefanić, P.; Ladan, I.; Caput Mihalić, K.; Jurkin, T.; Gotić, M.; Urlić, I. Synthesis and In Vitro Characterization of Ascorbyl Palmitate-Loaded Solid Lipid Nanoparticles. *Polymers* **2022**, *14*, 1751. [CrossRef]
161. Karthikeyan, A.; Senthil, N.; Min, T. Nanocurcumin: A Promising Candidate for Therapeutic Applications. *Front. Pharmacol.* **2020**, *11*, 487. [CrossRef]
162. da Silva Santos, V.; Ribeiro, A.P.B.; Santana, M.H.A. Solid Lipid Nanoparticles as Carriers for Lipophilic Compounds for Applications in Foods. *Food Res. Int.* **2019**, *122*, 610–626. [CrossRef] [PubMed]
163. Ramesh, N.; Mandal, A.K.A. Pharmacokinetic, Toxicokinetic, and Bioavailability Studies of Epigallocatechin-3-Gallate Loaded Solid Lipid Nanoparticle in Rat Model. *Drug Dev. Ind. Pharm.* **2019**, *45*, 1506–1514. [CrossRef] [PubMed]
164. Subroto, E.; Andoyo, R.; Indiarto, R.; Lembong, E. Physicochemical Properties, Sensory Acceptability, and Antioxidant Activity of Chocolate Bar Fortified by Solid Lipid Nanoparticles of Gallic Acid. *Int. J. Food Prop.* **2022**, *25*, 1907–1919. [CrossRef]
165. Mostafa, E.S.; Maher, A.; Mostafa, D.A.; Gad, S.S.; Nawwar, M.A.M.; Swilam, N. A Unique Acylated Flavonol Glycoside from *Prunus persica* (L.) Var. Florida Prince: A New Solid Lipid Nanoparticle Cosmeceutical Formulation for Skincare. *Antioxidants* **2021**, *10*, 436. [CrossRef] [PubMed]
166. Güney, G.; Kutlu, H.M.; Genç, L. Preparation and Characterization of Ascorbic Acid Loaded Solid Lipid Nanoparticles and Investigation of Their Apoptotic Effects. *Colloids Surf. B Biointerfaces* **2014**, *121*, 270–280. [CrossRef] [PubMed]
167. Silva, S.; Veiga, M.; Costa, E.M.; Oliveira, A.L.S.; Madureira, A.R.; Pintado, M. Nanoencapsulation of Polyphenols towards Dairy Beverage Incorporation. *Beverages* **2018**, *4*, 61. [CrossRef]
168. Shtay, R.; Keppler, J.K.; Schrader, K.; Schwarz, K. Encapsulation of (—)-Epigallocatechin-3-Gallate (EGCG) in Solid Lipid Nanoparticles for Food Applications. *J. Food Eng.* **2019**, *244*, 91–100. [CrossRef]
169. Radhakrishnan, R.; Kulhari, H.; Pooja, D.; Gudem, S.; Bhargava, S.; Shukla, R.; Sistla, R. Encapsulation of Biophenolic Phytochemical EGCG within Lipid Nanoparticles Enhances Its Stability and Cytotoxicity against Cancer. *Chem. Phys. Lipids* **2016**, *198*, 51–60. [CrossRef]
170. Ahangarpour, A.; Oroojan, A.A.; Khorsandi, L.; Kouchak, M.; Badavi, M. Solid Lipid Nanoparticles of Myricitrin Have Antioxidant and Antidiabetic Effects on Streptozotocin-Nicotinamide-Induced Diabetic Model and Myotube Cell of Male Mouse. *Oxid. Med. Cell. Longev.* **2018**, *2018*, 7496936. [CrossRef]
171. Ahangarpour, A.; Oroojan, A.A.; Khorsandi, L.; Kouchak, M.; Badavi, M. Antioxidant, Anti-Apoptotic, and Protective Effects of Myricitrin and Its Solid Lipid Nanoparticles on Streptozotocin-Nicotinamideinduced Diabetic Nephropathy in Type 2 Diabetic Male Mice. *Iran. J. Basic Med. Sci.* **2019**, *22*, 1424–1431. [CrossRef]
172. Gokce, E.H.; Korkmaz, E.; Dellera, E.; Sandri, G.; Bonferoni, M.C.; Ozer, O. Resveratrol-Loaded Solid Lipid Nanoparticles versus Nanostructured Lipid Carriers: Evaluation of Antioxidant Potential for Dermal Applications. *Int. J. Nanomed.* **2012**, *7*, 1841–1850. [CrossRef] [PubMed]
173. Neves, A.R.; Lúcio, M.; Martins, S.; Lima, J.L.C.; Reis, S. Novel Resveratrol Nanodelivery Systems Based on Lipid Nanoparticles to Enhance Its Oral Bioavailability. *Int. J. Nanomed.* **2013**, *8*, 177–187. [CrossRef]
174. Li, H.; Zhao, X.; Ma, Y.; Zhai, G.; Li, L.; Lou, H. Enhancement of Gastrointestinal Absorption of Quercetin by Solid Lipid Nanoparticles. *J. Control. Release* **2009**, *133*, 238–244. [CrossRef]
175. Farboud, E.S.; Nasrollahi, S.A.; Tabbakhi, Z. Novel Formulation and Evaluation of a Q10-Loaded Solid Lipid Nanoparticle Cream: In Vitro and in Vivo Studies. *Int. J. Nanomed.* **2011**, *6*, 611–617. [CrossRef] [PubMed]
176. Gokce, E.H.; Korkmaz, E.; Tuncay-Tanriverdi, S.; Dellera, E.; Sandri, G.; Cristina Bonferoni, M.; Ozer, O. A Comparative Evaluation of Coenzyme Q10-Loaded Liposomes and Solid Lipid Nanoparticles as Dermal Antioxidant Carriers. *Int. J. Nanomed.* **2012**, *7*, 5109–5117. [CrossRef]
177. Xie, S.; Zhu, L.; Zhao, D.; Wang, Y.; Wang, X.; Zhou, W. Preparation and Evaluation of Ofloxacin-Loaded Palmitic Acid Solid Lipid Nanoparticles. *Int. J. Nanomed.* **2011**, *6*, 547–555. [CrossRef]
178. Li, J.; Guo, X.; Liu, Z.; Okeke, C.I.; Li, N.; Zhao, H.; Aggrey, M.O.; Pan, W.; Wu, T. Preparation and Evaluation of Charged Solid Lipid Nanoparticles of Tetrandrine for Ocular Drug Delivery System: Pharmacokinetics, Cytotoxicity and Cellular Uptake Studies. *Drug Dev. Ind. Pharm.* **2014**, *40*, 980–987. [CrossRef]

179. Ravanfar, R.; Tamaddon, A.M.; Niakousari, M.; Moein, M.R. Preservation of Anthocyanins in Solid Lipid Nanoparticles: Optimization of a Microemulsion Dilution Method Using the Placket-Burman and Box-Behnken Designs. *Food Chem.* **2016**, *199*, 573–580. [CrossRef]
180. Trapani, A.; Mandracchia, D.; Tripodo, G.; Di Gioia, S.; Castellani, S.; Cioffi, N.; Ditaranto, N.; Esteban, M.A.; Conese, M. Solid Lipid Nanoparticles Made of Self-Emulsifying Lipids for Efficient Encapsulation of Hydrophilic Substances. *AIP Conf. Proc.* **2019**, *2145*, 020004. [CrossRef]
181. Tungmunnithum, D.; Thongboonyou, A.; Pholboon, A.; Yangsabai, A. Flavonoids and Other Phenolic Compounds from Medicinal Plants for Pharmaceutical and Medical Aspects: An Overview. *Medicines* **2018**, *5*, 93. [CrossRef]
182. Muflihah, Y.M.; Gollavelli, G.; Ling, Y.-C. Correlation Study of Antioxidant Activity with Phenolic and Flavonoid Compounds in 12 Indonesian Indigenous Herbs. *Antioxidants* **2021**, *10*, 1530. [CrossRef] [PubMed]
183. Subroto, E. Monoacylglycerols and Diacylglycerols for Fat-Based Food Products: A Review. *Food Res.* **2020**, *4*, 932–943. [CrossRef] [PubMed]
184. Subroto, E.; Indiarto, R. Bioactive Monolaurin as an Antimicrobial and Its Potential to Improve the Immune System and against COVID-19: A Review. *Food Res.* **2020**, *4*, 2355–2365. [CrossRef] [PubMed]
185. Feltes, M.M.C.; de Oliveira, D.; Block, J.M.; Ninow, J.L. The Production, Benefits, and Applications of Monoacylglycerols and Diacylglycerols of Nutritional Interest. *Food Bioprocess Technol.* **2013**, *6*, 17–35. [CrossRef]
186. Qushawy, M.; Nasr, A. Solid Lipid Nanoparticles (SLNs) as Nano Drug Delivery Carriers: Preparation, Characterization and Application. *Int. J. Appl. Pharm.* **2020**, *12*, 1–9. [CrossRef]
187. Ud Din, F.; Zeb, A.; Shah, K.U. Zia-ur-Rehman Development, in-Vitro and in-Vivo Evaluation of Ezetimibe-Loaded Solid Lipid Nanoparticles and Their Comparison with Marketed Product. *J. Drug Deliv. Sci. Technol.* **2019**, *51*, 583–590. [CrossRef]

antioxidants

MDPI

Review

Applications of Antioxidants in Dental Procedures

Fan Qi, Haofei Huang, Ming Wang, Weifeng Rong and Jing Wang *

School of Chemistry and Chemical Engineering, Shandong University of Technology, 266 Xincun Road, Zibo 255000, China

* Correspondence: wjing@sdut.edu.cn

Abstract: As people are paying more and more attention to dental health, various dental treatment procedures have emerged, such as tooth bleaching, dental implants, and dental restorations. However, a large number of free radicals are typically produced during the dental procedures. When the imbalance in distribution of reactive oxygen species (ROS) is induced, oxidative stress coupled with oxidative damage occurs. Oral inflammations such as those in periodontitis and pulpitis are also unavoidable. Therefore, the applications of exogenous antioxidants in oral environment have been proposed. In this article, the origin of ROS during dental procedures, the types of antioxidants, and their working mechanisms are reviewed. Additionally, antioxidants delivery in the complicated dental procedures and their feasibility for clinical applications are also covered. Finally, the importance of safety assessment of these materials and future work to take the challenge in antioxidants development are proposed for perspective.

Keywords: antioxidants; antioxidant delivery; dental procedures; tooth bleaching; dental implants; dental restorations

1. Introduction

Since the 20th century, the prevention and treatment of oral diseases have made great progress, and the occurrence of dental caries and oral inflammation have also dropped significantly [1]. It is reported that many oral problems are related to an imbalance of antioxidants and reactive oxygen species (ROS) in the body. In recent years, free radicals have been found to be related to the occurrence and development of dental diseases, and antioxidants have also been used in dental treatment [2].

Free radicals and ROS are the products of oxidative stress and have extremely oxidative properties. The main sources of free radicals in the oral environment are considered as the following: food (high fat, high calorie), alcohol and cigarettes, dental treatment (surgery, laser, ultraviolet, etc.), dental materials (adhesive, composite resin, etc.), and periodontal diseases [3]. The antioxidant capacity in the oral environment of each person is different. Oxidative stress occurs when the body's oxidative and antioxidant capacity is imbalanced and favors oxidation, which is also the main cause of oral and dental diseases. When reacting with antioxidants, free radicals will gain an electron and are converted into normal molecules [4], thereby reducing damage to the body.

Antioxidants prevent free radicals from requesting electrons from normal cells, and actively donate electrons to free radicals, thereby achieving the purpose of protecting normal cells. Antioxidants can also inactivate free radicals before they attack the body's cells, and they play a supporting role in the treatment of oral problems such as periodontitis [5]. In addition, some researchers found that the intake of antioxidants can effectively inhibit the growth and reproduction of oral cancer cells [6,7]. Antioxidants are typically divided into two types: endogenous and exogenous. Endogenous means that they can be produced by the human body, including superoxide dismutase (SOD), catalase (CAT), and reduced glutathione (GSH). Exogenous means that the human body cannot synthesize them. Commonly used exogeneous antioxidants are ascorbic acid (vitamin C), tocopherol (vitamin E), quercetin, tannic acid, and N-acetyl cysteine (NAC). The mechanisms of action and delivery form of some exogenous antioxidants are shown in Table 1. A variety of delivery methods, such as encapsulation and sol–gel technology, have emerged [8–10]. During the transition process, the antioxidant might decompose due to its instability, leading to a decreased effectiveness. Although an appropriate amount of ROS has a bactericidal effect, a large number of decomposed antioxidants can adversely affect the treatment of diseases [11]. From this point, the biocompatibilities of current antioxidants also need to be addressed.

Table 1. Mechanism of action and delivery of some exogenous antioxidants.

Antioxidants	Mechanism of Action	Selected Delivery Form	Ref.
Vitamin C	$C_6H_8O_6 + \bullet OH \rightarrow C_6H_6O_6 + H_2O$	Gel assembled from nanoparticles.	[12,13]
Vitamin E	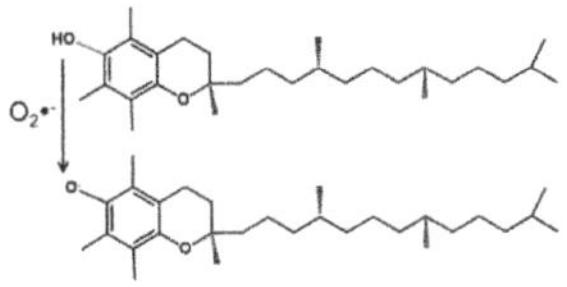	Responsive intelligent hydrogel.	[14,15]
Quercetin	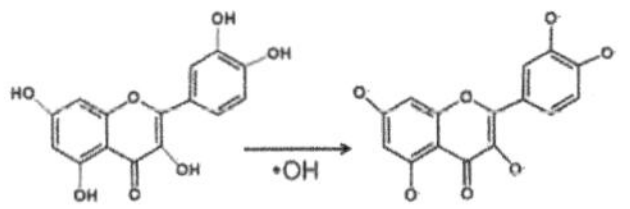	Quercetin-loaded nanoemulsion (QNE), polymeric nanoparticles, liposomes.	[16,17]
Oligomeric proanthocyanin complexes (OPCs)	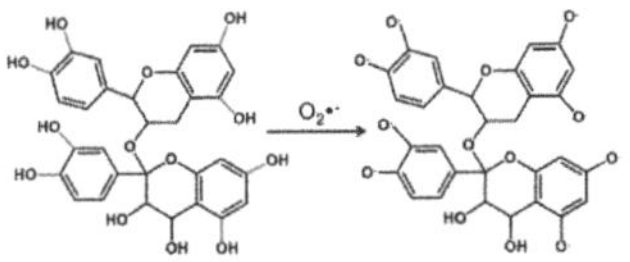	Solid, self-double emulsified drug delivery system (SDEDDS).	[18,19]

This review focuses on the involvement of antioxidants in dental procedures, such as dental bleaching, implants, and dental fillings. Types of antioxidants used to treat oxidative stress induced by dental treatments and restorations are covered, and the mechanism of action and delivery of antioxidants are also discussed. From the developmental perspective, the advantages and disadvantages of current antioxidants are evaluated, and future challenges are also proposed.

2. Reactive Oxygen Species (ROS) and Oxidative Damage

2.1. ROS in Oral Environment

ROS refers to an extremely powerful oxidant that includes free radicals and nonradical molecules [20]. In general, free radicals must be ROS, but ROS are not necessarily free radicals [21]. The atomic orbitals of free radicals contain unpaired electrons, which are very unstable and highly reactive.

ROS of physiological concentrations have positive effects [22]. In the medical field, the active oxygen produced by photolysis, photocatalysis, and photodynamic therapy is targeted for cancer therapy. In the dental field, an appropriate amount of ROS is used for the treatment of periodontal diseases and antibacterial photodynamic therapy of root canal disinfection. The hydrogen peroxide in tea and coffee is an example, which has a preservative effect [23]. In addition, an appropriate amount of ROS is also used as a dental bactericide for dental fillings [24]. Moderate amounts of free radicals are usually involved in immune responses and metabolism in certain parts of the body [25].

However, when stimulated, excess ROS may cause oxidative stress and, thus, disease. The most damaging radicals in the body include hydroxyl radicals, superoxide anion radicals, hydrogen peroxide, oxygen singlet, hypochlorite, nitric oxide free radicals, and peroxynitrite free radicals [4]. For an ROS, under aerobic conditions, a part of oxygen is converted into superoxide anion radicals and hydroxyl radicals through electron transfer;

another part of oxygen is converted into hydrogen peroxide through electron reduction and accepts a proton. These highly reactive free radicals mainly damage deoxyribonucleic acid (DNA), proteins, carbohydrates, and lipids in the nucleus and cell membranes [26].

Sources of free radicals in oral environments include normal metabolic processes in the body and some external sources, including X-rays, ozone, smoking, and dental treatments. Oral inflammation is the main source of inflammatory response and the increase of ROS in oral tissues, gums, and saliva [25]. ROS are produced by phagocytic cells, such as mitochondria, to fight microbial invasion. In this process, a large amount of bactericidal superoxide anions can be produced, and the process of superoxide anion elimination produces hydrogen peroxide [20]. While causing local damage to the oral cavity, the free-radical-rich gingival fluid mixed with saliva stimulates the production of ROS in other oral tissues [27]. Oxidative stress in the oral cavity is mainly related to infection and inflammation of the gums and other soft tissues, but other factors may also lead to oxidative stress. The sources of ROS are also relatively wide, mainly including food, cigarettes, alcohol, dental materials, and drugs [3]. When drinking alcohol, the amount of ethanol, acetaldehyde, and ROS in the oral environment will increase rapidly, and after a period of time, acetaldehyde and ROS will remain at high concentrations [28]. Surprisingly, free radicals are produced at every stage of alcohol metabolism, including alcohol dehydrogenase and mitochondrial enzymes, which oxidize to superoxide anion radicals and hydroxyl radicals, respectively [29]. Whether it a chronic alcohol intake or one dose, it will affect the homeostasis of the oral cavity, reduce the activity of enzymes, and cause an increase in ROS [30,31]. There are thousands of toxic substances and hundreds of pro-oxidants in cigarette smoke [32]. According to the research, burning of a cigarette produces tar and smoke, 35 milliliters of cigarette smoke contains 10^{15} free radicals, and 1 g of tar has 10^{17} [33]. These free radicals may further promote the production of oxidants in saliva, change its proteins, and reduce the activity of antioxidant enzymes [34]. In addition, it has been reported that high-fat, high-calorie-fed rats have increased ROS production and reduced antioxidant barriers in the oral cavity [35]. The main source of ROS in the oral environment is periodontitis. At the same time, the oral cavity is also exposed to ROS produced by various dental materials, and some dental procedures, such as bleaching, implants, fillings, crowns, veneers, orthodontics, and tooth extractions, may also produce ROS (Figure 1).

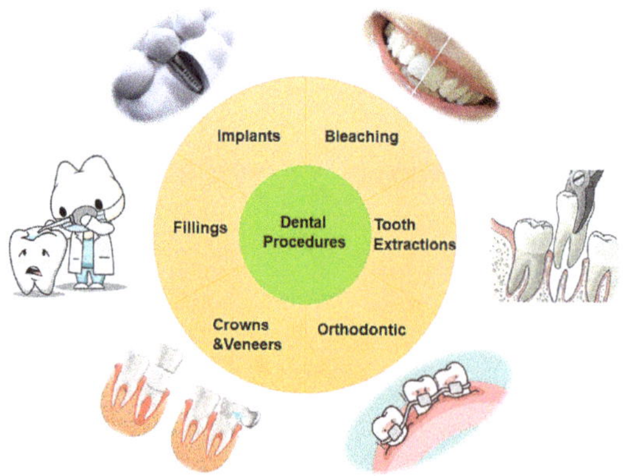

Figure 1. Sources of ROS production in dental procedures.

As people are paying more attention to dental health, various dental treatment procedures are becoming popular, which also means that the sources of ROS are more extensive than expected.

2.2. Oxidative Stress and Oxidative Damage

Oxidative stress, the phenomenon of excess oxidants, is caused by an imbalance in the production of free radicals in the antioxidant system [36]. Theoretically, oxidative stress can be divided into basal, low-intensity, medium-intensity, and high-intensity oxidative stress according to the content of oxidants [21]. Short-term oxidative stress may occur in tissue loss such as trauma, infection, and heat damage. These damaged tissues produce increased activity of phagocytic free-radical-generating enzymes, release free metal ions, destroy epoxidation phosphorylated electron transport chain, and produce excessive ROS [4]. It has already been proven that oxidative damage of cellular components such as proteins, lipids, and nucleic acids may occur when ROS production increases or antioxidant capacity decreases [37]. Oxidative stress corresponds to many diseases, including cardiovascular disease, cancer, and various kinds of inflammation. Oxidation of the lipid component of low-density lipoproteins is an important factor in atherosclerosis [38]. At the same time, a large number of free radicals react with DNA, such as strand breaking base modification and DNA protein cross-linking, and induce DNA damage, resulting in cell mutation and cancer.

In the course of dental procedures, oxidative stress and oxidative damage also occur. It has been shown that periodontal inflammation is a direct result of increased ROS and oxidative damage products in the oral cavity [25]. Except for the factors of alcohol consumption and nicotine exposure, dental procedures such as implants, bleaching, and fillings also lead to oxidative damages (Figure 2). When exogenous coupled with endogenous antioxidants are utilized, free radicals are scavenged to reduce the oxidative damage. Periodontitis is a chronic inflammation of periodontal tissue, which can lead to the loss of alveolar bone or even tooth loss when it is serious, and oxidative stress is a part of the pathogenesis of periodontal disease [39,40]. The usual treatment is to scrape the tissues related to root gouging, which can successfully treat most periodontal diseases [41].

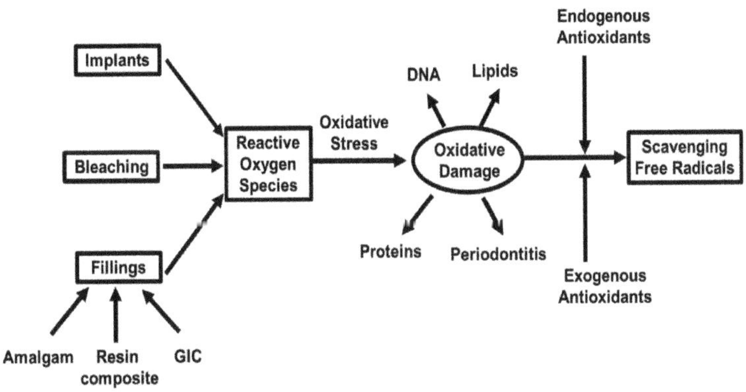

Figure 2. Schematic diagram of ROS production and clearance during dental procedures.

As for the oxidative stress phenomenon generated in dental procedures, antioxidants might be added to eliminate free radicals. Antioxidants are used to combat oxidative stress. Working mechanisms of antioxidants mainly include two types: one is the chain-breaking mechanism, that works through antioxidants to provide electrons to free radicals, so that free radicals become stable molecular structures without damage to normal cells; the other is to remove ROS or reactive nitrogen species (secondary antioxidants) by quenching chain-initiating catalyst [4]. Therefore, appropriate antioxidants must be chosen according to the species of free radicals. Among them, naturally extracted antioxidants are more popular.

3. Antioxidants Used in Dental Procedures

3.1. Tooth Bleaching

Tooth colors and structures might be affected by foreign pigments or drugs such as tobacco, tea, coffee, and so on. With the pursuit of aesthetics, tooth bleaching technology has attracted more and more attention. Tooth bleaching is the use of chemical principles, through the method of oxidative replacement by using oxidants, to replace the pigment in the tooth surface in order to achieve the purpose of tooth whitening. At present, the commonly used tooth bleaching agents are hydrogen peroxide and carbamide peroxide. In addition to a variety of bleaching substances, light sources such as allografts, lasers, light emitting diodes (LEDs), and ultraviolet lights can also be used to enhance bleaching [42].

Bleaching works by releasing ROS. The active ingredients of bleaching agents are 10–40% hydrogen peroxide or 10–22% carbamide peroxide [43], which whiten the tooth by using chemicals to oxidize organic pigments within the tooth structure. In the presence of metal ions such as iron ions, hydrogen peroxide can generate oxygen-derived free radicals, hydroxyl radicals, which have strong oxidation capacities [44]. In the process of tooth bleaching with hydrogen peroxide, hydroxyl radical plays the oxidative role. Hydroxyl radical does not affect the inorganic tissue of dentin, but does attack the organic components of dentin, thus achieving the purpose of whitening teeth [45]. As for carbamide peroxide, it is first decomposed into hydrogen peroxide in the mouth, and the bleaching mechanism is the same as described above. The heat generated by light sources is helpful to further activate the bleaching agents, and better bleaching effect is able to be obtained by better penetration of hydrogen peroxide into the tooth structure. However, deeper penetration of hydrogen peroxide may not only infiltrate the enamel and dentin, but also reach the dental pulp, which may lead to irreversible damage to tooth structures and pulp cells [46]. Soares et al. [47] demonstrated that pulp cells exposed to a certain concentration of bleaching gel were in a state of oxidative stress, the intensity of which was proportional to the contact time between the bleaching gel and enamel. Additionally, dental bleaching may cause tooth sensitivity and periodontal discomfort [48], and periodontal tissue damage may further cause root absorption, resulting in trauma or developmental defects in the cementum layer of the tooth neck [49]. If a nonvital tooth has been developed without response to electric pulp test, its discoloration can be managed by an internal bleaching. A clinical case report by Anugrahati et al. [50] demonstrated that the internal bleaching on a nonvital tooth was the best option to restore the function and aesthetics of the original tooth. At the same time, the hydroxyl radical is one type of oxygen-derived free radical and is considered to be extremely oxidizing, which can destroy connective tissue components, collagen, hyaluronic acid, etc. [51,52]. If hemoglobin is exposed to hydrogen peroxide, the iron in the hemoglobin molecule reacts with hydrogen peroxide, which produces hydroxyl radical (an oxygen-derived free radical), thereby destroying healthy hemoglobin [53]. Hydroxyl radicals are also able to alter DNA by strand breaks and damage cell membranes by lipid peroxidation [54]. When composite bonding is performed immediately after tooth bleaching, the bonding strength might be negatively affected [55]. The residue of peroxide in the bleaching procedure inhibits the polymerization and curing of adhesive resin materials [56]. The enamel pores and dentin can store peroxides, leading to a greatly increased concentration of peroxides on the enamel surface, which further prevents the complete curing of some resin materials and finally affects the effect of adhesive repair [57].

During tooth bleaching, oxidative stress occurs in the mouth due to the residual oxide caused by bleaching agents, causing damage to the human body, and also affecting the bonding to teeth after bleaching. The proper use of sealer base is the most direct approach to protect the periodontal area and limit the penetration to dental pulp. Even if sealer base has been applied, there are still risks that bleaching agents induce negative changes in tooth surfaces, such as reduction of microhardness, mineral loss, and surface roughness, where the residue oxygen radicals and peroxides after bleaching are considered as the main reason [58,59]. Antioxidants in saliva cannot remove these residual reactive oxygen species in a short time, and more than two weeks are needed to eliminate the effect [60]. Therefore, the use of antioxidants in the bleaching process is very important to neutralize the residual oxidants in the oral environment. Ascorbic acid is one of the most commonly used antioxidants, and cannot be synthesized by humans. Ascorbic acid mainly achieves the purpose of antioxidation by loosing two electrons and two protons to form L-dehydroascorbic acid [12]. Applying 10% ascorbic acid to the tooth surface after tooth bleaching is helpful to counteract the adverse effects of the adhesive bonding to the enamel [61], and ascorbic acid may also play the roles of polymerization promoter and co-initiator to have a positive effect on the adhesion of the composite resin to the tooth [62]. Garcia et al. [63] provided a one-year follow-up case report to further prove that immediate bonding after bleaching is trustable in dental clinics by using sodium ascorbate gel to avoid waiting time. However, a clinical trial by De Paula et al. [64] indicated that oral administration of ascorbic acid (500 mg, three times daily) was not a feasible approach to prevent bleaching-induced tooth sensitivity or reduce its intensity. Louzada et al. [65] investigated the anti-inflammatory potential of carvedilol gel in the pulp of rats after bleaching, where Carvedilol played the role of antioxidants. This histopathological study proved the effectiveness of Carvedilol in minimizing the damage of hydrogen peroxide, especially in deep resins of the dental pulp. Gupta et al. [66] assessed the antioxidant property of 10% amla extract on bond strength and color stability of power-bleached teeth, but, unfortunately, negative results were obtained. Vidhya et al. [18] reported another natural antioxidant of grape seed extract (oligomeric proanthocyanin complexes (OPCs)) which had neutralization effect on excessive free radicals of bleached tooth, and the effect was superior to ascorbic acid.The 5% OPCs and 10% ascorbic acid solutions had the ability to remove free radicals, and the effectiveness was 50 times that of 10% ascorbic acid [67]. As a natural plant metabolite, it has been proven safe in various clinical applications and dietary supplements as an antioxidant [68]. To improve the bioavailability of OPCs, Tian et al. [19] proposed a solid self-double-emulsified drug delivery system (SDEDDS) to deliver antioxidants. The double emulsification system is mainly composed of water-in-oil emulsion and hydrophilic surfactant, which can protect it from degradation and make it better absorbed by the small intestine [19,69].

3.2. Dental Implants

Periodontal disease leads to changes in the periodontal tissue, which in turn leads to the destruction of the alveolar bone. If it is not treated in time, tooth loss might be the consequence. Dental implantations are currently an effective method for the treatment of tooth loss [70]. Biomaterials used to make dental implants include metals, ceramics, carbons, polymers, and composites. Polymer materials are rarely used in implant dentistry and were only used to manufacture shock-absorbing assemblies placed between the implant and the superstructure [71]. As early as 1957, a Swedish surgeon studied bone healing and regeneration, and found that bone could grow together with titanium (Ti), and it could effectively be adhered to teeth without repulsion [72]. This also laid a foundation for the development of titanium dental implants. Since 1992, with the development of modern ceramics, ceramic surface treatments and ceramic-like elements have been incorporated into implants to further enhance osseointegration [73]. The titanium dental implants have attracted the most interest.

The process of dental implant implantation inevitably generates ROS. On one side, ROS are required for cell signaling and normal metabolism. On the other hand, excessive oxidative stress may lead to damage on DNA, ribonucleic acid (RNA), and proteins [74]. Tsarik et al. [75] reported that the oxide layer generated on the surface of titanium alloy implant may reduce the corrosion potential of the metal, while friction would lead to the rupture and corrosion of the titanium dioxide layer. From this point, the electrochemical reaction would occur. A large number of titanium ions were generated at the anode, and free radicals and hydrogen peroxide were generated as intermediate products. When titanium dioxide is corroded, hydrogen peroxide generated by electrochemical reaction will continue to react with titanium dioxide to form hydroxyl radicals [76]. Bressan et al. [77]

analyzed the effects of titanium (Ti) particles on mesenchymal stem cells (MSCs) and fibroblasts (FU), and the 3-[4,5-dimethylthiazol-2-yl]-2,5 diphenyl tetrazolium bromide (MTT) test was used to evaluate cell proliferation and generation of ROS. It was found that titanium particles reduced the cell survival time and increased the generation of ROS. Accompanied by oxidative stress, bone regeneration imbalance was induced. The process of implant placement may lead Ti particles to enter the tissue and cause inflammation. Therefore, tetracycline, doxycycline, chlorhexidine, hydrogen peroxide, and citric acid can be used to remove excess Ti particles, among which hydrogen peroxide, citric acid, and chlorhexidine are more effective [78]. In addition, Abdulhameed et al. [79] reported that titanium dioxide nanoparticles (TiO_2NPs) can induce oxidative stress, reduce osteogenesis, and damage the antioxidant defense system. After placement of a dental implant, friction and twisting can destroy the oxide layer on the surface, leading to an increase of ROS and an inflammatory, such as peri-implant (PI), infection may occur (Figure 3) [70,80]. Antioxidants such as ascorbic acid, polyphenols, and vitamin E are choices for treatment. PI and periodontal disease are manifested by soft tissue and bone damage, in which ROS play an important role in cell transmission, maintenance, and proliferation [81]. Dental implant materials are usually made of titanium or titanium alloys, and when exposed to oxygen, a layer of titanium oxide forms on the tooth surface to protect it [82]. In homeostatic conditions, ROS are involved in cellular maintenance, signal transduction, and repair of all tissues. However, if excessive ROS are accumulated, it can lead to oxidative stress, resulting in cellular damage and tissue destruction. Similarly, antioxidants protect immune cells by converting free radicals into waste products affected by the destructive effects of ROS.

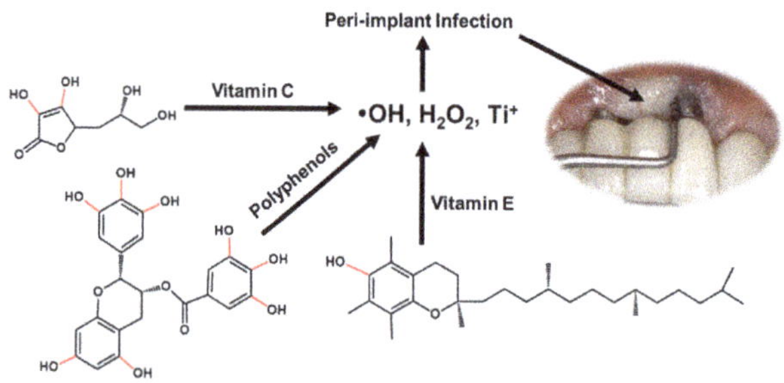

Figure 3. Antioxidants for the treatment of periodontitis during dental implants.

Typically, a certain amount of ROS is already present before the implant is implanted [83]. Antioxidants have a protective effect on periodontal tissue and can neutralize ROS to prevent tissue damage [84]. At present, antioxidants in the treatment of local inflammatory reactions, such as periodontitis, usually quickly disappear with reactive oxygen species and other free radicals. The lower treatment effect might correspond to the antioxidants delivery. When the inflammation is serious, there are redness, swelling, bleeding, wound split, and other conditions. Most of these antioxidants can be obtained from diets and supplements, and supplements can be taken in addition to the diets mentioned above [2]. Tannic acids are macromolecules consisting of a central glucose molecule linked to 10 surrounding gallic acid units [85]. Thus, tannic acids have a large number of functional groups but are still water-soluble and hydrolysable [86,87]. Huang et al. [88] modified the Ti implant surface with Ag nanoparticles incorporating tannic acid/nanoapatite composite coatings, and their antibacterial and antioxidative properties were highlighted. The slow release of tannic acid in this study is favorable to the persistent antioxidative activity of the dental implant. Maruyama et al. [89] investigated the effects of dentifrice containing green tea catechins using a rat model, and up to 8 weeks of follow-up proved the efficacy of green tea catechins to prevent periodontal inflammation by decreasing gingival oxidative stress. Quercetin is a natural flavonoid [9], and is an antioxidant that has both anti-inflammatory and antioxidant properties [90,91]. Catauro et al. [92] entrapped quercetin in a silica/poly(εcaprolactone)-based hybrid material by a sol–gel route to use as novel dental implant, and the hydrogen-bonded reactions between quercetin, silica, and polymer matrices were considered as the key to produce antiradical efficacy. Polyphenols are natural compounds with antioxidant and antimicrobial properties and aromatic benzene rings containing multiple hydroxyl groups [93,94]. The antioxidant activity of polyphenols scavenges free radicals by supplying hydrogen atoms from hydroxyl groups in the phenolic ring [94]. Additionally, polyphenols exert their antioxidant function through their ability to chelate iron and other metal ions, thereby preventing the catalytic oxidation of hydrogen peroxide and superoxide to hydroxyl radicals [95,96]. Polyphenolic compound curcumin can also lead to an increase in the level of the antioxidant enzyme glutathione peroxidase, which reduces the ROS level in cells [97]. Vitamin E is a common antioxidant with the highest concentration in human mitochondria. The main mechanism of action of vitamin E is to interact with superoxide in mitochondria, limit its formation, stabilize mitochondrial membrane, and remove antioxidants that have been generated [98]. Vitamin E could be added to implant formulas for antioxidative purposes, and a clinical study [99] indicated that adding low concentrations of vitamin E (less than 0.1%) did not affect the physical and mechanical properties and can prevent oxidation for up to 24 months post-implantation.

At present, antioxidants in the treatment of local inflammatory reactions, such as periodontitis, usually quickly disappear with ROS and other free radicals. The lower treatment effect might correspond to the antioxidants delivery. Ozawa et al. [100] reported a new material in which hydrogels containing nitrogen oxide radicals were injected into experimental rat models with PI and in vitro osteoblasts. These hydrogels can reduce the presence of ROS, inhibit hydrogen peroxide and lipid peroxidation, and can increase the retention time of antioxidants during treatment. After injection, the gel was assembled by nanoassembly, and the micelles containing nitroxide radicals were partially decomposed [13]. These redox nanoparticles usually remove extracellular ROS without affecting the normal cellular reactions. Therefore, the delivery of antioxidants by gel encapsulation is worth studying for the treatment of oxidative stress conditions such as periodontal diseases caused by dental implants.

3.3. *Dental Restorations*

Dental filling materials have been widely used as a means of dental restoration in recent years, mainly aimed at repairing teeth damaged by dental caries or trauma. There are three main types of filling materials, which are amalgam, dental resin composites, and glass ionomer cement (GIC) [101].

3.3.1. Dental Amalgam

Dental amalgam is one of the most widely used restorative materials in dentistry. Despite the continuous progress in the development of dental fillings, amalgam is still widely used due to its durability, low price, easy use, and other advantages [102]. However, there are still many disputes about the use of amalgam: the continuous release of mercury vapor in dental amalgam, the possible formation of organic mercury in the mouth, the impact of mercury exposure on human cell gene regulation, and the relationship between amalgam and Alzheimer's disease, Parkinson's disease, and other diseases [103]. The alloys currently used are 40 to 70% silver, 12 to 30% tin, and 12 to 24% copper. It may also include 0–4% indium, 0.5% palladium, and more than 1% zinc. Zinc prevents the oxidation of other metals in the alloy during manufacturing. The powder alloy is mixed with liquid mercury, then soft amalgam putty is poured into the alveolar bone to cure. Cured amalgam fillings are cheaper, stronger, and last longer than other types [103].

Mercury penetrates into the brain through the oral area and accumulates in the brain, thereby affecting the central nervous system [103]. Mercury in amalgams is responsible for the redox imbalance in the system. Mercury in amalgams usually exists in various oxidation states (Hg^{+} and Hg^{2+}) and is prone to react with cysteine and glutathione to form sulfide, which is methylated by bacteria to form highly toxic methylmercury (MeHg) or dimethyl mercury (Me_2Hg) and organic compounds [104]. The catalytic oxidation of mercury has also been the focus of attention. Similar to other metal ions, mercury interacts with most sulfhydryl (-SH) groups and produces living ROS, such as superoxide anion, hydrogen peroxide, and hydroxyl radical, thus inducing oxidative damage in tissues. Pizzichini et al. [105] conducted a clinical study towards the release of mercury from dental amalgam, and they found a significant negative correlation between total antioxidant activity (TAA) and mercury levels in females but not males. Another clinical study, by Lindh et al. [106], suggested that the metal exposure from dental amalgam did cause ill health, and the removal of dental amalgam coupled with antioxidant therapy were supportive to improve the quality of life in patients.

Amalgam restorative systems currently in use typically include encapsulated and predosed presentations, which are applied with isolation of the tooth by means of a rubber dam both for insertion and removal. Couple with the high-powered suction during operation, the possible toxic effect of amalgam is actually very limited. As for the potential mercury release and induced oxidative stress, an appropriate application of antioxidants is necessary. Cysteine, homocysteine, and GSH play the role of antioxidants in the body, and GSH maintains the oxidative balance of cells by quenching free radicals. As an important defense against oxidative stress, GSH increases the antioxidant capacity of mitochondria and protects mitochondria by resisting lipid peroxides produced by hydrogen peroxide, hydroxyl radicals, and mercury [107]. Due to the poor selectivity of GSH, it may not only remove toxic ions, but also eliminate the ions necessary for the human body.

Antioxidants such as vitamin C, vitamin B complex, vitamin E, and niacin are usually taken to supplement the treatment [106]. Fisk et al. [108] investigated the correlation of dental amalgam restorations supported by antioxidant therapy (vitamin B complex, vitamin C, vitamin E, and sodium selenite), and the systemic route was proved to be effective. Vitamin C as an antioxidant is discussed here. The antioxidant effect of vitamin C is manifested in the rapid reaction with O_2^-, HOO·, and OH to produce semi-dehydroascorbic acid, and can also restore the prototype of oxidized vitamin E [109] (Figure 4). Because a large amount of vitamin C may cause damage to the stomach and intestines, excess vitamin C is excreted with body fluids. Vitamin C has the advantages of antioxidation and antiaging, but the sustainability of vitamin C in light, oxygen, and heat is very low. In order to extend the shelf life of vitamin C, encapsulation technology is used to wrap it. Common packaging materials include liposomes, nanoparticles, and microcapsules [110]. Additionally, according to Gallusi et al. [111], dental amalgam was not as toxic as expected, and human clinical studies have shown no increased risk for systemic diseases or conditions compared with composite restorations. Therefore, a systemic route is applicable for the delivery of antioxidants.

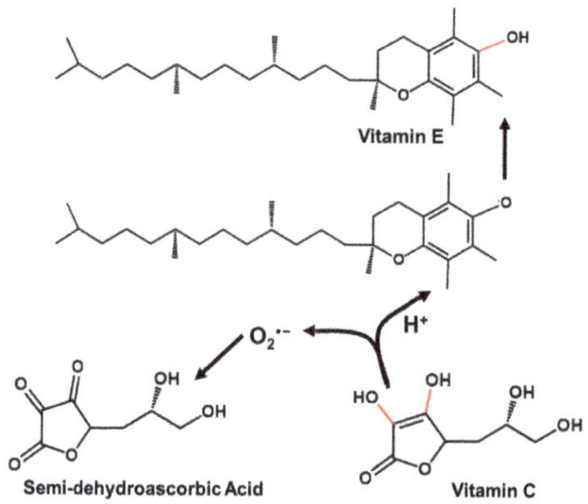

Figure 4. Antioxidative mechanism of vitamin C.

In practical clinical applications, the uses of dental amalgams are controversial at present. The Norwegian Ministry of Environment banned the use of amalgam on January 2008, but the Scientific Committee of European Commission did not follow this ban because all available direct restorative materials have drawbacks and potential biological side effects. Alkhudhairy [112] investigated the attitudes of dental practitioners working in Riyadh, Saudi Arabia, towards the use of dental amalgam, and the results were strongly gender-dependent. Male participants did not oppose the use of amalgam in their clinical practices, and did not consider it an occupational risk factor. However, female participants held significantly different options to those of males. Joshi et al. [113] limited their studies to males, and investigated the mercury level difference between dentists and nondental health professionals. No relationship was found between these two groups, and consumption of saltwater fish was considered as the primary exposure factor. A clinical report by Broadbent et al. [114] demonstrated that the decreased use of dental amalgam has been a global trend despite having no official policy. The tooth-colored direct restorations, particularly composites, have become the most frequently used filling materials in dental clinics.

3.3.2. Dental Resin Composites

In the last century, composite resin was introduced into dental repair as a filling material, such as for caries, and tooth structure damaged by erosion or fracture [115]. Resin composites are also widely used because of their good compressive strength and aesthetic properties. Dental resin composites are usually composed of two parts, a small part of polymerizable free radicals and a large part of inorganic fillers, which mainly include quartz, ceramics, and silica [116]. Commonly used monomers are 2-hydroxyethyl methacrylate (HEMA), bisphenol A-glycidyl methacrylate (Bis-GMA), and co-monomer triethylene glycol dimethacrylate (TEGDMA) [117]. These fillers and monomers are mixed in a certain proportion, and a certain initiator is added. After heat or light irradiation, they can be solidified. Finally, after grinding and polishing, the tooth repair is completed. However, the composite resin has potential toxicity in the process of polymerization and release, and some added compounds, such as monomers and initiators, may produce a certain amount of free radicals, and even lead to oxidative stress [118].

The polymerization process of composite resin is typically incomplete. The monomer HEMA released from the resin restorations may interact with living tissues in the oral environment, producing cytotoxicity, and the immune cell response and the function of odontoblast cells may be affected (Figure 5). It was also reported that apoptosis of odontoblast-like cells, undifferentiated pulp cells, or macrophages in mice repaired with composite resins depended on the degree of adhesion resin polymerization [119,120]. In addition, a low degree of conversion causes the unpolymerized monomers to be released into the oral environment, which may reduce the mechanical properties of the composite and accelerate the degradation. The generation of free radicals and ROS when applying dental composite materials is mainly related to the induction of monomers in the composite materials [119]. Methacrylate in dental resin may lead to the consumption of GSH, but NAC generated by GSH may alleviate this situation. Schweikl et al. [119] demonstrated that resin monomer damages mitochondria, consumes the antioxidant glutathione in cells, reduces its free radical scavenging ability, increases the production of ROS, and accelerates oxidative damage. Among them, epoxy resins and acrylic monomers are listed as important occupational sensitizers and have the potential of cross-reaction [119]. By 2021, the European Food Safety Authority (EFSA) had reduced the tolerable daily intake of bisphenol A to 0.04 ng/kg. If the amount of exposure is too high, it may lead to tooth sensitivity in clinic and even affect the health of the body [121]. When concentrations reach a certain amount, the composition of the composite may alter cytokine secretion in human monocytes. Recent studies also found that camphorquinone (CQ), as an initiator of composite resins, is also considered to be a compound that produces ROS. In addition, the use of ultraviolet curing in composite resin restoration is also an aspect in the production of ROS.

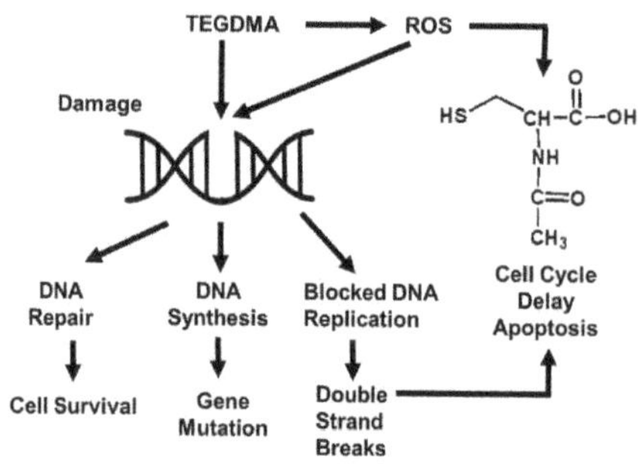

Figure 5. Damage to cell function by monomer HEMA released by resin restorations.

Antioxidants have been considered when using dental resin composites. It has been proven that antioxidant-added binders produce less ROS and are correspondingly less toxic [122]. Antioxidant polymers with molecules of natural antioxidants (e.g., quercetin and curcumin) have also been synthesized for attenuating material-induced oxidative stress [123]. GSH and NAC are antioxidants responsible for the reduction of DNA damage caused by CQ oxidation at relatively higher concentrations. The addition of NAC in resin-based materials favors the formulation of a new material in which the intrinsic cytotoxicity of the resin was potentially detoxified [124]. Flavonoids are powerful antioxidants that can scavenge free radicals in the body and have antibacterial and disinfectant properties.

Vitamin E is a common antioxidant, with the highest concentration in human mitochondria. Vitamin E also has the function that other antioxidants do not have, namely, regulating the activity of related enzymes. It can inhibit the activity of protein kinase C and inhibit the production of monocytes [125]. The absorption of vitamin E is mainly in the small intestine. Since direct oral administration may destroy the strong acid in the stomach and lose its activity, a functional ingredient delivery system is needed to retain its activity and improve stability [14]. Zhang et al. [15] mentioned a new oral delivery-responsive intelligent hydrogel in their research a few years ago. It forms a spatial network structure through macromolecules and can change its performance through environmental conditions or interface reactions [126]. Carboxymethyl starch is used as the carrier material, and the carboxyl group on the starch macromolecule is related to the hydration, swelling, and solubilization of the delivery carrier [14]. Another material of the hydrogel is xanthan gum, which is acid-resistant and antienzymatic. Research has shown that xanthan gum is helpful to delay the release, making vitamin E stay longer [127]. The microcapsules containing vitamin E were prepared by spray-drying the mixture of carboxymethyl starch and xanthan gum, and are able to reach the upper part of the small intestine and improve the bioavailability and efficiency of vitamin E [14].

3.3.3. Glass-Ionomer Cement (GIC)

GIC is a dental translucent cement, which is the product of the reaction of ion-leachable glass and polyacrylic acid aqueous solution [128]. In terms of performance, although it is not as perfect as resin composite material, it has a wider clinical application because it can control the performance according to changing the ratio [129]. The advantages of GIC are strong adhesion with teeth, low risk of tooth corrosion, and more realistic and beautiful color [130]. GICs are widely used in artificial crowns, orthodontic brackets, and cavity liner [131]. In order to further improve the mechanical strength, resin-modified GIC (RMGIC) was developed, and can be photocured by adding monomers [132]. The monomers used here are typically bis-GMA and HEMA [133]. The monomers added in RMGICs are the main source of free radicals, which may cause certain oxidative damages. When resin components, such as monomers and initiators, are added to the traditional GIC formula, the residual HEMA monomer easily spreads through the dentin tubules to the pulp cells, stimulating the production of free radicals. Meanwhile, the antibacterial substance fluoride added to the GIC will also bring certain cytotoxicity, which may cause pulp damage [134]. The clinical manifestations are pain when the teeth are irritated by heat and cold, or bleeding gums. Generally, vitamin E is used as an antioxidant, and its mechanisms of action and delivery are similar to those of the dental resin composites.

4. Conclusions and Perspective

As people are paying more and more attention to oral health, the details about dental procedures are also growing. This has greatly improved people's oral conditions and promotes the innovation and progress of dental materials. This article focused on the applications of antioxidants in dental procedures. For each dental procedure, the types of antioxidants used in dental treatment, the mechanism of action, and delivery of various antioxidants were reviewed. The challenges and safety assessment of these materials in the current field were also discussed.

In various dental procedures, antioxidants are highlighted for their significance in the process of scavenging free radicals and repairing damaged cells. However, determining how to select the most appropriate antioxidant according to a certain type of free radicals generated in dental procedures, how to deliver these antioxidants to maximize their effectiveness, and how to balance their toxicity and bioavailability still need further studies. Additionally, scientific trials that support the widespread use of various antioxidants in dental clinics are of limited validity. Future works focused on antioxidants delivery and bioavailability assessment are highly recommended. It is also urgently necessary to conduct clinical studies, especially the long follow-up period studies in dental clinics, to further confirm the appropriate antioxidative approach for human usage. The explorations of advanced applications of antioxidants in the dental field are still underway.

Author Contributions: Writing—original draft preparation, F.Q., W.R. and J.W.; writing—review and editing, H.H. and M.W.; funding acquisition, H.H., M.W. and J.W. All authors have read and agreed to the published version of the manuscript.

Funding: This research was funded by the startup fund from Shandong University of Technology (M.W. and J.W.).

Institutional Review Board Statement: Not applicable.

Informed Consent Statement: Not applicable.

Acknowledgments: H.H. would like to acknowledge the support from the Talent Introduction Plan for Youth Innovation Team in Universities of Shandong Province.

Conflicts of Interest: The authors declare no conflict of interest.

References

1. Rozier, R.G.; Pahel, B.T. Patient-and population-reported outcomes in public health dentistry: Oral health-related quality of life. *Dent. Clin. N. Am.* **2008**, *52*, 345–365. [CrossRef] [PubMed]
2. Carnelio, S.; Khan, S.A.; Rodrigues, G. Definite, probable or dubious: Antioxidants trilogy in clinical dentistry. *Br. Dent. J.* **2008**, *204*, 29–32. [CrossRef] [PubMed]
3. Ahmadi-Motamayel, F.; Goodarzi, M.T.; Hendi, S.S.; Kasraei, S.; Moghimbeigi, A. Total antioxidant capacity of saliva and dental caries. *Med. Oral Patol. Oral Cir. Bucal* **2013**, *18*, e553. [CrossRef]
4. Lobo, V.; Patil, A.; Phatak, A.; Chandra, N. Free radicals, antioxidants and functional foods: Impact on human health. *Pharmacogn. Rev.* **2010**, *4*, 118. [CrossRef] [PubMed]
5. Aksakalli, S. Antioxidants in dentistry: Review of literature. *Dentistry* **2013**, *4*, 1000181. [CrossRef]
6. King, M.; Chatelain, K.; Farris, D.; Jensen, D.; Pickup, J.; Swapp, A.; O'Malley, S.; Kingsley, K. Oral squamous cell carcinoma proliferative phenotype is modulated by proanthocyanidins: A potential prevention and treatment alternative for oral cancer. *BMC Complement Altern. Med.* **2007**, *7*, 22. [CrossRef]
7. Shirataki, Y.; Kawase, M.; Saito, S.; Kurihara, T.; Tanaka, W.; Satoh, K.; Sakagami, H.; Motohashi, N. Selective cytotoxic activity of grape peel and seed extracts against oral tumor cell lines. *Anticancer Res.* **2000**, *20*, 423–426.
8. Khalil, I.; Yehye, W.A.; Etxeberria, A.E.; Alhadi, A.A.; Dezfooli, S.M.; Julkapli, N.B.M.; Basirun., W.J.; Seyfoddin, A. Nanoantioxidants: Recent trends in antioxidant delivery applications. *Antioxidants* **2019**, *9*, 24. [CrossRef]

9. Catauro, M.; Papale, F.; Bollino, F.; Piccolella, S.; Marciano, S.; Nocera, P.; Pacifico, S. Silica/quercetin sol-gel hybrids as antioxidant dental implant materials. *Sci. Technol. Adv. Mater.* **2015**, *16*, 035001. [CrossRef]
10. Kim, Y.H.; Lee, D.W.; Jung, E.J.; Bae, J.T.; Lee, S.G.; Pyo, H.B.; Kang, K.H.; Lee, D.K. Preparation and characterization of quercetin-loaded silica microspheres stabilized by combined multiple emulsion and sol-gel processes. *Chem. Ind. Chem. Eng. Q.* **2015**, *21*, 85–94. [CrossRef]
11. Skibsted, L.H.; Dragsted, L.O.; Dyerberg, J.; Hansen, H.S.; Tjnneland, A.M. Antioxidants and health. *Ugeskr. Laeg.* **2006**, *168*, 2787–2789. [PubMed]
12. Englard, S.; Seifter, S. The biochemical functions of ascorbic acid. *Annu. Rev. Nutr.* **1986**, *6*, 365–406. [CrossRef] [PubMed]
13. Pua, M.L.; Yoshitomi, T.; Chonpathompikunlert, P.; Hirayama, A.; Nagasaki, Y. Redox-active injectable gel using thermo-responsive nanoscale polyion complex flower micelle for noninvasive treatment of local inflammation. *J. Control Release* **2013**, *172*, 914–920. [CrossRef] [PubMed]
14. Jiang, M.; Hong, Y.; Gu, Z.; Cheng, L.; Li, Z.; Li, C. Preparation of a starch-based carrier for oral delivery of Vitamin E to the small intestine. *Food Hydrocoll.* **2019**, *91*, 26–33. [CrossRef]
15. Zhang, Z.; Chen, L.; Deng, M.; Bai, Y.; Chen, X.; Jing, X. Biodegradable thermo-and pH-responsive hydrogels for oral drug delivery. *J. Polym. Sci. A Polym. Chem.* **2011**, *49*, 2941–2951. [CrossRef]
16. Das, S.S.; Sarkar, A.; Chabattula, S.C.; Verma, P.R.P.; Nazir, A.; Gupta, P.K.; Ruokolainen, J.; Kesari, K.K.; Singh, S.K. Food-grade quercetin-loaded nanoemulsion ameliorates effects associated with parkinson's disease and cancer: Studies employing a transgenic c. elegans model and human cancer cell lines. *Antioxidants* **2022**, *11*, 1378. [CrossRef]
17. Das, S.S.; Verma, P.R.P.; Singh, S.K. Screening and preparation of quercetin doped nanoemulsion: Characterizations, antioxidant and anti-bacterial activities. *LWT-Food Sci. Technol.* **2020**, *124*, 109141. [CrossRef]
18. Vidhya, S.; Srinivasulu, S.; Sujatha, M.; Mahalaxmi, S. Effect of grape seed extract on the bond strength of bleached enamel. *Oper. Dent.* **2011**, *36*, 433–438. [CrossRef]
19. Tian, Y.; Mao, X.; Sun, R.; Zhang, M.; Xia, Q. Enhanced oral bioavailability of oligomeric proanthocyanidins by a self-double-emulsifying drug delivery system. *Food Sci. Nutr.* **2020**, *8*, 3814–3825. [CrossRef]
20. Żukowski, P.; Maciejczyk, M.; Waszkiel, D. Sources of free radicals and oxidative stress in the oral cavity. *Arch. Oral Biol.* **2018**, *92*, 8–17. [CrossRef]
21. Lushchak, V.I. Free radicals, reactive oxygen species, oxidative stress and its classification. *Chem. Biol. Interact.* **2014**, *224*, 164–175. [CrossRef] [PubMed]
22. Sena, L.A.; Chandel, N. Physiological roles of mitochondrial reactive oxygen species. *Mol. Cell* **2012**, *48*, 158–167. [CrossRef] [PubMed]
23. Halliwell, B.; Clement, M.V.; Long, L.H. Hydrogen peroxide in the human body. *FEBS Lett.* **2000**, *486*, 10–13. [CrossRef] [PubMed]
24. Liu, F.; Hong, T.; Xie, J.; Zhan, X.; Wang, Y. Application of reactive oxygen species-based nanomaterials in dentistry: A review. *Crystals* **2021**, *11*, 266. [CrossRef]
25. Tothova, L.U.; Celec, P. Oxidative stress and antioxidants in the diagnosis and therapy of periodontitis. *Front. Physiol.* **2017**, *8*, 1055. [CrossRef] [PubMed]
26. Young, I.S.; Woodside, J.V. Antioxidants in health and disease. *J. Clin. Pathol.* **2001**, *54*, 176–186. [CrossRef]
27. D'aiuto, F.; Nibali, L.; Parkar, M.; Patel, K.; Suvan, J.; Donos, N. Oxidative stress, systemic inflammation, and severe periodontitis. *J. Dent. Res.* **2010**, *89*, 1241–1246. [CrossRef]
28. Waszkiewicz, N.; Chojnowska, S.; Zalewska, A.; Zwierz, K.; Szulc, A.; Szajda, S.D. Salivary hexosaminidase in smoking alcoholics with bad periodontal and dental states. *Drug Alcohol Depend.* **2013**, *129*, 33–40. [CrossRef]
29. Kimura, M.; Miyakawa, T.; Matsushita, S.; So, M.; Higuchi, S. Gender differences in the effects of ADH1B and ALDH2 polymorphisms on alcoholism. *Alcohol. Clin. Exp. Res.* **2011**, *35*, 1923–1927. [CrossRef]
30. Reznick, A.Z.; Klein, I.; Eiserich, J.P.; Cross, C.E.; Nagler, R.M. Inhibition of oral peroxidase activity by cigarette smoke: In vivo and in vitro studies. *Free Radic. Biol. Med.* **2003**, *34*, 377–384. [CrossRef]
31. Sim, S.S.; Choi, J.C.; Rhie, D.J.; Yoon, S.H.; Hahn, S.J.; Kim, C.J.; Kim, M.S.; Jo, Y.H. The involvement of phospholipase A2 in ethanol-induced gastric muscle contraction. *Eur. J. Pharmacol.* **2001**, *413*, 281–285. [CrossRef] [PubMed]
32. Domagala-Kulawik, J. Effects of cigarette smoke on the lung and systemic immunity. *J. Physiol. Pharmacol.* **2008**, *59*, 19–34. [PubMed]
33. Swan, G.E.; Lessov-Schlaggar, C.N. The effects of tobacco smoke and nicotine on cognition and the brain. *Neuropsychol. Rev.* **2007**, *17*, 259–273. [CrossRef]
34. Kanehira, T.; Shibata, K.; Kashiwazaki, H.; Inoue, N.; Morita, M. Comparison of antioxidant enzymes in saliva of elderly smokers and non-smokers. *Gerodontology* **2006**, *23*, 38–42. [CrossRef] [PubMed]
35. Kołodziej, U.; Maciejczyk, M.; Miąsko, A.; Matczuk, J.; Knaś, M.; Żukowski, P.; Żendzian-Piotrowska, M.; Borys, J.; Zalewska, A. Oxidative modification in the salivary glands of high fat-diet induced insulin resistant rats. *Front. Physiol.* **2017**, *8*, 20. [CrossRef] [PubMed]
36. Kopáni, M.; Celec, P.; Danišovič, L.; Michalka, P.; Biró, C. Oxidative stress and electron spin resonance. *Clin. Chim. Acta* **2006**, *364*, 61–66. [CrossRef]
37. Kna, M.; Maciejczyk, M.; Waszkiel, D.; Zalewska, A. Oxidative stress and salivary antioxidants. *Dent. Med. Probl.* **2013**, *50*, 461–466.

38. Esterbauer, H.; Puhl, H.; Dieber-rotheneder, M.; Waeg, G.; Rabl, H. Effect of antioxidants on oxidative modification of LDL. *Ann. Med.* **1991**, *23*, 573–581. [CrossRef]
39. TAAo, P. Parameter on chronic periodontitis with slight to moderate loss of periodontal support. *J. Periodontol* **2000**, *71*, 853–855.
40. Kornman, K.S. Mapping the pathogenesis of periodontitis: A new look. *J. Periodontol.* **2008**, *79*, 1560–1568. [CrossRef]
41. Muniz, F.W.M.G.; Nogueira, S.B.; Mendes, F.L.V.; Rösing, C.K.; Moreira, M.M.S.M.; de Andrade, G.M.; de Sousa Carvalho, R. The impact of antioxidant agents complimentary to periodontal therapy on oxidative stress and periodontal outcomes: A systematic review. *Arch. Oral Biol.* **2015**, *60*, 1203–1214. [CrossRef]
42. Junior, M.T.; Rodrigues, C.A.; Bernardes, V.L.; de Araujo, T.S.B.; Nicoli, G.A.; dos Reis Derceli, J. Dental bleaching and new possibilities: Literature review. *Health Sci. J.* **2018**, *12*, 600. [CrossRef]
43. Lertsukprasert, N.; Locharoenrat, K. Efficiency of tooth bleaching agent on staining and discoloration characteristics of nicotine stained dental enamel model. *BMC Oral Health* **2020**, *20*, 221. [CrossRef] [PubMed]
44. Dahlstrom, S.W.; Heithersay, G.S.; Bridges, T.E. Hydroxyl radical activity in thermo-catalytically bleached root-filled teeth. *Dent. Traumatol.* **1997**, *13*, 119–125. [CrossRef] [PubMed]
45. Kawamoto, K.; Tsujimoto, Y. Effects of the hydroxyl radical and hydrogen peroxide on tooth bleaching. *J. Endod.* **2004**, *30*, 45–50. [CrossRef] [PubMed]
46. De Moor, R.J.G.; Diachuk, A.; Verheyen, P.; Meire, M.A.; De Coster, P.J.; Keulemans, F.; De Bruyne, M.; Walsh, L.J. Insight in the chemistry of laser-activated dental bleaching. *Sci. World J.* **2015**, *2015*, 650492. [CrossRef] [PubMed]
47. Soares, D.G.; Basso, F.G.; Hebling, J.; de Souza Costa, C.A. Concentrations of and application protocols for hydrogen peroxide bleaching gels: Effects on pulp cell viability and whitening efficacy. *J. Dent.* **2014**, *42*, 185–198. [CrossRef]
48. Nathanson, D. Vital tooth bleaching: Sensitivity and pulpal considerations. *J. Am. Dent. Assoc.* **1997**, *128*, 41S–44S. [CrossRef]
49. Rotstein, I.; Torek, Y.; Misgav, R. Effect of cementum defects on radicular penetration of 30% H_2O_2 during intracoronal bleaching. *J. Endod.* **1991**, *17*, 230–233. [CrossRef]
50. Anugrahati, D.F.; Ernawati, R.; Irsya, W.; Sumur, Y.K.; Sukaton; Ismiyati, K. Management of non-vital teeth discoloration with the internal bleaching: A case report. *Indian J. Forensic Med. Toxicol.* **2021**, *15*, 1072–1076.
51. Curran, S.F.; Amoruso, M.A.; Goldstein, B.D.; Berg, R.A. Degradation of soluble collagen by ozone or hydroxyl radicals. *FEBS Lett.* **1984**, *176*, 155–160. [CrossRef] [PubMed]
52. Rowley, D.; Halliwell, B. Formation of hydroxyl radicals from hydrogen peroxide and iron salts by superoxide-and ascorbate-dependent mechanisms: Relevance to the pathology of rheumatoid disease. *Clin. Sci.* **1983**, *64*, 649–653. [CrossRef] [PubMed]
53. Gutteridge, J.M. Iron promoters of the Fenton reaction and lipid peroxidation can be released from haemoglobin by peroxides. *FEBS let.* **1986**, *201*, 291–295. [CrossRef] [PubMed]
54. Halliwell, B. Free radicals, reactive oxygen species and human disease: A critical evaluation with special reference to atherosclerosis. *Br. J. Exp. Pathol.* **1989**, *70*, 737. [PubMed]
55. Titley, K.; Torneck, C.D.; Ruse, N.D. The effect of carbamide-peroxide gel on the shear bond strength of a microfil resin to bovine enamel. *J. Dent. Res.* **1992**, *71*, 20–24. [CrossRef]
56. Dishman, M.V.; Covey, D.A.; Baughan, L.W. The effects of peroxide bleaching on composite to enamel bond strength. *Dent. Mater. J.* **1994**, *10*, 33–36. [CrossRef]
57. Titley, K.C.; Torneck, C.D.; Ruse, N.D.; Krmec, D. Adhesion of a resin composite to bleached and unbleached human enamel. *J. Endod.* **1993**, *19*, 112–115. [CrossRef]
58. Torres, C.R.G.; Koga, A.F.; Borges, A.B. The effects of anti-oxidant agents as neutralizers of bleaching agents on enamel bond strength. *Braz. J. Oral Sci.* **2006**, *5*, 971–976.
59. Oskoee, P.A.; Navimipour, E.J.; Oskoee, S.S.; Moosavi, N. Effect of 10% sodium ascorbate on bleached bovine enamel surface morphology and microhardness. *Open Dent. J.* **2010**, *4*, 207. [CrossRef]
60. Bulut, H.; Turkun, M.; Kaya, A.D. Effect of an antioxidizing agent on the shear bond strength of brackets bonded to bleached human enamel. *Am. J. Orthod.* **2006**, *129*, 266–272. [CrossRef]
61. Çakir, E.G.; Özcan, S.; Tulunoglu, I.; Üçtaşli, M.B.; Tulunoglu, O. Efficacy of In-office Bleaching on Microhardness of Permanent Teeth with Antioxidant Re-hardening. *Open Dent. J.* **2019**, *13*, 436–442. [CrossRef]
62. Ergün Kunt, G.; Yılmaz, N.; Şen, S.; Dede, D.Ö. Effect of antioxidant treatment on the shear bond strength of composite resin to bleached enamel. *Acta Odontol. Scand.* **2011**, *69*, 287–291. [CrossRef] [PubMed]
63. Garcia, E.J.; Mena-Serrano, A.; De Andrade, A.M.; Reis, A.; Grande, R.H.; Loguercio, A.D. Immediate bonding to bleached enamel treated with 10% sodium ascorbate gel: A case report with one-year follow-up. *Eur. J. Esthet. Dent.* **2012**, *7*, 154–162. [PubMed]
64. De Paula, E.A.; Kossatz, S.; Fernandes, D.; Loguercio, A.D.; Reis, A. Administration of ascorbic acid to prevent bleaching-induced tooth sensitivity: A randomized tripleblind clinical trial. *Oper. Dent.* **2014**, *39*, 128–135. [CrossRef]
65. Louzada, L.M.; Briso, A.L.F.; Benetti, F.; Vieira, L.B.; Jacinto, R.D.C.; Dezan-Júnior, E.; Cintra, L.T.A. Anti-inflammatory potential of a carvedilol gel in the pulpal tissue of rats after dental bleaching: A histopathological evaluation. *J. Investig. Clin. Dent.* **2019**, *10*, e1240. [CrossRef] [PubMed]
66. Gupta, S.; Shankar, P.; Bannimath, G.; Doddawad, V.; Annapoorna, B. Evaluation of antioxidant property of amla on bond strength and color stability of power bleached teeth: An in vitro study. *J. Pharm. Bioallied Sci.* **2021**, *13*, S1244–S1250.
67. Fine, A.M. Oligomeric proanthocyanidin complexes: History, structure, and phytopharmaceutical applications. *Altern. Med. Rev. Clin. Ther.* **2000**, *5*, 144–151.

68. Xie, Q.; Bedran-Russo, A.K.; Wu, C.D. In vitro remineralization effects of grape seed extract on artificial root caries. *J. Dent.* **2008**, *36*, 900–906. [CrossRef] [PubMed]
69. Qi, X.; Wang, L.; Zhu, J.; Hu, Z.; Zhang, J. Self-double-emulsifying drug delivery system (SDEDDS): A new way for oral delivery of drugs with high solubility and low permeability. *Int. J. Pharm.* **2011**, *409*, 245–251. [CrossRef]
70. Esquivel-Chirino, C.; Gómez-Landeros, J.C.; Carabantes-Campos, E.P.; Carmona-Ruiz, D.; Valero-Princet, Y.; Márquez-Correa, C.; Morales-González, J.A. The Impact of Oxidative Stress on Dental Implants. *Eur. J. Dent.* **2021**, *2*, 1–8. [CrossRef]
71. Triplett, R.G.; Frohberg, U.; Sykaras, N.; Woody, R.D. Implant materials, design, and surface topographies: Their influence on osseointegration of dental implants. *J. Long-Term Eff. Med. Implants* **2003**, *13*. [CrossRef] [PubMed]
72. Gaviria, L.; Salcido, J.P.; Guda, T.; Ong, J.L. Current trends in dental implants. *J. Korean Assoc. Oral Maxillofac* **2014**, *40*, 50. [CrossRef] [PubMed]
73. Crabb, C. History of dental implants. *Dent. Nurs.* **2006**, *2*, 398–399. [CrossRef]
74. Yanez, M.; Blanchette, J.; Jabbarzadeh, E. Modulation of inflammatory response to implanted biomaterials using natural compounds. *Curr. Pharm. Des.* **2017**, *23*, 6347–6357. [CrossRef] [PubMed]
75. Tsaryk, R.; Kalbacova, M.; Hempel, U.; Scharnweber, D.; Unger, R.E.; Dieter, P.; Kirkpatrick, C.J.; Peters, K. Response of human endothelial cells to oxidative stress on Ti6Al4V alloy. *Biomaterials* **2007**, *28*, 806–813. [CrossRef] [PubMed]
76. Lee, M.C.; Yoshino, F.; Shoji, H.; Takahashi, S.; Todoki, K.; Shimada, S.; Kuse-Barouch, K. Characterization by electron spin resonance spectroscopy of reactive oxygen species generated by titanium dioxide and hydrogen peroxide. *J. Dent. Res.* **2005**, *84*, 178–182. [CrossRef]
77. Bressan, E.; Ferroni, L.; Gardin, C.; Bellin, G.; Sbricoli, L.; Sivolella, S.; Brunello, G.; Schwartz-Arad, D.; Mijiritsky, E.; Penarrocha, M.; et al. Metal nanoparticles released from dental implant surfaces: Potential contribution to chronic inflammation and peri-implant bone loss. *Materials* **2019**, *12*, 2036. [CrossRef] [PubMed]
78. Delgado-Ruiz, R.; Romanos, G. Potential causes of titanium particle and ion release in implant dentistry: A systematic review. *Int. J. Mol. Sci.* **2018**, *19*, 3585. [CrossRef] [PubMed]
79. Abdulhameed, E.A.; Al-Rawi, N.H.; Omar, M.; Khalifa, N.; Samsudin, A.R. Titanium dioxide dental implants surfaces related oxidative stress in bone remodeling: A systematic review. *PeerJ* **2022**, *10*, e12951. [CrossRef]
80. Caton, J.G.; Armitage, G.; Berglundh, T.; Chapple, I.L.; Jepsen, S.; Kornman, K.S.; Mealey, B.L.; Papapanou, P.N.; Sanz, M.; Tonetti, M.S. A new classification scheme for periodontal and peri-implant diseases and conditions–Introduction and key changes from the 1999 classification. *J. Periodontol.* **2018**, *89*, S1–S8. [CrossRef]
81. Jazi, M.M.; Rodsari, H.R.S.P.; Mirmiran, F. Level of oxidative stress markers in peri-implant crevicular fluid and their correlation with clinical parameters. *J. Dent.* **2015**, *12*, 340.
82. Suárez-López del Amo, F.; Garaicoa-Pazmiño, C.; Fretwurst, T.; Castilho, R.M.; Squarize, C.H. Dental implants-associated release of titanium particles: A systematic review. *Clin. Oral. Implants Res.* **2018**, *29*, 1085–1100. [CrossRef] [PubMed]
83. Mouthuy, P.A.; Snelling, S.J.; Dakin, S.G.; Milković, L.; Gašparović, A.Č.; Carr, A.J.; Žarković, N. Biocompatibility of implantable materials: An oxidative stress viewpoint. *Biomaterials* **2016**, *109*, 55–68. [CrossRef] [PubMed]
84. Kaur, G.; Kathariya, R.; Bansal, S.; Singh, A.; Shahakar, D. Dietary antioxidants and their indispensable role in periodontal health. *J. Food. Drug. Anal.* **2016**, *24*, 239–246. [CrossRef]
85. Tardy, B.L.; Richardson, J.J.; Nithipipat, V.; Kempe, K.; Guo, J.; Cho, K.L.; Rahim, M.A.; Ejima, H.; Caruso, F. Protein adsorption and coordination-based end-tethering of functional polymers on metal-phenolic network films. *Biomacromolecules* **2019**, *20*, 1421–1428. [CrossRef]
86. Harmankaya, N.; Igawa, K.; Stenlund, P.; Palmquist, A.; Tengvall, P. Healing of complement activating Ti implants compared with non-activating Ti in rat tibia. *Acta Biomaterialia* **2012**, *8*, 3532–3540. [CrossRef] [PubMed]
87. Källtorp, M.; Askendal, A.; Thomsen, P.; Tengvall, P. Inflammatory cell recruitment, distribution, and chemiluminescence response at IgG precoated- and thiol functionalized gold surfaces. *J. Biomed. Mater. Res* **1999**, *47*, 251–259. [CrossRef]
88. Huang, D.; Lin, Q.; Zhou, Y.; Li, J.; Wei, Y.; Hu, Y.; Lian, X.; Chen, S.; Chen, W. Ag nanoparticles incorporated tannic acid/nanoapatite composite coating on Ti implant surfaces for enhancement of antibacterial and antioxidant properties. *Surf. Coat. Technol.* **2020**, *399*, 126169.
89. Maruyama, T.; Tomofuji, T.; Endo, Y.; Irie, K.; Azuma, T.; Ekuni, D.; Tamaki, N.; Yamamoto, T.; Morita, M. Supplementation of green tea catechins in dentifrices suppresses gingival oxidative stress and periodontal inflammation. *Arch. Oral Biol.* **2011**, *56*, 48–53. [CrossRef] [PubMed]
90. Catauro, M.; Bollino, F.; Papale, F.; Ferrara, C.; Mustarelli, P. Silica–polyethylene glycol hybrids synthesized by sol–gel: Biocompatibility improvement of titanium implants by coating. *Mater. Sci. Eng. C* **2015**, *55*, 118–125. [CrossRef]
91. Rathee, P.; Chaudhary, H.; Rathee, S.; Rathee, D.; Kumar, V.; Kohli, K. Mechanism of action of flavonoids as anti-inflammatory agents: A review. *J. Inflam. Allergy Drug Targets* **2009**, *8*, 229–235. [CrossRef] [PubMed]
92. Catauro, M.; Bollino, F.; Papale, F.; Piccolella, S.; Pacifico, S. Sol–gel synthesis and characterization of SiO2/PCL hybrid materials containing quercetin as new materials for antioxidant implants. *Mater. Sci. Eng. C* **2016**, *58*, 945–952. [CrossRef] [PubMed]
93. Re, R.; Pellegrini, N.; Proteggente, A.; Pannala, A.; Yang, M.; Rice-Evans, C. Antioxidant activity applying an improved ABTS radical cation decolorization assay. *Free Radic. Biol. Med.* **1999**, *26*, 1231–1237. [CrossRef]
94. Graham, H.D. Stabilization of the Prussian blue color in the determination of polyphenols. *J. Agric. Food Chem.* **1992**, *40*, 801–805. [CrossRef]

95. Boraldi, F.; Annovi, G.; Paolinelli-Devincenzi, C.; Tiozzo, R.; Quaglino, D. The effect of serum withdrawal on the protein profile of quiescent human dermal fibroblasts in primary cell culture. *Proteomics* **2008**, *8*, 66–82. [CrossRef] [PubMed]
96. Vroman, L.; Adams, A.L. Findings with the recording ellipsometer suggesting rapid exchange of specific plasma proteins at liquid/solid interfaces. *Surf. Sci.* **1969**, *16*, 438–446. [CrossRef]
97. Vroman, L.; Adams, A.L.; Fischer, G.C.; Munoz, P.C. Interaction of high molecular weight kininogen, factor XII, and fibrinogen in plasma at interfaces. *Blood* **1980**, *55*, 156–159. [CrossRef]
98. Chow, C.K.; Ibrahim, W.; Wei, Z.; Chan, A.C. Vitamin E regulates mitochondrial hydrogen peroxide generation. *Free Radic. Biol. Med.* **1999**, *27*, 580–587. [CrossRef] [PubMed]
99. Costa, L.; Carpentieri, I.; Bracco, P. Post electron-beam irradiation oxidation of orthopaedic Ultra-High Molecular Weight Polyethylene (UHMWPE) stabilized with vitamin E. *Polym. Degrad. Stab.* **2009**, *94*, 1542–1547. [CrossRef]
100. Ozawa, R.; Saita, M.; Sakaue, S.; Okada, R.; Sato, T.; Kawamata, R.; Sakurai, T.; Hamada, N.; Kimotoa, K.; Nagasaki, Y. Redox injectable gel protects osteoblastic function against oxidative stress and suppresses alveolar bone loss in a rat peri-implantitis model. *Acta Biomater.* **2020**, *110*, 82–94. [CrossRef] [PubMed]
101. Zieniewska, I.; Maciejczyk, M.; Zalewska, A. The effect of selected dental Materials used in conservative dentistry, endodontics, surgery, and orthodontics as well as during the periodontal treatment on the redox balance in the oral cavity. *Int. J. Mol. Sci.* **2020**, *21*, 9684. [CrossRef]
102. Al-Saleh, I.; Elkhatib, R. Effect of mercury (Hg) dental amalgam fillings on renal and oxidative stress biomarkers in children. *Sci. Total Environ.* **2012**, *431*, 188–196. [CrossRef] [PubMed]
103. Jirau-Colón, H.; González-Parrilla, L.; Martinez-Jiménez, J.; Adam, W.; Jiménez-Velez, B. Rethinking the dental amalgam dilemma: An integrated toxicological approach. *Int. J. Environ.* **2019**, *16*, 1036. [CrossRef] [PubMed]
104. Castoldi, A.F.; Coccini, T.; Manzo, L. Neurotoxic and molecular effects of methylmercury in humans. *Rev. Environ. Health* **2003**, *18*, 19–32. [CrossRef] [PubMed]
105. Pizzichini, M.; Fonzi, M.; Sugherini, L.; Fonzi, L.; Gasparoni, A.; Comporti, M.; Pompella, A. Release of mercury from dental amalgam and its influence on salivary antioxidant activity. *Sci. Total Environ.* **2002**, *284*, 19–25. [CrossRef] [PubMed]
106. Lindh, U.; Hudecek, R.; Danersund, A.; Eriksson, S.; Lindvall, A. Removal of dental amalgam and other metal alloys supported by antioxidant therapy alleviates symptoms and improves quality of life in patients with amalgam-associated ill health. *Neuro. Endocrinol. Lett.* **2002**, *23*, 459. [PubMed]
107. Jan, A.T.; Ali, A.; Haq, Q.M.R. Glutathione as an antioxidant in inorganic mercury induced nephrotoxicity. *J. Postgrad. Med.* **2011**, *57*, 72.
108. Frisk, P.; Danersund, A.; Hudecek, R.; Lindh, U. Changed Clinical Chemistry Pattern in Blood After Removal of Dental Amalgam and other Metal Alloys Supported by Antioxidant Therapy. *Biol. Trace Elem. Res.* **2007**, *120*, 163–170. [CrossRef]
109. Bendich, A.; Machlin, L.J.; Scandurra, O.; Burton, G.W.; Wayner, D.D.M. The antioxidant role of vitamin C. *Adv. Free. Radical. Biol. Med.* **1986**, *2*, 419–444. [CrossRef]
110. Abudu, N.; Miller, J.J.; Attaelmannan, M.; Levinson, S.S. Vitamins in human arteriosclerosis with emphasis on vitamin C and vitamin E. *Clin. Chim. Acta* **2004**, *339*, 11–25. [CrossRef] [PubMed]
111. Gallusi, G.; Libonati, A.; Piro, M.; Taranto, V.D.; Montemurro, E.; Campanella, V. Is Dental amalgam a higher risk factor rather than resin-based restorations for systemic conditions? A systematic review. *Materials* **2021**, *14*, 1980. [CrossRef] [PubMed]
112. Alkhudhairy, F. Attitudes of dentists and interns in Riyadh to the use of dental amalgam. *BMC Res. Notes* **2016**, *9*, 488. [CrossRef] [PubMed]
113. Joshi, A.; Douglass, C.W.; Kim, H.D.; Joshipura, K.J.; Park, M.C.; Rimm, E.B.; Carino, M.J.; Garcia, R.I.; Morris, J.S.; Willett, W.C. The relationship between amalgam restorations and mercury levels in male dentists and nondental health professionals. *J. Public Health Dent.* **2007**, *63*, 52–60. [CrossRef] [PubMed]
114. Broadbent, J.; Murray, C.; Schwass, D.; Brosnan, M.; Brunton, P.; Lyons, K.; Thomson, W. The dental amalgam phasedown in New Zealand: A 20-year trend. *Oper. Dent.* **2020**, *45*, 255–264. [CrossRef] [PubMed]
115. Krifka, S.; Spagnuolo, G.; Schmalz, G.; Schweikl, H. A review of adaptive mechanisms in cell responses towards oxidative stress caused by dental resin monomers. *Biomaterials* **2013**, *34*, 4555–4563. [CrossRef]
116. Klapdohr, S.; Moszner, N. New inorganic components for dental filling composites. *Monatsh. Chem.* **2005**, *136*, 21–45. [CrossRef]
117. Pratap, B.; Gupta, R.K.; Bhardwaj, B.; Nag, M. Resin based restorative dental materials: Characteristics and future perspectives. *Jpn. Dent. Sci. Rev.* **2019**, *55*, 126–138. [CrossRef] [PubMed]
118. Lavigueur, C.; Zhu, X.X. Recent advances in the development of dental composite resins. *RSC Adv.* **2012**, *2*, 59–63. [CrossRef]
119. Schweikl, H.; Spagnuolo, G.; Schmalz, G. Genetic and cellular toxicology of dental resin monomers. *J. Dent. Res.* **2006**, *85*, 870–877. [CrossRef]
120. Mantellini, M.G.; Botero, T.M.; Yaman, P.; Dennison, J.B.; Hanks, C.T.; Nör, J.E. Adhesive resin induces apoptosis and cell-cycle arrest of pulp cells. *J. Dent. Res.* **2003**, *82*, 592–596. [CrossRef]
121. Schmalz, G.; Widbiller, M. Biocompatibility of amalgam vs composite–A review. *Oral Health* **2022**, *2022*, 149–156.
122. Godley, B.F.; Shamsi, F.A.; Liang, F.Q.; Jarrett, S.G.; Davies, S.; Boulton, M. Blue light induces mitochondrial DNA damage and free radical production in epithelial cells. *J. Biol. Chem.* **2005**, *280*, 21061. [CrossRef]

123. Wattamwar, P.P.; Biswal, D.; Cochran, D.B.; Lyvers, A.C.; Eitel, R.E.; Anderson, K.W.; Hilt, J.Z.; Dziubla, T.D. Synthesis and characterization of poly (antioxidant β-amino esters) for controlled release of polyphenolic antioxidants. *Acta Biomater.* **2012**, *8*, 2529–2537. [CrossRef] [PubMed]
124. Att, W.; Yamada, M.; Kojima, N.; Ogawa, T. N-Acetyl cysteine prevents suppression of oral fibroblast function on poly(methylmethacrylate) resin. *Acta Biomater.* **2009**, *5*, 391–398. [CrossRef]
125. Ricciarelli, R.; Zingg, J.M.; Azzi, A. The 80th anniversary of vitamin E: Beyond its antioxidant properties. *Biol. Chem.* **2002**, *383*, 457–465. [CrossRef] [PubMed]
126. Davidov-Pardo, G.; McClements, D.J. Resveratrol encapsulation: Designing delivery systems to overcome solubility, stability and bioavailability issues. *Trends Food Sci. Technol.* **2014**, *38*, 88–103. [CrossRef]
127. Newton, A.M.J.; Kaur, B.; Indana, V.L.; Rajesh, K.S. Chronotherapeutic drug delivery of pectin vs. guar gum, xanthan gum controlled release colon targeted directly compressed propranolol Hcl matrix tablets. *SAJ Pharm. Pharmacol.* **2014**, *1*, 1–12.
128. Wilson, A.D.; Kent, B.E. The glass-ionomer cement, a new translucent dental filling material. *J. Appl. Chem.* **1971**, *21*, 313. [CrossRef]
129. Lohbauer, U. Dental glass ionomer cements as permanent filling materials? —Properties, limitations future trends. *Materials* **2009**, *3*, 76–96. [CrossRef]
130. Sidhu, S.K.; Nicholson, J.W. A review of glass-ionomer cements for clinical dentistry. *J. Funct. Biomater.* **2016**, *7*, 16. [CrossRef] [PubMed]
131. Park, E.Y.; Kang, S. Current aspects and prospects of glass ionomer cements for clinical dentistry. *Yeungnam Univ. J. Med.* **2020**, *37*, 169–178. [CrossRef] [PubMed]
132. Sidhu, S.K.; Watson, T.F. Resin-modified glass ionomer materials. A status report for the American Journal of Dentistry. *Am. J. Dent.* **1995**, *8*, 59–67. [PubMed]
133. Xie, D.; Brantley, W.A.; Culbertson, B.M.; Wang, G. Mechanical properties and microstructures of glass-ionomer cements. *Dent. Mater.* **2000**, *16*, 129–138. [CrossRef] [PubMed]
134. Siqueira, P.C.; Magalhães, A.P.R.; Pires, W.C.; Pereira, F.C.; Silveira-Lacerda, E.P.; Carrião, M.S.; Bakuzis, A.F.; Souza-Costa, C.A.; Lopes, L.G.; Estrela, C. Cytotoxicity of glass ionomer cements containing silver nanoparticles. *J. Clin. Exp. Dent.* **2015**, *7*, e622. [CrossRef] [PubMed]

MDPI AG
Grosspeteranlage 5
4052 Basel
Switzerland
Tel.: +41 61 683 77 34

Antioxidants Editorial Office
E-mail: antioxidants@mdpi.com
www.mdpi.com/journal/antioxidants